Contents

Cardiovascular Psychophysiology

current issues in
response mechanisms,
biofeedback,
and methodology

edited by

Paul A. Obrist
A. H. Black
Jasper Brener
Leo V. DiCara

ALDINE PUBLISHING COMPANY/chicago

First published 1974 by
Aldine Publishing Company
529 South Wabash Avenue
Chicago, Illinois 60605

ISBN 0-202-25116-0
Library of Congress Catalog Number 73-89517

Printed in the United States of America

Contributors

A. H. Black
Department of Psychology
McMaster University
Hamilton, Ontario, Canada

Jasper Brener
Department of Psychology
University of Tennessee
Knoxville, Tennessee

Rachel Keen Clifton
Department of Psychology
University of Massachusetts
Amherst, Massachusetts

David H. Cohen
Department of Physiology
School of Medicine
University of Virginia
Charlottesville, Virginia

Mary R. Cook
Institute of the Pennsylvania
    Hospital and
Department of Psychiatry
University of Pennsylvania
Philadelphia, Pennsylvania

Leo V. DiCara
Departments of Psychiatry and
    Psychology
University of Michigan Medical
    Center
Ann Arbor, Michigan

Rogers Elliott
Department of Psychology
Dartmouth College
Hanover, New Hampshire

Bernard T. Engel
Laboratory of Behavioral
    Sciences
Gerontology Research Center
National Institute of Child Health
    and Human Development
Baltimore City Hospitals
Baltimore, Maryland

Ralph P. Forsyth
Cardiovascular Research Institute
School of Medicine
University of California
San Francisco, California

William W. Hahn
Department of Psychology
University of Denver
Denver, Colorado

J. Alan Herd
Department of Physiology
Harvard Medical School
Boston, Massachusetts

James L. Howard
Department of Psychiatry
School of Medicine
University of North Carolina
Chapel Hill, North Carolina

Beatrice C. Lacey
Section of Behavioral Physiology
Fels Research Institute
Yellow Springs, Ohio

John I. Lacey
Section of Behavioral Physiology
Fels Research Institute
Yellow Springs, Ohio

Peter J. Lang
Department of Psychology
University of Wisconsin
Madison, Wisconsin

James E. Lawler
Department of Psychiatry
School of Medicine
University of North Carolina
Chapel Hill, North Carolina

Neal E. Miller
Rockefeller University
New York, New York

Paul A. Obrist
Department of Psychiatry
School of Medicine
University of North Carolina
Chapel Hill, North Carolina

Larry E. Roberts
Department of Psychology
McMaster University
Hamilton, Ontario, Canada

Neil Schneiderman
Department of Psychology
University of Miami
Coral Gables, Florida

Gary E. Schwartz
Department of Psychology
    and Social Relations
Harvard University
Cambridge, Massachusetts

David Shapiro
Department of Psychiatry
Harvard Medical School
Boston, Massachusetts

Bernard Tursky
Department of Political Science
State University of New York
    at Stony Brook
Stony Brook, New York

Introduction

This book is the result of a conference held at the University of North Carolina at Chapel Hill on May 1 to 3, 1972. The need for both a conference and a book concerning cardiovascular psychophysiology seemed apparent. Over the past decade, cardiovascular activity has received considerable attention in psychophysiological research, to the point that one past president of the Society for Psychophysiological Research suggested, somewhat facetiously, that the Society be renamed the Society for Cardiovascular Psychophysiological Research. The reasons for this interest in cardiovascular parameters are many. A very distinct impetus has been given to it by the work of the Laceys, and more recently by the work using operant and biofeedback procedures. As in any area of active investigation, there are growing pains—as exemplified by both methodological and conceptual controversy. It appeared to the organizers that the time was ripe to bring together a group of investigators who represent different problem areas as well as different conceptual and strategical orientations. If for no other purpose than to foster communication, and hopefully result in the clarification of issues and problems. The conference was also intended to serve as the basis for this publication, which is meant to provide a current picture of the state of the science.

The book, as was the conference, is structured around problem areas. Because of recent interest in the use of operant or biofeedback procedures in the modification of visceral events, 10 chapters are devoted to the description of research and airing of problems by a diverse group of researchers, using both human and animal preparations. Most of the research is basic although two chapters summarize the work in clinical application. Five chapters deal with research using primarily the classical conditioning paradigm or some variation thereof, not so much because of interest in conditioning per se, but because this simplest of behavioral paradigms offers an excellent vantage point for observing the interactional nature of cardiovascular and behavioral processes. An additional three chapters overview work which might be best subsumed under attentional and motivational processes, problem areas which continue to draw considerable effort.

The book also has five chapters devoted to methodological issues. One principle issue concerns the use of the curarized preparation, which recent evidence has shown to contain some unforeseen problems. Three chapters are devoted to measurement problems. One details currently available techniques for the indirect measurement of blood pressure, for which there is growing interest. Another surveys available techniques for chronic preparation with references cited for more detailed presentation of procedures. There is no question that the chronic preparation is a strategy that will be used more and more frequently. A third chapter overviews techniques for measuring the contractile force of the heart. It is beyond the scope of this book to be a methodological atlas. Rather, it is our purpose to emphasize current issues and make the reader aware of contemporary techniques.

Finally, two introductory chapters are devoted to an overview of cardiovascular physiology. One concerns central nervous system control, and the other overviews peripheral cardiovascular physiology and contemporary theories on hypertensive states. These are provided as only starting points or primers so that the reader may grasp some fundamentals of the physiology of the system. Such knowledge would seem to be necessary to the behaviorally-oriented researchers, yet often it is not provided in a book of this sort.

Admittedly, the chapters vary as to the scope and depth of their coverage; this was done intentionally. Some detail efforts of individual investigators, while others are more or less critical overviews of an area and still others provide some combination of these two.

The book is intended for investigators, teachers, and students at the advanced undergraduate and graduate levels. In order to make it useful for instructional purposes, the chapters on cardiovascular physiology and central nervous control of the heart have been added to provide the reader with a minimal working knowledge of the cardiovascular system. These chapters are adequately referenced so that the reader can obtain more detailed background information. The methodology chapters can also be useful to the student in providing an updated overview of available techniques.

Numerous organizations and people have contributed substantially to the organization of the conference and preparation of the book; for this we are very grateful. The conference was funded by the National Science Foundation, Grant GB-31624. Additional funding for various conference activities and for preparation of the book was provided by the Department of Psychiatry, Medical School, University of North Carolina, Morris A. Lipton, Chairman. Beckman Instruments and Aldine Publishing Company also enhanced the social atmosphere of the conference.

A special note of thanks is given to Professor Richard L. Solomon, University of Pennsylvania, for his role as a discussant at the conference. Numerous people associated with the Department of Psychiatry of the University of North Carolina have contributed both to the conference and preparation of the book. We wish to particularly express our gratitude to Ann L. Greer, conference coordinator and editorial assistant, and Virginia Hodson, secretary. Lastly, we wish to thank Eleanor B. Obrist for acting as conference hostess and general expeditor.

Cardiovascular Psychophysiology

I

Cardiovascular Function
and Measurement

The first section attempts to provide an overview both of cardiovascular physiology and some contemporary measurement techniques. The first chapter by Forsyth initially describes some fundamentals of cardiovascular physiology so that the reader, if necessary, can better grasp material in this as well as other chapters. Obviously such an overview has to be superficial, but it is well documented with references to more detailed publications. Forsyth then overviews current conceptualizations about both the hemodynamic basis of hypertension and the role environmental stress may have in the etiology of hypertension. There are a couple of reasons for the necessity of this latter overview. Hypertension involves a quantitatively significant number of the population, and it has been held that environmental stressors or factors are critical in the etiology of at least certain hypertensions. On the other hand, psychophysiologists commonly appear naive with regard both to the hemodynamics of hypertension as well as to the complexities of the proposed etiological factors. It is hoped that this review will foster efforts by psychophysiologists to become more biologically sophisticated when we deal with this complex process. It might also be noted that over the past decade a greater emphasis has been placed on the role of cardiac output in the etiology of hypertension, thus making hypertension not just due to a vascular abnormality. This is of significance since the neural-humoral processes controlling the heart and vascular may differ.

The second chapter by Cohen and MacDonald overviews the central nervous system (CNS) control of cardiovascular events. In a sense, a knowledge of CNS processes might be considered a necessary starting point in understanding cardiovascular behavioral interactions. Unfortunately our knowledge of CNS control is very primitive and at a point

3

where it bears only in a limited manner on contemporary work. Nonetheless, such a review seems necessary if for no other reason than that a review of this kind has not been undertaken in the past decade.

The remaining four chapters focus on several parameters of cardiovascular function, particularly measurement techniques. These are parameters, which have not, in comparison to heart rate, drawn as much attention in psychophysiological research probably because of the more complex methodology involved. Yet they are from a hemodynamic point of view significant parameters of cardiovascular functioning.

Vasomotor activity and the force of the cardiac contraction are discussed in two of the chapters in an attempt to at least provide an overview of contemporary work with these measures which the editors feel is a minimal necessity in a book of this type. Both chapters delve only limitedly into specific issues and research efforts. The chapter on vasomotor activity by Cook rather briefly overviews some of the psychophysiological issues which plethysmographic phenomenon have concerned. Just as importantly, it attempts to depict the biological complexity of plethysmographic events, an effort which has not been previously made in the psychophysiological literature. The chapter on force of contraction by Lawler first discusses the nature of the force of contraction and then some of the means by which it has been measured. A particular effort is spent on assessing the use of rate of change measures as indices of left ventricular performance. Such measures have received considerable attention in the cardiovascular physiology literature but have as yet drawn little attention in the psychophysiology literature. They are also controversial measures in that they are subject to influence by hemodynamic processes other than the force of contractions. Yet there is emerging evidence that they do have a certain degree of validity, and in turn may provide unique information of behavioral influences on hemodynamic processes.

The last two chapters are more strictly methodological. Tursky discusses several of the newer automated devices used in the indirect measurement of blood pressure. In the light of the current interest in blood pressure, it was deemed essential to update the reader on this methodology. The final chapter, also by Forsyth, presents an updated overview of the techniques that are available for the study of the chronic intact preparation. The study of the chronic preparation is one of the necessary directions of future work, and we now have available a technology which enables us to obtain a reasonably complete picture of hemodynamic events. Yet it is likely that many readers are not aware of this technology. Hopefully, while this chapter will familiarize them with the techniques available, other chapters will convince the reader of the necessity and legitimacy of a chronic preparation.

RALPH P. FORSYTH

Mechanisms of the Cardiovascular Responses to Environmental Stressors

INTRODUCTION

The mechanisms controlling systemic arterial blood pressure and the distribution of blood flow in different tissues in the body involve highly complex regulatory systems which are interdependent and interactive. Changes in any one system necessarily affect the others. The advantage of this "mosaic" (Page 1966) multilevel control is the flexibility the cardiovascular system has in the maintenance of arterial blood pressure within narrow limits, the preservation of blood flow to vital organs such as the heart and brain during emergency situations, and the ability to redistribute blood flow to tissues in accordance with their metabolic needs. A disadvantage of this complexity is the increased chance that the regulatory mechanisms can misfunction and, themselves, produce disease states. Indeed, hypertension is often called a "disease of regulation."

This chapter[1] partially reviews some current knowledge about the operative mechanisms of cardiovascular control and examines the physiology and pharmacology of spontaneous and experimental hypertension. Selective hypotheses and promising lines of research on the role of environmental factors in the development of hypertension will be discussed. Only selected references are given. Especially useful reviews are Burton (1965), Rushmer (1961), Folkow and Neil (1971), and Pickering (1968).

Research supported in part by N.I.H. Program Project Grants HL-06285 and GM-16496.

MECHANISMS OF CARDIOVASCULAR CONTROL

Heart and Blood Vessels

The cardiovascular system consists of the heart, the blood vessels, and the lymphatics. The heart is a muscular organ which acts as a pump; its chief role is to deliver oxygenated blood to tissues. The blood carries carbon dioxide and other waste products from tissues to the organs of excretion and detoxification (chiefly the kidneys, liver, and lungs). Measurements of systemic arterial or venous blood pressure, cardiac output, and total peripheral resistance are useful indices of cardiovascular function but often do not reflect important changes in the perfusion of individual organs. Ideally, measurements of organ blood flow should be made, as these are the primary variables of importance in cardiovascular function.

The heart is composed of two pumps in series; between these pumps is the pulmonary circulation which oxygenates blood and is also an important organ of metabolism (Figure 1.1). The heart's intrinsic mechanical contractile properties, such as the velocity of muscle-fiber shortening and the development of tension (expressed as the velocity-length relationship), as well as its rhythmicity and rate can be influenced by nervous and humoral factors and total peripheral resistance. These variables can be partially controlled experimentally by use of the preparation in which the heart of an experimental animal is removed and studied in vitro (Starling 1918). Results obtained with this type of preparation may not be applicable to the intact organism. In other preparations, the heart (or other organs) may be left in situ and denervated or perfused with donor blood in order to exclude the influences of the nervous, humoral, or peripheral resistance factors. These kinds of studies are important in examining the mechanisms involved in cardiovascular regulation, and they complement studies in intact preparations which are more "physiological" but less specific concerning the mechanism(s) involved.

Cardiac output, usually expressed in liters per minute, is the product of the stroke volume (amount of blood ejected per contraction) and the heart rate. The ventricle contracts in systole in response to electrical stimulation originating from automatic pacemaker cells in the sino-atrial node. Pressure builds up inside the ventricle, opening the aortic valve, and blood is driven into the systemic circulation and distributed to peripheral tissues. The peak pressure is called systolic pressure, normally about 130 to 140 mmHg. Normally only about half of the blood in the left ventricle is pumped during each contraction, but during exercise, for example, when the contractility of cardiac muscle is increased, as much as 80% can be pumped. As the left ventricle relaxes in diastole, it refills with blood from the left atrium. When systemic arterial pressure exceeds left ventricular pressure, the aortic valve closes and pressures within the left ventricle continue to fall to near zero mmHg (left ventricular end-diastolic pressure). Systemic diastolic pressure is normally about 70 to 80 mmHg, because of the elastic recoil properties of peripheral arteries. A similar process with much lower pressure (20 to 30 mmHg systolic) occurs in the right ventricle.

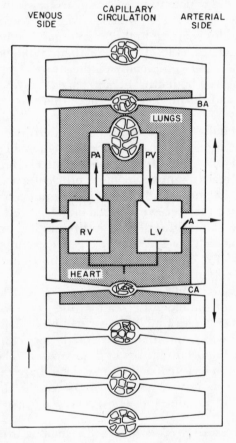

FIGURE 1.1 *A schematic diagram of the cardiovascular system. A=aorta; BA=bronchial artery; CA=coronary artery; LV=left ventricle; PA=pulmonary artery; PV=pulmonary vein; RV=right ventricle.*

The heart rate and the contractile properties of the heart are neurogenically controlled by both parasympathetic vagal and sympathetic influences. Factors affecting the stroke volume include the volume of venous return, the left ventricular end-diastolic filling pressure, the degree of contractility of the left ventricle, and the resistance opposing the ejection of the blood into the circulation. The heart supplies most of its own oxygen and nutritives via the peripheral circulation (coronary arteries); if the cardiac output is decreased and there is no compensatory regulation to increase blood flow to the heart, a progressive compromise of the pumping ability of the ventricles will occur.

Several mechanisms protect the heart and other vital organs in situations which threaten their oxygen supply. When systemic arterial pressure decreases, the hypotension evokes a strong sympathetic response, mediated by the baroreceptors, which evokes a redistribution of cardiac output favoring the heart and other vital organs at the expense of the kidney and skeletal muscle. The sympathetic influences also increase the pumping rate and contractility of the heart. These compensatory changes are observed both after hemorrhage (Forsyth, Hoffbrand, and Melmon 1970) and during anemia, where there is a reduced number of oxygen-carrying red blood cells (Hoffbrand and Forsyth 1971). Under these conditions, blood flow to the brain is maintained by sensitive local mechanisms which evoke vasodilatation in response to the anoxia (decreased PO_2) that follows inadequate cerebral blood flow.

Other organs react to anoxia by more efficient extraction of oxygen from the blood. The heart and skeletal muscle in exercise extract about 70% of the oxygen they receive (skeletal muscle at rest consumes about 33%), while the skin, kidney, and gastrointestinal tract receive disproportionate blood flow for their oxygen consumption. These last organs, of course, use blood to support other functions such as dissipating heat, producing urine, and absorbing nutrients.

As arteries branch and become progressively smaller, the pressure and the velocity of the blood decrease as the total cross-sectional area and resistance increase in rough approximation to Poiseville's law. The length and radius (to the 4th power) of the vessel and the viscosity of the blood are important factors in this equation. The arterial vessels are covered with innervated smooth muscle and are called "resistance" vessels. The venous return system, because of the thinner walls and lower pressures in venules and veins, serves a "capacitance" function hemodynamically.

The major pressure drop occurs in the smallest arterioles, the precapillary resistance vessels, which have muscularly cuffed sphincters at the entrance to capillaries. Changes in the radius (and thus the resistance) of these vessels and in the sphincter tension at the arterial and venous ends of the capillaries largely determine both the blood flow to that tissue and the hydrostatic (driving) pressure in the capillary. At this level, control is partly local, due to inherent myogenic activity of smooth muscle (the smooth muscle contracts in response to increased pressure within it) and to vasodilator metabolites; these influences attempt to maintain a relatively constant capillary blood flow over

a range of pressure, and are thus designated "autoregulatory." Neurogenic influences are also present via sympathetic innervation of the
smooth muscle covering arterial and venous blood vessels.

The basic work of transport between the blood and tissue is performed in capillaries which have no neural innervation. The hydrostatic pressure difference between the capillary and interstitial fluid
(about 15 mmHg) largely determines the amount of filtration that
occurs. For example, during hemorrhage or other states of low arterial
and, thus, capillary pressure, water is taken up from the tissues into
the vascular space. This increases blood volume, cardiac output, and,
finally, arterial blood pressure. The opposite will occur in states of high
capillary pressure due to either high arterial pressure or obstructed
venous return. In these cases, edema will occur in the affected tissue.
For example, during heart failure, when sympathetic stimulatory
mechanisms cannot compensate, the left ventricle is not able to pump
all the blood supplied to it by the right ventricle. Pressure increases
in the capillaries of the lungs and pulmonary edema occurs.

Other influences, such as the colloid-osmotic pressure difference in
the plasma and interstitial fluid which mainly affects absorption, will
affect transcapillary exchange. Local hormones, such as bradykinin,
kallidin, and histamine, in addition to their vasodilator action, increase
capillary permeability and diffusion of protein and water from the
blood to the tissues. This process also occurs in response to inflamma-
tion and other stimuli. Lymphatic vessels serve to return protein and
fluid from tissues to the vascular system.

Capillaries in various tissues are remarkably specialized in their structure and function. Capillaries in the central nervous system and in all
types of muscle, lung, fat, and connective tissue are covered by a continuous single layer of endothelial cells with an outer basement membrane, both of which restrict capillary exchange. Cerebral capillaries,
uniquely, have no (or very small) intercellular pores. This may be the
structural basis of the blood-brain barrier. On the other hand, capillaries in the renal glomeruli, glands, and intestinal mucosa have numerous intracellular openings (fenestrations) which facilitate exchange of
solvents and solutes. Bone marrow, liver, and spleen have no basement
membrane. The large intracellular holes or gaps allow transmural
exchange of very large molecules and even of whole blood cells.

Capillary exchange function is an important participant in the regulation of both extracellular fluid volume and cardiovascular events
(Mason and Bartter 1968; Gauer, Henry, and Behn 1970). The
described capillary function plays an important role in the amount of
blood in the venous circulation, which in turn influences the filling
pressures of the heart (right and left atrial pressure, and right and

left ventricular end-diastolic pressure and volume). Starling's law of the heart, although strictly applicable only in the isolated heart (i.e., neurogenic and hormonal influences can be mitigating), states that, up to a critical point, the energy of contraction of ventricular muscle is a function of the length of the muscle fiber. This same principle is the basis of the myogenic response. Thus, stroke volume will vary as the ventricular end-diastolic volume of each ventricle varies. This principle is essential to the maintenance of equal output from the right and left ventricles and to a stable distribution of blood volume between the systemic and pulmonary circulation (Hamilton 1955). The profound effects of the regulation of fluid volume which are also under both autonomic and hormonal control are central points in various models of hypertension and will be discussed below in greater detail.

The Autonomic Nervous System

The autonomic nervous system is comprised of sympathetic and parasympathetic divisions which supply innervation of glands, heart, and blood vessels. Afferent neural impulses originate from stretch and chemical transducers, as well as from the central nervous system (CNS). Preganglionic autonomic nerves have cholinergic (acetylcholine) transmission at their synapses, as do the postganglionic nerves of the parasympathetic nervous system (PNS). In most cases, norepinephrine (NE) is the transmitter in postganglionic nerve endings in the sympathetic nervous system (SNS). An example of this arrangement is shown in Figure 1.2. One important exception to this is sympathetic innervation of the adrenal gland, which is cholinergic. Recent important advances have been made in the pharmacology of neural transmission at the postganglionic sympathetic nerve endings where synthesis, storage, release, and reuptake of the neurotransmitter, NE, occur. Most clinical treatment of hypertension is now accomplished by interfering with SNS transmission either at the pre- or postganglionic level, concomitant with treatment with thiazide diuretic which deplete salt from the body and thus lower the blood volume. This type of combined treatment reduces blood pressure mostly by lowering cardiac output. This does not necessarily mean that the primary mechanism in essential hypertension is excessive SNS activity, although some investigators believe it can be an important factor (Dustan, Tarazi, and Bravo 1972).

The adrenergic (sympathetic) receptors are functionally classified in two types, the α and β receptors (Ahlquist 1948). Although this distinction is based purely on pharmacological evidence and has no direct anatomical support, the theory has proved useful in understanding the dose-related responses of the cardiovascular system to epinephrine. More recently, the discovery of independent α and β blocking agents (phentolamine and propranolol, respectively) has added considerable support to this theory (Moran 1970).

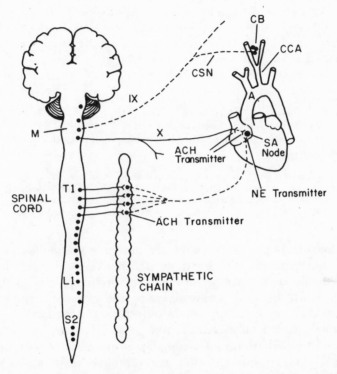

FIGURE 1.2 *A schematic diagram of the autonomic pathway serving the carotid baroreceptor reflexes. The IX and X nerves are parasympathetic; outflow from T_1 to T_4 is the efferent sympathetic innervation. The long dotted line represents the afferent neural connection from the baroreceptor to the medulla. The solid line represents the preganglionic autonomic nerves. The short dotted lines are the postganglionic autonomic nerves. A=aorta; ACH=acetylcholine; CB=carotid baroreceptor; CCA=common carotid artery; CSN=carotid sinus nerve; L=lumbar; M=medulla; NE=norepinephrine; S=sacral; SA=sino-atrial; T=thoracic; IX=glossopharyngeal nerve; X=vagus nerve.*

Phenylephrine and norepinephrine primarily stimulate α-receptors, while isoproterenol is the "purest" β-stimulator. Epinephrine at low doses is an α-stimulator; at high doses it additionally evokes β-like effects. Table 1.1 lists the cardiovascular effects of α and β stimulation. These drugs have a wide variety of clinical uses. For example, blocking agents can be used to screen patients with acute hypertensive episodes due to pheochromocytomas (chromaffin cell tumors in the adrenal medulla secreting excessive amounts of catecholamines). If blood pressure falls dramatically after injection of phentolamine, it can be assumed that the hypertension was due to excessive blood levels of NE or epinephrine.

TABLE 1.1   *Alpha and beta cardiovascular adrenergic function*

Alpha Stimulation
1. Constricts arterioles, mostly in skin, splanchnic bed, and kidneys
2. Inhibits insulin release

Beta Stimulation
1. Dilates arterioles, primarily in skeletal muscle and heart
2. Constricts veins and venules (maybe)
3. Inotropic and chronotropic actions on heart
4. Increased metabolic lipolysis, glycogenolysis, and insulin release
5. Dilates bronchial tree

NOTE: The net result of sympathetic stimulation is an increased cardiac output with a balanced pattern of total peripheral resistance changes; i.e., increases in resistance in skin, splanchnic bed, and kidneys while vasodilatation, occurs in skeletal muscle and heart. Metabolic effects include increased levels of blood sugar and plasma free fatty acids.

In dogs and cats, but apparently not in primates, a sympathetic cholinergic pathway independent of the classical SNS has been reported and anatomically verified. This system, originating in the motor areas of the cortex and bypassing the vasomotor center (VMC) in the medulla, is especially potent in inducing vasodilatation of resistance vessels in skeletal muscle (Uvnas 1954).

The most powerful, rapidly acting homeostatic mechanism in the cardiovascular system is the carotid baroreceptor reflex (Figure 1.2). At the bifurcation of the carotid artery, nerve endings (which form the carotid sinus nerve) sensitive to distortion or stretch are seated in an expansion of the vessel wall. These endings transduce pressure to neural pulses; the higher the pressure (from about 20 to 200 mmHg), the higher the frequency of the pulses in the visceral afferent fibers. Different receptors respond to different ranges of pressure. The carotid sinus nerve travels with the glossopharyngeal (1Xth) nerve to the VMC in the medulla. As pressure and afferent activity increases, the efferent arm of the reflex slows the heart through the motor nucleus of the vagus (Xth) nerve and decreases sympathetic influences on the peripheral vasculature. As pressure and then carotid sinus nerve activity decrease, efferent vagal activity is inhibited and sympathetic tone is increased which in turn accelerates heart rate (chronotropic effect), enhances atrial and ventricular contractility (inotropic effect), and increases peripheral sympathetic tone: Thus, this is a negative feedback system. Although parasympathetic drive influences the rate and contractile properties of the heart, it is believed that the peripheral vascular tone, as far as neural regulation is concerned, is completely controlled by excitation or inhibition of sympathetic outflow (see Heymans and Neil 1958); so post-ganglionic sympathetic nerves are often referred to as the "final common pathway" of peripheral neurogenic control.

There are also other stretch receptors in the cardiovascular system. A group of them are located on the aortic arch (aortic baroreceptors); their afferent fibers travel with the vagus to the VMC. Others whose functions are less well known are located in the walls of the descending thoracic aorta and the cerebral and pulmonary vessels, and in the atria and ventricular walls of the heart. There are also chemoreceptors which become functionally important during anoxia. Their prototype is the carotid body (also lying in the carotid bifurcation) which is densely innervated and has a rich blood supply. These receptors are stimulated by a reduced oxygen supply, increased carbon dioxide, or a lowered arterial pH—any of which leads to increased sympathetic drive which increases ventilation and blood pressure.

In the past decade, there has been increasing interest in the interaction of the CNS and the VMC in the medulla (Piess 1965). It is thought that supramedullary (especially hypothalamic) influences operate by modulating excitability of the VMC. For example, during electrical stimulation of pressor hypothalamic areas and pressor episodes related to emotional stress, at least part of baroreceptor function appears to be inhibited; heart rate as well as blood pressure remain high until the stimulus is stopped. However, the baroreceptor control of central sympathetic outflow remains functionally important during hypothalamic stimulation (Gebber and Snyder 1970). The threshold for regional vascular resistance changes in response to sympathetic stimulation appears to be lower than that needed to produce systemic changes. It is apparent that there can be physiologically important, sympathetically-mediated redistribution of cardiac output without major changes of systemic blood pressure, cardiac output or total peripheral resistance (Forsyth 1972).

Humoral Influences

Another important homeostatic mechanism originates in the kidney, which evokes a humoral, rather than a neural, response. The afferent stimulus probably originates from a stretch receptor in the afferent glomerular arteriolar wall, but some investigators believe the effective stimulus is a change in sodium concentration at the macula densa. In either case, a fall in blood flow (and/or pressure) in the renal artery evokes renin release into the plasma from the juxtaglomerular apparatus (Table 1.2). Renin, an enzyme, rapidly converts a substrate to angiotensin I which is then converted to angiotensin II. Angiotensin II influences the glomerular filtration rate (rate of fluid passing from the glomerular capillaries into the renal tubules) and the tubular reabsorption of sodium. Angiotensin also causes renal vasoconstriction; thus, it has a powerful influence on both renal circulation and renal function (McGiff 1968). In addition, circulating angiotensin can evoke aldosterone secretion from the adrenal cortex and can potentiate the effects of SNS activity and circulating catecholamines, presumably by substituting for NE in postganglionic nerve synapses (Zimmerman 1967). Angiotensin may also have a direct effect on the VMC in the brainstem, evoking a sympathetic discharge (Ferrario, Gildenberg, and McCubbin 1972). Many investigators feel that impaired renal function with even slightly elevated levels of angiotensin may be important in both the early labile phase of hypertension and in many cases of essential hypertension.

TABLE 1.2 *Pathway of the normal homeostatic control of fluid volume by the renin-angiotensin-aldosterone system*

Consequence	Sequence of Events	Consequence
IF		IF
DECREASED	Circulating blood volume and/or arterial pressure	INCREASED
DECREASED	Renal perfusion pressure Justaglomerular cell receptor (or sodium receptors in macula densa)	INCREASED
RELEASE	Renin production (substrate angiotensinogen)	INHIBITION
INCREASED	Angiotensin I (converting enzyme mostly in pulmonary circulation)	DECREASED
INCREASED	Angiotensin II (inactivated by angiotensinases)	DECREASED
INCREASED	Aldosterone	DECREASED
INCREASED	Sodium reabsorption from renal tubules	DECREASED
INCREASED	Circulating blood volume and/or arterial pressure	DECREASED

These mechanisms are important in the body's defense against hemorrhagic shock. As blood volume and pressure fall during bleeding, renin, angiotensin, and aldosterone are released. This constricts peripheral vessels, thus slowing the bleeding and increasing total peripheral resistance. At the same time there is both an increased sodium reabsorption from the renal tubules and an inhibition of diuresis which expand blood volume. Also, as previously mentioned, the lowered capillary (compared to interstitial) pressure promotes an increased vascular absorption of tissue water. Concomitantly, the baroreceptor response evokes increased sympathetic tone stimulating the heart's rate and contractility as well as a redistribution of cardiac output to vital organs. It is evident that this elaborate hormonal regulation is designed to maintain control of fluid volume which is of critical importance in cardiovascular control. As will be seen below, dysfunction of these regulatory mechanisms can cause or contribute to arterial hypertension.

The adrenal medullary catecholamines, epinephrine and NE, secreted in response to sympathetic stimulation, have important metabolic actions in liver, muscle, and fat as well as the previously mentioned effects on α- and β-cardiovascular receptors. Epinephrine, the more important of the two adrenal amines in man, increases glycogenolysis and the mobilization of free fatty acids and, thus, serves both as a homeostatic regulator of blood sugar levels and a mechanism for a source of "emergency" energy. The metabolic effects of these adrenal catecholamines appear to be more important than their direct effects on the heart and blood vessels, in that their direct cardiovascular effects in normal "physiologic" situations are, like those of angiotensin, relatively trivial (Celander 1954). However, the amounts of NE (in a separate "pool") released by sympathetic postganglionic nerve fibers are powerful influences in sympathetically mediated function.

Mineralocorticoids, such as desoxycorticosterone and aldosterone, are secreted from the adrenal cortex in response to adrenocorticotrophic hormone (ACTH) and other stimuli such as angiotensin. They cause the retention of sodium in the body and the loss of potassium, with attendant hemodynamic effects.

A number of other hormones, such as thyroxin and the prostaglandins, also have important metabolic and cardiovascular effects which will not be described here. Of particular interest is the role of the electrolytes, sodium and potassium, especially their extracellular/intracellular content in arteriolar smooth muscle cells. This interest was stimulated by the observation that the water content of arteries in hypertensive patients is often increased (Peterson 1963). This may be due to secondary effects of excessive mineralocorticoid production. The fact that diuretics potentiate the hypotensive effects of ganglionic blocking agents adds additional support for this point of view.

Central Nervous System (CNS)

The brain and the spinal cord comprise the CNS; its role in regard to cardiovascular regulation is more speculative than that of the peripheral nervous system, due to obvious technical problems. Detailed maps of many parts of the brain and spinal cord locate areas which evoke changes in blood pressure and, in some cases, blood flow to peripheral tissues when electrical or chemical stimulation is applied. Except for the hypothalamus and brain stem, little is known about CNS mechanisms of control. Head injuries, brain tumors, or poliomyelitis can lead to hypertensive episodes of varying duration.

The best understood function of the CNS is the neuroendocrine system regulated by the hypothalamic-pituitary axis. The hypothalamus secretes different polypeptide "releasing factors" into the portal hypophysial vessels which regulate the release of anterior pituitary hormones. These "stimulating" pituitary hormones have widespread metabolic effects which directly affect the function of the thyroid, adrenals, sexual organs, and somatic growth. The resultant hormonal outputs of these glands have direct feedback effect on their own release, either at the hypothalamic or pituitary level. Of most direct importance to the cardiovascular system is the hypothalamic release of the corticotropin-releasing factor which regulates ACTH release. ACTH promotes adrenal cortical release of cortisol and other glucocorticoids; it has a lesser effect compared to the stimulating action of angiotensin II, on mineralocorticoid secretion. Glucocorticoids are essential to survival in severely stressful situations; it is interesting that during such stressful situations, the negative feedback control of cortisol on ACTH release is overridden—allowing blood levels of cortisol to continue to increase, promoting increased carbohydrate, protein, and fat metabolism.

Vasopressin (antidiuretic hormone) is secreted by the posterior lobe of the pituitary in response to neural stimulation originating in or near the supraoptic nuclei of the hypothalamus. Near this area, osmoreceptor cells sensitive to the osmotic pressure of blood plasma are the receptors involved in this delicate feedback mechanism. Vasopressin causes retention of water by the kidney with a resulting increase of extracellular fluid and blood volume, and a reduced osmotic pressure; further vasopressin secretion is then inhibited. Hemorrhage, pain, trauma, and emotional stress increase the release of this hormone. The baroreceptors appear to have some influence on this system through direct neural connection.

The hypothalamus has multiple afferent and efferent neural connections which make the elucidation of its control difficult. It has been called the "head ganglion of the autonomic system" in that its multiple functions involve integrating many different stimuli and response systems. Limbic structures (hippocampus, amygdala, and septum) have direct neural pathways to the hypothalamus. Electrical and chemical stimulation (or ablation) of limbic areas can markedly affect autonomic function as well as feeding, sexual, and emotional response. Thus, it is believed that the limbic areas, as well as the cerebral cortices, have an important synergistic relationship with hypothalamicpituitary function.

The concepts about the function of the earlier mentioned VMC in the medulla have been challenged (Hilton 1966), especially the concept of discrete pressor (vasoconstriction) and depression (vasodilator) centers in the VMC. Since there are multiple neural inputs from cortical and limbic structures to the hypothalamus, it is likely that the integration of emotional behavior and voluntary movement with the appropriate cardiovascular responses is located at the hypothalamic level, while the integration of reflex stimuli from baroreceptors and chemoreceptors are handled in medullary areas. The hypothalamus, as previously noted, has important influences on baroreceptor efficiency (Wang and Chai 1965). The practical relevance of this function in hypertension is as yet unresolved, as is the extent of independent control by supramedullary structures.

There has been much work in CNS pharmacology in regard to cardiovascular control. Part of this interest is the continuing problem of defining the synaptic transmitter(s) in the CNS: Various candidates include acetylcholine and NE, as in the autonomic nervous system; as well as the NE precursor dopamine; serotonin; and gamma amino butric acid. All of these possible transmitters have been found in various concentrations and locations in the CNS, but their functional roles are not known.

Interest in this area has been spurred by the recent introduction of two clinically used drugs which can control hypertension apparently by acting in the CNS. These drugs, alpha-methyldopa and clonidine, appear to exert their hypotensive action by interfering with central mechanisms of blood pressure regulation; this in turn leads to a reduction of sympathetic tone (Henning 1969). Similarly, recent evidence using an experimentally bred strain of spontaneously hypertensive rats indicates that brainstem and hypothalamic levels of NE decrease as hypertension develops (Yamori, Lovenberg, and Sjoerdsma 1970). Although these studies remain controversial in many respects, it is apparent that pharmacological studies of the CNS may be as fruitful in understanding cardiovascular regulation as those in the peripheral nervous system.

Summary

The mechanisms of cardiovascular regulation can be conveniently grouped into two categories, local and remote control. At the local level (within each tissue) there are powerful homeostatic mechanisms which attempt to autoregulate blood flow. When pressure and/or blood flow is increased, arteriolar smooth muscle is stretched and exerts increased tone (myogenic forces). High pressure in tissue capillaries promotes filtration of fluid into the tissues decreasing blood volume, cardiac output, and blood pressure. High arterial pressure in the kidney increases the glomerular filtration rate and the production of urine, which also lowers blood volume. In states of low blood pressure and decreased blood flow, these processes are reversed. Ischemic tissues may also produce and release a number of vasodilator substances to attempt to increase their blood supply.

Remote mechanisms consist of the neurogenic and hormonal influences which also serve to maintain homeostasis. The most important neurogenic reflexes are the stretch receptors in the carotid sinus region, which evoke autonomic activity to modulate changes in systemic arterial blood pressure. An important exception may be the brain which has particularly powerful autoregulatory mechanisms. Different tissues have different densities of sympathetic innervation as well as different combinations of efferent receptors (alpha and beta). Thus, although the SNS discharges "en masse," it has different actions in different organs. The CNS also has powerful, but ill-defined, control over the autonomic nervous system.

Remote homeostatic hormonal influences have important interaction with the SNS; they are slower, but longer-acting compared to neurogenic influences. Glucocorticoids, mineralocorticoids, and catecholamines are released into the circulation from the adrenal gland in response to SNS stimulation and/or the hypothalamic—pituitary hormone system, and vasopressin is released from the posterior pituitary. Finally, stretch or chemical transducers in the kidney exert powerful homeostatic control of renal function and can, in certain situations, affect the whole cardiovascular system through activation of the renin-angiotensinaldosterone pathway.

MODELS OF HYPERTENSION

Naturally Occurring Hypertension

Essential Hypertension. It is variously estimated that between 80 and 95% of patients clinically diagnosed as hypertensive (an age- and sex-related norm with pressures above 140 to 150 mmHg systolic and/or 90 to 100 mmHg diastolic) have no known cause or etiology for the disease; thus, the term "primary" or "essential." There has been continuing disagreement (the Pickering-Platt controversy) over whether essential hypertension is a pathological disease process per se or merely the upper limits of a continuous distribution of pressures which are genetically determined (Pickering 1968). In either case, the consequences of continuous elevated pressures are real since they are associated with cerebrovascular accidents, congestive heart failure, coronary heart disease, and renal damage. Effective treatment dramatically reduces the risk of cardiovascular complications.

The natural history of untreated essential hypertension illustrates its progressive, long-term nature. In the early phases blood pressure may only transiently elevated, but it can fluctuate unusually in response to emotional or environmental stressors (the cold pressor and mental arithmetic tests are often used clinically). Strong familial influences on blood pressure are evident relatively early in life (Zinner, Levy, and Kass 1971), indicating that either very early environmental factors or genetic influences are responsible for a later predisposition to hypertension.

Blood pressure increases throughout adult life in almost all people. Some reports find that the slope of this statistical relationship is steeper in those persons whose blood pressure starts in the upper segment of the population distribution curve. As pressures increase, the severity of ocular funduscopic abnormalities (pathology in retinal vessels), enlargement of the left ventricle (hypertrophy of cardiac muscle), and electrocardiographic changes increase (Sokolow et al. 1966). If unchecked, a course of accelerated and finally malignant hypertension can ensue with further tissue damage, renal dysfunction, and early death.

In early labile hypertensive subjects, the cardiac output as well as heart rate and oxygen consumption are found to be elevated, although there is considerable variation in these findings (Eich et al. 1966). Many investigators have commented on the similarity of these findings with those in normal persons who have an emotional response, are exercising, or are preparing to exercise. This in turn has led to speculation that emotional or environmental factors are important in this early stage of hypertension.

The elevated pressures of patients with essential hypertension are, in general, entirely due to an increased total peripheral resistance; i.e., cardiac output is normal while systemic arterial pressures are high. The elevated resistance is thought to be reflected in every tissue of the body except skeletal muscle, but is unusually intense in the kidney (Pickering 1968). The mechanisms which act over years to change the hemodynamic pattern from one of an elevated cardiac output to one of a fixed increased peripheral resistance have been hotly debated and will be discussed in detail later.

There have been many attempts to define neurogenic and humoral deficits of dysfunction in essential hypertensive patients. Like research in the etiology of schizophrenia, reports of abnormal function in hypertension have difficulty in separating the cause and effect relationships; i.e., are the dysfunctions a cause of the hypertension or a result of it? The answer to this problem awaits either long-term studies in humans or a reliable experimental animal model which can be verified in man.

Renovascular Hypertension. The most common curable (as opposed to controllable) form of hypertension is renovascular hypertension caused by the obstruction of the blood supply, or other types of damage to one or both kidneys. Interest in this disease goes beyond the clinical, because the mechanisms understood concerning its etiology have led to important discoveries about renal function and the regulation of blood volume and blood pressure by the renin-angiotension-aldosterone system, as previously described. Goldblatt and his colleagues (Goldblatt et al. 1934) first demonstrated in dogs that persistent hypertension follows constriction of the renal artery which causes a decrease of pressure and flow as seen by the renin receptors. Thus, renovascular hypertension is often complicated by secondary aldosteronism. The high blood levels of aldosterone released by circulating angiotensin cause increased sodium retention, a decrease in body potassium stores, an expansion of blood volume, and an increased arterial pressure.

A similar mechanism with some variation occurs when the kidney becomes ischemic due to renal parenchymal disease (lesions of the glomerulus or other small intrarenal vessels). In either large or small vessel occlusion the renin receptor mistakenly interprets the fall in blood flow and pressure as evidence that the systemic arterial pressure and circulating blood volume are low.

Surgical removal of the diseased kidney or correction of the renal blood flow obstruction usually results in a fall of blood pressure to normal. In animals with chronic experimental renovascular hypertension produced by a clamp on the renal artery, the blood pressure can be lowered to normal when adequate blood levels of antirenin are induced, thus confirming the humoral nature of the disease.

Renin may have important action independent of its angiotensin-stimulating function. A recent study indicated that essential hypertensive patients with low renin levels have fewer complications than those with normal or elevated renin levels. (Laragh et al. 1972). Some investigators believe that "occult" renal disease is responsible for many cases of hypertension diagnosed as essential; however, pathological renal lesions have not been found in essential hypertensives who died of other causes unless they were in advanced phases of the disease.

Endocrine Hypertension. Cases of endocrine-evoked hypertension are rare, but they are important in understanding the role of the endocrine system in cardiovascular control. Three syndromes relating to raised blood levels of adrenal hormones and their subsequent hypertensive effects are well known. Cushing's syndrome refers to a constellation of symptoms, including hypertension, due to elevated blood levels of the glucocorticoid, cortisol, and caused by autonomous hypersecreting adenomas or hyperplasia in the inner layers of the adrenal cortex, or by hypersecretion of ACTH. The hypertension of Conn's syndrome is due to overproduction and release of the mineralocorticoid, aldosterone (primary aldosteronism); these tumors are found in the outer layers of the adrenal cortex. The third type of endocrine hypertension (pheocromocytoma) results from tumors in chromaffin tissue mostly in the adrenal medulla which release excessive amounts of catecholamines.

The ability of these tumors to secrete hormones depends on their size and function. Clinically, any sudden appearance of hypertension, especially in a younger person, should suggest the possibility of endocrine hypertension. Adenomas can be surgically removed, but this will not always lead to a lowered blood pressure—either because of an incomplete removal or because of the possibility that smooth muscle hypertrophy, hyperplasia, or renovascular sclerosis has begun.

Miscellaneous Secondary Hypertension. Common causes of increased systolic pressure are arteriosclerosis or atherosclerosis, especially in the older patient. In these conditions, the vessel walls have reduced diameter and become stiff and less compliant. Thus, a normal ejection of blood into the arterial tree will cause a higher systolic, but not necessarily an increased diastolic, pressure.

Other mechanical factors occasionally cause clinically interesting cases of hypertension. In aortic coarctation, usually seen in infants, the aorta is narrowed or constricted causing high pressure in those arterial vessels above the coarctation (the arms and head) and hypotension in those vessels below. In these circumstances regulatory mechanisms will oppose each other; the carotid baroreceptor would reduce sympathetic activity to the heart and blood vessels, while the renal receptors would engage the renin-angiotension-aldosterone system. Local influences at the capillary level would also be different depending on the pressure they received.

Experimental Models of Hypertension

Renovascular. As previously mentioned, this experimental model has been used since Goldblatt developed the original technique in 1934. Despite its prodigious use since then, several vexing problems remain to be solved. For example, there are apparent species differences. In the dog and rabbit—in contrast to the rat and, probably, man—the kidney contralateral to the occluded renal artery must be removed to produce the hypertension. In all these species, hypertension causes hypertrophy in the left ventricle and in small and medium-sized arteries throughout the body. Fibrinoid arteriolar necrosis, like that found in the malignant phase of human hypertension, is also present in animals with severe hypertension. The clamped kidney is spared in this regard in that it does not face the full force of the pressure load (see Pickering 1968). Recent research has indicated that, for unknown reasons, a different hemodynamic pattern occurs (with a worse prognosis) if the kidney contralateral to the clipped kidney is removed rather than being left in place.

In renal, as with essential, hypertension the carotid baroreceptors appear to be "reset" at the new high pressure level. That is, after a period of hypertension the carotid baroreceptors fire intermittently as when pressures were normal, rather than firing continuously. One explanation for this is that the arterial wall in the baroreceptor area, as elsewhere, hypertrophies and stiffens in response to the increased pressure and, thus, stretches less for a given pressure load. It has been also mentioned that supramedullary neural influences can change the threshold level of the baroreceptors.

Continuous infusions of renin or angiotensin will also create hypertension, although not to the same high levels produced by experimental renal artery stenosis. Often in patients and other animals with chronic renal hypertension, renin levels are not found to be elevated, although aldosterone usually is. Some investigators believe that renin is responsible for the early but not the later stages of hypertension, a hypothesis that has also been invoked in essential hypertension.

Salt and Mineralocorticoid Excesses. In the rat, but not in the dog or rabbit, hypertension can be created by introducing salt in the drinking water. Rats have been bred for their sensitivity to this response (Dahl, Heine, and Tassinari 1962), illustrating the possible genetic mechanism seen in essential hypertension. The importance of salt and potassium in arterial smooth muscle cells is also illustrated by the adrenal mineralocorticoid, desoxycorticosterone, which, unless the diet is salt-free, can produce hypertension in the rat. These results led to treatment of essential hypertension first with salt-free diets and, later, with the salt-depleting thiazide diuretics.

Neurogenic. Bilateral transection of the carotid sinus and aortic nerves produces a marked instability of arterial blood pressure with periodic hypertension. Since the important baroreceptor reflexes that buffer blood pressure changes are removed, any excitement will cause prolonged tachycardia and hypertension, and an increase in cardiac output; however, in patients at rest or during sleep, these measurements are usually at normal levels. Although this preparation is of some research interest, its relevance to essential hypertension is not as compelling as that obtained in renovascular or other salt-related models. Essential hypertensives do have functioning baroreceptors although they are reset and, perhaps, less efficient than those in normals. It is generally felt that the resetting occurs during the period of high blood pressure rather than before.

Recent evidence has indicated that bilateral electrolytic lesions of the nucleus tractus solitarii at the level of the obex (where afferent baroreceptor nerves terminate) abolish baroreceptor reflexes and produce an acute fulminating hypertension in unanesthetized rats (Doba and Reis 1973). The hypertension was shown to be due to intense sympathetic discharge and peripheral vasovonstriction mediated by alpha receptors. Stroke volume and cardiac output fell while heart rate was unchanged. Thus, the presumed complete removal of all inhibitory influences from systemic baroreceptors by these lesions produces a more dramatic neurogenic hypertension than the cutting of the carotid sinus and aortic nerves. This study suggests that baroreceptors, other than those in the ascending aorta and the carotid areas, play an important role in blood pressure regulation.

Genetic. At least three different strains of rats have been bred to show conclusively that genetic predisposition is an important cause of hypertension in this species. This evidence has led many investigators to interpret that the familial tendency of human hypertension is genetic in nature, at least in terms of predisposing the individual who also faces physiologic or environmental stressors. To date, however, the mechanism of this predisposition is not clear; it may relate to a supersensibility to salt intake, hyperresponsiveness to normal amounts of angiotensin or aldosterone, changes in the pharmacology of the CNS, or a variety of other mechanisms. There may, in fact, be a number of different genetically based defects which result in hypertension. The search for a single determinant of all essential hypertension is probably futile; a reasonable hope is to dissect out as many secondary causes as possible. Only a few decades ago, all hypertension was "essential."

Environmental and Psychological. It is clear that those environmental stimuli which produce behavioral reactions can have profound acute effects on circulation, as well as on other organ systems. In normotensive subjects, environmental stimulation results in a rise in cardiac output due to an increased heart rate (stroke volume remains normal; the increase in contractility and the fraction of blood ejected per stroke is balanced by a decreased left ventricular end-diastolic volume, which occurs because the heart rate increases, causing the filling time during diastole to decrease). There is usually little change in total peripheral resistance, since a balanced pattern of vascular resistance changes is maintained by neurogenic sympathetic stimulation. The vessels in the skin, kidneys, and splanchnic and gastrointestinal organs vasoconstrict while there is vasodilatation and markedly increased blood flow to skeletal muscle and the coronary and hepatic arteries (Brod 1960; Forsyth 1971) (Table 1.3). The same general pattern can occur during fainting, except that there is a more profound vasodilatation in skeletal muscle causing a net reduction in total peripheral resistance. Concommittantly there is a pooling of blood in the skeletal muscles, causing a decreased venous return and a lesser increase of cardiac output. Thus, arterial pressure will fall, instead of rising. Blood flow to the brain is reduced and fainting occurs. Environmental stressors also provoke a predictable pattern of endocrine responses (Mason 1968), which may contribute to the continued cardiovascular effects from an acute stressor.

TABLE 1.3 *Systemic measurements and the regional distribution of cardiac output in selected organs at rest and after twenty minutes of stress induced by operant avoidance schedules in five rhesus monkeys.*

	Rest	Acute Stress
MEAN SYSTEMIC ARTERIAL PRESSURE (mmHg)	102	128
CARDIAC OUTPUT (ml/min)	1070	1443
HEART RATE (beats/min)	145	190
STROKE VOLUME (ml)	7.4	7.6
TOTAL PERIPHERAL RESISTANCE [mmHg/(L/min)]	97	89
PERCENT OF CARDIAC OUTPUT DELIVERED TO:		
HEART	4.8	6.2
BRAIN	5.1	4.5
KIDNEYS	16.2	9.9
SKIN	7.1	5.2
SKELETAL MUSCLE	25.8	33.5
GASTROINTESTINAL TRACT	8.3	6.0
SPLEEN	2.4	1.8
PANCREAS	1.9	1.6
LIVER (HEPATIC ARTERY)	4.6	5.9

SOURCE: Forsyth, *Science, 147,* 546-48; reprinted with permission from *Science.* Copyright 1971 by the American Association for the Advancement of Science.

Although these acute changes are well documented, the chief difficulty has been to establish the connection between these normal acute rises in blood pressure and the occurrence of permanent hypertension. Three general types of research have been pursued to answer this question, with varying degrees of success, and there are still considerable differences of opinion as to the acceptability of this evidence and/or its applicability to man.

One approach has correlated the incidence of hypertension in subjects with the degree of "stress" these individuals have naturally encountered in their lives. The stress has been defined variously as certain occupations, combat experiences, or exposure to fearful situations. Many of the reported clinical observations in patients have been difficult to interpret or translate into generalities; even objectively perceived stress is handled differently by different people and is hard to quantitate.

A second type of research has reported (and some times denied) the presence of unique personality characteristics, measured with interviewing or psychological test techniques, in hypertensive or pre-hypertensive (labile) individuals. Since the assumed disease process itself probably evokes certain characteristic behaviors, the study of the pre-hypertensive personality is the more convincing. In this respect, it is essential to know if these individuals will actually develop hypertension. Thus, long-term studies are required before meaningful interpretations can be made.

Thirdly, a number of studies show that sustained high blood pressure can be produced in animals with the use of environmental stressors. Most of these studies have used strong sensory stimuli such as air blasts or noise, but others have successfully used operant conditioning techniques or more natural fear-producing experimental techniques as the stressor.

The details and the methods of these studies have been reviewed (McGinn et al. 1964; Harris and Forsyth in press; Henry, Meehan, and Stephens 1967; Cochrane 1971; Simonson and Brozek 1959). It is evident that additional support is needed in each of these areas of research to strengthen the case for the role of environmental or psychological influences in hypertension. There is little doubt, however, that in some individuals genetic influences will play an interactive or permissive role with environmental factors in the etiology of high blood pressure.

Summary

During the past 40 years a variety of causes of hypertension have been discovered; however, these known mechanisms account only for a small percentage of the total hypertensive population. More important clinically has been the development of potent antihypertensive drugs which can effectively lower blood pressure in a large number of patients, although the side effects of the treatment are often a problem. The search for the "ideal" therapeutic agent as well as for other curable forms of hypertension continues.

The strong familial influences evident in the development of essential hypertension have led many investigators to emphasize the genetic role in this disorder. As with other diseases (e.g., schizophrenia, ulcers, and diabetes), it is likely that genetic factors predispose individuals to different degrees. Thus, some individuals may develop hypertension "spontaneously" with or without a stressful environment. In others, genetic factors will interact with environmental factors; at the other extreme, environmental factors may have little lasting effect on blood pressure. Thus, psychological effects may be much like environmental stressors such as salt intake; perhaps salt-reactive individuals will turn out to be most affected by other stressors. It is obvious that there are many critical unanswered questions in this area.

HYPOTHESES CONCERNING ENVIRONMENTAL STRESSORS AND HYPERTENSION

It should again be emphasized that environmental factors will prove to be a primary etiology in only a subset of hypertensives. In other cases stressors may contribute to more basic genetic or physiological defects, as in coronary artery disease where the heart cannot cope with the increased oxygen demands evoked by stressful situations. Most of the hypotheses presented invoke a two factor model: One set of influences raises the pressures acutely engendering a second process which ultimately "fixes" the total peripheral resistance and blood pressure at a high sustained level. Obviously there is no conclusive evidence that any of these hypotheses are correct; but these theories are testable, and conclusions about their validity should be forthcoming.

Renovascular and/or Electrolyte Theories

Because the renovascular model has been most successful in creating experimental hypertension and because it occurs naturally, there has been strong interest in it as a mechanism for explaining environmental influences. This hypothesis is attractive because sustained neurogenic renal vasoconstriction is a well-known response to environmental stressors and to electrical stimulation of hypothalamic areas which mimic the cardiovascular reactions to stress and exercise (Feigl, Johansson, and Löfving 1964; Brod 1960; Forsyth 1970, 1971). Despite the fact that cardiac output is increased, there is reduced blood flow through the renal arteries, thus engaging the reninangiotensin-aldosterone system. These secondary influences cause renal retention of sodium with a resulting increased blood volume. Over a period of time, increased stiffness of arterioles would be expected to occur due to the increased vascular smooth muscle sodium content.

Individuals who experience chronic stress, who are genetically hyperresponsive to and/or who ingest excessive salt would be those who develop a fixed, rather than an acute, pressor response. Studies reporting that hypertensive patients have an abnormal response to a salt load (e.g., Ulrych, Hofman, and Hejl 1964) support this hypothesis, as do studies showing that systemic blood vessels of hypertensive patients (and normotensive children of hypertensive patients) are more reactive than vessels from normotensives to NE and other vasoactive substances (Doyle, Fraser, and Marshall 1959).

Since vessel radius is the most important determinant of flow resistance, even a small generalized swelling (edema) of arteriolar walls causes a marked increase in resistance. It has been estimated that a 13% swelling would increase flow resistance 54% (Tobian and Binion 1952). Also the sodium-induced stiffness would inhibit local vasodilatory responses.

Other theories are concerned with different aspects of the same initial mechanism. For example, the fact that essential hypertensives have "normal" renin and aldosterone blood levels in the face of increased systemic pressure may be abnormal. The higher pressures in the renal arteries should suppress renin production if the homeostatic mechanisms continue working. The fact that "normal" as well as elevated renin levels are reported to be associated with complications in essential hypertension illustrates this point (Laragh et al. 1972).

Similarly, even slightly elevated blood levels of angiotensin (and/or aldosterone) may contribute to a cycle of elevated pressures and lability. Beside its direct vasoconstricting effect on blood vessels, angiotensin, at very low levels, has been shown to potentiate the effects of SNS activity and circulating catecholamines. Long-term infusions of subpressor doses of angiotensin in both dogs and monkeys evoke enhanced pressor responses to environmental stimuli (McCubbin and Page 1963; Forsyth, Hoffbrand, and Melmon 1971). Thus, a vicious cycle could be created especially in those individuals particularly reactive to angiotensin. Repeated environmental influences set the renal hormone system in motion which then potentiates further neurogenic renal artery constriction. Eventually the arterial tree becomes edematous or hypertrophied in response to chronic mineralocorticoid excess, and the arterial pressure and the total peripheral resistance become fixed at a high level.

One other variant to this theme has been suggested. The possibility exists that hypertensives have a defect in the storage mechanism of NE in postganglionic sympathetic nerves which results in low NE stores and a failure to properly modulate NE release. Thus, an increased reactivity (vasoconstriction) to vasoactive substances occurring in some organs is aggravated by the increased sympathetic nerve discharge during stress (Mendlowitz et al. 1964).

Neurogenic Theories

The observation that CNS structures located above the VMC can acutely suppress the usual bradycardia when arterial pressure rises during episodes of environmental stress suggests a mechanism whereby continued stress might lead to a fixed hypertension. In an unknown manner, chronic stress might cause a permanent resetting or loss of efficiency of the reflex or, more likely, might interact with a dysfunction evoked by other physiological causes. It is thought that this reflex becomes less sensitive with increasing age, probably because the carotid sinus region is especially prone to arteriosclerosis and arterial degeneration. Similarly, some reports indicate that, with increasing arterial pressure, the reflex becomes less sensitive, as well as being reset (Sleight 1971). Increased pressure can, as in arteriosclerotic conditions, cause the arterial wall to become stiff and can reduce the sensitivity of the reflex, or it might damage the receptor elements.

Most investigators feel that this mechanism contributes to the pathological process, especially in older individuals, but that it probably is secondary to the rise of blood pressure due to other factors. Mineralo-corticoid influences would also increase the stiffness of the arterial wall by increases of salt and water content. It remains to be demonstrated that higher CNS influences activitated by stress can both initiate and maintain a resetting of the reflex. This question needs to be answered, and the cause-effect relationship between baroreceptor function and high blood pressure established (Horrobin 1966).

Failure of Skeletal Muscle Vasodilation

Of critical importance in the hemodynamic response to environmental stressors (and exercise) is the marked vasodilation in skeletal muscle, which along with the increase in cardiac output causes a substantial increase in muscle blood flow. This response is sympathetically medi-ated—in that electrical stimulation of hypouhalamic areas, which evokes a sympathetic discharge, mimics this response—and pharmacologic sympathectomy (with ganglionic blocking drugs) can abolish it (Brown 1969). Many authors have noted that the response "primes" the organ-ism for physical exertion (the heart is also overperfused), and that there may be psychosomatic implications because, in our society, most situations in which anxiety occurs are not followed by muscular exer-tion. (Some investigators have invoked this mechanism in associating measures of "repressed" hostility with hypertension.) The increased oxygen and glucose consumption that occurs in skeletal muscle during exercise has not been found during experimentally induced environ-mental stress (Brod, Hejl, and Ulrych 1963).

Since skeletal muscle comprises such a large portion of total body weight (even though blood flow per unit weight is low in resting con-ditions), even small changes in its resistance are important in determin-ing changes in total peripheral resistance and, thus, blood pressure. For example, unusual vasodilation in muscle can lead to hypotension and a fainting response even when the cardiac output is normal or increased.

Although the SNS is known to be primarily involved with this neuro-genic response, there are obviously other important control mecha-nisms which can influence or even change the direction of the re-sponse. For example, hemorrhage causes a baroreceptor-induced sympathetic response, but there is vasoconstriction, rather than vasodil-atation, in skeletal muscle. This response is teleologically appropriate, but the mechanism involved is unknown; the control of skeletal muscle blood flow is a puzzling problem. For example, electrical hypothalamic stimulation, exercise, and emotional stress lead to vasodilatation while hemorrhage and electrical stimulation of postganglionic sympathetic nerves evoke vasoconstriction in skeletal muscle. This discrepancy would be less troublesome if a sympathetic cholinergic pathway to skeletal muscle independent of the VMC could be demonstrated to exist in primates. The facts do suggest that SNS activity arising from hypothalamus and higher CNS structures evokes a very different response in skeletal muscle blood flow compared to that arising reflexly from the VMC.

The hypothesis is supported by the well designed study of Lund-Johansen (1967) who found that, at rest, the youngest hypertensive group, in contrast to normotensive controls, had a raised cardiac output (due to increased heart rate) and oxygen consumption, but a normal total peripheral resistance. The older groups of hypertensives (over 30 years of age) generally had a normal cardiac output and raised total peripheral resistance. Interestingly, the total peripheral resistance of hypertensives at all ages was higher during exercise compared to age-matched controls. The author interpreted these data as support for a reduced vasodilating capacity in the skeletal muscle of hypertensives.

Normotensive monkeys subjected to 72-hour operant conditioning schedules show a response similar to that seen in Lund-Johansen's hypertensive group (Forsyth 1971) (Figure 1.3). Initially blood pressures were increased due to increases in heart rate and cardiac output; there was a marked vasodilatation and increase in skeletal muscle blood flow. However, there were progressive decreases in cardiac output toward baseline levels during the 72-hour period, although blood pressure remained elevated. The calculated increase in total peripheral resistance was primarily caused by progressive vasoconstriction in skeletal muscle, after the initial vasodilatation, so that at the end of the stress period there was significant muscular vasoconstriction. Vessels in the kidney and gastrointestinal organs remained vasoconstricted throughout the experiment, while the coronary arteries remained dilated.

The evidence suggests that skeletal muscle cannot maintain its initial vasodilatation during chronic stress, and that the hemodynamic changes occurring over time correspond to what is seen in the progression of labile hypertension to a fixed essential hypertension in man. This evidence is only suggestive, and the mechanism involved in this response can only be clarified by further work. The best current guess is that local autoregulatory mechanisms in skeletal, but not cardiac, muscle can react to the increase in blood flow to reduce arteriolar diameter. Skeletal muscle might also be particularly sensitive to increased levels of catecholamines and/or mineralocorticoids, which would explain the vasoconstriction in continued, but not acute, stress and during hemorrhagic hypotension.

Nonspecific Mechanisms

Two hypotheses concern mechanisms which attempt to explain how the transition from a labile to a fixed hypertension occurs. Both theories recognize that blood pressure can be acutely elevated in a variety of ways but focus on a final common mechanism which can pathologically cause a permanent reduction in the arteriolar lumen and a fixed increase in total peripheral resistance.

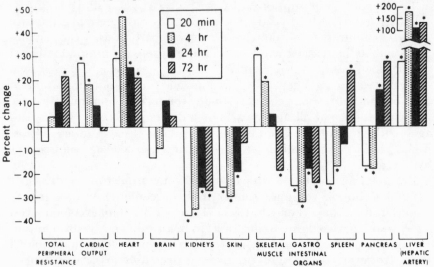

FIGURE 1.3 *Mean percentage changes compared to the baseline measurement, in total peripheral resistance, cardiac output, and regional fractions of cardiac output in five monkeys in nine major organs during the 72-hour stress period. The gastrointestinal tract includes the stomach, small and large intestines, and cecum. An asterik indicates significance levels of P<.05 Compared to control-group changes, by use of the Mann-Whitney U-Test. Inset denotes time after initiation of stress.*

SOURCE: Forsyth, *Science*, 1971, *173*, 546-548; reprinted with permission from Science. Copyright 1971 by the American Association for the Advancement of Science.

Autoregulation. As summarized by Guyton and his colleagues (Guyton et al. 1970), this hypothesis emphasizes the role of mechanically induced local blood flow regulation. For whatever reason, when cardiac output is increased, excessive blood perfuses some tissues which evokes a progressive myogenic vasoconstriction of peripheral blood vessels, raising the total peripheral resistance. Cardiac output is returned toward normal by changes in blood volume and baroreceptor influences. The important long-term effects are attributed to changes in renal resistance or impaired renal function which decrease the kidney's ability to excrete salt and water. Thus, a new equilibrium at a higher arterial pressure would be maintained because of increased extracellular fluid volume.

Parts of this theory fit with what is known to occur in many types of hypertension and with the two-factor theory many investigators favor. Thus, for example, the initial increase of renin and angiotensin in renovascular hypertension might initiate the hypertension through increases of blood volume and cardiac output, while local autoregulatory influences would sustain it. Although still controversial, there is evidence that in each of the models of hypertension discussed above and in genetic models where hypertension appears spontaneously there is an initial increase of cardiac output followed by a rise in total peripheral resistance. This would include, as discussed, the natural history of many cases of essential hypertension.

Hypertrophy. This hypothesis as expressed by Folkow (1971) and Folkow and Neil (1971) stresses structural changes in resistance vessels as the final common pathway to a sustained hypertension. Autoregulatory changes are seen as the more immediate response to increases in blood pressure, but long-range sustained peripheral arterial constriction would be caused by irreversible smooth muscle hypertrophy which would change the wall/lumen ratio of the arterial tree. Resistance vessels have been reported to so structurally adapt themselves to chronic pressure elevations over a relatively short period of time (Silvertsson 1970), much like the hypertrophy seen in the left ventricle after longer periods of hypertension.

This hypertrophy would not only raise resistance when the smooth muscle is relaxed, but would also result in exaggerated pressor responses to neurogenic and hormonal vasoconstrictor influences. The vasoconstriction in carotid sinus areas would result in a reset and less efficient baroreceptor system, while that in the renal vasculature would precipitate the release of renin, angiotensin, and aldosterone with their attendant effects. Thus, long periods of perfectly appropriate increased blood pressure responses to emotional stress might result in a fixed hypertension in particularly susceptible individuals.

Summary and Comment

There are a number of theories about how environmental stressors might lead to a fixed hypertension, but at the present time there is little convincing data to substantiate any or allow a choice among them. The basic research problem has been the long time periods needed to develop a sustained high blood pressure in experimental animals (or in humans) subjected to environmental stressors, in contrast to the more quickly acting effects of renal artery stenosis or carotid nerve section. The necessity of control groups also adds to the tedious nature of this research.

Despite these problems, there is probably no alternative to the development of a long-term experimental model in which relevant cardiovascular measurements can be made in conjunction with carefully defined and controlled environmental manipulations. Several such models using restrained monkeys have recently given early encouraging results (Benson et al. 1969; Forsyth 1969). The development of telemeteric devices should facilitate the use of unrestrained models in which more naturalistic types of environmental stressors can be evaluated. It is becoming increasingly clear that these kinds of long-term preparations will be of value to many biological disciplines as well as the psychophysiologist.

2

DAVID H. COHEN AND ROBERT L. MACDONALD

A Selective Review of Central Neural Pathways Involved in Cardiovascular Control

INTRODUCTION

As stated in a subsequent chapter (see Chapter 7, Cohen), we have been developing visually conditioned heart rate change in the pigeon as an experimental model system for cellular neurophysiological investigations of information storage and retrieval. A considerable portion of this experimental effort has been directed toward obtaining a detailed specification of the anatomical pathways that mediate the development of the conditioned heart rate response, particularly the descending pathways constituting the efferent segments of the system (Cohen in press). While the subsequent chapter deals at some length with the strategy and problems entailed by an analysis of the final common path for heart rate conditioning, the present paper will focus exclusively on the central neural pathways.

In attempting to identify these pathways, one possible strategy is through a combined physiological and anatomical analysis to first carefully map the major descending systems capable of influencing cardiovascular activity. Such a map then establishes a sound foundation

Part of the research reviewed here and the preparation of this paper have been generously supported by grants to D. H. Cohen from the National Science Foundation (GB-2767, GB-6850, GB-8008, GB-13816X), the Heart Association of Northeast Ohio, the National Association of Mental Health, and the Scottish Rite Committee on Research in Schizophrenia. Dr. Cohen's work is supported by Public Health Service Research Career Award HL-16579 from the National Heart and Lung Institute. A portion of this review was prepared by R. L. Macdonald as part of his doctoral dissertation in the Department of Physiology, University of Virginia.

for subsequently applying an approach in which the different major pathways are interrupted at various rostrocaudal levels and the effects on cardiovascular conditioning are assessed. This type of strategy has been applied in our program (Cohen 1969, in press), and the present chapter deals with the initial step in such an analysis, namely the definition of the major descending systems exerting control over cardiovascular activity. While the specific goal has been to identify these pathways in the pigeon, comparisons with other vertebrate classes are important for obtaining some perspective on the relevant central organization. However, since mammals have been the most intensively studied, considerably more information is available for these species, and, hence, the focus in this chapter will be upon the central neural control of mammalian cardiovascular activity. A detailed description of central cardiovascular control in birds may be found in Macdonald and Cohen 1971, and a fuller discussion of the pathways specifically mediating heart rate conditioning is available in an article by Cohen (in press).

General Organizational Features of Central Cardiovascular Control

During the course of normal cardiovascular function, the specific circulatory demands of all tissues must be fulfilled. In general, there are a variety of mechanisms to accomplish this, including adjustment of vascular smooth muscle tone in different portions of the vascular bed, change in myocardial contractility, and alterations of heart rate. While these effects can be exerted by a variety of control systems, including nervous, normonal, and local, in many tissues the local factors are overriding. Consequently, neural influences do not necessarily represent the dominant control system available to the animal. Nonetheless, it is an essential one and permits rapid adjustments to alterations in the external environment, as required by defensive behavior, and to alterations in the internal environment, as during hemorrhagic shock.

Historically, there have been two kinds of approaches to investigating central neural control of cardiovascular activity. The first has involved the stimulation or ablation of nervous tissue, with measurement of appropriate peripheral responses to indicate the state of the cardiovascular system following such intervention. Approaches of this nature have permitted the identification and classification of the central and peripheral neural structures concerned with cardiovascular control. Given this information, the second kind of approach, an analysis of peripheral responses to stimulation of specific areas of the nervous system, has then permitted characterization of how specific structures control cardiac dynamics or alter vascular function at the level of individual vascular beds.

A rather massive literature has resulted from the application of these approaches, much of it dealing with mammalian cardiovascular control.

After lengthy consideration, we felt that it was convenient to consider central cardiovascular control as primarily consisting of the following six major organizational features:

1. a medullary vasomotor center.
2. a medullary depressor center.
3. a descending "defense" pathway originating in the amygdala.
4. a descending "exercise" pathway originating in the motor cortex.
5. a "postural adjustment" pathway originating in the cerebellum.
6. supramedullary control of vasomotor reflex mechanisms.

This conceptualization will, in fact, provide the basis of the organization of the review to follow. While this will undoubtedly impose a certain interpretative quality on the discussion, we feel that this framework is a reasonable one and that it avoids a rather tedious structure-by-structure review.

Specific Comments on the Nature of the Review

As a preface to undertaking the actual review, it is necessary to establish some boundary conditions and to make a few definitional statements. Firstly, as indicated above, the emphasis is on an integrated presentation of major functional systems rather than upon an encyclopedic, structure-by-structure review. Further, no attempt is made at a totally comprehensive coverage of the literature; rather, selected studies are cited to document specific points. Also, certain topics are not discussed, such as peripheral control, and others, such as baroreceptor activity, receive only minimal attention. In this regard the reader is referred to a recent review by Korner (1971). Finally, the primary concern is with heart rate and systemic blood pressure, although we fully recognize the importance of eventually specifying total cardiovascular response patterns, including regional blood flow and other components of cardiac performance.

Some prefatory explanations regarding terminology are also in order. First, the term "pathway" will generally be used in a functional sense and, unless otherwise specified, is not intended to imply a specific anatomical connection. Second, pathways will often be described as "cardiovascular" or "cardiomotor." While convenient, this is oversimplified terminology, since it is not meant to indicate that any given pathway is *exclusively* cardiovascular in function. The pathways to be described almost certainly mediate more complex integrated behaviors, and the cardiovascular responses generally reflect the adjustments in cardiac performance and regional peripheral resistance demanded by such integrated activities as agonistic behavior, exercise, and postural change. A final point concerns the reference to these pathways at "motor." In the strictest sense, only the vagal and sympathetic pre- and postganglionic cardiac nerves are "cardiomotor," somewhat analogous to the motoneurons of the somatomotor system. However, in the somatomotor system central pathways only a few synapses from the motoneuron are frequently designated as "motor" pathways; similar license is taken in describing central cardiovascular pathways.

MEDULLARY CONTROL OF THE CARDIOVASCULAR SYSTEM

Cardiovascular Excitatory (Vasomotor) Center

Localization of pressor control. Most formulations of central cardiovascular control have been historically dominated by the postulation of a medullary vasomotor center. That the medulla is critical in the maintenance of mean arterial blood pressure has been recognized since early demonstrations that transections at medullary levels abolish vascular reflexes and produce a precipitous fall in blood pressure (Dittmar 1873; Owsjannikow 1871). In fact, such evidence constituted the primary basis for assuming an essential medullary vasomotor center, until Ranson and Billingsley (1916) showed a rise in mean arterial blood pressure following electrical stimulation at the apex of the ala cinerea (inferior fovea). Chen and his associates (Chen et al. 1936, 1937b) then essentially confirmed this finding, and further suggested that the vasomotor region be more generally considered as a medullary sympathetic center, since concomitant sympathetic responses were observed in various organs. (More recent work (e.g., Bach 1952) would appear to extend yet further the generality of this region to include respiratory and somatic effects as well.)

The subsequent application of stereotaxic techniques then represented a particularly important advance, in that it permitted systematic depth exploration of the medulla (e.g., Alexander 1946; Amoroso, Bell, and Rosenberg 1954; Kuo et al. 1970; Monnier 1939; Wang and Ranson 1939a). In one of the more extensive of such investigations, Wang and Ranson (1939a) demonstrated pressor responses with stimulation of the dorsal reticular formation throughout the pons and medulla, indicating a considerably greater extent of the vasomotor region than reported in the earlier surface stimulation studies. This implied that the more limited surface zone simply represented a portion of the active reticular zone which shifts dorsally toward the floor of the fourth ventricle at the level of the inferior fovea. In brief, the outcome of these pioneering efforts is the now classical view that a specific medullary vasomotor center is located throughout the dorsal reticular formation, and that this area constitutes a primary site of central vasomotor control. Not only do pressor responses follow its activation, but the maintenance of normal levels of arterial blood pressure depend upon its integrity. However, it must be pointed out that while medullary control is no longer disputed, its relative importance is still a point of contention for some (e.g., Khayutin and Lukoshkova 1970).

Without minimizing the importance of these earlier contributions, it is important to recognize that from a morphological viewpoint the medullary vasomotor region remains poorly localized. Perhaps the most detailed description is that of Bach (1952), indicating that in the rostral medulla the vasomotor region is found primarily in the dorsomedial reticular formation. At mid-medulla it shifts slightly to occupy a central and dorsomedial position, while at caudal medullary levels it is confined almost entirely to the dorsolateral reticular formation. However, more precise localization is still required, particularly in view of the rather ubiquitous nature of pressor points in the medulla. For example, there is general agreement regarding the existence of another pressor area located in the ventrolateral medulla (e.g., Bach 1952; Kuo et al. 1970; Rosen 1961a; Wang and Ranson 1939a), although it has been frequently suggested that this region is involved in relaying descending hypothalamic influences (e.g., Lindgren 1961; Magoun, Ranson and Hetherington 1938; Wang and Ranson 1939a). Regardless, the cardiovascular response patterns to stimulation of these dorsal and ventral medullary regions differ only with respect to vascular resistance in skeletal muscle, vasoconstriction following dorsal medullary activation, and active vasodilatation following ventral medullary stimulation. This can be particularly troublesome, since in species such as the bird (Macdonald and Cohen 1973) and the monkey (Kuo et al. 1970) the separation between these dorsal and ventral cardioactive zones may not be that distinct. In addition to this ventrolateral medullary zone, Calaresu and Henry (1970) have recently described a discrete accelerator-pressor area ventrolateral to the hypoglossal nucleus and including the nucleus intercalatus. The primary cardioactive nature of this area is suggested by evoked sympathetic discharges occurring at latencies of only 3 to 10 msec. However, this "parahypoglossal" region would appear to be located well outside the classically defined vasomotor center. Consequently, an eventual comprehensive description of medullary vasomotor control would require not only that the dorsal vasomotor region be more clearly delineated anatomically, but also that its relationship to other "vasomotor" areas in the medulla be clarified.

Influence of the pressor region on cardiac performance. Throughout the period in which the vasomotor center was being actively pursued, minimal attention was directed toward medullary control of cardiac performance, despite demonstrations that the sympathetic system (Hunt 1899) and the hypothalamus (Karplus and Kreidl 1909) influence heart rate and myocardial contractility. Thus, although central control of cardiac performance was acknowledged, considerable question remained as to its organization and extent. As Peiss (1960) has pointed out, the evidence suggesting a cardioacceleratory center was far from conclusive, its existence being inferred largely by analogy to the vasomotor center. Such ambiguity apparently provided the impetus for the investigative efforts of the late 1950s and early 1960s concerning the central control of cardiac dynamics.

In this context, Peiss (1958, 1960) denied the existence of a sympathetic cardioaccelerator region, arguing that the acceleratory responses elicited by stimulation of the dorsal medulla actually reflect activation of afferent pathways projecting to more rostral areas of the nervous system. The responses evoked by stimulation of the ventrolateral medulla were argued to represent activation of descending hypothalamospinal pathways. In a somewhat similar spirit, Manning (1965) concluded that the importance of medullary control had been overemphasized. This conclusion was based on his reported finding that increases in blood pressure, heart rate, and myocardial contractility occur with stimulation throughout the entire brainstem, and that the medulla is no more active than the hypothalamus, midbrain, or pons.

The vast majority of studies, however, have yielded results in marked disagreement with the conclusions of Peiss (1958, 1960) and Manning (1965). Among the more significant investigations emerging during this controversy was that of Wang and Chai (1962) which demonstrated cardioaccelerator sites in the dorsal medullary reticular formation and adjacent periventricular gray. With more intense stimulation, accelerator responses were also elicited from activation of the ventrolateral reticular formation. These results generated the position that the active dorsal medullary sites comprised a bulbar pressor and cardioaccelerator center, while the ventrolateral region contained a hypothalamic efferent system (Chai and Wang 1962). It is of particular significance that Wang and Chai (1962) were also able to elicit cardioacceleration with dorsal medullary stimulation in the decerebrate animal, since this is inconsistent with the interpretation by Peiss·(1960) that the heart rate changes are secondary to activation of ascending pathways.

With respect to myocardial contractility, Wang and Chai (1962) have also shown that pressor responses evoked by stimulation of the right medulla are frequently accompanied by marked cardioacceleration with only slight or moderate cardioaugmentation, while those elicited by stimulation of the left medulla are accompanied by marked augmentation and only moderate acceleration. This finding is consistent with the early conclusion by Hunt (1899) that the right cardiac sympathetics are primarily chronotropic and the left primarily inotropic, and it clearly extends this "lateralization" into the medulla. It has thus been concluded that the dorsal medulla, in fact, contains an important integrative mechanism for the central control of blood pressure (Chai and Wang 1962), heart rate (Wang and Chai 1962), and myocardial contractility (Chai, Share, and Wang 1963). Consequently, the cardioactive dorsal medullary region cannot in any sense be strictly characterized as a vasomotor or pressor center. In fact, it is undoubtedly inaccurate to consider it even as exclusively cardiovascular in view of the respiratory, somatic, and other autonomic responses which are evoked by stimulation at the same sites eliciting cardiovascular changes (e.g., Bach 1952; Chen et al. 1936, 1937b).

Cardiovascular Inhibitory (Depressor) Center

Localization of depressor region. While the existence of a medullary pressor or vasomotor area has been readily accepted, considerable controversy has surrounded the nature of a presumptive medullary depressor center. In Bayliss's (e.g., 1923) early theories of central cardiovascular control, he postulated the existence of both medullary vasoconstrictor and vasodilator centers. The vasodilator center was assumed to exert an inhibitory influence on the vasoconstrictor region, as well as to have a direct action on the tone of peripheral vascular beds through active vasodilator nerves traveling in the dorsal roots.

In their classic study, Ranson and Billingsley (1916) reported that stimulation at the area postrema just lateral to the obex produced a decrease in mean arterial pressure, and this, in conjunction with their identification of the pressor area, appeared to support the Bayliss notion of dual, tonically active vasomotor centers. However, Scott and Roberts (1924) and Scott (1925) presented conclusions inconsistent with this concept, arguing that the presumed depressor region was, in fact, a site where the afferent limb of the depressor reflex arc approaches the medullary surface, and that the portion of the arc being stimulated represents either the afferent vagal fibers or their terminations. More recently, Lindgren and Uvnäs (1954) have reported that destruction of a medullary area presumed to include the depressor region abolished depressor reflexes to sinus and vagus nerve stimulation while not affecting those elicited by peripheral nerve stimulation. This finding, of course, is consistent with that of Scott (1925) and supports his contention that the depressor area consists of afferent inhibitory fibers of the carotid sinus and vagal depressor nerves. However, with the exception of these studies evidence generally seems to confirm the existence of separate pressor and depressor medullary centers (e.g., Alexander 1946; Kuo et al. 1970; Lim, Wang, and Yi 1938; Wang and Ranson 1939a). Also noteworthy is the report of Lim, Wang, and Yi (1938) that modest bradycardia accompanies the depressor effect even in the vagotomized animal (see also Calaresu and Thomas, 1971).

Studies in recent years would appear to have rather conclusively established the existence of an independent depressor region, as well as having further delineated its extent. For example, the data of Porszasz and his colleagues [Porszasz et al. 1962] suggest that the depressor region consists of a rather small and well-defined area confined primarily to dorsal and ventral aspects of the paramedian reticular nucleus. Careful examination of this specific region by Calaresu and Thomas (1971) clearly confirm its depressor-decelerator nature.

With respect to the contention of earlier investigations (e.g., Lindgren and Uvnäs 1954) that the depressor effect is consequent to direct activation of baroreceptor afferent fibers, it is important to point out these were largely surface stimulation studies. Thus, it may well be that such a conclusion is legitimate for those experiments. However, given the recent evidence implicating the paramedian reticular nucleus as the major constituent of the depressor region, this alternative seems unlikely for a variety of reasons. Among these are: (1) The predominant baroreceptor influence on the paramedian nucleus is polysynaptic (Miura and Reis 1969), and this is primarily from the small contingent of myelinated carotid sinus nerve fibers (Miura and Reis 1972). In fact, paramedian nuclear lesions selectively eliminate the baroreceptor reflexes mediated by these myelinated fibers, while destruction of the intermediate nucleus solitarius is required to completely abolish reflex depressor responses. (2) Accumulating evidence of the convergence on the paramedian nucleus of various systems influencing cardiovascular activity, such as baroreceptor afferents and fastigiobulbar fibers (Miura and Reis 1971), suggests that this constitutes an independent region for the integration of cardiovascular responses. (3) Kirchner, Sato, and Weidinger (1971) have demonstrated that direct depressor region stimulation exerts a considerably stronger inhibitory effect on the early-spinal sympathetic reflex than baroreceptor activation, implying that depressor neurons are only partially recruited by the baroreceptor afferents, and this is further suggested by the electrophysiological evidence of Miura and Reis (1971). These, and other, lines of evidence would, in brief, seem sufficient to reject the notion that medullary depressor responses are secondary to activation of baroreceptor afferents and would appear to strengthen the case for an independent inhibitory area.

One rather troublesome feature that has been reported frequently with studies of the depressor region is the occurrence of pressor points in the same area (e.g., Bach 1952; Wang and Ranson 1939a), and it has often been concluded that this indicates considerable overlap between the pressor and depressor centers. However, a recent study by Calaresu and Thomas (1971) has very nicely demonstrated the somewhat surprising result that the paramedian region inhibits both the vagus and the sympathetics. Thus, whether cardioacceleration or cardiodeceleration follows paramedian stimulation is a function of the resting vagal outflow at the time of activation—high resting activity leading to evoked tachycardia and low resting activity to bradycardia.

Consequently, it now seems reasonable to conclude firmly that a medullary depressor-decelerator region does in fact exist, and that it is located largely in the area of the paramedian nucleus, a few millimeters rostral to the obex. However, as with the pressor region, further information is required concerning its precise locus and relationship to other medullary areas inhibiting cardiovascular activity, such as the dorsal medullary region including the dorsal motor nucleus of the vagus and the nucleus solitarius. Also, additional data are required to determine the general inhibitory properties of this region, particularly in view of the Calaresu and Thomas (1971) result suggesting that possibly the paramedian zone should be considered as generally inhibitory rather than depressor-decelerator.

Mediation of depressor effect. Regarding the mechanism underlying the depressor effect, recall that Bayliss (1923) postulated both a direct action on peripheral vascular beds, via dorsal root vasodilator fibers, and a sympathoinhibitory action, via inhibition of the vasopressor region. While there has been a consensus that the assumption of dorsal root vasodilator fibers is incorrect (Frumin, Ngai, and Wang 1953; Lim, Wang, and Yi 1938; Lindgren and Uvnäs 1954), there has not been complete agreement as to whether the depressor effect is mediated through inhibition of spinal preganglionic neurons or the vasomotor center. However, most recent evidence seems to favor the contention of direct spinal inhibition.

To review this evidence partially: Lim, Wang, and Yi (1938) demonstrated that the depressor response was unaffected by either midbrain transection, or transection between the inferior fovea and the obex. This would seem to imply that the depressor response is not mediated through the dorsal reticular pressor area. Further support is provided by their demonstrations of (1) the persistence of the depressor response following interruption of the descending pressor pathway in the upper cervical cord, (2) the existence of an independent spinal depressor pathway, and (3) the elimination of the depressor response by either sympathetic ganglionectomy or α-adrenergic blockade. Lim, Wang, and Yi (1938) thus conclude that the depressor center is sympathoinhibitory at the level of the sympathetic preganglionics, but they are careful to point out that their results do not exclude the possible participation of an inhibitory effect mediated through the pressor center as well. Based on transection experiments, Alexander (1946) has also obtained results consistent with the concept of a direct spinal inhibitory action. In fact, he concludes that the depressor region contains the cells of origin of a medullospinal pathway that tonically inhibits the sympathetic preganglionic neurons, an interpretation agreed with by Kirchner, Sato, and Weidinger (1971). Finally, Gootman and Cohen (1971) have reported quite convincing electrophysiological evidence for direct spinal action. In recording splanchnic potentials, they find that the latency to the excitatory responses upon stimulation of the pressor region is 10 msec longer than the latency to the inhibition of splanchnic activity upon stimulation of the depressor region, suggesting that at least the early depressor effect cannot be mediated through the pressor area.

Inconsistent with the direct spinal inhibition hypothesis are the findings of Porszasz et al. (1962). They report that undercutting the depressor region with a transection extending almost to the lateral margin of the olive just caudal to the obex did not alter resting blood pressure or depressor responses to either direct or vagal afferent stimulation. This would seem to imply that the depressor response is not dependent upon fibers descending along the midline, and, consequently, that the medullary depressor region must operate through inhibition of the pressor area.

In summary then, it remains to be resolved what the precise mechanism of the depressor effect might be, although the literature is suggestive of direct spinal inhibition constituting at least one component. However, it may well be that inhibition of the pressor region also occurs, such that both mechanisms are operative, an alternative that would be consistent with Bayliss's (1923) original formulation.

Cardiovascular Reflex Control

The concept of reflex regulation of cardiovascular function apparently originated in Ludwig's laboratory, as did the hypothesis of a medullary vasomotor center (Dittmar 1873; Owsjannikow 1971). Cyon and Ludwig (1866) first identified the depressor nerve, and some 58 years later Hering (1924) described the carotid sinus nerve. In addition, the vasomotor reflex responses to stimulation of peripheral somatic nerves had been established by Hunt (1899), thereby providing three afferent sources of cardiovascular reflex effects.

One of the pioneering investigations of the central organization of vascular reflexes was that of Chen and his co-workers (Chen et al. 1937a), in which they demonstrated that sciatic nerve stimulation evokes a wide variety of sympathetic responses in a pattern similar to that following activation of the medullary pressor center. Transection studies then indicated medullary mediation of these reflex effects, and it was proposed that the bulbar reflex center is probably coincident with the pressor region. Alexander's (1946) study supported this contention, and Lindgren (1961) subsequently extended the findings to include reflex effects of carotid sinus nerve stimulation. In this latter study the use of chronically decerebrate animals also secured the notion that the medullary reflex center in fact contains neurons rather than merely fibers en passage.

The concept of exclusive medullary mediation of vascular reflexes was accepted as dogma until Akers and Peiss, cited by Peiss (1960), reported that reflex acceleration following bilateral carotid occlusion in vagotomized animals was eliminated by mesencephalic transection. Subsequently, Manning (1965) described data purporting to show that acute destruction of the dorsolateral medullary reticular formation did not significantly alter the reflex adjustments to bilateral carotid occlusion or sciatic nerve stimulation. Furthermore, it was reported that decerebration reduced blood pressure and abolished vascular reflex responses. These studies consequently suggested that the participation of supramedullary structures in cardiovascular reflex organization and maintenance of basal blood pressure was more important than previously conceived. The specific implications were that cardioacceleratory reflexes may be mediated entirely at supramedullary levels, while other reflex alterations may be mediated at supramedullary levels if the dorsal-medulla is not intact, including the maintenance of basal blood pressure.

However, a series of convincing studies from Wang's laboratory failed to confirm these findings. First, Wang and Chai (1962) demonstrated cardioacceleratory reflexes to carotid occlusion and sciatic nerve stimulation in the decerebrate preparation. Second, Chai, Share, and Wang (1963) showed that reflex cardioaugmentation did not depend upon the integrity of supramedullary structures. Finally, Wang and Chai (1967) and Chai and Wang (1968) reported elimination of reflex responses to sciatic, carotid sinus, and depressor nerve stimulation following extensive dorsal medullary lesions, while the hypothalamically evoked pressor response was unaffected.

In brief, the above and other studies would seem to indicate that reflex cardiovascular responses to sciatic, carotid sinus, and depressor nerve stimulation are mediated at medullary levels. Further, they reaffirm the classical view that the reflex centers are geographically coincident with the medullary vasomotor centers, both pressor and depressor. However, this is not meant to imply complete coincidence at the individual neuronal level. Finally, supramedullary mediation of vascular reflexes independent of the vasomotor centers is moot—Manning (1965) supporting such a concept, and Wang and Chai (1967) and Chai and Wang (1968) denying it.

Final Comments on Medullary Control

Despite the fact that numerous papers were not discussed, the preceding sections have perhaps conveyed some idea as to the voluminous literature concerned with medullary control of cardiovascular activity. Clearly, substantial data have been accumulated, and an obvious question at this point concerns the major problems still requiring resolution. In our view there are three rather pressing issues, and these will constitute the topics for this closing section on medullary control.

First, the medullary cardiovascular centers require more precise anatomical delineation. That is, the specific neuronal populations comprising these control centers must be identified, since this would be instrumental in establishing a foundation for more precise investigations of supramedullary control. While some progress has been made in this regard through higher resolution stimulation studies, this approach is inherently limited. Microelectrode studies of single medullary neurons hold some promise (e.g., Humprey 1967; Przybyla and Wang 1967; Salmoiraghi 1962), but these too are limited until 'the efferent pathways from the medullary centers are sufficiently specified to allow the antidromic identification of medullary cardiomotor neurons.

Second, the intrinsic organization of the pressor and depressor centers, as well as their interrelationships, remain largely unspecified, and many moot points would undoubtedly be clarified were such information available. Largely due to the lack of precise identification of the relevant cardiomotor neurons, the analysis of such intrinsic organization is at a rather primitive stage. However, in recent years some rather intriguing results have been reported in this context, and, while the area is far too premature for systematic review, a brief illustration involving the depressor center might indicate the kind of direction recent efforts are following.

To begin with, Miura and Reis (1971) have established that the paramedian reticular nucleus includes at least two classes of neurons: those polysynaptically excited by carotid sinus nerve stimulation, primarily the myelinated fibers (Miura and Reis 1972); and those excited by fastigial stimulation. Further, there is a mutually inhibitory interaction between these two systems. In a different line of research, Calaresu and Thomas (1971) have found that the paramedian nucleus inhibits both cardioaccelerator and cardiodecelerator neurons, the sympathoinhibition possibly being exerted directly through a medullospinal pathway (Kirchner, Sato, and Weidinger 1971). Collating these various findings, Calaresu and Thomas (1971) propose a model in which the paramedian neurons excited by sinus nerve activation inhibit the cardioaccelerator neurons, and the paramedian neurons receiving fastigial input inhibit the cardioinhibitory neurons. (Also included in this model is the mutually inhibitory interaction between the two classes of paramedian neurons.) This kind of functional heterogeneity within the paramedian nucleus supports the earlier contention of Reis and Cuènod (1965) that the medullary neurons mediating baroreceptor reflexes are distinct from those involved in the tonic maintenance of arterial blood pressure. And a somewhat analogous dissociation has also been demonstrated at the level of the sympathetic preganglionic neurons (Jänig and Schmidt 1970). Thus, although the medullary centers for the maintenance of arterial blood pressure and the mediation of cardiovascular reflexes may be coextensive, as indicated in the preceding section, more recent evidence suggests a functional heterogeneity within these regions such that phasic and tonic systems are dissociated. While this kind of hypothesizing is obviously at its inception, it is clear that attacking the organization of the medullary centers at such a cellular level is both appropriate and essential at this time.

The third, and final, issue concerns identification of the way in which the medullary cardiovascular centers are coupled to the cardiovascular preganglionic neurons. This may well be one of the more critical unresolved problems, since such information would provide a basis for identifying with greater precision the specific neuronal elements constituting the medullary cardiovascular centers. The rationale for this statement is that, generally speaking, the greatest successes in delineating neural systems have derived from efforts that have begun at the periphery and progressed centrally in a systematic manner.

While this problem is currently under active investigation, the present emphasis has been primarily upon determining the funicular loci of the descending cardiomotor pathways in the spinal cord. In this regard four excitatory regions have apparently been identified by various workers: the dorsal columns near the midline (Illert and Gabriel 1972); the dorsal aspect of the lateral funiculus (Foreman and Wurster 1972; Illert and Gabriel 1972; Illert and Seller 1969; Kerr and Alexander 1964); a region ventromedial to the lateral corticospinal tract (Cicardo and Garcia 1958; Foerster and Gagel 1932; Johnson, Roth, and Cray 1952; Kell and Hoff 1952); and the ventral aspect of the lateral funiculus (Chen et al. 1937c; Wang and Ranson 1939b). The disagreement is rather disturbing, since, with the exception of the dorsal column region reported only by Illert and Gabriel (1972), each region has been described by the respective investigators as the exclusive localization of the descending excitatory spinal path. With respect to inhibitory pathways, study has been less intensive, and the available literature (Illert and Gabriel 1972; Illert and Seller 1969; Lim, Wang, and Yi 1938) indicates one such area in the ventromedial lateral funiculus. In addition, Illert and Gabriel (1972) describe a second area just lateral to the apex and head of the dorsal horn.

Thus, the precise localization of the spinal cardiomotor paths remains moot, although a reasonable consensus seems to exist regarding an excitatory region in the dorsal aspect of the lateral funiculus, with its most active portion being just dorsal to the dentate ligament. A similar consensus apparently holds for an inhibitory zone located in the ventrolateral aspect of the cord. However, as yet there is no information regarding either the cells of origin of these pathways, or the precise manner in which they gain access to preganglionic neurons.

Evidence would seem to indicate that there are no direct projections from long descending pathways or dorsal root fibers upon the spinal preganglionics, suggesting one or more interneuronal pools in the spinal grey through which visceral fibers must relay (Petras and Cummings 1972). Analogously, projections to the medullary cells of origin of the vagal cardioinhibitory fibers remain largely unspecified, and in many species it is still uncertain even as to the locations of these parasympathetic preganglionic neurons (see Chapter 7, Cohen; Cohen and Schnall 1970; Cohen, Schnall, Macdonald, and Pitts 1970).

SUPRAMEDULLARY CONTROL OF THE CARDIOVASCULAR SYSTEM

General Comments

That the medulla constitutes an essential locus for maintaining arterial blood pressure and mediating cardiovascular reflexes has been recognized for some time. Similarly, early investigators were also aware that supramedullary structures must play a major role in cardiovascular control. While the medullary preparation is capable of maintaining its internal milieu within reasonable tolerances if unperturbed, vascular adjustments to situations such as stress, exercise, sexual activity, feeding, and temperature and postural change are not possible. Consequently, the cardiovascular demands of a normal environment cannot be effectively met by the medullary animal. Given this, the emphasis in earlier investigations was upon demonstrating that supramedullary structures are, in fact, capable of altering cardiovascular function. As early as 1875, it had been shown that electrical stimulation of the cortex can influence heart rate and mean arterial blood pressure (Danilewsky 1875; Schiff 1875). Further, the classic experiments of Karplus and Kreidl (1909) established that hypothalamic stimulation evokes a broad range of autonomic responses including pupillary dilation, bladder contraction, gastro-intestinal peristaltic changes, salivation, and sweating as well as increases in mean arterial blood pressure, heart rate, and rate and depth of respiration. Subsequent efforts were then directed toward systematically identifying the supramedullary structures participating in cardiovascular control, and, more recently, toward specifying the nature of the cardiovascular adjustments that each mediates.

Illustrative Early Investigations

As an illustration of such efforts, it is worthwhile to briefly discuss selected findings of a few of the more classical systematic explorations that prevailed through the 1930s. These centered primarily around the organization of the hypothalamic regions, influencing cardiovascular activity, and their immediate outflow.

Beattie, Brow, and Long (1930) conducted a rather extensive study including both stimulation and anatomical approaches. On the basis of such data they concluded that a parasympathetic center could be localized to the anterior and tuberal regions of the hypothalamus, while a sympathetic center is found in the posterior hypothalamus. They further suggested that the major hypothalamic outflow followed a periventricular route to the central grey and adjacent areas, with a less extensive distribution in the rostral mesencephalic tegmentum. Kabat, Magoun, and Ranson (1935) challenged these findings on a number of grounds. First, they disputed the rostrocaudal hypothalamic organizational scheme, suggesting instead a mediolateral organization. This was based on their finding that stimulation of the lateral hypothalamus produces a variety of sympathetic responses, while most of the medial hypothalamus is unresponsive to stimulation. Although they were able to trace a depressor pathway from rostral telencephalon to rostral diencephalon, this pathway could not be followed caudal to the level of the anterior commissure, either because it mingled with a dominant pressor pathway or was interrupted synaptically in septal or preoptic areas. Second, they questioned the description of the hypothalamic outflow as being primarily confined to the central grey. This attack was more vigorous in the study of Magoun, Ranson, and Hetherington (1938) who applied a technique of locating a reactive point in the hypothalamus, making selective mesencephalic lesions, and then stimulating the hypothalamic point again and evaluating the response changes. Such an approach clearly indicated that descending hypothalamic connections are much more diffusely and widely represented throughout a large extent of the mesencephalic tegmentum than indicated by Beattie and his colleagues. This conclusion was a forerunner of the more contemporary view of the hypothalamic outflow as dividing at the caudal end of the mammillary bodies—one division projecting upon the central grey and adjacent areas, and the other maintaining a more ventral course through the mesencephalic tegmentum (e.g., Enoch and Kerr 1967; Nauta 1958). It also anticipated subsequent anatomical descriptions of the central grey as giving rise to diffusely radiating projections distributing throughout the midbrain tegmentum.

Dispute of this sort has not been uncommon in the area of central cardiovascular control, although the level of the nervous system that is the focus of contention has varied historically. As indicated in the introduction to this chapter, more recent emphasis has been upon attempting to integrate the cardioactive regions of the nervous system into "pathways" of some functional meaning, such as the "postural adjustment" pathway. This, although subject to more interpretive bias, is both more coherent and interesting, and it is for this reason that the subsequent discussion of supramedullary control will be cast in such a context rather than assuming the form of a structure-by-structure review.

"DEFENSE" AND "EXERCISE" PATHWAYS

Introduction

As indicated in the introduction, among the important organizational features of central cardiovascular control are a set of pathways concerned with mediating the cardiovascular adjustments demanded by various behaviors. The three to be specifically considered in this chapter are those involved with producing the integrated cardiovascular response patterns accompanying: (1) defensive or agonistic behavior, (2) preparation for exercise, and (3) postural change. The presumptive "postural adjustment" pathway will be discussed in the subsequent section. In this section the so-called "defense" and "exercise" pathways will be discussed together, since for many years they were not clearly distinguished in the literature and, consequently, their joint consideration is more efficient. It might be pointed out that this confusion was apparently engendered by the similarities in the cardiovascular response patterns occurring during exercise and defensive behavior, and by the participation of the hypothalamus in both systems.

The development of the relevant literature essentially began with the early identification of a sympathetic vasodilator system in muscle (Bülbring and Burn 1935). In an extensive series of investigations beginning in the late 1940s, this vasodilator system has been systematically and comprehensively explored by Swedish workers. It is these papers that constitute the starting point for discussion. Their specific relevance to the "defense" and "exercise" pathways will become more apparent as the discussion develops.

Characterization of the Vasodilator System

Uvnäs (1966) has characterized sympathetic vasodilatation as an active, neurally mediated decrease in vascular resistance confined primarily to skeletal muscle. Originally described in carnivores, recent evidence also indicates its existence in primates—although in primates it is not atropinesensitive (cholinergic) as it is in carnivores (Schramm, Honig, and Bignall 1971). While muscle vasodilatation is the defining characteristic of the system, a variety of concomitant cardiovascular responses are observed (Folkow, Haeger, and Uvnäs 1948; Folkow and Uvnäs 1948; Rosen 1961a, b). These include vasoconstriction of the high resistance vessels in other vascular beds, such as skin, intestines, and kidney, leading to a redistribution of circulating blood volume to the muscles. Cardioacceleration and cardioaugmentation also occur to effect an increase in cardiac output, these cardiac responses being primarily mediated by the sympathetic innervation of the heart with only a minor contribution from the adrenal medulla. Yet, despite this increased cardiac output, systemic arterial blood pressure remains largely unchanged, and, to foreshadow later discussion, it might be pointed out that this cardiovascular response pattern has striking similarities to that seen in the preparation for exercise.

This vasodilator system apparently arises from the motor cortex (Eliasson, Lindgren, and Uvnäs 1952) and descends polysynaptically to the spinal cord (Lindgren, Rosen, Strandberg, and Uvnäs 1956). The corticohypothalamic projection may be a direct one (Eliasson, Lindgren, and Uvnäs 1952), but since the hypothalamus remains active following chronic removal of the motor cortex Eliasson, Lindgren, and Uvnäs (1954) suggest that a synaptic relay occurs at this diencephalic level. This conclusion should perhaps be qualified, however, since sympathetic vasodilatation also follows amygdalar stimulation, and this structure, too, projects upon the hypothalamus.

Within the hypothalamus, the vasodilator points are concentrated in an area forming a horizontal band which extends from the anterior margin of the supraoptic region to the level of the mammillary bodies (Eliasson et al. 1951; Eliasson, Lindgren, and Uvnäs 1952). In the mesencephalon, the vasodilator pathway has been reported as localized in the basal parts of the superior colliculus and adjacent regions, and there appears to be a partial decussation of the pathway ventral to the central grey in the region of the dorsal tegmental decussation (Lindgren 1955). As will shortly be described in more detail, Abrahams, Hilton, and Zbrozyna (1960) contest Lindgren's (1955) description of the mesencephalic course of the pathway, arguing that it is actually located just dorsal to the cerebral peduncles. Schramm and Bignall (1971) have recently confirmed this finding, and both Abrahams, Hilton, and Zbrozyna (1960) and Schramm and Bignall (1971) have provided strong support for their position by combined lesion and stimulation studies showing elimination of the hypothalamically induced vasodilator effect after small lesions in the peduncular region.

At medullary levels vasodilator points are distributed principally in two regions: (1) an area coincident with the depressor center, and (2) a region 1 to 2 mm above the ventral surface of the medulla. However, an extremely important distinction between these two regions is that the vasodilatation elicited by stimulation of the ventrolateral medulla is not accompanied by bradycardia or hypotension, and is blocked by atropine. This is quite in contrast to the effects of stimulating the depressor region, where vasodilatation results from sympathoinhibition and is accompanied by cardiodeceleration and a fall in arterial blood pressure (Lindgren and Uvnäs 1953a,b, 1954). This ventrolateral medullary vasodilator area apparently forms a narrow longitudinal band above the ventral medullary surface, and it may be traced from the level of the restiform bodies to 6 to 7 mm caudal to the distal tip of the rhomboid fossa. Finally, Schramm and Bignall (1971) recently have confirmed the descending nature of the pathway at brainstem levels by demonstrating the persistence of the vasodilator response following interruption of the pathway just rostral to the stimulating electrode.

Thus, it now seems clear that the sympathetic vasodilator pathway originates in the motor cortex, at diencephalic levels traverses the hypothalamus, and subsequently courses through the brainstem ventrally and ventrolaterally to enter the spinal cord. An important remaining question, however, regards the possible synaptic interruption of the pathway. As stated above, the Swedish investigators argue that the descending cortical projection synapses in the hypothalamus. However, this must be considered uncertain in view of the amygdalar projection. There is more convincing evidence for a mesencephalic synaptic relay, since chronic supracollicular decerebration does not alter the response evoked by mesencephalic stimulation, and infracollicular decerebration abolishes the medullary response (Lindgren 1955). Also important in this regard have been the clear demonstrations that the sympathetic vasodilator pathway is entirely independent of the medullary pressor and depressor centers (Lindgren 1955; Lindgren and Uvnäs 1954; Schramm and Bignall 1971). Consequently, it would seem that this vasodilator pathway, of cortical origin, constitutes a rather direct route to the spinal cord, involving at most only a few synapses. However, the precise nature of the possible descending relays remains uncertain.

Possible Functional Significance of the Vasodilator System

Given at least a preliminary description of the sympathetic vasodilator pathway, an obvious question, and one which was raised quite early in the literature, regards its possible functional significance. In this respect two prominent speculations were advanced by the Swedish group. Eliasson and his associates (Eliasson et al. 1951) hypothesized first that this system is activated when a sudden increase in muscle blood flow is demanded for muscular effort, as in emergency situations. However, they were uncertain as to whether this vasodilator system would be activated in situations exclusive of emotional stress. Shortly after this, Eliasson, Lindgren, and Uvnäs (1952) were able to elicit the vasodilator response pattern in the dog without accompanying autonomic responses, leading to the hypothesis that the system may be more concerned with voluntary muscular activity. This associated the system with exercise independent of emotional stress. These two classes of speculation were, however, based entirely upon the associated autonomic response patterns observed in anesthetized animals.

As stated earlier, the cardiovascular response patterns during defensive behavior and exercise have many similarities, a finding which is hardly surprising in view of the muscular effort involved in agonistic behavior. In both cases sympathetic muscle vasodilatation is presumed to occur. The major differentiating characteristic appears to be that systemic arterial blood pressure increases during defensive behavior (Zbrozyna 1972), but not during preparation for exercise. However, as the severity of exercise increases arterial blood pressure does tend to rise, and, since the level of exercise during defensive behavior can be considerable, this may seriously qualify blood pressure as a discriminating feature. Further confounding the issue are recent reports (Adams, Baccelli, Mancia, and Zanchetti 1969) that the cardiovascular alterations occurring during naturally elicited fighting behavior are not identical to those evoked by electrical stimulation of the presumptive defense areas of the nervous system.

Consequently, the key to differentiating the proposed "exercise" versus "emotional stress" hypotheses would seem to lie in studying unanesthetized animals in which the behavioral correlates of stimulating a given area of the nervous system may be observed. At this point it becomes necessary to backtrack historically and to examine briefly the development of ideas centering about the control of cardiovascular adjustments during defensive behavior.

Sham Rage and the Defense Reaction

The behavioral pattern of sham rage has been recognized since the turn of the century (Woodworth and Sherrington 1904) and is well described in the classical studies of Cannon and· Britton (1925), Bard (1928), and Hess and Brügger (1943). The latter made the particularly important contribution of identifying a delimited hypothalamic region where electrical stimulation elicits organized behavior characteristic of emergency reactions, a region designated as the "defense area."

With such literature as a foundation, Abrahams, Hilton, and Zbrozyna (1960) subsequently characterized the cardiovascular components of the hypothalamically induced defense reaction, and, among their important findings, reported the occurrence of active muscle vasodilatation. This ostensibly supported the Eliasson et al (1951) hypothesis that the sympathetic vasodilator system is concerned with muscular effort demanded by stressful situations. However, the findings of Abrahams and his co-workers (1960) with mesencephalic stimulation led them to a somewhat different suggestion. Briefly, they demonstrated distinct response patterns following activation of three mesencephalic locations: the subcollicular region, central grey, and peduncular region. While defensive behavior accompanied subcollicular and central grey stimulation, no characteristic behavioral effects occurred with stimulation in the peduncular region. Their conclusion was that the hypothalamus, central grey, and subcollicular area are integrative centers for the defense reaction, while the peduncular vasodilator region is not. They further suggested that the efferent pathway for the active muscle vasodilator system described by the Swedish group traverses the peduncular region. (Recall that the Swedish group localized the pathway at mesencephalic levels in the subcollicular region.)

Further work regarding the localization of the "defense" pathway then centered around the amygdala, and Hilton and Zbrozyna (1963) demonstrated a characteristic cardiovascular response pattern with stimulation of the nucleus basalis, pars medialis, overlapping slightly with the adjoining pars lateralis and nucleus centralis. This is the same region in which the amygdalar defense zone was localized in earlier studies (e.g., Magnus and Lammers 1956; de Molina and Hunsperger 1959; Ursin and Kaada 1960). While the defense reaction can be elicited with stimulation of the stria terminalis, stimulation studies following interruption of the stria seem to indicate that it is afferent to the amygdala with respect to the defense reaction. This prompted Hilton and Zbrozyna (1963) to conclude that the ventral amygdalofugal pathway constitutes the relevant efferent system from the amygdala, and their stimulation results are consistent with this hypothesis. Moreover, anatomical data (e.g., Nauta 1961) clearly indicate that the amygdala has access to the entire rostrocaudal extent of the hypothalamus through this system.

Thus, the "defense" pathway appears to originate in a restricted portion of the amygdala, and continues to the hypothalamus via the ventral amygdalofugal pathway. From the hypothalamus the pathway continues into the mesencephalon and seems to be represented in the subcollicular tegmentum and central grey. Its subsequent course remains undescribed, however. A point of interest is that an apparently analogous system is also found in the avian brain, although the muscle vasodilatory component of the response has not been specifically investigated (Macdonald and Cohen 1973).

Review of the Pathways and Their Functional Significance

With studies of the behavioral correlates occurring during stimulation of the various cardiomotor pathways, data regarding their possible functional significance have begun to emerge. For example, in summarizing the hypothalamic regulation of the cardiovascular system, Hilton (1966) has concluded that the pathway traced by the Swedish group produces a redistribution of circulating blood volume to the skeletal muscles, without the behavioral and autonomic responses characteristic of the defense reaction. He suggests that this may reasonably be considered as a pathway mediating the cardiovascular alterations involved in "exercise" or the "preparation-for-exercise." This pathway, arising in the motor cortex, is apparently distinct from that originating in the amygdala and participating in the cardiovascular adjustments that accompany defensive behavior.

Although in many respects less precisely described, the broader functional significance of the so-called "defense" pathway is somewhat more obvious because of the striking nature of the correlated agonistic behavior. The absence of such decisive behavioral effects during stimulation of the presumptive "exercise" pathway makes its functional significance more obscure, although the lack of behavioral effects could be considered consistent with the proposed "exercise" function of the vasodilator pathway. However, there are various lines of evidence, some rather recent, which lend even more credence to this functional designation for the sympathetic vasodilator system described by the Swedish group. This section will be concluded with some brief comments in this context.

First, to reiterate an important point made earlier, the cardiovascular responses evoked by stimulation of the vasodilator system are quite similar to those observed during exercise (Smith, Rushmer, and Lasher 1960). Second, Clarke, Smith, and Shearn (1968) have demonstrated that stimulation of discrete areas in the motor cortex giving rise to movement of only one limb causes increases in muscle blood flow confined to that limb. Finally, Bolme and Novotny (1969), in a most interesting series of experiments, have shown that sympathetic vasodilatation occurs as a conditioned response in dogs trained to anticipate exercise, as well as constitutes a component of the orienting response. This provides clear evidence for sympathetic vasodilatation occurring during preparation for exercise and supports recent contentions (Bolme et al. 1967; Hilton 1968) that the sympathetic vasodilator system can mediate cardiovascular events preparatory to exercise quite independently of the defense reaction.

"POSTURAL ADJUSTMENT" PATHWAY

The marked cardiovascular adjustments that accompany postural change have been clearly documented for some time (See Gauer and Thron 1965). For example, in orthostasis (assuming an upright posture) the heart rate increases. But since this is paralleled by a decrease in stroke volume, the cardiac output is either unchanged or more frequently falls. While there may be a transient decrease in mean arterial blood pressure, rapid reflex compensation ensures either no net change or a slight increase under steady state conditions: This maintenance of mean arterial blood pressure in the face of reduced cardiac

output is apparently accomplished by a large increase in total peripheral resistance resulting from neurally mediated vasoconstriction. The
salient point to be derived from this brief description is that characteristic and predictable patterns of adjustment appear in response to
alterations in posture, thus implying an organized central control.

The question germane to this chapter then concerns the nature of
this central neural organization, beginning with the relevant pathways
that mediate these cardiovascular adjustments. It is of interest in this
context that some years ago Moruzzi (e.g., 1940) demonstrated cardiovascular effects following cerebellar stimulation. While this report
had little apparent impact at the time, more recently there has been
a rejuvenation of interest in the role of the cerebellum in cardiovascular control, particularly with respect to postural adjustments. This
seems to have been stimulated largely by the reports of Achari and
Downman (1970) and Miura and Reis (1970) that cerebellar stimulation
produces a rise in mean arterial blood pressure frequently accompanied by cardioacceleration and apnea. It is of interest that a similar
effect has been described in the bird, including the concomitant apnea
(Macdonald and Cohen 1971, 1973).

More specifically, the cardiac response pattern has been shown to
consist of cardioacceleration, cardioaugmentation, decreased stroke
volume, and no significant change in cardiac output (Doba and Reis
1972). The tachycardia apparently is mediated by both an increase in
sympathetic outflow and a release of vagal inhibition (Lisander and
Martner 1971) with no adrenal medullary contribution (Achari and
Downman 1970; Doba and Reis 1972). With respect to vascular
changes, a widespread systemic vasoconstriction that is neurally mediated appears to be responsible for the increase in mean arterial blood
pressure (Achari and Downman, 1970; Doba and Reis 1972), and
Lisander and Martner (1971) report that the vasoconstriction in skeletal
muscles and the intestines exceeds that in the renal and cutaneous vascular beds. Of particular significance in this context is the conclusion
of Doba and Reis (1972) that this response pattern evoked by cerebellar stimulation closely approximates that occurring during orthostasis,
prompting serious consideration of the cerebellum as an important
participant in the central organization mediating the cardiovascular adjustments to postural change. These same investigators provided rather
convincing evidence of this by demonstrating that the cardiovascular
responses to tilt are severely impaired following destruction of the cerebellar region from which cardiovascular responses are elicited with
electrical stimulation.

Thus, it may now be concluded that this cerebellar pressor system
is a major participant in organizing the cardiovascular adjustments
necessary to compensate for postural changes, and this consequently

provides a focal point for further investigations of the relevant central pathways. Unfortunately, little is known regarding the afferent pathways that are involved in initiating the cerebellar response, although it is quite likely that these will include a complex of somatic, vestibular, and baroreceptor systems.

Somewhat more information is available, however, with respect to the cerebellar outflow. First, the active cerebellar region from which cardiovascular responses are elicited appears to be confined to the ventromedial aspect of the rostral third of the fastigial nucleus (Miura and Reis 1970). The relevant cerebellofugal system then apparently includes both crossed and uncrossed fibers coursing through the restiform body, since restiform lesions abolish the cardiovascular responses to fastigial stimulation while destruction of the superior or middle cerebellar peduncles has no effect (Miura and Reis 1970). The brainstem representation of the pathway is not entirely clear, but it does appear to involve fastigiobulbar projections to the paramedian reticular nucleus. In fact, Miura and Reis (1970) claim that the response can be entirely eliminated by destruction of the dorsal and ventral divisions of the paramedian nucleus rostral to the obex. While lesions of the lateral vestibular nucleus also eliminate the response, this could well be due to interruption of fastigiobulbar fibers en passage. Therefore, it presently appears that the cerebellar pressor-accelerator pathway originates from neurons in a highly restricted region of the fastigial nucleus and follows the course of the fastigiobulbar fibers to the rostral portion of the paramedian reticular nucleus.

Since the paramedian nucleus has been identified as a major constituent of the medullary depressor center (e.g., Calaresu and Thomas 1971), some rather intriguing problems are raised by its relationship to the cerebellar pressor system, problems relating to the mechanism of the cerebellar pressor-accelerator effect. Regarding this mechanism, three views have been prominent. The first hypothesizes that the fastigiobulbar system inhibits the paramedian neurons and thereby disinhibits the sympathetic preganglionics. This alternative seems unlikely, however, since it has been established that stimulation of the nucleus fastigius excites, rather than inhibits, paramedian neurons (Miura and Reis 1971). Moreover, paramedian lesions produce no change in resting heart rate or blood pressure (Miura and Reis 1971), contrary to the view that the depressor center exerts a tonic sympathoinhibitory effect (Alexander 1946). Second, the fastigial system could operate through inhibition of the baroreceptor mechanisms. While there is ample evidence of mutual inhibition between baroreceptor and fastigial systems at the level of the paramedian nucleus (Miura and Reis 1971), the cerebellar response persists after elimination of the baroreceptor inputs (Achari and Downman 1970; Miura and Reis 1971). Third, it

is conceivable that the fastigiobulbar system directly excites sym-
pathoexcitatory and/or parasympathoinhibitory pathways via the paramedian nucleus. This would then imply that the paramedian region
is not purely depressor but heterogeneous, containing both "pressor"
and "depressor" neurons (Bach 1952; Wang and Ranson 1939a). While
recent evidence casts considerable doubt on the earlier simplistic view
of the depressor center (Calaresu and Thomas 1971), strong support
for this particular view of the fastigiobulbar mechanism is still lacking.

Consequently, the manner in which the cerebellar pressor-accelerator system influences preganglionic activity is still obscure, and it is
likely to remain so until the intrinsic organization of the medullary cardiovascular centers is more fully understood. Regardless, the recent
investigations of this system do seem to establish it as an important
component of the central control of the cardiovascular adjustments
occurring during postural change, and they, thereby, have provided
a focal point for further investigations to delineate the central pathways
mediating this neural control.

CENTRAL CONTROL OF CARDIOVASCULAR REFLEX ACTIVITY

In preceding sections the medullary mechanisms of cardiovascular
reflex activity and the supramedullary control of cardiovascular activity
in general have been discussed. However, these topics were treated
rather independently, reflecting the view which predominated for
many years that structures rostral to the pons neither participated in
the maintenance of mean arterial blood pressure nor influenced cardiovascular reflex activity. More recent evidence, on the contrary, has
now clearly established supramedullary structures as powerful mod-
ulators of such reflex activity. The existence of such central modulation
perhaps could have been inferred by analogy to the reflex modulation
in the somatomotor system, although such inferences are considerably
easier in retrospect. However, prior to supporting experimental evidence, Bard (1960) insightfully ventured such a suggestion, and a few
years later Hilton (1963) provided experimental validation by demonstrating that hypothalamic stimulation could inhibit baroreceptor
reflexes.

Following the establishment of the phenomenon by Hilton (1963),
Reis and Cuénod (1964) obtained evidence suggesting that supramedullary structures exerted tonic as well as phasic influences on reflex
activity. The critical feature of their study was the recognition of a
masking of tonic descending influences by the buffer nerves in the
intact preparation. These data then led to the conclusion that supramedullary structures do not on the whole exert any significant tonic
effects on vasomotor neurons involved in the maintenance of blood

pressure, but rather that they maintain the responsiveness of neurons involved in determining baroreceptor reflex excitability.

The nature of central reflex modulation has been elaborated to a considerable extent in subsequent studies, and this has included the determination of the classes of modulation that may obtain and the characterization of the role of given central structures in reflex modulation. Research of the first type has now established the existence of a wide range of modulatory effects and to some extent has elucidated the mechanisms involved. For example, not only may baroreceptor induced cardiodeceleration be inhibited by stimulation of such structures as the hypothalamus (Gebber and Snyder 1970; Hilton 1963) and cerebellum (Achari and Downman 1970; Moruzzi 1940), but activation of other structures such as the amygdala can facilitate the reflex bradycardia (Gebber and Klevans 1972). Thus, modulatory effects can be either facilitatory or inhibitory, and in certain instances cardiovascular responses to central stimulation are mediated exclusively through baroreceptor reflex modulation—for example, the septum (Gebber and Klevans 1972). In other cases, it has been found that structures presumed not to be cardioactive do, in fact, exert modulatory influences on cardiovascular reflexes as demonstrated by a conditioning-testing approach. Further evidence of the high degree of differentiation of central reflex modulation is provided by the demonstration that stimulation at certain hypothalamic sites can selectively inhibit vagally mediated reflex bradycardia without reducing the sympathoinhibitory reflex depressor response (Gebber and Snyder 1970). Moreover, Reis and Cuénod (1965) describe various sites facilitating or inhibiting the pressor response to carotid occlusion with no apparent effects on the depressor response to sinus stretch.

In any case, although the story regarding central reflex modulation is only at its inception, it is already clear that such central control is highly differentiated. As with central control of γ-efferent activity, it will obviously require considerable effort to establish in detail the geography of these central modulatory effects, since this necessitates a careful and systematic cataloguing of numerous central structures. While information is rapidly accumulating in this regard, a detailed review would be premature. It may in fact be the case that such a review must await a comprehensive description of the major descending systems generally influencing cardiovascular activity and specification of their functional roles. The "exercise," "defense," and "postural adjustment" pathways are but a start in this direction, and it has already been established that certain structures participating in these systems are involved in the reflex regulation of the baroreceptor reflexes. For example, stimulation of the hypothalamic defense area suppresses baroreceptor reflex inhibition of heart rate without influencing reflex vasomotor responses (Humphreys, Joels, and McAllen 1971; Lisander 1970), although the absence of an effect on vasomotor reflexes has recently been questioned (Coote and Perez-Gonzales 1972). Similarly, stimulation of the cerebellar pressor-accelerator system is reported to inhibit baroreceptor induced bradycardia (Achari and Downman 1970; Lisander and Martner 1971), but its effects on the reflex vasomotor responses are in contention (Lisander and Martner 1971; Miura and Reis 1971).

Perhaps the most salient point of this section is that the recognition of central reflex modulation is critical in any broad functional approach to central cardiovascular control. This is true not only with respect to the identification of central cardioactive structures and the description of their mechanisms of action, but also for any attempt to describe the role of a given pathway in any detail. In this latter respect, it might be pointed out that central reflex modulation is of particular significance for certain issues raised at this symposium, since it is almost certainly involved during conditioned cardiovascular responses. The fact that in many species the conditioned response includes both cardioacceleration and increased blood pressure suggests a possible uncoupling of the heart rate and arterial blood pressure responses through inhibition of baroreceptor mechanisms. Consequently, a detailed description of the central mechanisms producing the conditioned response dynamics must clearly take account of possible central reflex modulation.

CONCLUDING COMMENTS

In closing, we would once again stress the selective nature of this review. As stated earlier, our attempt has been to focus on the medulla and certain of the more extensively described descending systems for which information regarding their broader functional significance is available. In part this strategy was dictated by the nature of this symposium, since we felt that a review of central control that, where possible, related specific cardiomotor pathways to behavior would be more germane to cardiovascular psychophysiology. However, even independent of that consideration, this broader view of central control appears to have imposed an order and perspective on the more recent literature that was not present in the earlier studies emphasizing comprehensive, structure-by-structure analyses. It must be recognized, though, that this more contemporary approach relies critically upon the information derived from such earlier studies.

Unfortunately, a review of this nature necessarily omits many important investigations. For example, cardiovascular reflexes were not discussed in any detail, except insofar as they had direct bearing on the consideration of medullary and supramedullary control. Also, only the "defense," "exercise," and "postural adjustment" pathways were considered, with no mention of pathways involved in mediating the cardio-vascular adjustments accompanying such behaviors as thermoregulation, feeding, and sexual activity. Perhaps more disconcerting is the omission of various areas of the nervous system where stimulation clearly elicits cardiovascular responses but which do not fit as yet into any clear functional system. Among the more serious of such omissions is the presumptive depressor-decelerator pathway arising in the anterior cingulate gyrus (Löfving 1961). Stimulation of this pathway has profound inhibitory effects on the cardiovascular system, including marked vagal bradycardia and profound sympathoinhibition which together yield severe hypotension.

Some comment is also merited regarding the functional designations of the various descending systems as "defense," "exercise," and "postural adjustment" pathways. The evidence supporting these designations has been discussed along with the description of each pathway. However, it is essential to point out that, while suggestive, such evidence is not yet decisive, and we have assumed a certain liberty in assigning connotative names to these pathways. The question is less one of whether these pathways are participating in the cardiovascular components of the designated behavior. The uncertainty more likely concerns the uniqueness of each system. For example, does the cerebellar pathway participate in cardiovascular adjustments *only* during postural change, or is it also involved during other kinds of behaviors as well? Are the "defense" and "exercise" pathways mutually exclusive except at the level of the final common path, or do they interact and possibly share neuronal elements at pontine or bulbar levels?

Questions of this nature then raise the general issue of interactions between the various cardiomotor pathways, and, if such interactions obtain, under what conditions are they synergistic or antagonistic? This is of particular importance within the context of cardiovascular conditioning. In most of the commonly applied paradigms a nociceptive stimulus is employed as the unconditioned stimulus, and this could well produce involvement of the "defense" pathway as part of the motor system mediating the conditioned response. However, since muscular effort is an important component of the response, anticipation of defensive behavior could also involve participation of the "exercise" pathway. Supporting this argument is the important study of Bolme and Novotny (1969) in which it is demonstrated that sympathetic muscle vasodilatation can be conditioned in anticipation of either exercise or the occurrence of a nociceptive stimulus. In any case, a tentative classification of cardiomotor pathways into such functional categories provides, in our view, effective working guidelines for elucidating the central pathways mediating conditioned cardiovascular responses, particularly those constituting the motor segments of the system (Cohen in press).

MARY R. COOK

Psychophysiology of Peripheral Vascular Changes

INTRODUCTION

We commonly speak of an individual becoming purple with rage, red with embarrassment, pale with anger, gray with fear, or blue with cold. Such phrases reflect, at least in part, accurate observations of the state of the circulation in the face, and they suggest that peripheral vascular changes might provide unique information about the relationships between emotion, behavior, and physiological change. The exciting findings of Sokolov and of Kelly and his co-workers are recent examples supporting this view. Sokolov (1963) has reported that innocuous stimuli can be distinguished from those having painful or threatening qualities by measuring the direction of vasomotor changes in the forehead. Kelly and his colleagues (e.g., Kelly and Walter 1968), using a different approach, have demonstrated a close relationship between forearm blood flow and anxiety level, and, in addition, have reported that treatment with Librium not only improved the subjective symptoms of anxiety, but also decreased resting forearm blood flow (Kelly,

The preparation of this paper, as well as the substantive research conducted at the Unit for Experimental Psychiatry, was supported in part by Contract DADA 17-71-C-1120 from the United States Army Medical Research and Development Command, by Grant 5 RO1 MH 19156-02 from the National Institute of Mental Health Public Health Service, and by a grant from the Institute for Experimental Psychiatry. Special thanks are due Harvey D. Cohen for many hours of helpful discussion during the preparation of this paper, and to Frederick J. Evans, Charles Graham, Emily Carota Orne, Martin T. Orne, and David A. Paskewitz for critical reading of the manuscript. Bette Newill and Deborah E. Seeley provided invaluable assistance in preparation of the manuscript and data analysis.

Brown, and Shaffer 1970). Observations such as these have generated wide interest, for they point toward techniques which not only allow psychological state to be evaluated, but also provide information about the ways in which psychological variables interact with cardiovascular functions.

The present paper will attempt to bring together several lines of research which have contributed to our understanding of the psychophysiology of the peripheral vascular system in the intact human, alert and interacting with his environment. Physiological mechanisms, relationships with other autonomically-controlled variables, stimulus and task variables affecting responsivity, and areas where crucial information is lacking will be discussed. It should be emphasized that the purpose here will not be to provide an exhaustive review of the literature; rather, the focus will be on the principles and mechanisms elucidated by a wide range of investigations. Studies are therefore discussed only insofar as they illustrate or clarify basic issues.

THE PLETHYSMOGRAPHIC RESPONSE

Because he works with the alert, intact human being, the psychophysiologist tends to be restricted to those measures which can be obtained without subjecting the individual to stress or physical discomfort. The plethysmograph owes its widespread popularity as a psychophysiological measure as much to this factor as to the nature of the information which it provides.

Plethysmographic techniques essentially measure changes in the volume of a given body part. Since most of the tissues which contribute to such volume are constant, changes in volume are used as an indirect index of changes in the amount of blood contained within the part. Such volumetric changes reflect the transient difference between the flow of blood into the part and the flow of blood out of the part (Burch 1954a), and are consequently dependent on both the arterial and venous sides of the vascular bed.

Plethysmographic changes are of two types. The rapid component, usually referred to as pulse amplitude or pulse volume, is the manifestation of the pumping action of the heart as modified by peripheral vascular mechanisms. There is also a slower component, which reflects the overall engorgement of the area, and which is referred to as blood volume. As can be seen in Figure 3.1, both components of the plethysmographic tracing are sensitive to stimuli from the environment. The upper tracing shows the rapid component, pulse amplitude (PA), while the middle tracing is the slower component, blood volume (BV). These tracings were obtained by placing a photoplethysmographic transducer on the finger, and recording the BV component with direct coupling at low gain, and the PA component (AC) at high gain. Binaural presentation of 95 dB, 1000 Hz tones served as stimuli. For purposes of comparison, the lower tracing shows mean blood flow as recorded with a radiant heat-measuring device.

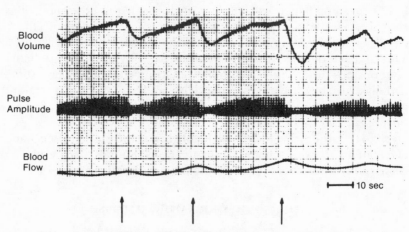

FIGURE 3.1   *Blood volume, pulse amplitude and blood flow responses from the finger to a 95 dB, 1000 Hz tone. Arrows mark the onset of stimulus presentation.*

The plethysmographic response has a latency of 1.5 to 4 seconds, and usually reaches its peak 7 to 10 seconds after stimulus onset. Recovery time is quite variable, and may depend on the demands of the stimulus on the individual. It should be noted that correlations between the PA and BV components of the response are usually low. Other characteristics of the response have been discussed in detail by Lidberg, Schalling, and Levander (1972).

Because both the venous and arterial sides of the cutaneous vascular bed are under sympathetic control, the plethysmograph provides a measure of sympathetic nervous system (SNS) activity, even though it does not provide information about the relative influence of different component vessels in the vascular bed. This information is often quite useful in psychophysiology. However, the specificity of the SNS, and the fact that the venous and arterial sides of the vascular bed may respond quite differently, suggest that more detailed information is needed. Ideally, we would like to measure arteriolar tone, venous tone, and the distribution of blood between the true capillaries and other vessels, in order to relate these variables to the behavior and psychological state of the subject. The question of the extent to which plethysmographic data can be used to obtain this sort of information is an extremely important one.

Arteriolar and venous contributions to the plethysmographic response

While the usual plethysmographic tracing reflects both flow into the part and flow out of the part, by occluding the venous outflow and observing the rate of increase in the volume of the part, it is possible to obtain an indirect estimate of blood flow, and so long as blood pressure is reasonably constant, of arteriolar tone. This technique, known as venous occlusion plethysmography, has become the standard against which other noninvasive methods of measuring blood flow are evaluated. The method, however, provides only intermittent measures of flow, and psychophysiologists have continued to seek a simpler, more continuous measure.

It was suggested many years ago that PA is highly correlated with arteriolar tone, and therefore with blood flow, while BV reflects venous changes. Some evidence was presented supporting this hypothesis, and it is now assumed by many investigators that pulse amplitude changes can be interpreted in terms of changes in blood flow. Such an interpretation seems to be an oversimplification of the physiological mechanisms involved in the plethysmographic response, and the evidence for and against the use of PA as a measure of blood flow deserves careful consideration.

Burton (1939) reported that, for an individual subject under baseline conditions, a high correlation ($r = .88$, $p < .01$) exists between blood flow as measured by the venous occlusion technique and volumetric PA at the time of blood flow determination. No such relationship with BV was found, and Burton suggested that the venous system primarily determined the BV component.

Hertzman and his colleagues, in a series of papers (Hertzman, Randall, and Jochim 1946, 1947; Hertzman 1948), have shown that resting PA also reflects blood flow when the photoplethysmograph is used. While the relationship within subjects was appreciable, it was considerably less with across subject comparisons. The differences reported, however, could well have been a function of slight differences in the placement of the transducers, or the pressure with which they were applied. For an individual subject under resting conditions, therefore, a linear relationship between basal PA and blood flow seems to exist. However, such a relationship does not necessarily imply that decreased PA in response to psychological stimuli is caused exclusively by a reduction in blood flow. Many different lines of research have provided evidence that venous changes are involved in such responses, and that the position of the limb relative to the heart is one of the variables determining the extent of the venous contribution.

Effects of limb position

In 1937, Turner, Burch, and Sodeman demonstrated that raising the arm above heart level increased PA but decreased BV. Lowering the arm had the opposite effects. Both volumetric and photometric data were reported, and were in agreement. The authors hypothesized that the observed increase in PA was a function of the decreased resistance of the arterioles necessary to maintain physiologic levels of pressure and flow in the elevated capillary bed. The BV decrease was seen as a function of both the draining of the veins due to hydrostatic pressure and decreased venous tone. Increases in the distensibility of the capillaries and venules in the elevated position, and the effects of venous pressure on the changes in PA in the depressed position were emphasized. Goetz (1950) observed similar effects in the toes of the elevated limb, but reported that the phenomenon was not dependent on SNS innervation, since it was still obtained after sympathectomy.

Gaskell and Burton (1953) reported a series of experiments in which both changes in volume and changes in blood flow as measured by the venous occlusion technique were observed. Plethysmographs were placed on the toes of both feet in order to make simultaneous comparisons between a limb at heart level and a lowered or elevated limb. The volumetric observations of increased PA and decreased BV when the limb was elevated, and decreased PA with increased BV when it was lowered, were replicated. Blood flow, however, was found to be greatest with the limb at or near heart level. Similar responses were observed in a sympathectomized limb, supporting the earlier observation by Goetz (1950) that the changes were independent of the SNS. Spontaneous responses in the digit at heart level were constrictive, but in the elevated toe they appeared as dilations; under these circumstances, blood flow in the elevated toe also showed a transient increase.

In a study by Holling and Verel (1957), carried out on the muscular forearm site, the elevated arm again showed greater PA and reduced BV. Blood pressure changes were consistent with changes in hydrostatic pressure, but only slight variations in venous pressure were seen. When venous occlusion was applied to the elevated arm, a longer period of time was necessary before the characteristic inflow curve was seen. Flow was reduced when the arm was elevated, and the greater the elevation, the greater the reduction in flow. Nutritive blood flow, however, did not seem to decrease. Even after the arm was elevated for as long as 2 hours, no reactive hyperemia was observed. Occlusion of the brachial artery with sufficient pressure to reduce apparent flow in the control arm to the level seen in the elevated arm, however, was followed by clear-cut reactive hyperemia.

There are three plausible explanations for the breakdown in the relationship between PA and blood flow when the limb is not at heart level. First, blood flow determinations might be inaccurate. Even if flow in the elevated digits were the same as flow in digits at heart level, differences in venous filling might result in apparently different degrees of blood flow when measured with the occlusion technique. When the arm is elevated, the veins tend to be much less filled. Since the pressure-volume relationship within the veins is not linear, this might reduce the apparent rate of inflow. Holling and Verel's observation that the characteristic inflow curve was delayed in the elevated arm supports this interpretation. Similar problems exist in using the venous occlusion technique to measure flow in a dependent limb. The venous vessels are engorged, and pressure capable of breaking past the occlusion cuff is quickly built up. Consequently, the extent to which results were affected by such artifacts needs to be determined using other methods for blood flow determination.

A second plausible explanation was proposed by Gaskell and Burton (1953). They postulated a veni-vasomotor reflex which, when the veins in an area are engorged, acts on the arterioles to reduce blood flow. Such a reflex would explain reduced blood flow in a dependent limb. In the elevated limb, reduced flow would come about as a function of reduced pressure. The lack of reactive hyperemia in an arm which has been elevated for a long time, however, mitigates against this explanation unless it is further postulated that it is only flow through the arterio-venous anastomoses (AVA) which is reduced. While the hypothesized veni-vasomotor reflex is adequate to explain flow changes, it does not deal adequately with volumetric changes.

Finally, venous filling decreases when the arm is elevated, suggesting an alternative explanation for decreased blood flow concomitant with increased PA. Reduction of venous filling increases the distensibility of the vascular bed. The pressure wave associated with each heart beat would, therefore, distend the vessel walls more under low venous tone than under high venous tone, thus increasing the observed PA (Burki and Guz 1970). Decreased BV in the elevated limb could then be explained by the reduced flow into the area and the increased flow out of the area due to hydrostatic pressure differences. Conversely, in the limb below heart level the veins are engorged, and because of the pressure-volume characteristics are less distensible, explaining the reduced PA. Reduced flow in such a situation could then arise from either decreased arterio-venous pressure differences or the veni-vasomotor reflex.

Effects of raising venous pressure

The findings discussed above suggest the important role of venous pressure in plethysmographic phenomena. Several studies have artificially increased venous pressure and observed the effects on the plethysmographic response to a variety of stimuli. For example, Capps (1936) raised the venous pressure in the hand to 70 mmHg by means of a wrist cuff. He reported that this effectively prevented venous constriction without markedly affecting inflow—an interpretation which would hold only in the absence of a veni-vasomotor reflex. Under these conditions, a pinch did not produce the usual vasomotor response. Gaskell and Burton (1953) reported that under similar conditions of venous engorgement, spontaneous responses were much reduced in frequency. Abramson and his colleagues (Abramson 1967; Abramson and Ferris 1940; Abramson and Katzenstein 1941) replicated these findings, although they found that a very strong noxious stimulus would still elicit a response. These results have been interpreted to indicate that, in the hand, the normal response to moderate psychic stimuli is primarily due to venous constriction, which has lesser effects on volume at high venous pressures.

Effects of temperature

Another approach to the question of whether PA is a reliable reflection of blood flow is to alter the environment in such a way as to differentially affect the venous and arteriolar vessels. Determinations are then made of the effect on PA, BV, and blood flow responses to stimuli known to affect these variables under normal circumstances. Wood and Eckstein (1958) demonstrated that, when a subject is comfortably warm, the veins are maximally dilated. Arterioles dilate further when a heat load is applied, and can greatly increase blood flow. When a subject is cooled, both arterioles and veins are affected, although there is a time difference in the constrictions of each system. These relationships were used to indirectly investigate the venous contribution to the plethysmographic response (Cook, 1970). If it is hypothesized that resting PA is a reliable indication of blood flow, then heating the subject during a rest period should result in increased PA, and cooling in decreased PA. Since timelocked changes in PA have been demonstrated which are independent of experimental manipulations, the results of heating and cooling were compared with a control group maintained at constant temperature. Under these conditions, the control group showed a significant decrease in PA. The subjects who were cooled also showed a decrease, which was reliably greater than that of the controls. The heated subjects had significantly greater PA than the control group, suggesting that heat, in fact, had a dilating effect on PA. The hypothesis that resting PA reflects blood flow was therefore supported.

To the extent that plethysmographic responses depend on the venous system, pulsatile response amplitude should be little affected by increased temperature, but markedly reduced by cooling. If the hypothesis is incorrect, and arteriolar flow changes are the primary mechanism, heat should increase response amplitude and cold decrease it. The venous hypothesis was supported in the present experiment. Both hot and control groups showed a decline in response amplitude, and the groups were not significantly different. The cold subjects, on the other hand, showed a decline in response amplitude which was significantly greater than that seen in the other two groups. These alterations in response amplitude were found not to be a function of changes in base level. The findings support the hypothesis that pulsatile response amplitude, but not resting level, is to a large extent dependent upon the state of the venous vessels.

Hemodynamic analysis

The experiments discussed above suggest that the plethysmographic response is largely dependent on venous change, and that the distensibility of the low pressure vessels, which act as a hydraulic capacitor, must be considered. During the systolic portion of the pulse beat, inflow increases, and will transiently distend these vessels in accordance with their compliance. A greater degree of compliance will result in a larger increase in volume during systole and, hence, a larger PA. Evaluation of the role of venous tone in determining PA could be carried out by determining the amplitude of the pulse associated with each heart beat for blood pressure, flow, and volume. These data are not presently available. However, a preliminary investigation, using a measure of mean flow, has been conducted (Cook 1970). During the course of each of the experiments, points in time were selected for which mean flow was identical, and correlations then computed between PA and mean pressure taken from the carotid artery using the technique described by Wiggers (1952). All points were selected from periods during which tones of various intensity were being presented. High positive correlations, which would be expected if changes in venous tone were not involved in the plethysmographic response, were observed in only 2 of 12 subjects. The results for the remaining 10 subjects seem clearly to require changes in venous tone. These data are only preliminary, and much more accurate measurement techniques must be used before one can conclude that the hypothesis is supported. The results, nevertheless, indicate that variations in blood flow cannot entirely account for PA changes, even when variations in blood pressure are taken into account.

Summary

The effects of alterations in limb position, of changes in venous pressure, and of alterations in environmental temperature suggest that plethysmographic responses to psychological stimuli cannot be explained solely on the basis of changes in blood flow. A preliminary analysis of the relationship between pressure, flow, and plethysmographic response supports this conclusion. Evidence has been presented which supports the hypothesis that venous changes are important determinants of the plethysmographic response; the contribution of the venous system to PA in the finger appears to be primarily a function of changes in the distensibility of the vessels, rather than of outflow changes. Changes in outflow rate may well be reflected in the BV component of the response.

EFFECTS OF "NONPSYCHOLOGICAL" EVENTS
ON THE PLETHYSMOGRAPHIC RESPONSE

Location of the transducer

The location of the transducer has profound and sometimes startling effects on the observed plethysmographic recording. Using volume plethysmographs on the fingers, which contain no muscle, and on the forearm, which is mostly muscle, it can readily be demonstrated that the typical response to a psychological stimulus is increased volume in the muscle and decreased volume in the skin. It is not too surprising that vascular beds serving such distinct types of tissue as skin and muscle should differ. What is more intriguing is that different areas of skin produce response patterns which differ from each other both qualitatively and quantitatively. No systematic mapping of the skin using appropriate controls has been carried out. The results of several studies taken together, however, indicate that responses from different areas may reflect the distribution of the various types of vessels in the area under the transducer, and, therefore, provide indirect information about the contribution of such vessels to the overall response.

When recorded from the finger, responses are usually monophasic; when recorded from the thenar eminence, however, a brief increase in volume is often seen immediately after stimulus onset, followed by the typical volume decrease. If placed on the forearm over a large vein, the plethysmograph often fails to record PA at all; when not placed over a vein, pulsations associated with each heart beat are observed, even in the skin of the arms and legs, although the amplitude is much reduced.

Even greater differences are seen when sites on the head are used. In 1939, Hertzman and Dillon reported that changes in the forehead were often independent of those on the hand, both in timing and direction. Auditory stimuli resulted in decreased volume in the finger and either increased volume or no change in the forehead; the cold pressor test produced finger constriction and a slight decrease in BV in the forehead. However, a subsequent study (Hertzman and Roth 1942), with the plethysmograph placed in the center of the forehead, failed to show volume decreases in response to startle, the cold pressor test, or a deep breath. When cold was applied directly to the forehead, a slow and gradual constriction was seen, but there was no evidence of the rapid, reflex-like constriction seen in the hand to the application of cold.

Luria and Vinogradova (1959) used a site over the region of the bifurcation of the temporal and frontal arteries. Subjects were instructed to press a button every time they heard the word "cat." Subsequently, the word elicited a dilation in the forehead. When shock was paired with the word, however, further presentations elicited a constriction in the forehead. Findings such as these led Sokolov (1963) to postulate that orienting and defensive responses could be differentiated by observing the direction of change of cephalic vasomotor responses. Although these results have since been questioned by other investigators, reliable responses to auditory stimuli have been found from several sites on the forehead (Cohen and Johnson 1971a; Cook 1971a; Keefe 1970; Raskin, Kotses, and Bever 1969a, 1969b; Weinman 1967; Weinman and Manoach 1962). The center of the forehead usually gives the largest PA, while sensitivity to stimulation is often greater over the temporal artery (Cook 1971a).

Since even small changes in the location of a transducer can materially affect the plethysmographic tracing, it is important to keep in mind the region from which recordings are made when comparing conflicting experimental results. These observations suggest the need for systematic stimulus-contingent mapping of the body with respect to both base levels and response amplitudes.

Environmental temperature

In the skin, an increase in temperature usually results in increased PA, while decreased temperature reduces both PA and BV. Since the cutaneous circulation is known to play an important role in temperature regulation, the mechanisms have been studied extensively. Several reviews of the effects of temperature on the cutaneous circulation are available (Barcroft 1960; Greenfield 1963; Hertzman 1959; Thauer 1965). When environmental temperature increases above the "comfortably warm" level, blood flow in the skin of the hand also increases; the rate of this increase is partly a function of the starting temperature. In the palm, heat vasodilation appears to be entirely a function of reduced sympathetic tone, and in fact can induce vasodilation equivalent to that seen with a complete nerve block. In the forearm, and in other areas where vasoconstrictor tone is minimal, heat vasodilation occurs which does not appear to be a function of reduced constrictor activity. Whether active vasodilator fibers are responsible for this, or whether it is a result of bradykinin formation associated with thermoregulatory sweating, is not clear. Cutaneous veins, however, seem to be maximally dilated at a moderate temperature (32° C) (Alexander 1963; Capps 1936; Webb-Peploe and Shepherd 1968).

As environmental temperature decreases below the comfortably warm level, blood flow through the skin is markedly reduced. In the resistance vessels of the hand, this is accomplished very quickly. The digital artery also constricts, but the onset of the constriction is delayed and the effect much more gradual (Hertzman and Roth 1942). Reduction of environmental temperature also produces marked venoconstriction (Alexander 1963; Burch 1954b; Page et al 1955; Webb-Peploe and Shepherd 1968). Wood and Eckstein (1958) have shown that, on going from a warm to a cool environment, arterial constriction usually precedes venous constriction. When going from a cool environment to a warm environment, venous tone first returns to control levels. The need to maintain reasonably constant environmental temperature during plethysmographic studies is clear from these data.

Local temperature

In addition to the changes which take place when the body is exposed to a changing environment, vaso- and veno-motor responses can be induced by local temperature change. When a warm stimulus is applied to a portion of the body, cutaneous blood flow increases in that area, and may, after several minutes, increase in other areas of the body normally under strong sympathetic constrictor influence. Local cold induces constriction at the site of application and also in other areas. The venous response to local temperature change is not quite so clear. Nachev, Collier, and Robinson (1971) have reported that local cooling results in constriction of the veins in the area cooled, but that no response is seen in the opposite side of the body. The effect of heating also was localized to the area of stimulation. Page et al. (1955), however, have reported responses in an isolated venous segment to immersing the opposite foot or hand in cool water. Since the measurement techniques used by the two studies were quite different, and since in the experiment of Nachev et al. the limb was elevated, it is difficult to evaluate the results. The venous effects of local temperature change seen in other areas may be part of the "orienting" response. Thus, immersing the foot in cold water might result in venoconstriction in both sides of the body, while immersing the foot in warm water would result in local venodilation and contralateral venoconstriction. Supporting this hypothesis, Sokolov (1963) and Zimny and Miller (1966) have shown that brief application of either hot or cold stimuli initially results in decreased volume as observed plethysmographically. With repeated presentations, however, the response to the warm stimulus changes to increased volume, while decreased volume is maintained to the cold stimulus.

Increased environmental temperature can reduce the venous response to other stimuli. Capps (1936) and Zitnik, Ambrosioni, and Shepherd (1971) have reported that local heating also reduces the response, but only in the area heated. If this is in fact the case, the reduction of response amplitude may be a function of increased venous engorgement in that area, rather than a result of decreased sympathetic output. Elevating the limb slightly might therefore augment the response so that it more resembles that from the unheated areas.

Respiratory effects

Fluctuations associated with the normal breathing cycle are rarely seen from the hands and feet, but are common when the transducer is placed on the ear lobe or the forehead (Burch 1954a; Sokolov 1963). When the subject engages in a respiratory maneuver, however, responses are greater from the hands and feet. Deep breaths or Valsalva's maneuvers are known to elicit reductions in PA and BV in the hands and feet, and increases in these measures in skeletal muscle (Abramson 1967; Bolton, Carmichael, and Stürup 1936). The amplitude of the response varies with the depth and speed of the inspiration (Stern and Anschel 1968), and the response occurs whether the maneuvers are spontaneous or carried out on request.

Sharpey-Shafer (1965) and Richards (1965) reviewed the effects of respiratory maneuvers on the component vessels in the vascular bed. When an individual takes a deep breath or performs other respiratory maneuvers such as hyperventilation, the blood flow in the skin of the hands decreases; no evidence is available about other cutaneous areas. Sudden deep inspiration produces venoconstriction, but with repeated breaths the response habituates (Burch, 1960). Both procaine (Burch, 1960) and a sympathetic ganglionic blocking agent (Merritt and Weissler, 1959) abolish the response. Hyperventilation also produces consistent venoconstriction, which is much reduced or abolished by ganglionic blockage. Page et al. (1955) found the Valsalva's maneuver to be more effective in eliciting venoconstriction than hyperventilation; in their experiment, two subjects with dysfunctions of the SNS lost consciousness during performance of Valsalva's maneuver. The maneuver blocks forward flow from the large veins due to changes in thoracic pressure; on cessation of the maneuver, blood pressure decreases markedly, and venous constriction is observed. In the sympathectomized patient this venoconstriction is absent, and venous return to the heart may well be inadequate (Sharpey-Shafer 1965).

The widespread effects of respiration on the behavior of blood vessels point to the desirability of monitoring respiration during plethysmographic studies so that responses which are the result of spontaneous changes in respiration can be excluded from analysis.

EFFECTS OF STIMULUS VARIABLES

The most frequent task imposed upon the subject in a psychophysiological experiment is the passive reception of stimuli. Often the subject is instructed that he will hear or see or feel a series of stimuli, but that it is not necessary for him to do anything other than attend to them. The qualities of the stimuli are then varied, and the effect on vasomotor behavior observed. The interesting thing about such circumstances is that subjects do respond to the stimuli. Why, when a bell is rung, do the blood vessels of the hand constrict?

The only model which deals explicitly with the effects of these "unconditional" stimuli is that of Sokolov (1963). He divides responses to unconditional stimuli into three classes: the orienting, the adaptive, and the defensive. Orienting responses are nonspecific, and quickly habituate. Any change in the environment, i.e., the onset or termination of a stimulus, variation in its intensity, or changes in any other parameter, may result in an orienting response. If the stimulus is repeated, the response will eventually habituate.

Adaptive responses appear after habituation of the orienting response, and represent the attempt of a specific system to cope with a specific stimulus. For example, Zimny and Miller (1966) have shown that, when a cold stimulus is applied to a finger, the blood vessels in the skin of that finger contract. If the stimulus is warm, the vessels dilate. Adaptive responses show little habituation.

The defensive response is elicited by stimuli which are very intense or psychologically threatening, and does not appear until habituation of the orienting response has occurred. The distinction between orienting and defensive responses is potentially very important. On the autonomic level, Sokolov based the distinction on the behavior of cutaneous blood vessels in the fingers and forehead. Defensive responses can also be distinguished from orienting responses by virtue of the failure of the defensive response to habituate. Although Sokolov does not discuss the mechanisms of the defensive response, it can be assumed that it is highly specific, since inhibition of all autonomic behavior does not occur.

Sokolov maintains that the cutaneous vasomotor orienting response always consists of vasoconstriction in the finger and vasodilation in the forehead. He suggests, as did Hertzman and Dillon (1939), that forehead vasodilation reflects a concomitant increase in blood supply to the brain, which heightens perceptual sensitivity. The defensive response, on the other hand, always results in constriction of forehead vessels, thus reducing the blood supply to the brain, allegedly desensitizing it, and protecting it from over-stimulation. While such an explanation seems highly unlikely given our present understanding of neural mechanisms, Sokolov's model provides an excellent framework within which to consider the stimulus variables most frequently investigated in psychophysiological research—intensity, repetition, and autonomic conditioning paradigms.

Stimulus intensity

Sokolov's model predicts that the amplitude of vasoconstriction in the fingers will increase with increasing stimulus intensity. Such a relationship appears to hold for the intensity of shocks (Hovland and Riesen 1940), white noise (Uno and Grings 1965), tones (Cohen and Johnson 1971a; Cook 1970), and depth of inspiration (Stern and Anschel 1968). Often the relationship is nearly linear; for example, Cook (1970) has reported that linear trends accounted for 89 to 95% of the variance in PA, BV, and blood flow responses to seven tones ranging from 65 to 125 db.

According to Sokolov's model, stimuli which are alerting, arousing, or novel can be distinguished from those which are painful or psychologically threatening on the basis of forehead BV changes. He reported (1963) that with a volume plethysmograph placed over the temporal artery, increases in BV were observed when novel or alerting stimuli were presented, and decreases when the stimuli were painful or threatening. A number of replications of this phenomenon have been reported from Russian and European laboratories (e.g., Figar 1965). In these studies, no attempt was made to combine people into groups and perform statistical tests; the individual differences between persons, rather than being a source of error, were considered a source of information.

American attempts to study the distinction between orienting and defensive responses have typically been based on a rather different type of psychophysiological experiment. Using photoplethysmographic transducers placed over the brow or in the center of the forehead, they have tried to document a lawful relationship between stimulus intensity and the defensive response. In such studies, parametric analysis of plethysmographic responses from rather large groups of people has been carried out. Such attempts to document the defensive response have been unsuccessful (e.g., Cohen and Johnson 1971a; Raskin et al. 1969a,b).

Even with the photoplethysmograph placed over the temporal artery, results achieved on the basis of group data have been less than impressive. For example, Cook (1970) measured the beat-by-beat response to the first presentation of 65, 95, and 125 db stimuli for 30 subjects. A significant decrease in forehead BV was observed in response to the first presentation of the 125 db stimulus, and a small but insignificant increase to the 65 and 95 db stimuli. From these averaged-across-subjects responses, average latency to peak was determined, and the responses to three presentations, each of seven stimuli ranging in intensity from 65 to 125 db, were scored; thus for the overall analysis, only the pre-stimulus value and the BV at the sixth post stimulus beat were measured. Using this method of data reduction, no significant intensity effect was observed. Thus when data analysis is based on photoplethysmographic recordings, and when rigid latency-to-peak criteria are used to measure and combine the responses of several persons, the forehead BV response does not seem to distinguish between moderate and intense auditory stimuli, even with the transducer placed over the temporal artery.

The methods of analysis used in the studies reported above are not truly appropriate to test Sokolov's model with regard to orienting and defensive responses. It is well known that people differ markedly in their subjective responses to auditory stimuli. The extremely loud acid-rock music which is intensely pleasurable for some persons is just as intensely painful for others. A 100 db stimulus might therefore be expected to result in forehead BV decreases for some persons, and increases for others. Such an outcome would obviously reduce considerably the likelihood that stimuli of different intensities would produce significantly different BV responses. Visual examination of polygraph records from the Cook (1970) study suggested that such individual differences were in fact having a profound effect on the data. For most subjects, some stimuli elicited either an increase in BV or no change, while others elicited a large BV decrease. A sub-sample of 10 subjects was therefore selected at random for more intensive analysis.

Very conservative criteria for response occurrence were used; a change in BV was considered to be a response only if it began 1 to 4 seconds after stimulus onset and was larger than any BV change occurring spontaneously during the rest period immediately prior to stimulus presentation. With such restrictions, 45% of the 210 stimuli presented failed to elicit a response. Thirty-four percent resulted in dilations and 20% elicited constrictions. The distribution of these responses as a function of stimulus intensity is shown in Figure 3.2 and individual data in Table 3.1. There was no evidence that the defensive response "developed" after habituation of the orienting response, although perhaps too few presentations were given for such a phenomenon to occur. As indicated in Table 3.1, no subject showed a dilation to a stimulus to which he had previously constricted. For an individual subject, the transition from dilation to constriction, if it occurred, occurred smoothly. The data agree with Sokolov's conclusion that forehead BV changes indicate, for an individual subject, whether or not a stimulus is painfully intense or psychologically threatening.

Similar conclusions have recently been reached by Hare (1973) based on recordings of PA from the center of the forehead. He grouped subjects into three groups on the basis of their heart rate response to slides of homicide victims; moderate decelerators (N = 28), decelera-

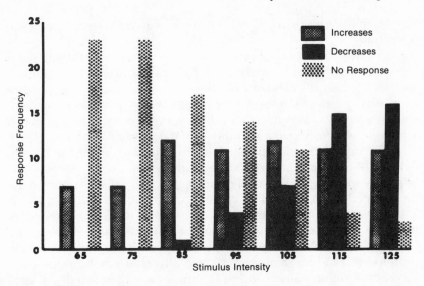

FIGURE 3.2 *Relationship between stimulus intensity and frequency of increases, decreases and no response in blood volume recorded from the area of temporal artery.*

TABLE 3.1   *Individual differences in cephalic vasomotor response**

S	Stimulus Intensity						
	65	75	85	95	105	115	125
1	+	+ −	=	−	−	−	−
2	+	+	+	+	+	+	+
3	+	+	+	+	+	+	+
4	=	=	=	−	−	−	−
5	+	+	+	+	+	+	.+
6	=	=	=	=	=	+	+
7	+	+	+	+ −	−	−	−
8	=	=	+	+	+ −	−	−
9	=	=	=	+	+	−	−
10	=	=	=	=	+	−	−

*Determination of direction of response is based on the evoked response curve over three stimulus presentations, and not on individual responses. Constrictions are indicated by (−), dilations by (+), biphasic curves by (+ −), and no response by (=).

tors (N = 12), and accelerators (N = 9). The cephalic responses of accelerators were then compared to those of decelerators. Accelerators responded to the slides of homicide victims with constriction, and decelerators with dilation. The decelerators also showed smaller PA responses from the thumb than did the accelerators, although skin resistance responses did not differentiate the groups. In a further study of the defensive response, Hare (1973) found that Ss who expressed strong fear of spiders responded with reduced forehead volume to slides of spiders more frequently than Ss who expressed little or no fear of spiders.

Since in the Cook study the transducer was placed over the temporal artery, and in the Hare study over the frontal artery, one obvious hypothesis is that the dilations observed were a function not of vaso-motor activity but of changes in blood pressure known to occur con-comitantly with vasoconstriction in the fingers. To test this hypothesis, 12 subjects were selected randomly from the original sample (Cook 1970), the only restriction being that recordings of carotid pulse and forehead BV be clear and contain a minimal amount of artifact. The recordings were examined to determine whether, when systolic pres-sure changed, a corresponding change could be observed in forehead BV. Of the 41 changes examined, 35 (85%) showed corresponding changes in forehead BV. No such relationship was found between fin-ger BV and carotid pulse, where the correspondence was 37 percent.

In another random sample of 12, the effects of carotid pulse pres-sure on PA from the forehead and the finger were examined. For each subject, 15 samples of each variable were taken, one sample every 25 seconds, and correlations computed. Eight of the 12 subjects showed stronger positive relationship between carotid pulse and forehead PA than between carotid pulse and finger PA. For five of the subjects, the correlation was significant ($p < .05$). While some of the variance is explained in this way, changes in pulse pressure do not seem to account entirely for changes in forehead PA. The relationship between changes in systolic pressure and changes in forehead BV also explains some, but not all, of the variance in the measure. The analyses provide some support for the hypothesis that cephalic dilation is dependent upon blood pressure change, but do not explain the constrictions observed at high stimulus intensities.

Another hypothesis is suggested by Gaskell and Burton's (1953) find-ing that, in the elevated limb, responses were dilatative, while in the limb at heart level they were constrictive. This difference was inter-preted as evidence that the state of the venous vessels is a major deter-minant of the vascular response observed. The situation is clearly analogous to cephalic responses, and the hypothesis deserves further consideration.

Neither of these suggested mechanisms accounts for the constriction observed with painfully intense stimuli. If the dilations observed are in fact found to be a function of increased blood pressure, the con-strictions could be explained as the result of constrictive sympathetic discharge to the skin of the head, which with very intense stimulation overrides the blood pressure increase usually observed. The extent to which differences in arteriolar and venous behavior could explain the data is not known, but evidence quoted previously indicates that the arteriolar portion of the response is greater with highly intense stimulation.

While Sokolov's model predicts stimulus intensity relations well when vascular responses are measured from the finger, results from the forehead are variable, and tend to depend both on the location of the transducer and on individual differences. A number of speculations about the physiological mechanisms of the response from the temporal artery have been put forth, but none seem truly adequate. Unfortunately, no data are available about the relationship between stimulus intensity and vasomotor changes in the muscle.

Vascular responses promise to provide useful data about the effects of stimulus intensity, both because the response is highly sensitive to such effects (Uno and Grings 1965; White 1964) and because of its potential applicability in the study of individual differences.

Stimulus repetition

Under most circumstances, cutaneous plethysmographic responses habituate more slowly than other autonomic components of the orienting response (e.g., Furedy 1969; Johnson and Lubin 1967; Koepke and Pribram 1967). Rate of vasomotor habituation depends upon a number of factors, such as the response component measured, the definition of habituation, the nature of the stimulus, and the state of the subject. While few studies have been concerned directly with the variables affecting vasomotor habituation, certain promising leads have developed.

Although habituation rate depends in part on whether PA or BV is the dependent variable, the relationship is by no means clear. In studies where only one component of the response is monitored, statistically significant habituation has been observed more frequently for BV than for PA. Recent studies by Levander, Lidberg, and Schalling (1969) and by Ginsberg and Furedy (1972) have, however, reported faster PA than BV habituation. The extent to which habituation of the two components can be differentially affected by such variables as site of measurement, arm position, and stimulus parameters is not known, but deserves careful investigation.

The use of different criteria to define habituation also has a disproportionate influence on whether an investigator concludes that vasomotor habituation has or has not occurred. The most commonly used definitions of habituation are: (1) percent of the sample of subjects who respond to a given stimulus; (2) the number of presentations of the stimulus necessary to reach a stated number of consecutive no-response trials; and, (3) a significant decrease in response amplitude. Even when applied to the same set of data, these definitions yield different apparent rates of habituation, and indicate different relationships between rate of habituation and stimulus intensity (Cook 1971b). Great care must therefore be taken in selecting the most appropriate definition of habituation for a given study. Clearly the investigator cannot select, post hoc, that measure of habituation which provides the best support for the hypothesis being tested.

Sokolov's model predicts that as stimulus intensity increases habituation rate decreases. This hypothesis has received some support (e.g., Cook 1971b; Uno and Grings 1965), but the relationship does not appear to be a strong one. Evaluation of the relationship must await the development of a more adequate experiemental design.

The nature of the stimulus and its relevance to the subject also require consideration. If sufficient presentations are given, habituation can usually be demonstrated to simple stimuli which require little or no overt response on the part of the subject. The dependence of the phenomenon on the relevance of the stimulus is well illustrated by a recent study by Bernstein and his colleagues (Bernstein et al. 1971). Habituation of PA responses to a stationary geometric pattern was demonstrated. When the figure showed apparent movement away from the subject, increased response amplitude was at first observed, but it rapidly habituated. If, on the other hand, the apparent movement was toward the subject, the plethysmographic response also increased, but significantly less habituation was observed.

The state of the subject appears also to be a relevant variable. Plethysmographic habituation is retarded in brain damaged persons (Davidoff and McDonald 1964), in persons with high scores on paper and pencil tests of anxiety (Jackson and Barry 1967; Koepke and Pribram 1967), and during sleep (Johnson and Lubin 1967). The study of individual differences in habituation to stimuli which vary qualitatively seems to hold more promise for understanding of the relevant relationships than does the study of group habituation to quantitatively varied stimuli, such as auditory intensity. For some persons habituation occurs gradually, while for others it is an all-or-none phenomenon. Unger (1964) has observed similar patterns of vasomotor habituation. Further research to determine whether pattern of habituation (i.e., gradual versus all-or-none) as a covariant would improve the relationship between psychological factors and plethysmographic habituation needs to be carried out.

Conditioning and stimulus generalization

While discussion of conditional vascular responses is beyond the scope of this paper, conditioning using either classical or operant techniques has been reported, and subjects who demonstrate such conditioning generally are able to verbalize the conditioned stimulus-unconditioned stimulus (CS-UCS) relationship, and also show larger orienting responses than subjects who do not develop a conditioned response (Baer and Fuhrer 1970; Raskin 1969; Shean 1968). Conditioning so developed shows stimulus generalization similar to that seen for electrodermal responses (Acker and Edwards 1964; Lang, Geer, and Hnatiow 1963; Luria and Vinogradova 1959; Raskin 1969). Furedy and Gagnon (1969) reported that the electrodermal response was more sensitive to stimulus differences in a differential conditioning paradigm than either BV or PA. They reported that the two components of the plethysmographic response were equally sensitive to stimulus differences, but the correlation between them was very low. In general, studies of vascular conditioning and of stimulus generalization have given us little unique information, either with regard to the vascular system or to the principles of autonomic conditioning. Conditional vascular responses have been reviewed extensively by Figar (1965).

EFFECTS OF PERFORMANCE TASKS

We are beginning to have an understanding of vascular responses of the skin when the subject is quietly receiving stimulation of various types. Sokolov's model holds reasonably well, although the mechanisms underlying the model are certainly not clear, particularly with reference to the response of the forehead. Does such a model also hold when the person is actively engaged in a task? Sokolov stated that, when a stimulus acquires signal value, the habituation to that stimulus is very much delayed. That this is the case has been demonstrated. However, there is some evidence to suggest that the type of task in which the subject is engaged has a strong influence upon the patterning of physiological responses observed. Such specificity has been repeatedly observed in the electrodermal system (Edelberg 1972), and it is suggested that such specificity also exists for plethysmographic responses.

Cognitive tasks

By far the most common task in vascular research is mental arithmetic. In 1940, Abramson and Ferris demonstrated that both volume and flow in the forearm increased in response to mental arithmetic, while in the hand volume and flow decreased. Blair and his co-workers (Blair et al. 1959) showed increased forearm blood flow in response to mental arithmetic. Increases in volume and flow in muscle and decreases in the skin of the hand in response to cognitive stimuli have been repeatedly demonstrated since that time. The effect of cognitive stimuli on forearm blood flow is greater than the effect of shocks (Rosenberg 1970) or of imagining a stressful scene (Gelder and Mathews 1968). Little comparison with other autonomic nervous system measures has been made.

Perceptual tasks

Very little relevant data using perceptual tasks has been reported, and there is clear need for information in this area. In an unpublished experiment, we examined PA, BV, and blood flow responses from the finger when subjects were required to note the position of a rapidly moving pointer when a tone was sounded. Five trials were given. The results of this experiment are shown in Figure 3.3. Both blood flow and BV responses habituated, but PA responses did not change significantly as a function of trials.

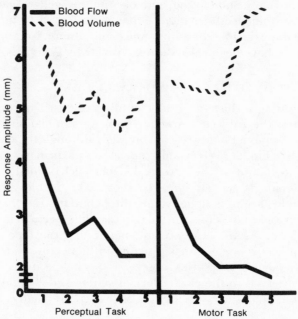

FIGURE 3.3   *Habituation curves for blood flow and blood volume under two task conditions.*

Motor tasks

Tasks involving vigorous exercise result in increased blood flow to the muscle (Barcroft 1963) and increased tone in the cutaneous veins of both hand and forearm (Nachev et al. 1971; Page et al. 1955; Rowell et al. 1971a,b). Unfortunately, the mechanisms underlying increased muscle blood flow during exercise are not understood; metabolic factors seem to be responsible, but the role of sympathetic nervous system dilator fibers is not clear (Barcroft 1963). Constriction of cutaneous veins during exercise appears to be neurally controlled, and can be reduced or abolished by heating the subject (Rowell et al. 1971a,b; Zitnik et al. 1971). Whether this response reduction is a function of reduced sympathetic discharge or of reduced sensitivity of the vessel is not clear, and it may be that both factors are involved. In all these studies, psychological and emotional factors are considered artifacts, so that their role in exercise is not understood. It should be noted that the increased venous tone observed when exercise begins may decline during the exercise period, suggesting that psychological factors play an important role.

In the psychophysiological laboratory, motor tasks are usually much less strenuous than in physiological studies. Typically subjects are asked to close a micro-switch, depress a lever, or turn a knob. While there is plentiful heart rate and electrodermal data on motor tasks of this type, few vasomotor studies have been done. In a preliminary attempt to look at some of the relevant variables, we asked subjects to close a switch as quickly as possible upon hearing a tone. Five trials were given. Blood flow in the finger declined as a function of trials, but BV increased, producing a pattern quite different from that seen during a perceptual task presented to the same subjects (see Figure 3.3).

While data with regard to the effects of specific tasks on vaso- and venomotor responses are meager, the available information supports the hypothesis that differences in response patterns will provide important information about the psychophysiological function of vascular changes. This interpretation is given additional support by a recently completed experiment. Because it is observed primarily in the hands and feet, it has been speculated (Cook 1970) that the response contributes to increased tactile sensitivity, not on the level of the central analyzer, but at the level of the sensory receptors. This point of view does not contradict that of Sokolov, but is complementary to it. Edelberg (1961) presented evidence that decreased tactile threshold to a vibratory stimulus accompanies vasoconstriction, and that the relationship between tactile sensitivity and autonomic discharge was greater for finger PA than for electrodermal measures. A preliminary investigation of this relationship has recently been completed. Fourteen subjects were asked to identify a series of smooth figures presented against a sandpaper background, using only their sense of touch, and their basal PA and BV levels during the task were expressed as a percent of those during the rest period immediately prior to the task. A Spearman's rank order correlation of .77 ($p < .01$) was found between performance on the task and the change in PA, indicating that the greater the decrease in PA, the better the performance on the test. The relationship between performance and BV change, however, was .29 and insignificant.

Another study supporting the idea that patterns of vascular response differ as a function of task requirements was recently completed by Williams et al. (1972). Subjects were given information intake (reading words presented blurred, backward, and upside down on a screen) and mental arithmetic tasks, as well as an interview. Blood pressure, forearm blood flow, finger PA, and heart rate were recorded and submitted to multivariate analysis of variance to compare the patterns of cardiovascular responses during these tasks. Patterns were found to differ among the three conditions at the .0001 level. During the word task, finger PA showed a 60% constriction, forearm blood flow decreased insignificantly, and heart rate increased to 10 to 15%. During the mental arithmetic task, however, finger PA showed a smaller constriction, forearm blood flow a 50% increase, and heart rate also showed a 20% increase. Measures taken during the interview were intermediate between these two tasks. The results suggest that forearm blood flow, as well as heart rate (see Chapter 26 Lacey and Lacey), distinguishes between the intention to note and detect external stimuli and the intention to ignore or reject such events.

The data presented above strongly support an adaptive, patterned vasomotor response in the conscious human actively interacting with his environment, and point out the relevance of further studies in which the response required of the subject rather than the stimulus is the independent variable.

SUBJECT VARIABLES

Surprisingly little is known about the effects of subject variables on vascular responses. Subjects have often been treated as physiological preparations, ignoring both individual differences and the state of the individual with regard to such important variables as the subject's motivation, attention, state of arousal, and perception of the experimental situation. Even such commonly reported variables as sex and age have had little attention in vascular studies. The few available investigations, however, have demonstrated the importance of these variables in vascular psychophysiology.

Chronic anxiety

Anxiety has been investigated more than any other subject characteristic. Ackner (1956a) has reviewed the effects of emotional states on the peripheral vasomotor system. He demonstrated (1956b) that while no differences in finger PA were found between anxious patients and normal controls in the waking state, sleep induced by Seconal resulted in large differences. The patients showed much greater increases in PA during sleep than the normal controls; there was, in fact, no overlap between the groups.

Kelly (1966), noting the greatly increased blood flow in the forearm as a function of psychological stimuli, hypothesized that forearm blood flow should distinguish between anxious patients and controls. This hypothesis has been confirmed in a series of studies. Hospitalized patients suffering from chronic anxiety had resting forearm blood flow twice as high as that of a group of control subjects, and this observation has been repeated on a number of samples. During a brief period of stressful mental arithmetic, however, no difference was found between the two groups (Kelly and Walter 1968). When compared with patients having psychiatric diagnoses other than anxiety, blood flow was found to be significantly higher for the chronic anxiety patients. As anxiety decreases—due to medication, psychiatric treatment, or neurosurgical techniques—forearm blood flow also decreases (Kelly et al. 1970). Kelly and his co-workers have pointed out that heart rate also distinguishes patients suffering from chronic anxiety. Since heart rate is much easier to measure than forearm blood flow, the extent to which it is useful as an index of anxiety needs further investigation. Clearly it is sensitive to differences between groups of patients and controls (Kelly and Walter 1968), and to stressful tasks in normal subjects (Mathews and Lader 1971). Heart rate, however, seems less sensitive to clinical improvement achieved with tranquilizers than forearm blood flow (Kelly et al. 1970), and this finding should be more extensively explored.

Patients with phobic anxiety do not differ from normal controls in resting forearm blood flow or in response to mental arithmetic, but discussing or imagining the feared situation does increase flow in these patients (Harper et al. 1965; Gelder and Mathews 1968).

Field dependence

Field dependence seems to be a very promising psychological variable in vascular research. In 1967, Luborsky reported significant correlations between PA from the finger and the Rod-and-Frame Test, and between BV and the Embedded Figures Test. More recently, Silverman and McGough (1971) have measured venous tone in field-dependent and field-independent subjects. During rest, field-dependent subjects showed higher venous tone than field-independent subjects, and the venous tone of the field-dependent subjects increased with successive determinations, while that of field-independent subjects did not. During presentations of words, venous tone of field-dependent subjects decreased, while that of field-independent subjects increased; during mental arithmetic, both showed a small increase.

State of arousal

While it is generally assumed that vascular tone and vascular responses both increase with increased arousal, the evidence for this relationship is confounded with changes in other variables, such as whether the subject is performing a task, or the amount of stress induced by the experimental situation. Ackner (1956b) has shown that PA increases during barbiturate-induced sleep. Johnson (1970) has reported that spontaneous fluctuations in PA are more frequent during REM sleep than during other stages, but that evoked responses are smaller during REM. Plethysmographic responses during sleep are very resistant to habituation (Johnson and Lubin 1967), and are more sensitive to auditory stimuli than other autonomic measures (Johnson 1970).

Situational emotional states

Anxiety as a function of the experimental situation typically produces increased blood flow in the forearm, decreased volume in the hand, and increased venous tone (Ackner 1956a; Blair et al. 1959; Burch 1960; Duggan, Love, and Lyons 1953; Vanderhoof and Clancy 1962). Even such moderate stressors as difficult mental arithmetic result in increased forearm flow (Allwood et al. 1959). Some attempts have been made to describe patterns of vascular response during emotions other than anxiety. For example, Averill (1969) used films designed to elicit sadness or mirth, and compared finger PA changes with those elicited by a control film. While the sad film was distinguished from the control film, the effect was not a strong one.

It is surprising to find that emotion-induced changes in the circulation of the face have not been investigated. This is probably due both to the problems of making accurate measurements in the face and to the difficulty of inducing valid emotional states in a laboratory situation. Increased technical skills and application of social psychological techniques to psychophysiological studies will hopefully make such research possible.

CONCLUSIONS

The author's view that understanding the physiological mechanisms of a system is crucial to understanding psychophysiological relationships is undoubtedly apparent. Physiological mechanisms underlying the plethysmographic response have been considered in some detail. It is clear that the venous system makes an important and often ignored contribution. The qualitative and quantitative differences observed when different tissues and regions are monitored indicate the complexity of the system, but also point to its potential usefulness as a psychophysiological tool.

We now have techniques by which to monitor changes in flow, volume, and venous tone in the limbs of man, and we can relate these changes to the state of the subject, the stimuli to which he is attending, and the demands of the task which he is performing. The few studies available suggest that the peripheral vascular system is more sensitive to emotional and task-related factors, and less sensitive to stimulus contingencies, than some other common psychophysiological measures. New information is continually becoming available about the situational and emotional determinants of different patterns of vascular response. We may soon be able to move from primarily empirical research to testable theoretical positions which integrate our knowledge of vascular physiology with our information about human emotion and behavior.

4

JAMES E. LAWLER AND PAUL A. OBRIST

Indirect Indices of
Contractile Force

INTRODUCTION

A parameter of cardiovascular function that has received little attention in the psychophysiological literature is the forcefulness or vigor of the cardiac contraction, or contractile force (CF). There are at least two reasons why attention should be directed to its measurement. First, mounting evidence demonstrates that most increases in heart rate (HR) are due more to a release of vagal tone than to an increase in sympathetic activity. Thus, HR increases cannot unequivocally be due to increased sympathetic activity. Second, it appears that sympathetic influences manifest themselves more clearly on CF than on HR (Obrist et al. 1972b). Therefore, it would seem that the concomitant measurement of HR and CF would yield a greater understanding of the interplay between the sympathetic and parasympathetic nervous systems in control of the heart than either measure alone.

THE CONCEPT OF CONTRACTILE FORCE

The heart has three available mechanisms for changing CF: (1) the Frank-Starling mechanism; (2) a change in contractility; and (3) a change in synchrony. The Frank-Starling mechanism (the "law of the heart") states that, within limits, the heart pumps whatever volume of blood flows into it. Thus, if venous return to the heart is increased

This chapter is based in part on research supported by research grant MH-07995 to Paul A. Obrist, Ph.D., and training grant 5-T02-MH 11107-04, both from the National Institute of Mental Health, United States Public Health Service.

on a given beat, the ventricle will stretch and the following contraction will be more forceful. Such a change involves only the extent of cardiac muscle fiber contraction.

A change in contractility, on the other hand, involves an alteration in the rate at which individual cardiac muscle fibers contract. Since it is impossible to measure the contractility of these thousands of muscle fibers, changes in contractility must be inferred from indirect indices. Most of these indices utilize the rate at which some measureable CV parameter changes with respect to time. Thus, for example, Sonnenblick emphasizes changes "in the rate of force development . . . from any initial muscle length" (Sonnenblick 1962, p. 978) as a suitable index of a change in contractility.

Changes in the synchrony of ventricular contraction have been observed during sympathetic stimulation (Randall and Priola 1965). Because the ventricle is richly covered with sympathetic fibers, it might be expected that sympathetic stimulation would reach virtually all of the ventricular surface at the same time, as opposed to normal conduction through the Purkinje system, which, though quite rapid, first stimulates areas closest to the Bundle of His. Thus, sympathetic stimulation causes the entire ventricle to contract more simultaneously, leading to a more forceful contraction.

Although CF can be modified by extrinsic (i.e., neural-humoral) sympathetic influences on both contractility and synchrony of contraction, it is also influenced by intrinsic (inherent) hemodynamic mechanisms. The Frank-Starling mechanism is one example of such intrinsic control. There are at least two other intrinsic mechanisms which can influence CF through their influence on contractility. These are the Anrep effect and the Bowditch effect both of which have been demonstrated in the heart deprived of innervations. The Anrep effect can be demonstrated in the denervated heart when the aortic pressure suddenly rises. The heart at first responds by increasing its CF through the Frank-Starling mechanism. That is, the ventricle at first cannot maintain its stroke volume in the face of the increased resistance. Because of this, more blood comes into the ventricle than exits. The ventricle swells, and the following beats show an increase in CF due to this stretch of the ventricular muscle. Within a few beats, however, the amount of ventricular stretch decreases, yet the heart maintains a constant stroke volume, thus demonstrating an increase in contractility, i.e., a more complete emptying without greater ventricular stretching. The Bowditch effect shows similar increases in contractility several beats after a sudden increase in HR.

There has been considerable debate about the saliency of intrinsic control in the intact preparation. For example, Rushmer (1962, 1965) has stated that the only time the law of the heart operates in normal circumstances is during postural changes. In general, it appears that the closer one approaches the ideals of the heart-lung preparation through anesthetics, blocking agents, etc., the more relevant the law of the heart becomes. However, its role in normal cardiac adaptation appears secondary to the influence of the innervations on the heart. Similarly, the saliency of the Anrep and Bowditch effects on normal cardiac function has not been fully elucidated and may be secondary to the innervations.

MEASUREMENT

In the intact preparation CF can only be evaluated indirectly through its effect on ventricular performance. Of the various techniques, rate of change measures seem to hold the most promise. These measures, such as the rate of change or slope of the pressure pulse wave, use the time derivative rather than the magnitude of change. An inherent problem with any indirect measure is to ascertain the respective influence of intrinsic and extrinsic control mechanisms.[1] The remainder of this chapter will briefly describe several rate of change measures now in use, both invasive and noninvasive, and present some data indicating their validity in depicting the influence of sympathetic activity on CF.

Invasive Techniques

The primary invasive measures have involved rate of change in work (power), in blood flow (acceleration), in force of contraction, and in pressure (dP/dt). According to Rushmer, Smith, and Franklin (1959, p. 605), power "is the rate of doing work and can be computed for a pump by multiplying the rate of change of volume by the internal pressure." The rate of change of volume can be obtained from an electromagnetic blood flow probe. Intraventricular pressure can be obtained via an implanted catheter or Teflon needle. The transduced signals from these two devices can then be fed into an analog multiplier circuit whose output will be instantaneous power. The integral of this signal over one beat would yield stroke work.

Although the index is feasible in the intact animal, its sensitivity appears to be lower than that of other indices. For example, Noble, Trenchard, and Guz (1966) examined the saliency of various rate of change measures as indices of CF and found that stroke power was less sensitive to pharmacological agents which increase contractility than other indirect indices. Noble et al. (1966) have focused primarily on maximum acceleration of blood into the ascending aorta as an index of the contractile state of the left ventricular muscle. They demonstrated that maximum acceleration showed a greater percentage change to the myocardial stimulating effects of intracoronary injections of calcium and isopropylnoradrenaline than did stroke power, peak power, or maximum differentiated left ventricular pressure in resting dogs.

In an attempt to obtain a measure of CF in the intact, conscious dog which would be relevant to psychophysiological problems, Obrist et al. (1972b) examined rate of change of: (1) the acceleration of blood in the aorta; (2) aortic pressure (dP/dt); and, (3) the force of ventricular contraction. For this purpose, a classical conditioning paradigm was used and sympathetic influences evaluated pharmacologically. The maximum acceleration of flow had a great deal of electronic noise which precluded an evaluation of the sensitivity of this measure. However, both aortic dP/dt and the rate of change of the ventricular contraction were found to be sensitive to sympathetic influences on left ventricular performance. For example, comparison of the two measures in five Ss demonstrated a marked degree of concomitance in both magnitude and patterns of change over the 25-second period quantified on each trial. This is important since these indices measure two different aspects of ventricular performance. In addition, the rate of change of contraction might be considered a more direct means of assessing CF. As such, it can be used as a yardstick for comparing less direct indices.

That the increases in both rate of change measures in anticipation of and to the unconditioned stimulus (UCS) were influenced by sympathetic excitation of the myocardium was indicated by the attenuation of these increases by beta-adrenergic blockade. Less direct evidence indicating the validity of the measures was the association of large unconditioned increases of the indices of CF with an elevation of systolic blood pressure (SBP), an effect one might expect if the heart were beating more vigorously. This possibility was verified by the attenuation of both measures with beta-adrenergic blockade.

Another approach to evaluating the validity of these rate of change measures is illustrated in a more recent study (Lawler 1973) in which the facilitation of aortic dP/dt by intrinsic influences associated with preload, i.e., the Frank-Starling mechanism, and afterload was evaluated in a chronic dog preparation using a Sidman avoidance paradigm. Preload refers to the end diastolic volume of the ventricle or the volume of the ventricle just prior to the onset of the contraction. It is a direct function of filling time and/or venous return. Preload was assessed from HR, since the longer the R-R interval or the slower the HR the greater the filling time. As such, if preload was facilitating dP/dt, then HR and dP/dt should be inversely related or negatively correlated. Afterload refers to the aortic diastolic pressure or aortic head pressure which must be acceeded by intraventricular pressure before blood can be ejected by the left ventricle. A decrease in afterload could come about either because of the lengthening of the R-R interval, in which case the aortic diastolic pressure passively follows the lengthening of the cardiac cycle, or because of a decrease in total peripheral resistance. Afterload was assessed from diastolic blood pressure (DBP). As with HR, a facilitating influence on dP/dt would be indicated by an inverse relationship or negative correlation between dP/dt and DBP. In this study no attempt was made to evaluate sympathetic influences on dP/dt through beta-adrenergic pharmacological blockade. However, some indication of a sympathetic influence would be indicated if dP/dt were positively correlated with SBP at the same time it was shown not to be influenced by intrinsic mechanisms.

For this purpose, intercorrelations were obtained between aortic dP/dt, HR, DBP, and SBP on each of five dogs in both the resting state and during avoidance. Under each condition, 240 seconds or more of activity were sampled systematically over the one hour resting and one hour avoidance periods during an early training session, and the correlations between measures were obtained using values for each second.

A facilitating intrinsic influence of HR and DBP on dP/dt was suggested in four of the dogs. However, it appeared to be a function of how reactive the blood pressure was to the avoidance procedure and whether the dog was in a resting or avoidance condition. During rest in the two most reactive dogs, small but significant, negative correlations were found in 3 of 4 comparisons between aortic dP/dt and both HR and DBP (range $-.08$ to $-.21$). However, during avoidance, these measures were all positively and significantly correlated (range, $+.20$ to $+.68$).

In the two least reactive dogs, DBP was negatively and significantly correlated to aortic dP/dt during both rest and avoidance (range, $-.17$ to $-.38$). Heart rate, on the other hand, was negatively correlated in two comparisons and positively in another. In the fifth dog, aortic dP/dt was positively and significantly correlated to DBP and HR during both rest and avoidance.

In one of the more reactive dogs, the correlations were also obtained on the last day of Sidman avoidance. As compared to the rest period just prior to the early training sessions where aortic dP/dt was negatively correlated only to DBP ($-.24$), both HR and DBP were negatively correlated with aortic dP/dt ($-.72$ and $-.73$, respectively). At this point, the dog was less reactive cardiovascularly and was successfully avoiding all shocks during the avoidance hour. A similar observation was made during one of the rest periods early in training. In this period, the dog changed from a quiescent to a more reactive state both cardiovascularly and somatically. The correlations between aortic dP/dt and both HR and DBP changed from $+.12$ to $-.42$ for HR and from $-.24$ to $+.26$ for DBP.

Finally, SBP was directly related to both dP/dt and HR primarily when intrinsic influences were minimal, i.e., when dP/dt was directly correlated with HR and DBP. For example, in the two most reactive dogs during the early training days the correlations were all positive and significant. However, during avoidance they ranged from +.53 to +.63, but during rest they dropped, ranging from +.20 to +.41. In the two less reactive dogs, SBP was inconsistently correlated with both measures during rest and avoidance (range −.33 to +.30) with only 4 of 8 being significant. Similarly, in the one dog where additional correlations were carried out during periods of minimal and maximal reactivity, the size and direction of the correlations with SBP were similar to those between dP/dt and both HR and DBP.

Overall, these data indicate that aortic dP/dt can be facilitated by intrinsic mechanisms involving decreases in HR and DBP when the dog is less reactive. However, the magnitude of the correlations, with two exceptions, was small—accounting for less than 10% of the variance. The data also indicate that when the dog is more reactive cardiovascularly, no such intrinsic facilitating influence is observed. Rather, the large positive correlations between measures including SBP suggest an appreciable sympathetic influence. Therefore, the use of dP/dt with invasive procedures indicates a certain validity of the measure as an index of sympathetic influences on left ventricular performance. Obviously, more work is needed. The present data indicate that these indirect measures of CF, particularly dP/dt, may provide the most practical and valid means to assess sympathetic activity, providing some means is available to assess intrinsic influences.

Noninvasive Techniques

The noninvasive techniques most often suggested in the literature include the ballistocardiogram (BCG), the vibrophonocardiogram (VPC), finger plethysmography, and the use of externally-measured pulse waves from major arteries. Although the BCG appears to detect changes in CF caused by pharmacological intervention (e.g., Starr 1965), there are distinct disadvantages which would seem to preclude its use. For example, Ss must be lying down and immobile in order to obtain artifact-free readings. Such restrictions would preclude its utility in most psychophysiological settings.

The VPC is based on the external measurement of sound at the body's surface. One method of measuring the VPC involves the placement of a capacitance microphone at the fourth interspace on the left side. It has been demonstrated (Agress et al. 1964) that the output from such measurements bears a close resemblance to intraventricular dP/dt, and thus would seem to be a good index of CF. However, Obrist et al. 1973c, failed to obtain artifact-free readings in all but one S. As with the BCG, the requirement that the S sit motionless would seem to preclude meaningful use in psychophysiological settings.

Another device which could presumably be used as an index of contractility is the rate of change of the pulse wave derived from plethysmographic techniques. However, this method appears to be an unreliable index of CF. Changes in the pulse wave seem to be related more to vascular tone than to CF. For example, data from Obrist, Wood, and Perez-Reyes (1965) showed little relation between the amplitude of the directly measured radial pulse and the finger plethysmograph. In addition, Obrist et al. (1973b) found little relation between the plethysmographic slope and pharmacological manipulations. Therefore, this technique appears rather insensitive to CF changes.

The last major non-invasive technique involves obtaining the maximum slope of the pulse wave from a major artery, particularly those nearest the heart (e.g., the carotid). Data indicate that these indices may be sensitive to changes in CF (e.g., Starr and Ogawa 1962, 1963; Ambrosi and Starr 1965; Obrist et al. 1973b). All but the last of these studies is concerned with the use of slope as an index of cardiac malfunction, and virtually nothing is said about an index of CF, nor is any attempt made to quantify relationships. One exception to this is Starr and Ogawa (1963). Normative data are summarized for nearly 200 Ss, and a strong negative correlation (−.45) was found between the maximum brachial slope and age. The authors concluded that these results were due to changes in CF with age. The authors also report a great deal of similarity between externally and internally measured slopes of the brachial pulse wave.

In the study by Obrist et al. (1973b), the slope of the carotid pulse wave was transduced by a low frequency microphone. Radial slope was also obtained with a miniature pressure transducer. The carotid slope was consistently more sensitive to the experimental manipulations. Utilizing a stressful reaction time task in young adults, a pronounced increase in slope was found just prior to shock administration for slow performance. Several lines of evidence indicate that the increases in carotid slope were influenced by sympathetic influences on left ventricular performance. These are summarized in Chapter 8. But as in the study by Lawler (1973) using avoidance procedures in dogs, these data suggest a facilitating influence of DBP on dp/dt.

SUMMARY

In light of the evidence that sympathetic influences on the heart are more clearly depicted by the force rather than the rate of contraction (see Chapter 8), it becomes imperative that we develop techniques to assess CF. The problem is technically difficult since CF is influenced by both intrinsic hemodynamic events and extrinsic neural-humoral processes. Furthermore, there are no direct means of assessing CF. Therefore, one has to resort to indirect procedures utilizing manifestations of CF on hemodynamic events. Several lines of evidence suggest that rate of change measures of aortic blood flow, aortic pressure, or the carotid pulse wave may provide reasonably sensitive and valid indices of sympathetic influences on CF. However, further work is needed in evaluating these measures, since some data indicate that intrinsic influences play a significant role in the response of the intact preparation to environmental stressors.

NOTE

1. Indirect measures of CF which rely on rate of change of the acceleration of blood or of blood pressure in the aorta, as well as the extracorporeal measurement of the rate of change of the arterial pulse wave, are not only sensitive to intrinsic and extrinsic influences on CF, but to alterations in diastolic blood pressure associated with changes in peripheral resistance. In this case, changes in diastolic blood pressure can act directly to modify the rate of change measures. This problem is discussed later in this chapter. Another complicating factor is the influence decreases in blood pressure can have on extrinsic control of CF through baroreceptor reflex mechanisms. That is, decreases in blood pressure can act reflexively to trigger sympathetic excitation (see Obrist, Lawler, Howard, Smithson, Martin, and Manning 1973c). Although in this case we are dealing with extrinsic control of CF, the increase in CF is secondary to another hemodynamic event, i.e., the drop in blood pressure, and not directly initiated by central nervous system (CNS) activity associated with behavioral processes. It is assumed that this direct CNS control is more relevant to psychophysiological endeavors.

5

BERNARD TURSKY

The Indirect Recording of
Human Blood Pressure

INTRODUCTION

The indirect measurement of human blood pressure has been of clinical and experimental interest since the development of the air inflated arterial occluding cuff. This development, combined with the use of one of several methods of identifying systolic and diastolic blood pressure by detecting the beginning and end of turbulent flow in a superficial artery, led to the development of manual methods of measuring human blood pressure. This methodology has provided the careful physician with a reasonably accurate clinical measure of his patients' blood pressure.

In recent years, three major developments in the area of cardiovascular therapy and research have led to the need for the development of more automated error-free blood pressure measurement and recording techniques. These were:

1. The realization by clinicians of the life saving possibilities of the continuous monitoring of systolic and diastolic blood pressure from patients who have suffered acute cardiovascular disfunctions;
2. The recognition by epidemiologists of the increased incidence of hypertension in the general population, thus creating a need for more accurate and rapid screening instruments (Rochmis, 1969);
3. The growing interest in the use of biofeedback techniques to attempt to alter human cardiovascular functioning by instrumental means (Engel and Hansen 1966; Shapiro et al. 1969; Brener and Kleinman 1970).

The author's research is supported in part by NIH Program Project Grants HL-06285 and GM-16496.

The growth of interest in these techniques required the development of instruments that could provide recognition and reinforcement of momentary changes in blood pressure, and could monitor the more global changes in systolic and diastolic pressure.

Many attempts have been made in recent years to develop automated instrumentation for the determination of error-free blood pressure measurement in man (Lywood 1967; Geddes 1970). Although much effort has been expended on the recognition and reduction of errors in measurement caused by human mistakes (Rose 1965; London and London 1966) and by instrumentation problems (Rose, Holland, and Crowley 1964; Geddes, Spencer and Hoff 1959), very little has been done to compensate for the errors in measurement related to the beat-to-beat variability in arterial pressure.

This chapter will briefly review the automated techniques for human blood pressure recording, discuss in detail some of the problems introduced by beat-to-beat blood pressure variability, and describe some recent techniques that have been developed to overcome these problems; thereby making it possible to achieve a more accurate indirect measure of human blood pressure.

AUTOMATED BLOOD PRESSURE RECORDING METHODS

Many instruments have been devised to automatically record human blood pressure (Lywood 1967), and the successful ones for the most part have mimicked the manual sphygmomanometers. Several manufacturers of multichannel physiological recording instruments (Grass Instrument Co., Quincy, Mass.; Beckman Instruments Inc., Schiller Park, Ill.) provide special purpose amplifiers with built-in aneroid manometers, at a moderate price, that permit the recording of a sphygmomanometric measure of blood pressure at frequent (approximately 3-minute) intervals. More automatic devices are also available (Narco Bio Systems Inc., Houston, Texas; Lexington Inst., Waltham, Mass.) that use electrically operated solenoid valves to automatically inflate and deflate the blood pressure cuff. In all instances the cuff pressure is displayed on a calibrated strip chart recorder, and a suitable microphone or other detection device is attached to the arm, under or distal to the cuff, to detect the Korotkoff (K) sounds or arterial pressure pulsations. A procedure similar to the manual recording process is then followed. The cuff is automatically pumped up to occluding pressure and then slowly deflated to a fixed rate (2 to 4 mmHg/sec). The K sounds are picked up by the microphone, amplified, and displayed by superimposing them on the pressure record. It then becomes a simple matter to read the systolic pressure as the pressure level at which the first K sound occurs, and the diastolic pressure as the pressure level at which the last sound occurs. It is difficult, however, to electronically detect the more subtle muffled sound that is used to identify diastolic pressure in the manual procedure. Sophistication in solid state and digital electronic circuitry has enhanced the recording instrumentation by devising methods of eliminating artifacts (King 1967) and by improving the transducers used to pick up the identifying signals. Blood pressure recording equipment that utilizes several sophisticated transduction methods to determine systolic and diastolic blood pressure levels has been designed. These methods are:

1. The use of the Doppler effect to ultrasonically detect arterial wall motion (Ware 1966; Stegall, Kardon, and Kemmerer 1968). This principle has been incorporated into an automatic sphygmomanometer manufactured by Hoffman La-Roche Inc. of Cranbury, New Jersey.
2. The use of upper arm electrical impedance plethysmography (Geddes et al. 1964). This has been utilized by the Medical Systems Division of the North American Phillips Corp., New York, N. Y., to detect systolic and diastolic blood pressure levels by measuring changes in arterial flow.
3. The use of the recognition of a time delay or phase shift in signals between two side-by-side occluding cuffs on the upper arm (Ware 1965). The systolic pressure is detected by noting the first downstream volume change, and diastolic pressure is defined as the pressure at which there is a cessation of the time delayed signal. This instrument is manufactured by Instrumentation Associates, New York, N. Y.

Other systems have been devised to increase the reliability and accuracy of blood pressure measurements. However, no matter which transducer or pressure system is used, the basic problem of natural beat-to-beat fluctuations in blood pressure creates errors of measurement that make it impossible to insure that any single reading of systolic and diastolic pressure can reliably reflect a patient's typical blood pressure.

DIRECT AND INDIRECT BLOOD PRESSURE MEASUREMENT

Human blood pressure can be directly recorded by coupling a cannula that has been inserted into a major artery to a pressure-sensitive transducer. These instruments produce an electrical output proportional to the change in pressure produced by each heart cycle. This voltage can be recorded on a calibrated strip chart recorder. While this method is accurate, it is not feasible to use it for the casual measurement of clinical pressure. The indirect measurement of clinical human blood pressure is accomplished in most instances by use of an auscultatory sphygmomanometer. This instrument is used to raise the pressure in an inflatable cuff to a level that occludes the flow of blood in the superficial arteries—brachial and radial. A mercury or aneroid manometer attached to the cuff is used to register the pressure in the cuff. Gradual reduction of the pressure in the cuff at a steady, slow rate through a controllable valve permits the flow of blood in the arm to start when the pressure in the arteries exceeds the pressure in the cuff. Korotkoff (1905) discovered that turbulence in the arteries under the occluding cuff could be detected by listening with a stethoscope below the cuff for characteristic sounds produced by turbulence in the arteries as the cuff was slowly deflated. The manometer pressure when the first K sound is detected is noted as being representative of the systolic pressure (Phase I). As the cuff continues to slowly deflate, a K sound is heard in conjunction with each heart cycle (Phases II and III), until the diastolic pressure level is approached. At this time a muffling of the K sound occurs (Phase IV). With further deflation, the K sound disappears (Phase V), and the cuff is at a pressure lower than diastolic.

It has been clearly demonstrated (Burton 1967; Roberts, Smiley, and Manning 1953; Holland and Humerfelt 1964) that auscultatory blood pressure measurements, when compared to simultaneously recorded intra-arterial pressures, consistently underestimate systolic and Phase V diastolic pressure by approximately 10 mmHg, while overestimating Phase IV (muffling) diastolic pressure by about the same amount.

These differences in measurement can be explained by examining the details of the typical clinical bleed-down cuff procedure. In this instance the cuff pressure is reduced from an occluding level at a steady rate while the patient's pressure varies (Figure 5.1) from beat-to-beat. Since the auscultatory systolic pressure can only be determined by the detection of a K sound when turbulence is present in the artery, and this event can only occur when the cuff pressure is lower than the true systolic level of the detected pressure wave, it becomes clear that *all* comparisons at systolic level using bleed-down auscultatory methods must result in a noticeably lower systolic determination than that produced by direct recording of the same pressures. Similarly, the asucultatory determination of Phase V diastolic pressure relies on detection of the disappearance of the K sound when turbulence has ceased in the arteries. This can only occur when the cuff pressure is lower than the true diastolic pressure of the detected arterial pressure wave. Again it is clear that each auscultatory determination must be noticeably lower than its intra-arterial comparison at the diastolic Phase V level.

Conversely, the Phase IV auscultatory determination relies on detection of the muffled sound which is above the true diastolic pressure of each detected pressure wave, thereby insuring that Phase IV measurements must be consistently higher than comparable direct measures.

VARIABILITY OF HUMAN BLOOD PRESSURE

Since blood pressure is not a static measure, it is important to examine the extent of beat-to-beat variability. Tursky, Shapiro, and Schwartz (1972) demonstrated that the magnitude of the natural variation in sys-

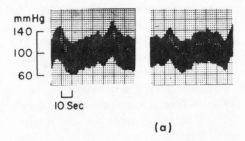

(a)

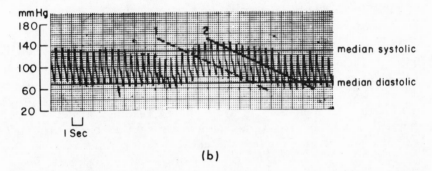

(b)

FIGURE 5.1 *Sample intra-arterial recordings from one patient. a. Two samples of intra-arterial pressure waves demonstrating the great variability of beat-to-beat systolic and diastolic blood pressure. b. Intra-arterial recording from same patient showing in detail the beat-to-beat variability. Diagonal lines 1 and 2 are two imaginary cuff deflations starting a few seconds apart to demonstrate the possible discrepancies between such determinations.*

tolic and diastolic blood pressure can be extremely large. Figure 5.1a shows two sample intra-arterial blood pressure recordings from one patient that demonstrate the variability of systolic and diastolic blood pressure that can occur in a 1-minute interval. Figure 5.1b is an intra-arterial recording from the same patient showing 50 pressure waves in detail. In this instance both the systolic and diastolic pressures have a range of 30 mmHg. It becomes apparent that a single sphygmomanometric determination of blood pressure can result in any combination of systolic and diastolic pressure, depending on the time of initiation and the rate of deflation of the cuff. To demonstrate this point, two parallel imaginary cuff deflations have been superimposed on the intra-arterial record starting a few seconds apart. The first results in a reading of 124 mmHq systolic and 90 mmHq diastolic; the second, taken a few seconds later, reads 144 mmHq systolic and 60 mmHq diastolic. For these 50 heart cycles, both determinations differ from the median blood pressure which is 128 mmHq systolic and 68 mmHq diastolic.

Clearly, measures of blood pressure based on a single beat-to-beat interval can result in a false assessment of the patient's typical pressure. The clinical aspects of this problem were experimentally examined by Armitage and Rose (1966) who compared single with multiple sphygmomanometric readings and found large variations both within and between subjects. They concluded that studies based on a single measure of blood pressure would result in frequent misclassification of individuals, exaggeration of the prevalence of hypertension, and a masking of genuine irregularities.

REDUCTION OF MEASUREMENT ERRORS
DUE TO BEAT-TO-BEAT VARIABILITY

A solution to the problem of error in blood pressure measurement caused by beat-to-beat variability is to develop a procedure that can yield stable average systolic and diastolic levels for a number of successive or closely spaced pressure measurements by taking into account beat-to-beat fluctuations. The averaging of readings made by hand operated or automatic sphygmomanometers is unsuitable because such readings can only provide intermittent data that is time consuming to collect and less reliable for the purpose of computing averages. Therefore, it is important to devise measurement techniques that can provide frequent determinations of systolic and diastolic pressure without causing an inordinate amount of discomfort to the subject.

SERVO CONTROLLED TRACKING SYSTEMS

One recording method that offers the possibility of frequent determinations of systolic or diastolic pressure is to use an instrument that can track pressure on an intermittent basis. Green (1955) designed a systolic pressure follower that used a servo system to increase the pressure in a finger cuff every time a pulse was detected distal to the cuff. Pressure in the cuff was increased through a valve until the pulse was extinguished, at which time the valve was closed and the cuff pressure was allowed to leak off until the pulse reappeared. This caused the valve to open and again admit air until occluding pressure was reached. This cycling procedure permitted the recording of a number of systolic pressure levels in the time usually required to record a single sphygmomanometric pressure.

Several servo controlled blood pressure tracking systems have been recently developed by investigators involved in the study of instrumental conditioning of cardiovascular functions. Brener and Kleinman (1970) developed a finger cuff blood pressure tracking system. The occluding cuff which was applied proximally to the left index finger measured slightly less than the circumference of the finger. Con-

sequently, about ¼ inch of the dorsal side of the digit remained unoc-
cluded to permit venous return. This technique obviated discomfort
caused by blood pooling, which is experienced in continuous systolic
monitoring when the limb is completely occluded. A crystal pulse sensor was fixed to the finger distal to the cuff. Each time a pulse was
detected by the sensor, the pressure in the cuff was increased by
approximately 5 mmHg. The cuff pressure was bled off at a rate of
approximately 3 mmHg per second in the absence of a pulse; that is,
when the cuff pressure exceeded the systolic pressure. This bleed rate
was adjusted to the subject's heart rate to maximize the rate of blood
pressure determinations. As a result, the cuff pressure oscillated about
the subject's systolic pressure and provided absolute systolic blood pressure readings every two to three heart beats without any reported
ischaemic discomfort.

The output of this system was subject to two major sources of error.
Firstly, the pressure recorded at the finger is considerably higher than
pressures taken closer to the heart; and secondly, the actual pressure
value in the cuff at any moment was an approximation (+5 mmHg)
of the subject's systolic blood pressure rather than an actual determination.

In view of these problems it was decided to develop a blood pressure
monitor that did not suffer from these deficits. This new instrument
employs standard brachial arm cuffs and monitors diastolic blood pressure from one arm and systolic blood pressure from the other arm.
Only one determination is made every three or four beats, but the
determination is a true reading of blood pressure rather than an
approximation. In the systolic determination a cuff inflates rapidly to
a pressure that is greater than *S*s systolic pressure. When it reaches
a preset value (approximately 160 mmHg for normals), the cuff goes
into a slow deflation mode. The pressure continues to drop at a slow
rate until a microphone detects a K sound; at this instant the pressure
in the cuff is read and held by a track-and-hold memory. The cuff
then deflates rapidly to atmosphere and the cycle recommences. In the
diastolic mode the cuff inflates rapidly to some value just less than the
subject's diastolic value (approximately 50 mmHg in normals), and then
goes into a slow inflation mode until the first K sound is detected. At
this point the cuff pressure is read and held by a track-and-hold memory, and the cuff is deflated to atmosphere. The entire cycle takes only
about 3 seconds in either mode, and both can be run simultaneously
using one arm for systolic monitoring and the other arm for diastolic
monitoring.

Miller and Dworkin (see Chapter 16) reported the use of a sensitive
servo controlled blood pressure system that was designed to track diastolic blood pressure on a semi-continuous basis. This system utilized

the fact (Tursky, Shapiro, and Schwartz 1972) that the relationship between the K sound and the systolic and diastolic pressure was a continuous monotonic, though highly nonlinear, function. This indicated the possibility of developing a servo mechanism which would establish a criterion Korotkoff sound level arbitrarily designated "the last diastolic sound," and would maintain the cuff pressure at a level determined by that sound intensity. The system which was finally developed and which has been in use for approximately three years depends on a number of known characteristics of the Korotkoff sound to achieve reliable tracking. These characteristics are: (1) that the peak energy of the K sound is contained in the 27 to 38 Hz band; (2) that in a given subject, the time relationship between the appearance of the Korotkoff sound at a fixed peripheral point (e.g., the brachial artery near the anti-cubital fossa) is fixed—generally on the order of 200 to 300 msec; and, (3) that gross motor movements create noise in the same order of magnitude and frequency as the K sound. These artifacts tend to extend over several hundred milliseconds and must be detected prior to the occurrence of an expected K sound to allow the system to bypass these contaminated heart cycles.

Electrodes detect the QRS complex which is amplified and discriminated through a series of filters and transformed into a logic pulse which activates the anti-noise gate, a sampling period immediately prior to the Korotkoff sound sampling interval. If the Schmitt trigger is not activated during the occurrence of this gate, then the channel is assumed to be "quiet," and the Korotkoff sound sample interval is initiated. The sound is detected with a crystal microphone, amplified, and filtered; the root mean square value is extracted and integrated over a time constant of about 60 msecs. The use of the integrated signal produces greater stability than peak detection in that the signal level is dependent on the total power contained in the sound and is less dependent on small changes in frequency. The sound is then transferred to one of two alternate sample-and-hold amplifiers which store a DC level equivalent to the RMS integrated value through the duration of the sampling cycle. In the servo amplifier this value is compared with the reference equivalent to the last diastolic sound, and a servo velocity is determined to adjust the difference to zero during the succeeding cycle. If the sound intensity is too low, the servo increases the cuff pressure; if it is too high, it decreases the cuff pressure. With proper damping the system tracks ±½% of the diastolic level within a time period of less than two cardiac cycles.

In spite of its complexity the system has performed reliably on a day-to-day basis for two years. Its principal shortcoming is that it requires a continuously inflated cuff, which, if maintained for more than 2 or 3 minutes, results in venous pooling, edema, and a certain amount of discomfort. Consequently, although the system tracks continuously, it can only do so for short periods of time, thereby limiting training procedures employing this system to 3-minute training intervals alternated with 3-to-5 minute rest periods. Probably by using two systems alternately between two different limbs, continuous tracking would be possible. The outstanding feature of the system is its immunity to noise and movement artifacts; this we find to be essential for any system used in instrumental conditioning.

CONSTANT CUFF-PRESSURE SYSTEM

Tursky, Shapiro, and Schwartz (1972) recently reported on a blood pressure recording system that measures systolic or diastolic pressure by establishing the median or average pressure for a number of successive beats of the heart. This system, shown in a block diagram (Figure 5.2), is described in detail in the original report. The original system was designed and produced in our laboratory. Digital logic modules were used to program and control the various events in the measurement procedure. An integrated commercial version of this system has been developed and is now being marketed by Lexington Instruments of Waltham, Massachusetts. This instrument evolved from the need for a method of providing feedback to subjects concerning relative changes in blood pressure on each heart cycle and rewarding them for altering their median pressure in the desired direction (Shapiro et al. 1969). This procedure has been used successfully in a number of systolic and diastolic blood pressure conditioning studies (Shapiro, Tursky, and Schwartz 1970a, b; Schwartz 1972; Benson et al. 1971). This measurement procedure is based on the idea that when a cuff is inflated and held at constant pressure, the Korotkoff sound will be present or absent as a function of the variation in blood pressure in the artery with each beat. When the pressure applied to the cuff is greater than the systolic pressure, the brachial artery is occluded and no Korotkoff sound can be detected. When the cuff pressure is lower than systolic, but higher than diastolic pressure, a Korotkoff sound will be picked up on every heart cycle. If the constant pressure applied to the cuff is adjusted upward so that a Korotkoff sound is detected on 50% of a given number of heart beats, the cuff pressure defines the median systolic pressure. The same procedure can be implemented at the diastolic level by use of an appropriate method for detecting the muffling (Phase IV) or the disappearance (Phase V) of the K sound.

Since the procedure for electronically isolating the muffled Korotkoff sound (Phase IV) is more difficult, the diastolic data in the present paper are based on the last sound (Phase V). At this level, when the applied cuff pressure is lower than Phase V diastolic, the cuff does not impede blood flow in the artery, and no Korotkoff sound will be detected. If the constant pressure applied to the cuff is adjusted upward so that a sound is detected on 50% of the prescribed number of heart cycles, the cuff pressure is by definition equal to the median diastolic pressure (Phase V). This procedure provides: (a) the ability to assess variations in systolic and diastolic pressure for each heart cycle; and, (b) the ability to derive automatically an average measure of systolic or diastolic pressure for a given number of heart cycles. These attributes satisfy the basic requirements for the accurate measurement of average systolic and diastolic pressure for clinical use, as well as the requirements for the ability to shape and reinforce momentary fluctuations of blood pressure in operant conditioning studies.

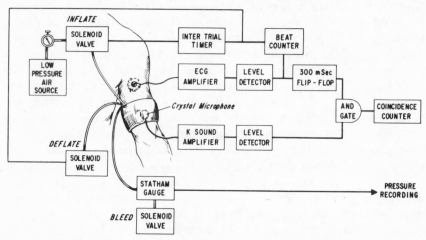

FIGURE 5.2   *Block diagram of automated constant cuff-pressure system.*

To evaluate the sensitivity of this method, a test was run on six subjects. For each subject a standard blood pressure cuff was pumped up to above systolic pressure and reduced in steps of 2 mmHg to below diastolic pressure. On each determination the cuff pressure was held constant for 50 heart beats, and the percentage of K sounds to heart cycles (R to K coincidence) was recorded. Figure 5.3 is a sample record of two consecutive constant cuff pressure inflations, 2 mmHg apart in pressure, recorded at the systolic level. The cuff pressure was reduced by 2 mmHg in the second trial, resulting in a R to K coincidence increase from 5 (10%) in the first trial to 25 (50%) in the second trial. Figure 5.4 (solid line) demonstrates the function generated by averaging the (R to K) percentage data of six subjects. On the average, a 2 mmHg increase in cuff pressure at the median systolic level reduced the average percentage of coincident (R to K) sounds from 59% to 29%, and a decrease of 2 mmHg increased it to 76%. Similar changes were observed at the diastolic level. Each individual subject produced approximately the same function. These results demonstrate the sensitivity of the constant cuff-pressure system; at median systolic or diastolic pressure a change of 2 mmHg alters the coincidence (R to K) rate by about ±25%, thus insuring that median pressure can be accurately measured to within a 2 mmHg.

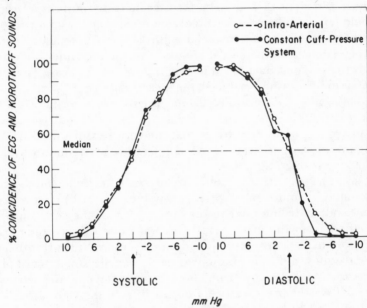

FIGURE 5.3   *Typical polygraph record of two consecutive constant cuff-pressure trials at the systolic level. Cuff pressure is reduced by 2 mmHg in the second trial. R to K coincidence increase from 5 (10%) in the first trial to 25 (50%) in the second trial.*

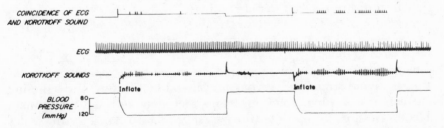

FIGURE 5.4   *Percent change in R to K coincidence around systolic and diastolic levels for constant cuff-pressure system (N=6) as cuff pressure is reduced in 2 mmHg steps from above systolic to below diastolic pressure. This function is compared to data from intra-arterial records (N=5) treated in a similar manner.*

A further assessment of the accuracy of the constant cuff-pressure system was made by comparing the data generated in the laboratory (Figure 5.4, solid line) to a similar treatment on intra-arterial recordings from five patients. These intra-arterial data were treated in a manner similar to that used in the laboratory. Starting at the highest pressure level recorded for each subject, an imaginary cuff pressure was reduced in steps of 2 mmHg. At each step the number of waves that would have produced a Korotkoff sound at that constant pressure lever were counted, and a percentage of these waves to total calculated. These percentages were plotted (Figure 5.4, broken line) and compared to the original data. In this case a 2 mmHg increase from the median systolic pressure reduced the percentage of K sounds from 56% to 28%, and a decrease of 2 mm in cuff pressure increases the percentage to 70%. The striking similarity between the two sets of curves in Figure 5.4 demonstrates that median pressure measured by this system can be as accurate as median pressure arrived at by averaging intra-arterial readings.

The accuracy of the constant cuff-pressure method can best be demonstrated by simultaneously recording intra-arterial pressure from one arm, and recording median pressure by use of the constant pressure method from the other arm. This was done by recording from a 50-year-old male patient who was admitted for a right heart catheterization to diagnose a possible pulmonary artery aneurysm. Arterial pressure was recorded directly from the brachial artery of the left arm, and median systolic pressures were obtained from the right arm using the constant cuff-pressure method. Five sets of 32 consecutive pressure waves were recorded several minutes apart. The intra-arterial data were treated as previously described to obtain the mean and median for each determination. In comparing the two measures they were found to be less than 2 mmHg apart—demonstrating that this method of obtaining median systolic pressure is as accurate as averaging a similar number of intra-arterial readings.

PORTABLE BLOOD PRESSURE RECORDING

The fluctuations in a patient's blood pressure as he progresses through the stress and strain of everyday life should be of value in diagnosing the extent of his hypertension. It has been demonstrated that human blood pressure is reduced during sleep, but rises and fluctuates dramatically during REM periods (Snyder, Hobson, and Goldfrank 1963). However, little is known about the fluctuation of blood pressure due to everyday life stresses.

While it is possible for patients to carry a sphygmomanometer and, with proper training, learn to record their blood pressure at intervals during the day, this procedure must rely upon the accuracy of the patient which might be impaired by the stress of the situation in which he is recording. To overcome this problem, portable automated blood pressure recording equipment that records blood pressure in a manner similar to the commonly employed auscultatory indirect method was developed (Hinman, Engel, and Bickford 1962). The system consists of a standard blood pressure cuff inflated by use of a bulb, a crystal microphone to record Korotkoff sounds, a frequency modulated pressure transducer, and a light portable tape recorder controlled by a pressure switch. The patient manually pumps up the cuff, but the maximum pressure and the deflation rate are electronically controlled. Cuff pressure and the superimposed K sounds are recorded on tape and decoded by means of an electronic demodulator at a central location. Recent improvements in this equipment, such as the use of a light-weight Cassette recorder, have decreased the size and improved the portability of this system which is now being manufactured by the Remler Company of San Francisco, California.

CONCLUSIONS

This chapter describes several automated techniques used in the recording of human blood pressure. The problems introduced by momentary and long-term variability are discussed, and solutions to these problems related to improved methods of measurement are suggested. While these methods improve the possibility of the accurate determination of human blood pressure, it is important to keep in mind the fact that all methods of physical measurement that impinge on the system to be measured must alter to some extent the measure of interest. R. C. Davis (1957) compared the recording of blood pressure to the measurement of electrical potentials, and clearly stated the importance in both cases of insuring that the recording instrument does not alter the measure by loading the system. The ideal instrument for the noninstrusive determination of blood pressure would be a transducer that could be taped to the skin over a superficial artery and that would accurately sense both the level and fluctuations of blood pressure without altering the pressure. Many attempts have been made to develop such devices using strain gages and various types of crystal pickups as transducer elements. In all instances these instruments have failed to produce an accurate measurement of true pressure level, but they have provided useful information about fluctuations in pressure.

It is hoped that the increasing interest in the epidemiological roots of hypertension and the therapeutic possibilities of the use of biofeedback techniques to treat this disease will add incentive for Biomedical engineers to develop the ideal nonobtrusive blood pressure monitor.

6

RALPH P. FORSYTH

Techniques for Long-Term Direct Measurements of Cardiovascular Variables

INTRODUCTION

The decision to use a long-term preparation for cardiovascular studies should be considered carefully, because such studies demand a major commitment by both the investigator and the institution in which the work is to be done. The investigator should be aware that the use of unreliable or unvalidated measurement techniques will make any data, however interesting, unacceptable for publication. Thus, the first step in any investigation is to select the most appropriate measurement technique and validate it in the preparation and under the conditions which will be used in the experiment.

This chapter will not attempt to specify the details of using the various techniques, although basic references to their use will be given. Rather, some of the advantages and disadvantages of the most commonly used techniques will be outlined, along with some discussion of the basic principles involved in their use. It should be understood that the successful application of any of these techniques will involve considerable practice and ingenuity on the part of the investigator. I recommend that the investigator who desires to use ·an unfamiliar technique should arrange to visit a laboratory using the method. Whenever possible, he should actually participate in the surgery and the use of equipment; there is no substitute for practical experience in learning the many small details that can often make the difference between success and failure.

There are a number of special problems in obtaining direct measurements in human subjects. Human experimentation committees must give approval for all procedures and, of course, expert medical care must be obtained. Under such circumstances, permission can often be obtained for acute catheterization procedures, but rarely can more extensive procedures be justified on volunteer subjects. In special circumstances, however, measurements can often be obtained in patients who are undergoing surgery or study in cardiac catheterization laboratories or intensive care units. Often cooperation can be obtained from renal transplant teams who are doing extensive workups on potential donors or recipients. Such fortuitous circumstances can be useful in obtaining measurements in humans, and this population can sometimes be used for validating indirect measurement techniques.*

CHOICE OF EXPERIMENTAL MODEL

There are two main considerations for the selection of species aside from the financial and space problems associated with buying and housing experimental animals. In general, up to a point, the larger the animal the better. In small animals, such as rats, the blood vessels are so small that there is difficulty in drawing blood and measuring an accurate blood pressure with catheters. Also, smaller animals do not tolerate blood loss well because of their small blood volume, and a variety of problems associated with hypovolemia and anemia may ensue if any bleeding occurs or even if a number of blood samples have to be drawn.

The second consideration is the type of protection needed for any indwelling catheters, wires, or other devices that have been implanted in the animals for measurement. Unless a restraint system can be used, in which the animal can live comfortably for the duration of the experiment, the catheters or wires have to be left directly under or on top of the skin so they can be connected without unduly disturbing the animal. For dogs and cats, comfortably fitted harnesses can be arranged so that the ends of wires and catheters cannot be disturbed by the animals. Small battery operated pumps can be installed in the harness to give constant or intermittent flushing to the catheter, or the catheters can be filled with heparin daily. Primate restraining chairs are commercially available in which virtually all sizes of monkeys can comfortably live for months at a time while their catheters can be continually or intermittently flushed.

Thus, if at all possible, medium-sized species, such as rabbits, cats,

* Editors' Note: Although not published yet, a book entitled *Chronically Implanted Cardiovascular Instrumentation*, E. P. McCutcheon (Ed.), New York, Academic, 1972, will have been marketed in late 1972. From the publisher's description this volume appears relevant.

dogs, or monkeys, should be selected for the experimental preparation. Before the surgery is performed, a good deal of planning should be given to the protective devices or restraint that will be used to protect the implanted devices.

Before and during the experimental procedures, it is important to monitor the animals' vital signs. Blood samples also need to be analyzed periodically for hematocrit, white blood cell counts, blood gases, and pH to insure that the preparation is free from infection and has good respiratory and cardiovascular function. Veterinary facilities must be available for any suspected health problems and for insuring that the animals are in good health before surgery. There are usually enough problems to be encountered without starting with a sick animal, and, in the long run, it is cheaper to spend some time and effort ensuring that the stock animals are healthy. Further care must be taken for the protection of any personnel working with the animals. Of particular concern are the handling of biological fluids and excretory products, as well as the safety regulations involved during surgery and autopsy and the proper treatment of bites and scratches.

In summary, the chief value of long-term work is the ability to make reliable, valid, and relevant cardiovascular measurements in healthy animals, free from the mitigating effects of anesthesia, pain, infection, or undue emotional stress. Meticulous care must be taken to assure that these conditions are adhered to, both for the success of the experiment and the safety of the investigators. Since each long-term experiment involves a large investment in time and effort, it is shortsighted to economize on the best available species to be used, the proper measuring equipment, or the efforts to ensure that the animal remains in good health. In short, long-term experiments should not be undertaken unless the proper facilities and equipment are available.

BLOOD PRESSURE

Direct measurements of blood pressure involve catheterization of the blood vessel. For acute measurements vessels near the skin surface are used for entry sites, e.g., the brachial or femoral artery or vein. In these cases extensive cutdowns are not needed, and usually a needle can be directly inserted into these vessels and a catheter inserted through the needle and pushed centrally. The needle is then removed leaving the catheter in place.

In long-term experiments, however, it is necessary to cut down on deeper vessels so that the catheter can be stabilized by ties around the blood vessel and the catheter, as well as be anchored into surrounding muscle. The iliac artery and vein (either the common, internal, or external branches) appear to be ideal for most species in that a retroperitoneal approach can be made which reduces the incidence of infection. At least 2 cm of the vessel need to be stripped of all adventitia, and any collaterals should be tied off and cut. The arterial catheter should not be pushed past the renal artery, to avoid compromising renal flow. Details of such surgery have been reported (Werdegar, Johnson, and Mason 1964; Forsyth and Rosenblum 1964). It is important to use a polyvinyl, rather than polyethylene, catheter since the former is more supple and does not kink easily. If the catheter cannot be flushed regularly it is helpful to siliconize the catheter.

Pressures in the left and right ventricles can also be continuously recorded. Catheters can be placed in the right atrium or ventricle from either the iliac or jugular veins; the easiest approach to the left ventricle is from the common carotid artery. As soon as the catheter tip reaches either of the ventricles, the pulse pressure will increase. If a recorder is not available during surgery, the experimenter can watch a pulsating bubble in the catheter to determine when the ventricle is reached. Fluoroscopic determination of the actual location should then be made, so that the catheter can be straightened out—to insure that the catheter tip is not embedded in the trabeculae and is far enough down in the ventricle that it cannot subsequently flip out. Mattress suturing is useful in anchoring catheters into muscle so that the catheter and vessel are protected from inadvertant pulling. The catheters can be directed subcutaneously to the desired point of leaving the skin.

With initial surgical help these types of catheterization procedures can be easily learned; success or failure of long-term measurement is usually dependent on other factors, such as the competency of the restraint system and the ability to flush the catheters regularly with heparinized saline to prevent clotting.

The actual recording of pressure is most often accomplished by connecting a strain gauge to the fluid-filled catheter. Pressure at the catheter tip is transmitted to a diaphragm in the gauge. Strain-sensitive wires are attached to the diaphragm in such a way that the resistance of the wire is directly related to the movement of the diaphragm. This resistance is part of a Wheatstone bridge circuit; when pressure changes, the bridge is unbalanced producing an electrical recording signal which, when properly amplified and calibrated, is a direct reflection of the pressure in the vessel. Useful discussion of the physical principles of such measurements are given by Linden (1963) and Franke (1966).

Catheters are now commercially available in which the diaphragm is located in the tip of the catheter so that pressure can be directly measured without problems of flushing (e.g., Bio-Tec Instruments, Pasadena, California). This kind of system has not yet been widely used but should facilitate the ability to telemeter the blood pressure signal and, thus, reduce the amount of restraint needed and the necessity to flush the catheter. However, having an indwelling catheter for infusion or blood withdrawal is essential for most experiments.

CARDIAC OUTPUT

Although there have been many methods devised to measure the cardiac output (Hamilton 1962), only two methods are practical in the long-term unanesthetized preparation. One is the Stewart-Hamilton indicator dilution method; an indicator, most often a dye (Evans blue or Cardio-green), is injected into the right heart or left ventricle while a sample of arterial blood is continuously withdrawn at a constant speed through a cuvette which measures the concentration of the dye. If the dye is well mixed with the blood leaving the left ventricle and does not leave the vascular space in significant amounts, the cardiac output can be calculated from the amount of dye injected and the average concentration in the peripheral arterial blood during the passage time. The principle is the same as measuring the volume of water in a reservoir; if a known amount of indicator is added and allowed to mix, the concentration of the indicator in a measured sample is inversely related to the total amount of water. The main problem in the cardiovascular system is that the dye indicators recirculate before the sampled concentration curve reaches zero. Thus, extrapolation of the downslope of the concentration curve, rather than the recorded curve, must be used. Other substances such as isotopes or slugs of hot or cold saline can also be used as indicators.

The main disadvantage of this technique is that estimations of cardiac output can only be made intermittently. This method is reliable but there is controversy as to its accuracy, especially at high flow rates (Jacobs et al. 1969). Other useful reports of its use and limitations have been reported by Zierler (1962), Oriol, Sekelj, and McGregor (1967); and Saunders et al. (1970).

Electromagnetic or ultrasonic flowmeters can be used to record continuously the amount of blood flowing in the ascending aorta; thus, except for coronary flow, the total cardiac output is measured. Theoretically, this measurement is superior to the indicator-dilution technique in that it is direct and continuous. In practice, there are often serious calibration problems, and the placement of the probe involves much more extensive surgery than the catheterization procedures. Since the probe must fit snugly around the pulsating aorta, there are often problems with ruptures and aneurysms. However, with patience and care these devices can be used successfully, although they often limit the period during which observations can be made.*

*Editor's note: A procedure which reduces the incidence of ruptures and aneurysms

The electromagnetic flowmeter, as developed by Kolin (1960), is based on the principle that blood, because it has electrolytic properties, generates an electric potential proportional to the volume of flow as it passes through an electromagnetic field. In commercial flowmeters, the electromagnetic field is created with either square or sine wave pulses, and the output signal is obtained from pickups located at right angles to the created electromagnetic field.

The ultrasonic flowmeter is based on the Doppler principle. The velocity of blood flow within the probe is directly proportional to the speed of propagation of an ultrasonic sound source which is located some distance upstream and at right angles to the recording electrodes (Franklin, Ellis, and Rushmer 1959). Since the diameter of the probe is known, the blood velocity can be converted directly to absolute flow measurements.

TOTAL BLOOD VOLUME

Various forms of the indicator-dilution principle, as previously mentioned, can be used to measure total blood volume as well as cardiac output. Some of the indicators used, such as Evans blue dye or radioactive iodinated serum albumin, mix with blood plasma; after thorough mixing, the plasma concentration can be measured by determining the optical density of the blood plasma with a spectrophotometer, or the amount of radioactivity with a scintillation counter. The amount of the indicator leaving the vascular space can be corrected for by taking several plasma measurements at regular intervals and extrapolating them to the time of injection. After the plasma volume is determined a hematocrit estimation is used to calculate total blood volume.

Hemoglobin in red blood cells can also be tagged with various markers such as carbon monoxide or radioactive chromium. These tagged cells are then injected into the experimental subject, allowed to mix, and sampled to allow estimation of the cellular component of the blood volume. Details of all these procedures and discussion of their accuracy are given by Erlanger (1921); Reeve et al. (1953); Lawson (1962); and Zierler (1962).

REGIONAL BLOOD FLOW

The most popular direct measurement of individual organ blood flow in the long-term unanesthetized preparation is with the electromagnetic or ultrasonic flowmeter. As previously described, chronic probes

on the ascending aorta involves the following. (a) The inner diameter of the probe should be slightly greater than the outer diameter of the aorta so that the probe initially fits somewhat loosely. (b) Either the probe or the aorta should be completely encapsulated with *Dacron* curtain mesh material. Do not accept substitutions. The Dacron acts to stimulate fibrotic growth, which in turn acts both to anchor the probe so that it fits snugly and to reinforce the wall of the aorta. (see Obrist et al. 1972b) can be fitted around almost any artery larger than 1 or 2 mm in diameter and 3 or more mm in length. Probes smaller than 4 or 5 mm in diameter, however, are as yet impractical for long-term recording. It takes at least a week after the implantation before the transducer is firmly fixed on the vessel and good flow recordings can be obtained. Serious problems in estimating absolute flow values occur if the probe causes the vessel to kink or otherwise obstructs flow.

Successful long-term measurements (up to six weeks or more) have been reported with flowmeters on both the ascending and descending aorta, left circumflex coronary, pulmonary, mesenteric, renal, and iliac arteries. Flow in larger venous vessels can also be recorded. Telemetry of these signals is also technically possible (Van Citters and Franklin 1969).

Recently, catheter-tipped flow transducers have been commercially manufactured. The catheter, which has a velocity transducer in the tip, can be placed in the desired blood vessel and continuous measurements of velocity recorded. The accuracy of these devices has not as yet been verified and careful validation is required.

Blood flow can also be measured in a number of organs using the Fick principle, which states that the amount of a substance taken up by an organ (or the total body) per unit of time is equal to the arterial level of the substance minus the venous level times the blood flow. Determination of the cardiac output in humans is often done using this principle with oxygen as the tracer. Thus, cardiac output (in L/min) is equal to the measured oxygen consumption (ml/min) divided by the arterial-venous oxygen difference across the lung (ml/L). Using various modifications of this principle, blood flow to such organs as the brain, kidney, and liver can be estimated (Kety 1960; Kramer, Lochner and Wetterer 1963).

In recent years there have been efforts to develop techniques in which the simultaneous distribution of the cardiac output to all major organs can be measured without the extensive surgery and problems involved with placement of multiple flowmeter probes. One of the earliest attempts used the intravenous injection of [86]rubidium (or [42]potassium) which was thought to be taken up in all peripheral organs (except for the brain) in a direct relationship with the regional organ blood flow (Sapirstein 1958). Only one measurement could be made with this method, however, as the animal had to be killed for radioactivity counting directly after the injection. Subsequently, it was also reported that the tissue uptake of this isotope is not solely dependent on blood flow, since the extraction ratio changed in various conditions (Love 1964).

An improved technique to measure the simultaneous distribution of cardiac output at up to five different observation times has been more recently developed (Rudolph and Heymann 1967; Kaihara et al. 1968).

In this method carbonized microspheres, which can be obtained in different sizes, are labeled with different gamma emitting radionuclides. Batches of microspheres with the same label are injected into the left atrium or left ventricle where they mix and are carried with the blood until trapped in arterioles in peripheral organs. Thus, the amount of radioactivity in each organ is directly related to its blood flow. Different isotope labels are used at the different measurement times; since the energy spectrum of each of the isotopes is constant, the amount of each of the isotopes in each organ can be calculated after the tissues are dissected and counted with a gamma scintillation counter and a pulse height analyzer.

If the cardiac output is measured at the time of the microsphere infusion, blood flow to each organ can be calculated as the percentage of the cardiac output received by each organ times the absolute cardiac output. Resistance in each organ can be determined by dividing the driving pressure to that organ (in most organs the mean arterial minus the mean venous pressure) by the calculated blood flow. Estimates of the reliability and validity of this technique have been reported for the rabbit (Neutze, Wyler and Rudolph 1968) and the monkey (Hoffbrand and Forsyth 1969).

With minimal amount of surgery catheters can be placed in the left ventricle, descending aorta, and the vena cava so systemic blood pressure, cardiac output, and regional organ blood flows can be obtained with this technique in the conscious animal. The catheters also allow for easy sampling of arterial and venous blood, and drug infusions can be made over extended periods of time. Disadvantages include the inability to make continuous measurements of cardiac output and regional blood flow, which are possible with flowmeters. Maintenance of the catheters also involves more elaborate restraint techniques in comparison to the use of flowmeters, and telemetering is not possible.

COMMENT

Techniques for measuring other aspects of cardiovascular function, such as ventricular contractility and volume, are also available. Some of these techniques are described elsewhere in this book (see Chapter 4 Lawler).

In many experiments other physiological measurements or interventions are desired in conjunction with recordings of the cardiovascular parameters. It is feasible to implant indwelling catheters in the bladder, the common bile duct, the lymph vessels, and in different parts of the gastrointestinal tract for long-term infusion of various materials and/or collection of biological fluids. Although every added catheter or implanted measuring device adds a cumulating chance of misfortune, it is possible and often desirable to be able to study an increased range of physiological events simultaneously.

It appears evident that these kinds of long-term measurements of biological function in the healthy, unanesthetized animal are a promising direction in psychophysiological research. The described invasive techniques allow a much more relevant and a wider range of biological function to be measured than the more commonly used indirect measurements. Use of these techniques should encourage the experimental psychologist to learn more about the physiological aspects of his research problem and help to facilitate communication between these disciplines.

II

Cardiovascular Function — Experimental Studies

This series of chapters primarily concerns the evaluation within some simple behavioral paradigm of the relationship either among hemodynamic events or between hemodynamic events and somatic and sudomotor activity. It is the purpose of this biological strategy to provide some perspective on the interactive nature of cardiovascular and behavioral events—a perspective which goes beyond establishing some concomitance between some one parameter of cardiovascular activity and the manipulation of behavioral processes. As is obvious, this interactive process is complex, and if nothing else warns us against oversimplistic concepts relating cardiovascular and behavioral processes. One conclusion that can be drawn from this work is that we are beginning to obtain a better idea of hemodynamic processes and the peripheral neural control of these processes.

The first chapter by Cohen overviews current work evaluating the role of the neural innervations in the control of heart rate, and details the strategy which is necessary in specifying the control mechanisms. The chapter by Obrist et al., is also concerned with neural control but that of both heart rate and contractile force and how these events relate to somatic activity. In the chapters by Roberts and Schneiderman, heart rate also is the primary focus. An effort is made to understand the relevance of heart rate to behavioral processes through assessing the interrelationship between heart rate and sudomotor and somatic activity in one case, and heart rate and blood pressure in the other. Finally, the chapter by Herd et al., details one specific effort which evaluates the role of the sympathetic nervous system on the maintenance of an experimental hypertension. It should be noted that this effort implicates the vasculature as the primary contributor to the effects seen. These data are not necessarily inconsistent with the proposed influence of cardiac output, if as proposed, cardiac output contributes early to the development of the hypertension.

7

DAVID H. COHEN

Analysis of the Final Common Path for Heart Rate Conditioning

INTRODUCTION

Some years ago we initiated a program to develop a vertebrate model system that would be effective for cellular neurophysiological studies of learning (Cohen 1969). For a variety of reasons visually conditioned heart rate change in the pigeon was selected (Cohen and Durkovic 1966), and during the intervening years we have been developing this system along numerous experimental lines to allow rigorous investigation of neuronal discharge characteristics during conditioning. A major portion of this experimental effort has been directed toward specifying in some detail the anatomical pathways that mediate the development of the conditioned heart rate response, particularly the descending or "cardiomotor" pathways that constitute the efferent segments of the system. It is this last aspect of the program that bears most directly upon issues of relevance to this conference.

The present chapter deals specifically with one component of these motor pathways, namely the final common path(s) in the Sheringtonian sense. Since the central "cardiomotor" pathways eventually converge upon the sympathetic and/or parasympathetic preganglionic cardiac neurons, it is important to delineate this more peripheral motor segment of the pathway as a prelude to investigations of other central

The research reviewed in this paper that is from the author's laboratory has been generously supported by grants from the National Science Foundation (GB-2767, GB-6850, GB-8008, GB-13816X), the Heart Association of Northeast Ohio, the National Association of Mental Health, and the Scottish Rite Committee on Research in Schizophrenia. Dr. Cohen's work is supported by Public Health Service Research Career Award HL-16579 from the National Heart and Lung Institute.

structures. This is dictated by a more general strategy of analyzing "conditioning pathways" from peripheral to central structures to insure coupling to either the sensory or motor periphery at all times (Cohen 1969, in press). In the ensuing discussion of the final common path, with respect to heart rate conditioning in particular, the emphasis is on the fundamental questions and modes of approach. Experimental material to support given arguments is included in a rather selective manner.

ANALYSIS OF POSSIBLE CONTRIBUTIONS TO
THE CONDITIONED HEART RATE RESPONSE NOT
MEDIATED THROUGH THE EXTRINSIC CARDIAC NERVES

Unlike the final common path for somatomotor activity, heart rate may be modified by sources other than the extrinsic cardiac nerves, for example, by circulating levels of catecholamines. A further complication is imposed by the dual, sympathetic and parasympathetic, cardiac innervation—although this is probably no more complex than the final common path for an integrated movement involving a number of muscles. Finally, in contrast to somatomotor activity, heart rate may be affected by the occurrence of other responses, as clearly illustrated by heart rate and blood pressure interactions.

Consequently, the analysis of the final common path for the conditioned heart rate response must deal with a number of questions, the first of which is whether any component of the response is mediated by sources other than the extrinsic cardiac nerves, such as conditioned hormonal release. This, of course, must be considered for each different experimental preparation, since there may not only be marked species differences, but details of the experimental paradigm may also be instrumental in determining whether or not such components are involved. A somewhat trivial illustration is provided by manipulating the duration of the conditioned stimulus. With stimulus durations of only a few seconds, it is highly improbable that a conditioned hormonal response would be involved in most species. While with durations of 10 seconds or longer, this may be a significant factor in the longer latency components of the heart rate response.

In a program directed toward the investigation of central neural mechanisms of heart rate conditioning, it is an obvious advantage to have an experimental preparation in which the final common path consists exclusively of the extrinsic cardiac nerves. The attractive corollary of this is that, given adequate technology, the conditioned heart rate response can, in principle, be reliably predicted from the discharge characteristics of the extrinsic cardiac nerves. However, as indicated above, it cannot be taken a priori that the final common path consists of only the extrinsic cardiac nerves. There are few, if any, conditioning paradigms in which only a single response develops (e.g., Cohen 1969), and generally a conditioned stimulus elicits an organized ensemble of responses that may well interact with each other to varying degrees. If concomitant responses, such as respiratory and arterial blood pressure, feed back to influence the heart rate response via the nervous system, then any interactions may well be mediated through the extrinsic cardiac nerves, and a tight coupling between neuronal activity and the conditioned response may still be possible. If, on the other hand, any interactions are mediated through such sources as conditioned release of a hormone acting directly on the heart, then a potentially serious problem arises, since there may thus be components of the heart rate response that are considerably more difficult to account for in a neurophysiological analysis.

While there has been an acute awareness of the interactions of heart rate with other conditioned responses (e.g., Black 1965; Obrist and Webb 1967; Schneiderman et al. 1969), experimental efforts to determine whether there are any contributions mediated exlusive of the extrinsic cardiac nerves appear to have been limited to the study of Cohen and Pitts (1968). Perhaps an important reason for this is the difficulty encountered in cardiac denervation and the maintenance problems presented by the bilaterally vagotomized animal. However, such studies are prevalent in the exercise literature, indicating that the problems are not insurmountable (e.g., Donald and Shepherd 1963; Gasser and Meek 1914; Robinson et al. 1966; Samaan 1935).

To summarize the findings of the one existing study (Cohen and Pitts 1968), it was demonstrated that no conditioned heart rate response could be established in animals with bilateral vagotomy and β-adrenergic blockade. Thus, for visually conditioned heart rate change in the pigeon it may be tentatively concluded that the extrinsic cardiac nerves are required if any heart rate conditioning is to occur. However, it is essential to recognize two important points in this regard. First, the use of a β-adrenergic blocking agent to eliminate sympathetic influences would also prevent the effects of any substances capable of acting on β-adrenergic receptors, such as catecholamines. This qualification can be eliminated by experiments involving surgical cardiac denervation, and the development of this technique for the pigeon (Macdonald and Cohen 1970) has allowed experiments which, on a very tentative basis, suggest no hormonal effects. Second, the conditioned stimulus duration in the Cohen and Pitts (1968) experiment was 6 seconds, and it is possible that conditioned hormonal release could affect the heart rate at a longer latency. For example, cardioacceleration in response to an intense auditory stimulus has a latency of less than one second in the intact cat. And following denervation, a response still occurs but with latencies on the order of 12 seconds, suggesting catecholamine mediation (Bond 1943). A similar result holds for heart rate changes in response to exercise (Donald and Shepherd 1963). Since the pigeon has an extremely rapid circulation time, one would anticipate that an analogous effect would occur with even shorter latency.

ANALYSIS OF INTERACTIVE EFFECTS MEDIATED THROUGH THE EXTRINSIC CARDIAC NERVES

Given an experimental preparation in which it is established that the extrinsic cardiac nerves constitute the exclusive final common path, it may be desirable, although not absolutely necessary, to describe the influences of other concomitant responses on the conditioned heart rate response. An advantage of this is that, in principle, it could allow one to develop a model system which is free of interactive effects, considerably simplifying the analysis of the central pathways. At the least, it provides some ideas as to the dynamics of the "primary heart rate response"—that is, the conditioned heart rate response free of interactions with accompanying conditioned responses (Cohen 1969). The importance of this is that there may well be experimental situations in which the heart rate response is largely or entirely secondary to some other conditioned response, such as a change in arterial blood pressure. In such instances the heart rate response would provide a less attractive model for investigating central pathways mediating conditioning.

As mentioned previously, there has been longstanding discussion of this problem of response interactions (see other chapters in this volume for examples), and it may be of some value to review selectively the literature dealing with the responses that have been of greatest concern, namely blood pressure, respiration, and movement. Potential hormonal effects on heart rate have been mentioned in a preceding section; however, it is also possible that conditioned hormonal release could affect heart rate via the nervous system. The lack of literature in this regard and the probable long latencies of such effects (which depend in part upon circulation time) dictate against a discussion of this variable. However, to cite but one highly speculative possibility, it is conceivable that a conditioning paradigm producing constriction of the renal artery may affect heart rate through the renin-angiotensin system, with angiotensin exerting its effect by acting directly upon the nervous system (Panisset, Biron, and Beaulnes 1966; Scroop and Lowe 1968).

Blood Pressure

A number of conditioning studies in a variety of species have included measurements of both heart rate and arterial blood pressure (e.g.,

Antal and Gantt 1970; Dykman, Mack, and Ackerman 1965; Hein 1969; Yehle, Dauth, and Schneiderman 1967), and it has often been reported that both conditioned blood pressure and heart rate responses develop concomitantly. Such correlational evidence raises two questions: (a) are the heart rate responses totally secondary to conditioned blood pressure changes; and, (b) even given a negative answer to this question, does the occurrence of a concomitant blood pressure response affect the dynamics of the conditioned heart rate change?

With respect to the first question, whether the blood pressure response results from altered cardiac output or a conditioned change in peripheral resistance, secondary heart rate changes could occur through baroreceptor reflex mechanisms. This case would generally apply in situations where the heart rate and blood pressure responses are opposite in direction, as in the rabbit (Schneiderman et al. 1969). That the heart rate response is not entirely secondary to blood pressure changes is suggested by the sporadic reports that, despite their close temporal coupling, trials do occur on which a heart rate response is observed without an accompanying change in blood pressure (e.g., Yehle, Dauth, and Schneiderman 1967). More direct evidence is provided by studies employing α-adrenergic blockade, since these clearly demonstrate that conditioned heart rate changes can occur independent of blood pressure responses (Obrist, Wood, and Perez-Reyes 1965; Schneiderman et al. 1969).

With respect to the second question, although heart rate change is not necessarily dependent upon conditioned blood pressure responses, their frequent temporal correlation provides the opportunity for blood pressure changes to affect the dynamics of the conditioned heart rate response through baroreceptor reflex mechanisms. The case in which one might anticipate the most marked interaction is when the heart rate and blood pressure responses are opposite in direction, as in the pressor-decelerator response pattern of rabbits and humans. Yet Obrist, Wood, and Perez-Reyes (1965) found no evidence for such interaction in the human, while Schneiderman et al. (1969) clearly showed that in the rabbit the pressor response contributes to the evoked bradycardia. Thus, even given common response patterns, interactive effects can apparently differ between species.

This raises the rather interesting question of how the absence of a heart rate and blood pressure interaction can obtain, given the powerful baroreceptor mechanisms. A possible answer is provided by the now ample literature indicating that certain neural structures influencing heart rate and blood pressure are capable of inhibiting the baroreceptor reflexes (Antal 1967; Hilton 1962; Moruzzi 1937; Reis and Cuénod 1965). In view of this, the possibility must be seriously entertained that at least in some conditioning situations in certain species the central pathways mediating the heart rate and blood pressure conditioned responses concomitantly inhibit the baroreceptor reflexes to effect an uncoupling of the two responses. Such a phenomenon might be most marked in situations where the blood pressure and heart rate responses are in the same direction, as in the pressor-accelerator response pattern of the dog (e.g., Katcher et al. 1969) and pigeon (Cohen unpublished data) or the depressor-decelerator response pattern of the cat (Hein 1969). Unfortunately, α-adrenergic blocking experiments have not yet been undertaken on these species.

In any case, it is clear that a full understanding of the nature of the conditioned cardiovascular response ideally requires measurement of a number of cardiovascular parameters (e.g., Smith and Stebbins 1965). Unfortunately, this is frequently prohibitive; regardless, it is essential that any generalization be made within the context of the integrated pattern of cardiovascular changes. In the specific case of interactive effects between heart rate and blood pressure responses this issue may be circumvented to a large extent if, for a given conditioning model, it can be rigorously demonstrated that blood pressure changes do not alter the conditioned heart rate response. This might be evaluated first by employing α-adrenergic blocking agents. If this suggested no heart rate-blood pressure interaction during the conditioned stimulus presentations, subsequent studies could be directed toward testing baroreceptor reflex activity during the conditioned response period.

Clearly what is required is a broader survey of species and conditioning paradigms in this context. From the viewpoint of an investigator specifically concerned with a heart rate conditioning model system, the ideal preparation would be one in which there are no conditioned changes in peripheral resistance, and in which any blood pressure changes that might occur are a consequence of changes in cardiac dynamics—since this would provide a model in which the extrinsic cardiac nerves exclusively constituted the final common path. Furthermore, an uncoupling of heart rate and blood pressure responses through inhibition of the baroreceptor reflexes is a particularly attractive possibility, since this would eliminate any concerns regarding response interactions and feedback.

Respiration

As with blood pressure, there have been numerous reports of concomitant development of conditioned heart rate and respiratory responses (e.g., Cohen and Durkovic 1966; Fitzgerald and Walloch 1966; Gantt 1960; Hein 1969; Obrist and Webb 1967; Wood and Obrist 1964). The possibility that heart rate responses are entirely secondary to respiratory changes (See Smith 1954) appears no longer to be an issue, since conditioned heart rate responses have been obtained in (1) pharmacologically immobilized animals that are artificially ventilated (e.g., Black, Carlson, and Solomon 1962); (2) experimental situations where respiration is controlled (e.g., Obrist, Webb, and Sutterer 1969); and (3) animals where no respiratory change was demonstrable (e.g., Smith and Stebbins 1965). This position is summarized in a recent paper by Obrist, Sutterer, and Howard (1972a) where it is concluded that conditioned respiratory and heart rate responses are concomitant peripheral manifestations of a common central mediating process.

However, the issue of whether the occurrence of conditioned respiratory changes affects the heart rate response is far from resolved. It is clear that any such interactive effects are neurally mediated, since Cohen and Pitts (1968) demonstrated that in animals with bilateral vagotomy and ß-adrenergic blockade conditioned respiratory responses comparable to those of control animals developed; yet, there was no evidence of any conditioned heart rate response. The literature dealing with the nature of possible respiratory-heart rate interactions has been somewhat controversial, the confusion in part deriving from differences in experimental designs among discrepant studies.

There have been two direct approaches to resolving this problem: control of respiration by instruction and training in human experiments, and pharmacological immobilization with artifical ventilation in animal experiments. With respect to the human controlled respiration experiments, the literature has recently been nicely reviewed by Obrist et al. (1972a). To recapitulate briefly the major findings, Westcott and Huttenlocher (1961) in a variety of paced respiration conditions were unable to demonstrate the deceleratory heart rate response generally described in human heart rate conditioning studies; however, they did obtain an acceleratory response. Deane (1964) and Headrick and Graham (1969) were unable to replicate the Westcott and Huttenlocher (1961) findings; and Wood and Obrist (1964) convincingly demonstrated that respiration did not affect the deceleratory conditioned heart rate response, but did affect an early acceleratory component. In experiments where respiration was suspended, rather than paced Smith (1966) and Zeaman and Smith (1965) reported elimination of the deceleratory response. However, in a direct comparison of paced and suspended respiratory conditions Obrist et al. (1969) could find no effect on the deceleratory response, and they raise some serious methodological questions regarding the Smith (1966) and Zeaman and Smith (1965) studies.

Therefore, the details of conditioned heart rate and respiratory interactions in the human studies remain an open question. However, Obrist and his colleagues present a rather convincing case that any interactive effects are not marked and may be confined to only the early accelerative component of the response. It is conceivable that a sizable inspiratory response at the start of the conditioned stimulus period could produce such a transient acceleration (Levy, DeGeest, and Zieske 1966).

Concerning pharmacological immobilization and artificial ventilation—the other approach to this problem—there have been many fewer studies (e.g., Black 1965; Black, Carlson, and Solomon 1962; Katcher et al. 1969). These experiments have largely been limited to the dog in which the conditioned heart rate response is generally cardioacceleration, although Black (1965) also describes deceleratory as well as biphasic responses. In a rigorous direct comparison of the dynamics of the heart rate response in curarized and non-curarized dogs, Black (1965) concluded that there is no difference in the form or stability of the response following curarization. Comparisons of the relative magnitudes of the responses were precluded by baseline rate differences between curarized and non-curarized groups. At face value this would seem to indicate that in the dog neither respiratory nor somatic responses interact with the heart rate response. However, as discussed elsewhere in this volume, the use of neuromuscular blocking agents raises certain problems that must be seriously considered before such a conclusion can be definitively accepted.

In summary, the literature at present suggests that there are no remarkable interactions between respiratory and heart rate conditioned responses in either human or animal studies. While it may be possible to design experiments to force such interactions, at most they probably play only a minor role in most heart rate conditioning paradigms. What small interactive effects may obtain are going to be difficult to describe rigorously, given the present methodology. Although pharmacological immobilization is the most promising approach in this regard, as described elsewhere in this volume, it raises a number of technological problems that must be surmounted before possible subtle effects of this nature can be resolved.

Movement

Of the various responses under consideration, somatomotor activity has received the greatest attention as a potentially confounding factor in heart rate conditioning, although the intensity of this concern is somewhat puzzling given that none of the classically described cardiovascular reflexes would provide a mechanism for such an interaction between movement and heart rate. The relevant literature dealing with this "cardiac-somatic linkage" is sizable and perhaps partially reflects a longstanding concern with the relationship between learned skeletal and autonomic responses, and the possible mediation of conditioned autonomic activity by learned somatic events. It was such somatic activity that Smith (1954) emphasized in arguing that conditioned heart rate change may be entirely an artifact. The concern with this issue has been strongly reinforced by the tight coupling that has repeatedly been found between heart rate change and movement. Obrist and his colleagues have presented an extensive series of papers documenting this coupling (e.g., Obrist and Webb 1967), and much of this work has recently been summarized by Obrist et al. (1970b) and Obrist et al. (1972a). Further support has appeared in the cardiovascular physiology literature with numerous reports of heart rate, blood pressure, and blood flow changes concomitant with muscular contraction (e.g., Clarke, Smith, and Shearn 1968; Freyschuss 1970).

As with respiration, sufficient evidence now seems to have accumulated to force the consensus that heart rate changes are by no means entirely secondary to conditioned somatomotor activity—in the sense that feedback from muscular activity is not a necessary and sufficient condition for the occurrence of the heart rate response. There are a variety of correlational observations that support this position. First, Perez-Cruet and Gantt (1959) report that in a situation where both conditioned heart rate and somatic responses occur, the heart rate response has a shorter latency than somatic activity. Second, in a variety of circumstances, trials have been observed where heart rate change was unaccompanied by any apparent movement (e.g., Cohen and Durkovic 1966; Jaworska, Kowalska, and Soltysik 1962; Yehle, Dauth, and Schneiderman 1967). Finally, Gantt (1960), Obrist and Webb (1967), and Bruner (1969) indicate that conditioned heart rate responses are acquired prior to the development of a conditioned leg flexion.

More definitive are the numerous studies demonstrating heart rate conditioning in animals that have been pharmacologically immobilized (Black 1965; Black, Carlson, and Solomon 1962; Black and Lang 1964; Gantt 1960; Hein 1969; Katcher et al. 1969; Schneiderman et al. 1969; Yehle, Dauth, and Schneiderman 1967). In certain of these studies high doses of d-tubocurarine have been used, and the occurrence of a conditioned heart rate change under these circumstances would seem to negate conclusively the argument that such responses are secondary to conditioned somatic activity. Unfortunately, since this has been the principal issue, there has been less concern as to whether or not there may be more subtle interactive effects where concomitant movements can affect the dynamics of the heart rate response. As stated earlier, the cardiovascular reflex literature suggests no obvious mechanism for such an interaction. However, at this time it is not possible to exclude definitively neurally mediated cardiovascular effects following activation of mechanoreceptors, such as those in joints and muscle.

The primary study dealing directly with such interactive effects is that of Black (1965), in which the performance of immobilized and non-immobilized animals was compared in some detail. Based on such data, Black (1965) has concluded that immobilization with d-tubo-curarine affects neither the form nor the stability of the conditioned heart rate response, magnitude differences being unassessable because of baseline differences between experimental and control groups. Thus, the existing data certainly indicate that there is little if any interaction between cardiac and somatomotor conditioned responses resulting from feedback—"overt chaining" in the terminology of Black and de Toledo (1972)—although the final word with respect to this topic is not yet available.

The evidence at hand would seem to be more consistent with the contention of Obrist et al. (1972a) that the cardiac and somatic events are independent but possibly mediated by a common central process —"central chaining" in the terminology of Black and de Toledo (1972). The literature concerning central control of the cardiovascular system provides some support for this contention, since it may be argued rather convincingly that the concept of a "cardiovascular pathway" per se is somewhat misleading and that "cardioactive" regions are in actuality more complexly organized to mediate a patterned set of autonomic and somatic responses appropriate for some integrated behavior such as in defense or excerise. However, it is important to recognize that, in the present context, "central chaining" is a qualitatively different problem from serial interactive effects based upon feedback. In the latter case the concern is with the possibility of a confounded heart rate response, while "central chaining" represents a problem in central neural organization where the goal would be to determine the sites of convergence and divergence of the relevant autonomic and somatic pathways.

ANALYSIS OF VAGAL AND SYMPATHETIC CONTRIBUTIONS TO THE CONDITIONED HEART RATE RESPONSE: SELECTIVE DENERVATION AND PHARMACOLOGICAL BLOCKADE

Given a preparation in which the extrinsic cardiac nerves constitute the final common path and possible interactive effects mediated through this path have been characterized, the subsequent major analytic steps are to determine: (1) whether both the vagi and cardiac sympathetics contribute to the conditioned heart rate response; and (2) if so, what are their relative contributions. This is a particularly interesting problem, and its resolution for a given species and paradigm is instrumental in establishing a foundation for the analysis of the relevant central pathways.

To gain a first approximation to describing the relative contributions, the traditional approach has been to investigate the effects on heart rate conditioning performance of different combinations of surgical cardiac denervation and/or pharmacological blockade. While this approach has certain limitations that will be discussed later, it is capable of providing important preliminary information if applied appropriately. As a prelude to raising these issues, following is a review of the literature directed toward this problem.

Since the relative vagal and sympathetic contributions are reflected in the dynamics of the conditioned heart rate response and there are rather striking differences among species and experimental situations, it is perhaps best to group the existing studies on the basis of the nature of the response. First, studies dealing with the pigeon and dog will be considered, since both demonstrate conditioned cardioacceleration. In the pigeon, Cohen and Pitts (1968) examined conditioning performance of animals following unilateral vagotomy, bilateral vagotomy, or ß-adrenergic blockade. In brief, the findings were that conditioned cardioacceleration in bilaterally vagotomized birds was significantly below that of control animals, although substantial conditioning still occurred.

In contrast, ß-adrenergic blockade markedly reduced conditioning performance, with almost no conditioned cardioacceleration occurring until later in training. Response latency was prolonged by bilateral vagotomy, while a short latency heart rate change could still occur following ß-adrenergic blockade. Although less conclusive, there was also a suggestion that right vagotomy affected performance more seriously than left vagotomy. Concerning differentiation, successful performance was obtained in birds with either bilateral vagotomy or ß- adrenergic blockade, but the differentiation took longer to establish with only the excitatory cardiac innervation. These results led Cohen and Pitts (1968) to conclude that early in training the principal contribution to the magnitude of the conditioned response is mediated by the cardiac sympathetic nerves, while the shortest latency component is mediated by the vagi. However, as training progresses there is an increasing vagal contribution, emphasizing the dynamic nature of the relative contributions.

In the dog, there have been no studies in which both sources of cardiac innervation have been examined, attention being directed to either the vagi or sympathetics in any given experiment. Dykman and Gantt (1956) reported that atropinization diminished the response and prolonged its latency. This led to the conclusion that the response was mediated by both extrinsic cardiac nerve supplies and that the shortest latency component was vagally mediated. Moreover, on the basis of the response amplitudes they suggested that while both the sympathetics and vagi were involved, the response was largely vagally mediated. In the remaining studies only the sympathetic cardiac innervation was studied. The work of Obrist and his colleagues supports the notion of the conditioned cardioacceleration being primarily vagally mediated with only a minor sympathetic contribution. Obrist and Webb (1967) found no rate effects with ß-adrenergic blockàde, and Obrist et al. (1972a) reported only small to moderate response decrements. Of particular interest in the latter study was the finding that ß-adrenergic blockade had a severe attenuating effect on the conditioned change in contractility, prompting the hypothesis that, in the dog, rate changes are primarily vagally mediated and contractility changes are sympathetically mediated. Katcher et al. (1969) also suggest that both the vagi and sympathetics are involved, based on the effects of cardiac sympathectomy. But in contrast to the conclusions of Dykman and Gantt (1956), Obrist and Webb (1967), and Obrist et al. (1972a) they suggest that the cardiac sympathetics are the most critical.

Other relevant studies include a description by Bond (1943) of the cardioacceleratory startle response to an intense auditory stimulus in the dog (and cat). In that study various combinations of surgical cardiac denervation were investigated. The conclusions were that the response is largely sympathetically mediated, although there was also a vagal contribution. This study stands alone in concluding that the shortest latency component of the response was both sympathetically and vagally mediated. Finally, the literature suggests that cardioacceleration consequent to exercise is both vagally and sympathetically mediated. However, release of vagal inhibition is generally argued to be the primary contributor (e.g., Freyschuss 1970; Robinson et al. 1966) with an increase in sympathetic outflow occurring at more strenuous levels of exercise (e.g., Robinson et al. 1966).

Therefore, in situations where the conditioned response is cardioacceleration it appears that both the cardiac sympathetics and vagi contribute, and where the data are available it would seem that the shortest latency component of the response is vagally mediated. Regarding response magnitude, in the pigeon it is felt to be largely sympathetically mediated, at least in earlier stages of training (Cohen and Pitts 1968), while in the dog there is some disagreement. Katcher et al. (1969) claim the cardiac sympathetics are most instrumental, consistent with Bond's (1943) position for the startle response. However, Dykman and Gantt (1956), Obrist and Webb (1967), and Obrist et al. (1972a) feel the primary component is release of vagal inhibition, consistent with the mediation of heart rate adjustments during exercise.

The literature is rather more consistent regarding preparations which show conditioned cardiodeceleration, as in the cat, rabbit, and rat. Hein (1969) has reported that atropinization abolishes the bradycardia response in the cat, and Schneiderman et al. (1969) report a similar finding for the rabbit. Vagotomy in the cat produces an analogous effect, and it is further claimed that surgical intervention of the cardiac sympathetics in no way affects the conditioned response (Flynn, 1960). Thus, for the cat and rabbit there is a consensus that the conditioned cardiodeceleration is vagally mediated with no sympathetic involvement. Fitzgerald, Martin, and O'Brien (1973) report that in the rat atropinization severely attenuates the deceleratory response, and they attribute the small residual bradycardia to sympathoinhibition. However, it may also be possible that this small residual response could be attributed to only partial vagal blockade in a small percentage of their experimental animals, since they report that approximately 14% of the rats evaluated for completeness of vagal blockade showed pronounced cardiac slowing to vagal stimulation. Consequently, at present there is no evidence inconsistent with the hypothesis that in all animals showing decelerative conditioned responses the mediation is entirely vagal with no sympathetic involvement.

The final situation to be considered is that in the human, where the conditioned heart rate response is a biphasic acceleration-deceleration, the deceleratory component being the more prominent. It has been reported (Obrist et al. 1965) that atropinization abolishes the decelerative component, indicating it is vagally mediated. Furthermore, this unmasks a small acceleratory component that is apparently sympathetically mediated. The initial acceleration, however, may be secondary to respiration, as discussed earlier. Consequently, in the human both the vagi and sympathetics contribute to the response, with the vagal contribution being predominant.

To summarize briefly, the conditioned bradycardia seen in the cat, rabbit, and rat appears to be exclusively mediated through the vagi. On the basis of existing literature it is doubtful that there is any sympathetic contribution. The deceleratory component of the human response also seems to be vagally mediated, although there is evidence for a masked sympathetic component suggesting involvement of both cardiac innervations. In animals showing acceleratory responses, it is also generally concluded that both nerve supplies contribute to the response, and the literature is not in complete agreement with respect to the predominant contribution.

There are two groups of problems that must be considered in evaluating studies of the above sort. The first concerns limitations fundamentally inherent in the approach and therefore applicable to all studies. The second is a group of specific methodological problems that vary from study to study. With regard to the basic approach, while it has produced fascinating results and in certain instances given a first approximation to the relative contributions of the extrinsic cardiac nerves, the elimination of one source of cardiac innervation may well alter the contribution of the remaining nerve supply. Moreover, the approach does not have sufficient resolution to permit a precise, quantitative description of the specific efferent contributions. Therefore, serious questions can always be raised concerning results obtained with this approach, although it should be clearly recognized that it provides a valuable foundation for subsequent, more precise studies employing different techniques.

The second group of problems includes a number of issues of varying generality. First, since the two cardiac innervations are not independent, and eliminating one may well affect the behavior of the other, it becomes important in any study of relative contributions to examine the effects of removing each nerve supply. This has not been done in most studies, either the sympathetics or vagi having been investigated, but not both. The only exceptions are the reports of Cohen and Pitts (1968) and Flynn (1960). Thus, in the controversial literature regarding the dog there have been no reports involving blockade or elimination of both nerve supplies; this would clearly be of importance and interest.

Second, if it has not been previously established that the extrinsic cardiac nerves constitute the exclusive final common path for the heart rate response, then one can conceivably be misled. For example, suppose there is a catecholamine response that feeds back to affect the heart rate in a situation where the response is primarily a vagally mediated acceleration. In such a case, atropinization or vagotomy would not affect the catecholamine component and it could thus be incorrectly concluded that the cardiac sympathetics play a substantial role. This, of course, does not apply to experiments in which the response is totally abolished by the experimental procedure, as in the studies of Flynn (1960), Hein (1969), and Schneiderman et al. (1969).

Third, difficult analytic problems are raised by baseline differences among experimental groups, this being most acute following bilateral vagotomy or atropinization in certain species. For example, in the study of Cohen and Pitts (1968) bilateral vagotomy produced marked increases in baseline heart rate which appeared to produce a striking attenuation of the conditioned cardioacceleration. However, an analysis of covariance, designed to correct for group baseline differences, indicated that the differences from the control group were much less than they appeared prior to correction. Moreover, in the same study it was shown that the negative correlation that generally obtains between a given animal's baseline rate and conditioned response magnitude was largely attenuated by bilateral vagotomy. Therefore, even if it is possible to avoid analytic problems resulting from baseline differences, one may still be faced with an altered baseline-conditioned response relationship that is more difficult to treat, another reflection of the fundamental limitation of this general approach.

Fourth, the relative contributions may differ at various points in training (Cohen and Pitts 1968). In the pigeon, the sympathetics predominate early in training with an increase in the relative vagal contribution occurring later in training. This is perhaps relevant to the discrepancy between the findings of Katcher et al. (1969) and those of Obrist et al. (1972a). In the former study, the dogs were sympathectomized prior to training, and it was concluded that the conditioned cardioacceleration was primarily sympathetically mediated, analogous to the findings for early training in the pigeon. In contrast, the Obrist et al. (1972a) study involved ß-adrenergic blockade of the sympathetic influences in trained dogs, and this resulted in minimal attentuation of the heart rate response, leading to the conclusion that the response must be primarily vagally mediated. A similar finding would have been the case for the pigeon had ß-adrenergic blockade been employed after training. This again illustrates the necessity for investigating both sources of cardiac innervation in any given study, and additionally it emphasizes that the dynamic nature of the relative contributions over the course of training must be clearly recognized.

A final point concerns the use of pharmacological blockade relative to surgical denervation, each having its advantages and limitations. Surgical denervation has the attractive feature of being free of difficulties involving central drug effects. However, it is not reversible, can be confounded by postoperative recovery time, may involve difficult maintenance problems, and often involves section of fibers other than cardiac efferents (e.g., vagal afferent fibers in cervical vagotomy). The pharmacological approach obviates many of these difficulties but clearly is not free of problems. There will always be concern regarding possible central effects of blocking agents such as atropine and propranolol, although normal development of another response such as respiratory rate provides some control for this (Cohen and Pitts 1968). In many instances it may be quite difficult to induce a complete block at dose levels that are free of central effects. In any case, the evaluation of all data in this area must take such potential problems into account.

In conclusion, the approach of selectively eliminating extrinsic cardiac nerve influences has yielded important and interesting results. However, in view of the numerous problems involved, it must be considered only a first approximation to answering the major questions regarding relative sympathetic and vagal contributions. A more rigorous, though demanding, approach is to record the activity of single vagal cardioinhibitory and sympathetic cardioacceleratory neurons in the intact animal, the topic of the following section.

ANALYSIS OF VAGAL AND SYMPATHETIC CONTRIBUTIONS TO THE CONDITIONED HEART RATE RESPONSE: THE ACTIVITY OF SINGLE CARDIAC PREGANGLIONIC OR POSTGANGLIONIC NEURONS

As suggested above, the next logical experimental step in characterizing the final common path is to record the activity of single cardiac preganglionic or postganglionic neurons, both vagal and sympathetic, in the context of conditioning. In many respects this approach perturbs the system substantially less than selective elimination of the extrinsic cardiac nerves. Further, it allows a more precise, quantitative description of the dynamics of the vagal and sympathetic contributions, including estimates of their response latencies. Such estimates may be more accurate indicators of the actual input-output time across the system, since peripheral delay times are eliminated. Finally, in principle this approach permits one to characterize cardiac vagal-sympathetic interactions, which in turn could allow more precise predictability of the dynamics of the conditioned heart rate response. Information such as the above would then be fundamental to interpreting discharge changes in more central pathways that descend to influence the cardiac preganglionic neurons.

Given acceptance of this premise, the subsequent steps in analyzing the final common path are (a) the anatomical localization of the medullary cells of origin of the vagal cardioinhibitory fibers and the spinal cells of origin of the sympathetic preganglionic cardioaccelerator fibers; and, (b) the development of stringent electrophysiological criteria for the identification of these neurons in the intact animal. The first step involving anatomical localization could conceivably be finessed by the direct recording of preganglionic fiber activity in the periphery, as has been done for single vagal cardiac efferents by Jewett (1964), and for single sympathetic preganglionic fibers by Beacham and Perl (1964). However, in a conditioning context, recording from the relevant cells of origin has certain advantages over such fiber recordings. Methodologically, there is less probability of damage to the cardiac innervation, and the cellular recording situation is more amenable to the chronic or semi-chronic requirements for conditioning. Moreover, localization of the relevant cells of origin must still be undertaken for anatomical investigations of the descending pathways influencing these neurons and for subsequent intracellular studies if they are required at some point.

With respect to the localization of the medullary cells of origin of the vagal cardioinhibitory fibers, a recent review of the literature (Cohen and Schnall 1970; Cohen et al. 1970) suggested that the text-book description confining them to the dorsal motor nucleus of the vagus is rather oversimplified. For example, over the past few years data from the cat tend to contradict this supposition (Achari, Down-man, and Weber 1968; Calaresu and Pearce 1965a,b; Gunn et al. 1968; Kerr 1969) and in contrast tend to support a longstanding suggestion (e.g., Bunzl-Federn 1899) that the vagal cardioinhibitory neurons are located in the region of the nucleus ambiguus. However, in other species—such as the monkey (Mitchell and Warwick 1955); rabbit (Getz and Sirnes 1949); and pigeon (Cohen and Schnall 1970; Cohen et al. 1970)—it appears that these cells are, in fact, in the dorsal motor nucleus. Finally, in some cases, such as the dog, the vagal cardioinhibitory neurons are found in both the dorsal motor nucleus and the region of the nucleus ambiguus (Gunn et al. 1968). This would seem to constitute reasonably firm evidence of marked species differences with respect to the degree of ventrolateral migration of these vagal cardioinhibitory neurons from the glossopharyngeal-vagal cell column (Cohen and Schnall 1970).

One implication of such differences for electrophysiological analyses of the final common path for heart rate conditioning is that the cells of origin of the vagal cardioinhibitory fibers must first be definitively localized for each species of interest. Where such information is not available, it is essential that preliminary localization studies be completed as a prelude to electrophysiological experiments. In this regard, it is important to recognize that solution of the localization problem requires a combined anatomical and physiological approach. As an initial step, one must identify the distribution of neurons giving rise to vagal fibers innervating the heart, a traditional approach being the mapping of the distribution of neurons showing retrograde degenerative changes following section of the vagal cardiac branches (e.g., Cohen et al. 1970; Mitchell and Warwick 1955). However, this approach does not indicate whether these are in fact cardioinhibitory neurons (see Kerr, 1969). Consequently, it is also important that one electrically stimulate within the region of distribution of degenerating neurons to determine if cardiodeceleration can be obtained having the same properties as the bradycardia found upon stimulation of the peripheral vagus nerve (e.g., Cohen and Schnall 1970). The only species in which both the distribution of chromatolytic neurons following cardiac vagotomy and the responses to electrical stimulation have been described is the pigeon (Cohen and Schnall 1970; Cohen et al. 1970); in this case the cells of origin of the vagal cardioinhibitory fibers are found in the lateral aspect of the dorsal motor nucleus of the vagus, approximately 0.5 to 1.0 mm rostral to the obex.

Concerning the localization of the sympathetic preganglionic cardioacceleratory neurons, the anatomical problem is in some respects less difficult. It is generally agreed that in most mammalian species these neurons are concentrated in the intermediolateral cell column of the thoracic spinal cord (e.g., Truex and Carpenter 1969), although more recent anatomical evidence indicates that preganglionic neurons may also be found scattered as far medially as the central canal (Petras and Cummings 1971). It is of interest that the more medial positions of the sympathetic preganglionic neurons correspond to the regions where these cells are found embryologically (Crosby, Humphrey, and Lauer 1962); and in certain species, such as the pigeon, the preganglionic neurons remain in this position in the adult animal forming a well-defined column dorsal and dorsolateral to the central canal (MacDonald and Cohen 1970). Consequently, it may be said with some confidence that the preganglionic neurons influencing heart rate are located in identified nuclear groups at specified levels of the spinal cord—for example, the upper three thoracic segments of the pigeon (MacDonald and Cohen 1970) and the upper six thoracic segments of many mammals (e.g., Truex and Carpenter 1969). However, it is still not resolved whether these cardioacceleratory neurons represent a unique and independent population of cells, or whether the neurons influencing heart rate also project upon postganglionic neurons innervating other thoracic structures. It is still a distinct possibility that all preganglionic neurons at upper thoracic levels in fact project upon postganglionic cardioaccelerator neurons.

Even given the rigorous anatomical localization of the cells of origin of cardiac preganglionic fibers for a particular species, it is still necessary to develop electrophysiological criteria for identifying these neurons in the intact preparation. There has been some progress in this regard for the cardiac vagal efferent fibers of the dog (Iriuchijima and Kumada 1963; Jewett 1964; Katona et al. 1970), while few conclusive criteria have been established for identifying the cardiac sympathetic preganglionic cells. These problems require clear solution before microelectrode analyses of the final common path for heart rate conditioning can be seriously undertaken. They are therefore problems deserving of substantial effort, not only for analyzing conditioning mechanisms, but also for understanding neural control of the heart in general. Moreover, subsequent studies of the influences of the various descending "cardiomotor" pathways, including those involved in heart rate conditioning, require investigations of the synaptic influences on the preganglionic cardiac neurons which, of course, demand rigorous localization and electrophysiological identification of these cells.

CONCLUDING COMMENTS

In outlining an approach to describing the final common path for heart rate conditioning a number of analytic steps have been proposed. The first involves the determination of whether or not the response in any given paradigm and species receives any nonneural contributions, that is, contributions exclusive of the extrinsic cardiac nerves. Although of great importance, this has been largely ignored in the literature. Given a preparation in which it has been demonstrated that the extrinsic cardiac nerves do in fact constitute the exclusive final common path, it is next appropriate to evaluate whether both the cardiac sympathetics and vagi are involved in mediating the response, and, if so, what are their relative contributions. A first approximation to this question can be obtained by applying the approach of selective denervation and/or pharmacological blockade, although this approach has a number of limitations. At some point it becomes necessary to study directly the discharge characteristics of both vagal and sympathetic preganglionic cardiac neurons during the conditioning procedure, and this requires two preliminary steps: (a) anatomical localization of these neurons, and, (b) development of electrophysiological criteria for their identification. Completion of such an analysis then places one in a position to characterize in some detail the motor output during heart rate conditioning. While it is unlikely that these preganglionic neurons participate directly in the requisite information storage, a full description of their discharge characteristics during conditioning would provide invaluable detailed performance information and would considerably facilitate the interpretation of neurophysiological data from more central structures.

Regarding the analysis of possible interactive effects between the heart rate response and concomitant conditioned responses, this is best studied in a preparation where it has already been established that the extrinsic cardiac nerves constitute the final common path, such that one knows a priori that any interactive effects are neurally mediated and expressed through the extrinsic cardiac nerves. While this line of research is not critical to the analysis of the final common path, its successful completion would insure greater control over the response and thereby would yield more accurate predictability.

As stated earlier, completion of an analysis of the final common path is important in a number of respects as a prelude to investigating more central aspects of the motor pathways involved in heart rate conditioning. While it is beyond the scope of this chapter to discuss such central pathways, a general experimental strategy for their identification has been discussed elsewhere (Cohen 1969, in press; Cohen and MacDonald, Chapter 2).

8

PAUL A. OBRIST, JAMES L. HOWARD,
JAMES E. LAWLER, RICHARD A. GALOSY,
KATHLEEN A. MEYERS, AND CLAUDE J. GAEBELEIN

The Cardiac-Somatic
Interaction

INTRODUCTION

Our purpose for studying the relationship between cardiovascular and
somatic activity[1] is to shed some light on the biological mechanisms by
which behavioral and cardiovascular processes interact. The necessity
to resort to such a biological-mechanistic strategy is indicated by the
ever increasing body of evidence which indicates that the relationship
between behavioral and cardiovascular events is quite complex and not
understandable at a conceptual level which links cardiovascular changes
in some direct-unidimensional manner to behavioral processes such as
motivational or affective states. The complexity of the problem is
perhaps best illustrated by the variety of heart rate changes that have
been observed in simple behavioral paradigms with heart rate sometimes increasing, decreasing, or changing in a biphasic or even triphasic
manner with regard to direction of change. There has been some effort
to understand these heart rate effects by recourse to concepts dealing
with the organism's receptivity to environmental events. For example,
decreases in heart rate have been associated with the facilitation of
organism-environmental interaction, such as with orienting responses
in one context (Graham and Clifton 1966) and with attention to
environmental events in another (Lacey and Lacey 1970), while heart
rate increases have been proposed to be associated with defensive
reflexes or rejection of environmental intake. While there is evidence
which indicates a certain validity to these positions (e.g., Chapter 26,

This chapter is based on research supported by Grant 07995, National Institute of
Mental Health, United States Public Health Service.

Lacey and Lacey), there is still other evidence which is not consistent with them (see Chapter 25, Elliott; Elliott 1972; Hahn 1972, for overviews). To us a biological strategy which focuses on the extrinsic neural-humoral mediating mechanisms which evoke cardiovascular effects would facilitate the resolution of such inconsistencies as well as act to delineate the nature of the interaction between behavioral and cardiovascular processes in general. The justification for such a biological strategy should become apparent in the following sections of this chapter. They boil down to the point that we are dealing with a very complex biological system both in regard to the function it serves and in the manner it is controlled in achieving this function. For example, we shall present data which shows—over a 30-second period commencing with the preparatory signal of a stressful reaction task—a complex display of heart rate changes which to us is uninterpretable with regard to behavioral significance without consideration of the role of the cardiac innervations and of the relationship of these heart rate changes to somatic activity.

We initially resorted to a more biological strategy in an attempt to explain the anticipatory deceleration of heart rate observed in humans during aversive conditioning, because behavioral concepts such as those concerning the learning process were inadequate. These first efforts concerned whether these heart rate changes could be understood as secondary to some other peripheral biological change such as an elevation of blood pressure which, acting via baroreceptor reflex mechanisms, slowed heart rate. These experiments seemed to negate any such peripheral explanation. They did indicate that biologically the heart rate decrease was due to a momentary increase in vagal or parasympathetic restraining effects which masked sympathetic activity and in turn suggested that the effect was due to a direct influence of central nervous system processes on the heart (Obrist, Sutterer, and Howard 1972a). It was somewhat fortuitously that the relationship between heart rate changes and somatic activity was studied. Nonetheless, from this work emerged a consistent picture with regard to a concomitance between heart rate and somatic activity.[2] The effect has been seen in adult humans, children, dogs, and cats, and in several experimental paradigms such as simple reaction time and classical aversive conditioning. The concomitance is seen with regard to direction of change, i.e., heart rate and somatic activity either both increasing or decreasing, as well as in regard to magnitude of the effects. The increase or decrease in heart rate and somatic activity can be either phasic as when it is associated with the anticipation of stimulus events or tonic as with base levels in different age groups of children. That this concomitance between heart rate and somatic events probably reflects a biologically substantive relationship between each type of event is suggested by the consistency with which experimental manipulations influence both effects. For example, in human Ss manipulating the conditioned stimulus-unconditioned stimulus (CS-UCS) or interstimulus interval (ISI) during classical aversive conditioning (Obrist 1968) influences the magnitude and duration of the anticipatory decrease in both heart rate and somatic activity. While under similar circumstances, manipulation of one parameter of somatic activity, respiration, consistently affected both heart rate and one other parameter of somatic activity (Obrist, Webb, and Sutterer 1969). When a reasonably systematic quantitative evaluation of the concomitance between heart rate and somatic activity has been undertaken, the consistency and magnitude of the relationship is pronounced (Obrist and Webb 1967; Obrist 1968; Obrist, Webb, and Sutterer 1969; Obrist et al. 1970a; Webb and Obrist 1970).

The purpose of this chapter is to examine further the cardiac-somatic interrelationship. This will involve first summarizing our own recent work as well as that from other laboratories which demonstrate a relationship between each type of event. Second, the issue of the independence of cardiac and somatic activity will be discussed, focusing on some of our recent data, which for the first time demonstrate a divorcement of heart rate as well as cardiac contractility from somatic activity. Finally, some of the issues, problems, and implications of these various lines of research will be discussed in an attempt to provide a critical perspective on the cardiac-somatic interaction.

RECENT EVIDENCE ON CARDIAC-SOMATIC COUPLING

Three of our recent studies have involved procedures, the intent of which was to manipulate or modify somatic activity and thus provide conditions to evaluate further the extent to which either tonic or phasic changes in heart rate were modified. One study was developmental in which four age groups of children (4, 5, 8, and 10-year-olds) as well as an adult reference population were subjected to a simple reaction time task (RT) with a fixed foreperiod (Obrist et al. 1973a). A developmental strategy was resorted to because it appeared to be a natural means to manipulate both background somatic activity as well as the facility to inhibit task-irrelevant somatic activity. The expectation was that younger children would show higher levels of background activity, i.e., be more restless, and have less facility to inhibit such activity. A reasonably consistent picture emerged. The younger Ss showed higher background or base levels in 3 of 4 somatic measures as well as in heart rate. All groups showed the phasic decrease in somatic activities and heart rate that has been previously found associated with responding. This was important because had an independence of cardiac and somatic activity been found at the younger age levels, it would definitely have weakened the notion that the cardiac and somatic effects are biologically integrated events. That is, one would expect both events to show parallel developmental changes if they are biologically integrated events. However, the age groups were not differentiated with regard to the magnitude of the phasic cardiac deceleration and two of the somatic measures, an effect apparently related to the large base level differences.

A second study (Sutterer and Obrist 1972) was intended to manipulate somatic activity by superimposing an aversive conditioning procedure on an operant bar-pressing baseline (a conditioned emotional response or CER) where dogs had been trained to bar press for food. In order to manipulate somatic activity, three conditions were used involving two operant schedules as well as two intensities of the UCS, in the expectation that in two conditions the CER would inhibit bar pressing, and hence somatic activity, but would increase somatic activity in the third condition. Although the desired somatic effects were not always found, the direction of the heart rate changes during the 15-second CS-UCS were consistent with the direction of the somatic changes. For example, in one dog when the CER was imposed on a variable interval (VI) 30 baseline and then a differential reinforcement of low rates (DRL) baseline using a lower intensity UCS—bar-pressing and general somatic activity both decreased and heart rate decelerated. However, when the intensity of the UCS was increased to the level used with the VI schedule, and the CER then superimposed on the DRL baseline, general activity and heart rate both increased even though bar pressing remained suppressed. It was not uncommon for bar pressing and general activity to go in opposite directions during the ISI. In such cases, heart rate changes always were directionally consistent with general activity (Black and DeToledo 1972). As in previous work, there was little evidence that somatic (general activity) and cardiac effects were independent, i.e., directionally out of phase.

A third study concerns the cardiac-somatic interrelationship in human Ss using operant procedures to modify heart rate (Obrist et al. 1973b). The necessity for this effort was indicated by the fact that little systematic work has been reported under these conditions on the evaluation of somatic effects. An avoidance paradigm was used in which a strong shock could be avoided and a monetary bonus obtained on any 1 of 33 60-second trials if heart rate changes reached criterion. A shaping procedure was used with feedback given on a beat-by-beat basis when criterion was met. Any influence of somatic activity was evaluated by manipulating through instructions the extent subjects controlled somatic activity. Also, four measures of somatic activity were obtained and quantified so as to assess the extent somatic activity was in fact controlled and/or associated with the effects of the contingency on heart rate. Five groups of subjects were run. In two groups—one reinforced for increasing and the other for decreasing heart rate—somatic activity was maximally controlled by the use of paced respiration and instructions. These are referred to as the maximum control groups. In two more groups—again one reinforced for increasing and another for decreasing heart rate—no effort was made to control somatic changes. In a fifth group, reinforced for increasing heart rate, an attempt was made to control minimally somatic activity but just through the use of instructions. This was done because when no control was used and heart rate was reinforced for increasing, very large increases in somatic activity were found, and it was thought desirable to have a condition which was between maximal and no control of somatic activity. Also, the type of instruction used here was similar to previous studies, thus, making this group more comparable to work of other investigators.

The results indicate in a reasonably consistent manner that the contingency had a similar effect on heart rate and somatic activity, although there was observed in one group an influence of the contingency which was specific to heart rate. When the effects of the contingency on heart rate were evaluated with regard to the instructional control of somatic activity, the magnitude of the base-S_D level differences was a function of instructional control, particularly in the three groups reinforced for increasing heart rate (see Figure 8.1). Base-S_D level heart rate increases were largest with no instructional control of somatic activity, and smallest with maximal control. When heart rate was reinforced for decreasing, neither experimental group demonstrated a pronounced effect, there being only a small deceleration of heart rate on the later trials. An analysis of the somatic changes revealed that three of the measures, i.e., general activity, chin electromyogram (EMG), and respiration, were—like heart rate—directly a function of instructional control in the three groups reinforced for increasing heart rate. The largest base-level-S_D level increases were found with no instructional control, and the smallest with maximum control (see Figure 8.2).

However, on the fourth somatic measure, i.e., eye movements and blinks, an effect of the contingency was found in the two groups reinforced for decreasing heart rate (see Figure 8.3). In all groups, on the first trial block, there was a decrease in occular activity during the S_D, an effect likely associated with fixating on the visual feedback stimulus. Thereafter over the remaining trial blocks, these base-S_D level decreases became progressively greater in the two groups reinforced for decreasing heart rate, with the decrease being significantly larger in the group with no instructional control. In the three groups reinforced for increasing heart rate, the base-S_D level decreases observed on the first

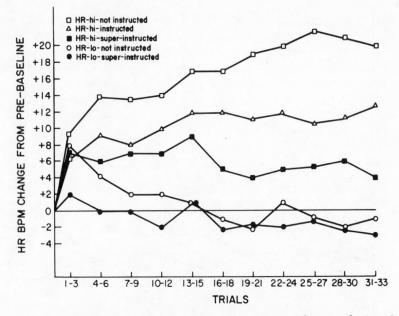

FIGURE 8.1 S_D *Control of Heart Rate. Heart rate changes during S_D as determined by difference between $\bar{x}$ base level heart rate just prior to start of each trial and $\bar{x}$ heart rate during 60 second S_D of each trial.*

NOTE: Data averaged over blocks of 3 trials.

NOTE: HR-hi in legend indicates *increases* in heart rate reinforced
HR-lo in legend indicates *decreases* in heart rate reinforced
Non instructed in legend indicates no control of somatic activity attempted
Instructed in legend indicates minimal control of somatic activity attempted
Super instructed in legend indicates that somatic activity is maximally controlled

trial block became progressively smaller, but not consistently with instructional control, in that the minimal instructional control group showed the largest effect.

Finally, as another means to assess the influence of instructional control on both heart rate and somatic activity, base-S_D level differences between heart rate and each of three somatic measures were correlated in each trial block. The correlations were obtained separately for the two groups with maximum instructional control and the three groups with either minimal or no instructional control. In both instances, the groups were combined. With maximal instructional control, no significant correlations could be found on any trial block. However, with either minimal or no control, heart rate was found to be positively and significantly correlated with each somatic measure but only after the first three trial blocks, i.e., nine trials, where acquisition effects were most pronounced.

The only evidence in these five groups that the contingency may have had a specific effect on heart rate independent of somatic activity

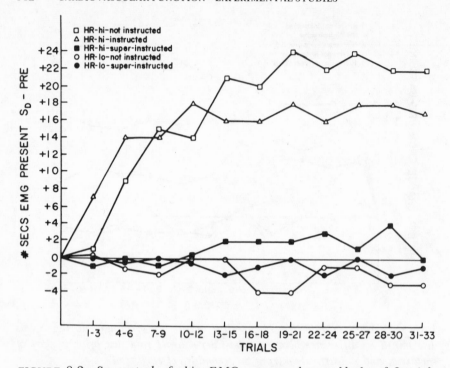

FIGURE 8.2 S_D *control of chin EMG*—*averaged over blocks of 3 trials.*
Legend symbols and derivation of S_D *control values same as in Fig. 8.1.*
   NOTE: General activity was also measured and quantified—and showed similar effects
as chin EMG. Respiration was also quantified in regard to the number of trials which
showed increases or decreases in frequency and amplitude. These results also paralleled
changes observed in chin EMG and general activity.

is suggested by the difference in base-S_D level heart rate observed in
the two groups with maximum instructional control. That is, heart rate
was significantly more accelerated in the group reinforced for increasing heart rate, but on none of the somatic measures other than eye
movements were these groups differentiated. However, there was also
observed on the first trial block that all five groups accelerated heart
rate during the S_D. Yet the groups were not significantly differentiated
on the magnitude of this heart rate effect, nor did it appear related
to increases in somatic activity. Thus, the acceleration of heart rate
observed in the group with maximal instructional control and reinforced for increasing heart rate may have reflected, not an effect of
the contingency, but just a perpetuation of this early trial effect. For
this reason, two additional groups of subjects were run in which feedback and shock avoidance were given randomly or noncontingently
with respect to any aspect of the subject's activity. In one group, somatic activity was maximally controlled by instructions and in the other
minimally controlled. As compared to the experimental groups, on

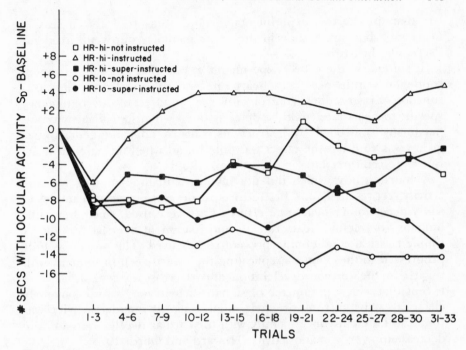

FIGURE 8.3   *S_D control of eye movements and blinks averaged over blocks of 3 trials. Legend symbols and derivation of S_D control values are the same as Fig. 8.1.*

NOTE: All groups show a decrease in occular activity on the early trial which is likely associated with fixating on visual feedback signal. The contingency thereafter modifies this effect and in a direction consistent with heart rate changes particularly where somatic activity was not controlled.

both heart rate and two of the somatic measures quantified, an effect of the contingency specific to heart rate was indicated in the experimental group with maximal control of somatic activity and reinforced for increasing heart rate. This initial acceleration of heart rate to the S_D was found to attenuate rapidly in the noncontingent group with maximal instructional control. Heart rate was significantly less accelerated over the trial blocks than in the experimental group with maximum control reinforced for increasing heart rate, while there were no significant differences on the somatic measures between these two groups. On the other hand, this noncontingent group was not differentiated on heart rate from the experimental group with maximal control reinforced for decreasing heart rate. The noncontingent group with minimal control, although demonstrating an accelerated heart rate over the trial blocks, was significantly differentiated on both heart rate and somatic measures, from the three experimental groups with either minimal or no control. On all measures, the base-S_D level differences were less than in the two experimental groups reinforced for increasing heart rate, but larger than in the experimental group reinforced for decreasing heart rate.

In summary, these two experiments reveal that the reinforcement contingency influences both heart rate and somatic activity and as a function of instructional control. However, an effect of the contingency specific to heart rate could be demonstrated when somatic activity was maximally controlled by instructions, once a noncontingent control group was run, but the effect was only found when increases in heart rate were reinforced.

A fourth study, which did not involve a manipulation of somatic activity, represented our first efforts to develop an animal model to study deceleratory heart rate effects. Cats were used, since they—like humans—decelerate heart rate in anticipation of aversive stimuli. A simple classical conditioning procedure was used. This work has only progressed to the point of replicating the effects seen in humans with regard to the cardiac deceleration and decrease in somatic activity, except that a new parameter of somatic activity was assessed, namely electrical activity from the pyramidal tract. Pyramidal activity was found to fade out concomitantly with the cardiac deceleration and the decrease in overt somatic activity (Howard and Obrist 1973).

A relationship between heart rate and somatic activity has been reported now by a number of other investigators. These studies have used several different behavioral paradigms and experimental strategies, as well as several different mammalian species. These data are briefly summarized in Table 8.1. In the column of the table labeled "Direction of Effects," increases indicate that both somatic and cardiac rate changes increase, while decreases indicate the converse in each type of measure. Where both types of directional changes are indicated for a given study, it indicates that both type of effects were seen. For example, Roberts and Young (1971) report a decrease in general somatic activity and heart rate when averaged over all trials and subjects, in rats with a CER procedure. Yet when a trial-by-trial analysis was done, there were trials in which somatic activity increased as did heart rate.

There are aspects of the data reported in these experiments which should be noted since they supplement our own data and provide a broader perspective on the cardiac-somatic relationship. First, cardiac and somatic activity have been assessed under conditions which involve a broader range of stimulating conditions, such as naturally-elicited fighting behavior in cats (Adams et al. 1968, 1969); threats from a predator in wild rodents (Hofer 1970); and the use of self-induced alterations in consciousness (Wallace 1970). Second, experimental manipulations have been used, which again suggest that the concomitance of

TABLE 8.1 *Summary of Studies on Cardiac-Somatic Effects*

Author(s)	Specie	Conditions	Somatic Measure	Direction of Effects
Adams et al. 1968, 1969	Cat	Naturally elicited fighting	EMG	Decreases-Increases
Belmaker et al. 1972	Human	Operant cond.- HR	Muscle Tension	Increases
Black and DeToledo 1972	Rat	Classical cond.- aversive	General activity- EMG	Decreases
Black and DeToledo 1972	Dog	Operant cond. of somatic activity	Bar pressing	Increases-Decreases
Black and DeToledo 1972	Dog	Operant cond. of hippocampal theta	Animal curarized	Increases-Decreases
Chase and Harper 1971	Cat	Operant modification of EEG	EMG- Eye movements- Respiration	Decreases
Cohen 1972	Human	Operant conditioning HR & EMG	Respiration EMG	Increases
Cohen and Johnson 1971	Human	Classical cond. aversive	EMG	Increases-Decreases
Freyschuss 1970	Human	Isometric tension in fore arm	EMG	Increases
Goesling and Brener 1972	Rat	Operant cond. of general activity	General activity	Decreases-Increases
Hein 1969	Cat	Classical cond.-aversive	EMG- Respiration EMG	Decreases
Hofer 1971	Wild Rodent	Natural stressors Open field preditors	General activity EMG	Increases-Decreases
Holloway and Parsons 1972	Human	Reaction time	Respiration EMG	Increases-Decreases
Jennings et al 1971	Human	Reaction time	EMG	Increases-Decreases
Johns 1971	Human	Operant cond.	Respiration	Decreases-Increases
Roberts 1971	Rat	Classical conditioning aversive	General activity	Increases-Decreases
Vanderwolf and Vanderwart 1970	Rat	Food deprivation	General activity	Increases
Wallace 1970	Human	Transcendental Meditation	O_2 consumption	Decreases
Wells 1972	Human	Operant conditioning	Respiration	Increases

cardiac and somatic effects is biologically substantive in that a consistency is observed between heart rate and somatic activity when the latter is manipulated either directly or by modifying the electrical activity of the brain (Goesling and Brener 1972; Black and DeToledo 1972; Chase and Harper 1971; Cohen and Johnson 1971b). For example, Chase and Harper, using appetitive reinforcement, operantly modified 12 to 14 cps electrical activity from the sensorimotor cortex in cats, a type of electrical activity usually associated with behavioral inactivity. They found concomitant with bursts or trains of such electrical activity both somatic quiescence and a pronounced cardiac deceleration. The importance of this study is that it demonstrates an integration of cardiac and somatic effects upon manipulation of cortical activity, an effect which is quite necessary in establishing whether cardiac and somatic events have a common central mediating mechanism. Also, the observation that heart rate is modified in the curarized state upon the operant modification of hippocampal theta (Black and DeToledo 1972), indicates that the heart rate changes are not dependent on the occurrence of somatic activity, but rather that the heart rate changes are initiated by central processes associated with the initiation of somatic events. Also consistent with the possibility of a common central nervous system (CNS) initiating mechanism is the observation by Freyschuss (1970) who found in human Ss an increase in heart rate upon the instruction to make an isometric muscular response in one arm, even though the response could not be executed because the arm muscles were curarized.

Several studies have been unable to demonstrate an influence on heart rate of experimental manipulations which were independent of somatic effects, even though the experimental procedures and methods of data quantification used should have delineated such differential influences (Roberts and Young 1971; Adams et al. 1968, 1969; Vanderwolf and Vanderwart 1970; Black and DeToledo 1972; Goesling and Brener 1972). For one of the first times in psychophysiological studies, O_2 consumption has been measured (Wallace 1970) which may prove to be the most reliable method we have to assess total somatic involvement. Finally, one of the most complete pictures of hemodynamic events, in addition to heart rate, is provided in the studies by Adams et al. (1968, 1969). Here cardiac output, total peripheral resistance, muscle and visceral blood flow, and blood pressure were assessed in cats as they first prepared and then engaged in a brief episode of fighting with another cat who initiated the attack. The effects observed are consistent with the metabolic requirements of each situation. When the cats prepared for or anticipated being attacked, they usually were inactive. This was associated with a decrease in heart rate, cardiac output, and blood flow, i.e., vasocontriction, in both the viscera and muscles of the hind leg. When the cats responded to the attack, heart rate and cardiac output increased, visceral blood flow still remained decreased, but muscle flow increased—providing the cats used those muscles in fighting back. Blood pressure, interestingly, did not show particularly consistent changes with it oscillating with respect to the baseline between small decreases and increases.

CARDIAC-SOMATIC UNCOUPLING

Although the evidence just presented quite consistently indicates a coupling of heart rate to somatic activity in a variety of behavioral paradigms, it is commonly assumed that behavioral processes can influence the heart independent of somatic activity. Such an assumption has been implicit in several areas of psychophysiological research, ranging from the use of heart rate as an index of emotional and motivational states (Gantt 1960; Malmo and Belanger 1967) to the more recent work on response contingent reinforcement (Miller 1969). However, there is little definitive evidence which either demonstrates an uncoupling of heart rate from somatic activity or the relevant biological and behavioral parameters which might be involved. Therefore, we have initiated experiments which are intended to determine if cardiac and somatic effects can be uncoupled, and then to determine the means both biologically and behaviorally by which the effect is brought about. The work up until now has progressed sufficiently to justify a summary of results.

In our previous work in which both aversive and nonaversive behavioral paradigms were used and in which heart rate could not be demonstrated to be independent of concomitant somatic effects, it appeared that the primary neural influence on heart rate was mediated through the vagal innervation (Obrist et al. 1970a). On the other hand, there is evidence which suggests that sympathetic influences on the heart might be more independent of somatic activity (Obrist et al. 1970b). However, in the light of several other lines of evidence (Obrist et al. 1970b) it appeared that sympathetic influences might be more clearly manifested through the force rather than the rate at which the heart beats. Thus, the initial experiments were intended to evaluate just this latter question, concerning the manner in which sympathetic influences are manifested, and were not concerned with the question of somatic influences. For this purpose, dogs were chronically prepared so as to measure contractility and then exposed to a simple classical aversive conditioning procedure.[3] Sympathetic influences were evaluated by the use of beta-adrenergic pharmacological blockade. It was found that contractility was more completely attenuated than was heart rate when sympathetic influences were blocked, thus indicating that contractility would provide a more unequivocal index of sympathetic influences (Obrist et al. 1972b).

The next experiments have involved human Ss (Obrist et al. 1973c). The first study sought to determine, with the use of aversive conditioning procedures, whether anticipatory sympathetic effects on contractility could be observed where previously vagal excitatory influences had been noted to dominate sympathetic influences on heart rate (Obrist, Wood, and Perez-Reyes 1965) which were concomitant with decreases in somatic activity (Obrist 1968). In this context, an independence of contractility and somatic effects was considered most convincingly demonstrated if reliable changes in each measure were demonstrated, but were in the opposite direction—contractility increasing, somatic activity decreasing (see Obrist et al. 1970b). Although this initial effort was only piloted on a small sample of Ss, no sympathetic influence could be observed on contractility. That is, there were no anticipatory increases in contractility when heart rate and somatic activity was decreasing.

On the basis of other considerations, all of which indicated that sympathetic influences might be observed if a more stressful task were used, human Ss were next exposed to a reaction time task using monetary rewards for fast performance and the threat of strong shock if performance was too slow. This task was made more stressful than simple aversive conditioning by requiring very fast reaction times with the S never certain whether he would receive shock until it was actually administered eight seconds after execution of the response, and by not allowing the S to have any prior experience with the shock until the first time he received it after a less than criterion response (Elliott 1966a). In previous aversive conditioning studies, Ss had always been exposed to the shock prior to conditioning since they set their own shock levels. Because an increase in contractility was seen in the pilot Ss, this study was then carried out in a sample of 33 Ss, in 11 of whom the sympathetic innervation was blocked pharmacologically. This was done in order to determine the extent to which sympathetic influences were responsible for the contractility changes, as well as to determine possible sympathetic influences on heart rate.

The data for heart rate and contractility changes are summarized on a second-by-second basis for both experimental groups in Figures 8.4 and 8.5. These data represent changes from the baseline in each 30 seconds following the ready signal, the first 8 seconds representing the preparatory interval (PI); the next 8 seconds (9 to 16) representing the period the S is waiting for the shock; and the next 14 seconds (17 to 30) representing the period following where shock is administered, but omitting all trials on which shock was actually givenm On the measure of contractility, i.e., rate of change or slope of the carotid

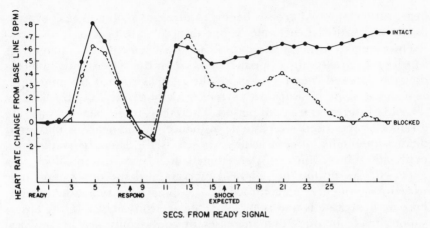

FIGURE 8.4   *Second-by-second changes in heart rate during a stressful reaction time task with the sympathetic innervation of the heart intact and pharmacologically blocked.*

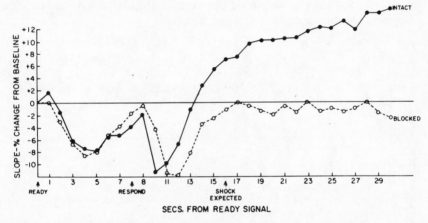

FIGURE 8.5   *Second-by-second changes in cardiac contractility during a stressful reaction time task with the sympathetic innervation of the heart intact and pharmacologically blocked.*

pulse wave, no sympathetic excitatory influence is apparent until just before shock is expected, at which point the slope of the pulse wave progressively increases until the end of the measurement period. The effect of sympathetic blockade was to block these slope increases completely. On the other hand, heart rate showed a triphasic effect up to the point where the slope increases were observed, which appears of vagal origin in that it is of the same magnitude and latency regardless whether the sympathetic innervation is intact or not. However, coincident with the increase in slope near where shock is expected,

heart rate in the two groups begins to diverge. With an intact sympathetic innervation, heart rate begins to accelerate becoming progressively larger up through the end of the measurement period, an effect
which now parallels the slope increase. When the sympathetic innervation was blocked, heart rate gradually returns toward baseline, and,
as with the slope measure with sympathetic blockade, is at baseline by
the end of the measurement period. Therefore, these data demonstrate
a rather pronounced sympathetic influence on the heart as measured
by the slope index of contractility whose onset is associated with shock
expectation but which is perpetuated well past where shock was
expected. As important, is the observation that once sympathetic
excitatory influences on contractility are observed, a sympathetic influence on heart rate is now seen. The data are consistent with the observations made in dogs that increases in contractility are unequivocal
indices of sympathetic excitation than is heart rate. Yet they also
demonstrate more forcefully than in this previous study that heart rate,
once the sympathetics become active, also is influenced. Therefore, the
data permitted an evaluation of the relationship between sympathetic
influences on the heart and somatic activity.

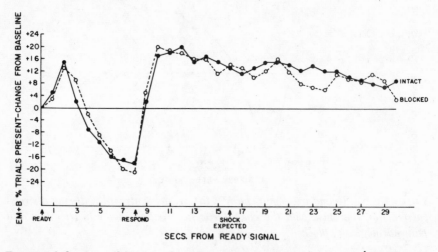

FIGURE 8.6   *Second-by-second changes in eye movements and blinks during
a stressful reaction time task with the sympathetic innervation of the heart intact
and pharmacologically blocked.*

For this purpose, a second-by-second analysis was carried out on
three measures of somatic activity, i.e., general activity, chin EMG, and
vertical eye movements and blinks. All three measures show comparable trends in both experimental groups. This is illustrated for eye
movements in Figure 8.6. As with heart rate, there is an initial triphasic

effect which parallels the heart rate changes. That is, in the early part of the PI, there is an increase in somatic activity and then a decrease which anticipates responding. Immediately following the execution of the task, there is another increase in somatic activity. Thereafter, and just prior to where shock is expected, all three somatic measures begin a gradual decrease toward base level. It is at this time that sympathetic effects become manifest with both heart rate and contractility showing a gradually increasing amount of activity up through the end of the measurement period. For example, between the average amount of activity in the three seconds terminating with the second where the UCS would occur and the average in the last three seconds of the measurement period, heart rate is observed to increase by 60% and contractility by 126%, while somatic activity between these two time periods averaged over all three measures decreased by 35%. Additionally, when the sympathetic innervation was intact, heart rate was significantly and positively correlated (r (21) = + .49, p < .02) with a summated measure of somatic activity in the three seconds just prior to UCS onset where the second-by-second curves had diverged little. However, during the last three seconds of the measurement period, where the second-by-second changes for somatic and cardiac activity have diverged, there is no correlation (r (21) = − .21, p > .10). Therefore, we seemed to have observed in the latter part of the measurement period a pronounced sympathetic effect on both heart rate and contractility which by two criteria, i.e., direction of change and correlation of the magnitude of effects, are unrelated to somatic activity.

There are two other observations to be noted. First, for the first time, we have not observed a deceleration of heart rate to anticipate shock. Although heart rate tends to decrease slightly where shock is expected, it is well above the baseline in both experimental groups. This effect likely involves both a loss of vagal inhibition associated with somatic activity and the onset of synergistic sympathetic activity. Second, sympathetic effects were greatest on the early trials, and dissipated as the experiment progressed. In some Ss, it was so great on the first trial that its full magnitude couldn't be quantified because the upper calibration range on the recording equipment was not set high enough.

In summary, these data indicate that an uncoupling of heart rate from somatic activity can be observed once sympathetic influences on the heart were evoked. It might be recalled that in the study previously described using operant procedures to modify heart rate, a similar independence of heart rate and somatic activity was observed in all seven groups of subjects on the early trials, and that this effect was perpetuated by the contingency in only one group where somatic activity was maximally controlled and heart rate reinforced for increasing. Although it has not as yet been determined whether these heart rate effects do in fact reflect sympathetic influences, the effects seen and the situation used are comparable enough to suggest that the uncoupling of heart rate from somatic activity is a replicable effect.

ISSUES, PROBLEMS, IMPLICATIONS

The issue of mediation.

A point of view in psychophysiological research has been that to the extent visceral events are related to striate muscular activity they have little significance to behavioral processes in the sense that they have been referred to as artifact (Smith 1967) or errors of measurement (Lazarus 1966). Considerable effort has been made particularly in the area of operant research to control for this "irrelevant" influence of somatic activity on autonomic events such as through the use of the curarized preparation. Recently, this point of view has come under criticism in a couple of respects, all of which suggests the need to reexamine the mediation issue (Black 1972a; Obrist et al. 1970b).

Although somatic activity has been viewed as a possible mediator of cardiovascular events, it has never been explicitly stated what the biological mechanism or process is. It would appear that mediation could be viewed biologically in two ways. One, the occurrence of some somatic event literally causes a cardiovascular change through afferent feedback mechanisms. There is some validity to this position biologically. For example, proprioceptive feedback from the striate musculature seems to exert an excitatory influence on both hypothalamic and cortical activity (Gellhorn 1964). Also, during exercise, metabolic byproducts significantly contribute to local vasodilatory activity in the exercising musculature (Bard 1968) and may also influence cardiac output (Kao and Ray 1954).

Another means by which mediation can be viewed is that the central nervous system exerts a direct influence on cardiovascular activity in that upon the initiation of change in somatic activity, there is a simultaneously initiated cardiovascular adjustment. That is to say both somatic and cardiac changes are initiated and controlled by the same CNS processes. The best evidence of this type of common CNS mediating mechanism is the data indicating that cardiovascular changes that are normally concomitant with somatic activity can be still observed even when the somatic changes are prevented from occurring by curarization (Rushmer and Smith 1959; Freychuss 1970; Delgado 1960; Lofving 1961; Hoff, Kell, and Carroll 1963; Black and DeToledo 1972; Goesling and Brener 1972). In this context, the cardiovascular events associated with somatic activity can be viewed as a visceral counterpart of the somatic event, in which case neither peripheral event, i.e., somatic or cardiac, causes the other but rather that they are concomitant events. The point to be made is that curarization is an effective control for somatic mediation only in regard to the first type of mediating mechanisms involving proprioceptive and metabolic effects resulting from the occurrence of somatic activity. The relative contribution of each of these types of mediational process is not known. Nonetheless, the evidence is sufficient to suggest that cardiovascular changes associated with somatic activity are significantly influenced by the direct CNS control of cardiovascular events. Thus, to the extent such direct central control of cardiovascular changes does exist, curarization is an irrelevant control for somatic mediation. On the other hand, to control somatic mediation when it involves the direct CNS control of cardiovascular changes presents problems. That is, we do not have at our disposal any direct means to block or prevent the initiation of somatic activities, such as with cortical lesions, without simultaneously influencing cardiovascular changes, because the two types of events likely involve very similar neural structures (Hoff et al. 1963). This does not deny that cardiovascular changes cannot be influenced by CNS processes which are not involved in the control of somatic activity. Thus, we must resort to methods which more indirectly control for somatic influences such as training subjects to control their somatic musculature (see Chapter 12, Black; Black and DeToledo 1972; Webb and Obrist 1967; Sutterer and Obrist 1972).

Mediation from a different perspective.

One can argue that the issue of mediation should be put in a different perspective in that one should also exploit, not just control or ignore, the relationship between cardiovascular and somatic activity.

Behavioral significance of coupling. In those behavioral paradigms where heart rate and somatic activity are found to be related, a consideration of the cardiac-somatic relationship offers several advantages. First, a biological basis for the cardiac rate changes is provided. That is, coupling of cardiac and somatic activities can be viewed biologically as involving the metabolic functions of the cardiovascular system. Alterations in metabolic requirements, such as O_2 consumption, are met by alterations in cardiac output, for which heart rate is a significant determinant (see Obrist et al. 1970b). This metabolic function is obvious with extensive somatic acts, such as exercise. The fact that cardiac and somatic events are interrelated in certain behavioral paradigms where the alterations in heart rate and somatic activity are very minimal, e.g., a simple RT task, suggests even more strongly that these two systems can be rather precisely integrated. That is, the cardiovascular system and somatic musculature can be so finely tuned or coupled that the least alteration in somatic activity will be accompanied by an equally discrete alteration in heart rate. In turn, these biological considerations suggest how we might view the behavioral relevance of heart rate. To the extent that heart rate is so attuned to alterations in somatic activity, it would appear that we have available in the action of one muscle, the heart, an index of the activity of the striate musculature. This offers an advantage considering the number of muscles in the body and the difficulty one would face in trying to assess striate activity. It follows then that, to the extent that knowledge of the activity of the striate musculature is important to our understanding of behavioral processes, heart rate may be a useful biological tool. Specifically, a case can be made that the phasic decreases in heart rate and task-irrelevant somatic activity which are associated with responding in the simple reaction-time task are biological manifestations of momentary or phasic alterations in attention. This is indicated by the fact that in adults performance speed is directly related to the magnitude of these decreases in phasic cardiac and somatic activity (Obrist, Webb, and Sutterer 1969; Obrist et al. 1970a; Webb and Obrist 1970).

In this context it might be noted that another and complementary position concerning the significance of heart rate to behavioral research, has been offered by Elliott (1969, 1970b, 1972) who proposes that ". . . heart rate accelerates in a situation in which there are action-instigating elements, and not where there are not, even when both kinds of situation could be described as emotion provoking or arousing" (Elliott 1969, p. 222). Although Elliott has not until recently (Chapter 25, Elliott) evaluated somatic activity per se, for example by measuring EMG, he has evaluated the effects on tonic levels of heart rate of manipulations which alter the necessity for subjects making some behavioral response. For example, tonic levels of heart rate were found to be inversely related to task difficulty in a perceptual task involving color naming (the Stroop Test) but directly related to the rate at which the subject verbally responds (Elliott 1969).

Another reason to consider the relationship of heart rate and somatic activity within this psychobiological perspective, is that it provides limits as to what one might expect heart rate to tell us about behavior. That is to say, heart rate, to the extent it is coupled to somatic activity, will provide uniquely useful information about behavior only if the activity of the striate musculature is relevant to behavioral processes. For example, if it can be shown that an emotional response, such as fear, is associated with behavioral immobility (e.g., Hofer 1970) then heart rate might provide the simplest and most reliable index of such an emotional state. On the other hand, if the relationship between the musculature and behavioral processes is unknown, unpredictable, or irrelevant, then heart rate would provide little or no useful information. Such an awareness of this limitation might act to avoid futile efforts

in using heart rate as an index of behavioral processes, such as is illustrated by the work with conditioned emotional responses where heart
rate had been viewed as a unidimensional index of emotional processes
(See Rescorla and Solomon 1967).

One of the problems we are faced with in regard to the behavioral
relevance of either phasic or tonic heart rate effects concerns the
sensitivity of heart rate as an index of striate muscular activity and
associated behavioral states. One approach has been to determine
whether phasic changes in heart rate associated with responding in a
RT task are sensitive to manipulation of attentional states. The results
of two recently reported studies would seem to indicate so. In each
case the phasic heart rate deceleration was largest when attentional
requirements were greatest as manipulated by the certainty of whether
the respond signal would be presented (Higgins 1971) and the requirement either to abstain from responding (Higgins 1971) or delay
responding (Jennings et al. 1971). That is either the more uncertainty
the subject had as to which of the two signals would be presented, i.e.,
the respond or no respond, or the requirement upon making the discrimination whether to respond immediately or delay responding, were
both associated with greater cardiac deceleration. There have also been
other reports which suggest, although less convincingly, that such
phasic heart rate changes are modified by manipulation of attentional
states (Eason and Dudley 1970; Sroufe 1971a).

As to the problem of the sensitivity of heart rate to changes in phasic
somatic activities per se, there is evidence indicating that under certain
conditions heart rate is less sensitive than some somatic indices to manipulations of behavioral states. For example, in the RT paradigm, we
have found that with an irregularly presented 2-second PI, the heart
rate deceleration is considerably less than with the longer PI's while
the magnitude of the somatic decreases is almost as great as with long
PI's (Obrist et al. 1970a). Also within the RT paradigm where we
evaluated cardiac and somatic effects developmentally (Obrist et al.
1973a), the magnitude of the phasic decrease in heart rate was not
related to age, while the magnitude of the phasic decrease in one aspect
of somatic activity, i.e., eye movements and blinks, was. Assuming that
older Ss were better able to attend, then occular activity in this situation
has to be considered a more sensitive index than heart rate of the
momentary shifts in attentional states associated with performance. In
these situations, the decreases in heart rate and somatic activity are reliable effects and directionally consistent. Thus, it does not appear that
cardiac and somatic changes are uncoupled.

What is suggested is that there are other considerations to be made
not directly concerned with nonsomatic mediated behavioral influences
on heart rate. For example, with a short 2-second PI, the small heart

rate changes might reflect an inherent lag in neural influences on heart rate that is not apparent with somatic activity (Smith 1945; Lofving 1961). In the developmental study, the coupling of heart rate and somatic activity seems to be manifested more consistently with regard to more extensive somatic acts, such as body movements. That is, phasic decreases in two other parameters of somatic activity, i.e., general activity and chin EMG, although reliable changes, were like heart rate, unrelated to age. On the other hand, all three measures showed consistent age related base level differences. One can conclude then that the magnitude of the phasic heart rate changes appears related to the magnitude of the phasic differences in these more extensive somatic acts. Thus, the influence of age on base level seems to place a restriction on the use of phasic changes under these conditions other than for occular activity.

Another potential restriction on the sensitivity of heart rate is in situations where an increase in task relevant somatic activities is essential for efficient performance. In this case, increases in task relevant somatic activity would influence heart rate to accelerate which in turn might either attenuate or override any deceleratory effects associated with an inhibition of task irrelevant activity. In our previous work the influence on heart rate of task relevant somatic activity appears minimal. For example, no anticipatory increases in EMG were found during the PI of an RT task on the responding muscles of the arm (Webb and Obrist 1970).[4] In summary, although it appears under certain circumstances that heart rate can be a sensitive index of somatic activities and associated behavioral states, there are other conditions in which heart rate does not appear to provide useful information about the biological substrate of such behavioral processes. What is needed are more parametric studies which will hopefully detail in a more systematic manner the relative merits of this biological event.

Coupling and nonsomatic influences. A second major reason to consider the cardiac somatic relationship is that it might provide the necessary starting point with which to evaluate how cardiovascular activity is influenced by behavioral processes independently of somatic activity. If one is interested in such nonsomatic influences, then it is important to determine the extent somatic influences are present or relevant. In a sense, it is like controlling for error variance. However, there is a possibly even more important reason to consider somatic influences. Even though cardiovascular activity may in a given situation or condition appear independent of somatic activity, somatic influences may still be relevant in other ways. For example, the manner by which the cardiovascular system is integrated so as to perform its metabolic function may place restraints on just what pattern of cardiovascular change one observes. That is to say, the manner by which nonsomatic influences are manifested cardiovascularly is not random or haphazard, but may be directed by the manner the cardiovascular system responds to somatic influences. For example, an exercise like adjustment—i.e., increased heart rate and cardiac output and, when measured, increased muscular blood flow—has been found in both normotensive and hypertensive subjects when stressed by a difficult conceptual task (Brod 1963), and in the resting state in individuals diagnosed as having a hyperkinetic circulatory state (Frohlich 1969). Such effects have led Brod et al. to conclude ". . . that the common denominator in all these situations for this type of hemodynamic response is either strenuous muscular exercise or preparation for muscular exercise" and, in regard to hypertension per se, that ". . . that hemodynamic basis of the increase in blood pressure in essential hypertension might be considered a fixation of this preparation for muscular action" (Brod, et al. 1962 P. 347). Thus, a knowledge of the manner by which cardiovascular and somatic events are integrated also seems to provide a direction to look for the basis for such cardiovascular events.

What remains uncertain is how biologically the cardiovascular system can mobilize for muscular activity and yet the organism doesn't execute such acts. Several possibilities are suggested in this regard. For one thing, the organism may in fact resort to subtle or covert somatic activities, such as muscular tensing, which interact with the acute stress to precipitate or trigger an exercise-like cardiovascular response. A second possibility is that the organism needs only to anticipate recourse to activity as a means to cope with the stress such as Elliott (1969) has suggested. This is in contrast to resorting to immobility such as passivity or helplessness, i.e., where the organism views the situation and stress as inescapable and feels nothing can be done about it. A third possibility, particularly when considering more chronic conditions such as hypertension, is that cardiovascular activity was coupled to somatic activity some time in the past history of the organism, but gradually became uncoupled due to a selective inhibition of somatic activity resulting in a cardiovascular effect which Brod et al. (1962) refers to as a fixation for muscular action. Granted these proposals are highly speculative as well as imprecisely formulated in regard to critical stimulus and biological parameters. But it suggests a direction—namely to determine whether somatic activity or the anticipation of such act as necessary precursors or triggers.

In this regard, there is a little relevant evidence. For example, in early or labile hypertensive states, the elevated pressure is commonly associated with an increased pumping action of the heart and a normal peripheral vascular resistance. That somatic activity might influence such hemodynamic events is suggested by the evidence that O_2 consumption is elevated in such individuals (Lund-Johansen 1967; Sanner-stedt 1966; Julius and Conway 1968; Gorlin et al. 1959; Ogden and Shock 1939). Also in the stressful RT task previously described, in which an independence was observed between cardiac and somatic activities, there is one bit of evidence which bears on this triggering notion. This is that although heart rate during the latter three seconds of the measurement period is unrelated to concomitant somatic activity, it is positively correlated to somatic events occurring just prior to shock onset (r (21) = + .57, p < .01). This indicates that subjects who demonstrated the largest change in somatic activity just prior to where they expected the shock showed the largest cardiac rate changes 15 seconds later, even though heart rate and somatic activity at this later time appear unrelated. The possibility that the exercise-like cardiovascular response is common to situations where the organism is actively trying to cope with stress rather than resorting to immobility or giving up is suggested by our recent data from the chronic dog preparation during aversive conditioning (Obrist et al. 1972b).

Here, pronounced sympathetic effects are commonly seen only on the first conditioning day where the dog appears to be trying to escape the situation. As conditioning progresses, sympathetic effects on the heart become minimal and most of the dogs appear resigned to the inescapable nature of the situation, usually remaining quite immobile except for some postural changes as they anticipate the UCS. This does not appear to be just adapting to the UCS, since UCS intensity is commonly increased and the dog appears bothered by the UCS. What is suggested then, is that the influences of nonsomatic processes on the heart are not completely independent of somatic influences, but act through them in such a manner that the resulting pattern of cardiovascular changes is in part determined by the manner in which the cardiovascular system is integrated biologically with metabolic processes. Furthermore, somatic activity or the anticipation of such may somewhere either in the past or immediate history of the organism act as necessary precussors or triggers of this exercise-like cardiovascular response.

Other issues

The biological bases for those instances where the two parameters of cardiac function appear independent of concurrent somatic effects is not particularly clear. One can only say that at least in one instance it does involve sympathetic influences on the heart. Currently, we are determining, through the direct measurement of blood pressure, whether the sympathetic effect is not secondary to a hypotensive episode which might act to facilitate sympathetic discharge and, in the case of the contractile measure, additionally facilitate the rate of change of the pulse pressure. Data so far available indicate that there are phasic decreases in blood pressure, but they appear inconsistently related to the slope and heart rate changes. Also in regard to sympathetic influences, it would appear that they are more readily apparent on other parameters of cardiovascular activity, such as vasomotor activity, than on heart rate and contractility. In turn, this raises the question as to what extent are parameters like peripheral blood flow and blood pressure coupled to somatic activity. There is no question that blood flow through muscles will increase during muscular activity. However, blood flow through muscles can also increase during acute stress even in the absence of measurable changes in metabolic activity (Brod 1963).

Similarly, visceral blood flow has been found to decrease both in anticipation of and during fighting in cats regardless whether the cats are quiet or active (Adams et al. 1968, 1969). It would also appear that cutaneous blood flow bears a similar lack of relationship to somatic activity, although somatic influences do not appear to have been evaluated in any systematic manner in this latter case. In any event, there is sufficient data to conclude that vasomotor activity is not consistently related to somatic activity.

Whether vasomotor changes, however, will provide more useful information about nonsomatically linked behavioral influences then heart rate would appear problematical. The picture here is also somewhat cloudy. For example, in our recent work where direct recordings of blood pressure were obtained during a stressful RT task, a somewhat paradoxical effect on blood pressure was observed. During the PI there is consistently observed a small phasic elevation of both systolic and diastolic pressure, in association with an acceleration of heart rate. However, during the period commencing where shock is expected and lasting for as long as 15 to 20 seconds there is sometimes observed a rather marked decrease in blood pressure. The depressor effect is usually preceded by an acceleration of heart rate and an increase in the slope measure of contractility. Also when shock is administered the depressor response tends to be even larger, having been seen in several instances to drop in excess of 50 mmHg. Such blood pressure effects suggest that the vasomotor activity is modified in at least two different manners by the experimental situation. That is, first there is likely an increase in peripheral vascular resistance during the PI, and then a decrease associated with the depressor response. Regardless of what might be going on somatically, blood pressure and vasomotor activity, like heart rate, do not respond to stress in a simple unidimensional manner.

In the light of this paucity of current evidence as to the biological basis of cardiac-somatic uncoupling, there would appear to be merit in resorting to more behavioral concepts in order to understand how behavioral influences are mediated biologically. From the perspective of the stimulus conditions in the two experiments in which we have seemingly uncoupled heart rate from somatic activity, three inter-related parameters are suggested to be important. First, it is likely that a greater degree of stress was involved in contrast to previously used behavioral paradigms where cardiac and somatic effects did not appear independent. Assuming this to be the case, and that biologically we are dealing primarily with sympathetic effects, it would appear that sympathetic influences on the heart are normally very minimal, at least in the normal young adult and healthy mongrel dog (Obrist et al. 1972b). Second, sympathetic influences on the heart appear to involve acute stress which is reasonably short lived in the sense that sympathetic influences are more apparent in the early phases of the experiment, i.e., the early trials. Third, this pronounced dampening of sympathetic activity appears to be lessened only when the organism is placed in situations where it is uncertain about how aversive the stressful stimuli will be and how he can cope with the task requirements. Once such uncertainties become minimal, then sympathetic influences are less. These speculations have similarities to the more traditional concept relegating sympathetic influences to emergency functions. They differ in that, with respect to the heart, such sympathetic influences are only mobilized with rather intense, acute stress, which is brought about by the subject's uncertainties.

These data, indicating an independence of cardiac and concurrent somatic effects, seem to argue all the more convincingly that in our prior studies, which demonstrate a coupling of heart rate and somatic activity, somatic influences are the primary biological mediating mecha-nism. The fact that the data suggest that it requires a rather intense degree of stress involving sympathetic influences to demonstrate an independence of cardiac and somatic activities suggests that, in less stressful behavioral paradigms involving vagal influences on heart rate and where cardiac-somatic coupling is observed, nonsomatic influences are very minimal. This is an important point because there is some evidence (Cohen, M. J. 1972; Elliott 1972; Jennings et al. 1971; Schwartz and Higgins 1971; Obrist 1968; Obrist et al. 1973a) suggest-ing some degree of independence between cardiac rate and somatic effects under less stressful conditions. But in each of these situations the data are hardly as convincing of an independence of the systems in that the magnitude of the changes are small and commonly not a reliable effect or that somatic activity was either not evaluated or only incompletely so.

There is a problem of reliably assessing somatic activity, particularly in adults, and behavioral paradigms which neither require nor provoke movements. For example, in a simple RT task we find some adults who show very little if any base level somatic activity as measured by general activity or chin EMG. Thus, any decrease in somatic activity on these measures is very small or absent. Yet, heart rate can be observed to decelerate although not as much as when there is somatic activity present during the base level (see Obrist 1968). However, we have not been inclined to view this as indicating an independence of heart rate and somatic activity, because of the variety of other evidence under these conditions which indicate a relationship between these two events. Rather we have been inclined to look at it as due to the limited reliability of any one somatic measure and to the fact that heart rate may under certain circumstances more sensitively reflect these inhibitory states. Also, the evidence from the recent RT stress study and operant study seems to argue more convincingly for cardiac-somatic uncoupling under these conditions and not in the previous studies because of the nature of the effects, i.e., the evidence in regard to the reliability, direction, and magnitude of the effects as well as the correlation data.

To reiterate, what we propose on the basis of available data with regard to cardiac-somatic coupling is that heart rate is quite invariantly linked to somatic activity in behavioral situations which involve minimal sympathetic influences on the heart. Such situations likely represent most that are used in typical psychophysiological studies. Whether behavioral processes under such circumstances can influence heart rate independently of somatic activity, will probably be difficult to determine because of the subtlety of such influences. Unless appreciable sympathetic influences can be evoked, then heart rate can likely be best viewed as an index of somatic activities which make heart rate a useful biological parameter only to the extent it is important to know whether somatic activities have been modified.

NOTES

1. The parameter of cardiovascular activity most commonly assessed in the research to be reviewed is heart rate. Thus, cardiac as used in the text most commonly refers to heart rate. However, recently other parameters of cardiovascular function, such as cardiac contractility and blood pressure, have been assessed and appear to relate to somatic activity in a more complicated manner, if at all. When cardiac is used in reference to these parameters, it shall be indicated. Somatic as used in the text refers to the activity of the striate musculature.

2. The somatic events that have been evaluated range from rather extensive acts, referred to as general activity exemplified by struggling and postural shifts, to rather subtle events involving localized and specific groups of muscles exemplified by mouth movements, swallowing, and eye movements and blinks. The particular type and amount of activity found depends on the subject and condition. For example, adult humans in a reaction time task usually show very little activity other than eye movements and blinks. On the other hand, adult humans have been found to show a high incidence of general activity during an operant task when increases in heart rate were reinforced. Where

a phasic decrease in somatic activity occurs as in the preparatory interval of a reaction time task, and in the CS-UCS interval during aversive conditioning, the effect usually involves all types of activity measured and might be likened to a momentary state of suspended animation. It would also appear that the decrease in somatic activity observed to anticipate responding in a reaction time task is task irrelevant activity.

3. These first experiments were also concerned with determining the reliability and sensitivity of the force of contraction measures. An indirect technique was used which involved a rate of change measure (Rushmer 1964) using any one of three manifestations of left ventricular performance, i.e., the rate at which blood is accelerated in the aorta, the rate at which the left ventricle contracts, and the rate at which the aortic blood pressure climbs from diastole to systole. The latter measure was evaluated because it was the only one that might be applicable to human Ss (see also Chapter 4, Lawler). These rate of change measures are henceforth referred to as slope.

4. Lacey (personal communication) has pointed out that increases in muscle tension in the arms preparatory to responding in a RT task have been reported. Also we have observed during aversive conditioning that when Ss are required to tap with their hands gently but continuously, tapping increases in intensity in anticipation of the UCS, even though heart rate decelerates and task-irrelevant somatic activities decrease (Obrist et al. 1969). In this instance, the magnitude of the anticipatory cardiac deceleration was smaller than has been previously found, suggesting that in this situation as well as in the RT task the influence of somatic activities somehow summate, and that the deceleratory heart rate effect reflects a dominance of inhibitory over excitatory processes.

9

LARRY E. ROBERTS

Comparative Psychophysiology of the Electrodermal and Cardiac Control Systems

INTRODUCTION

Psychophysiologists have long believed that the activities of the autonomic nervous system are regulated to an important degree by neural processes that have specific functions in behavior. However, the nature of these functions and the extent of their control over various forms of autonomic nervous system activity are a matter of considerable dispute. In the present chapter, I shall refer to the study of behavioral processes that regulate autonomic responding as the study of the "functional organization" of the autonomic nervous system.

The study of functional organization should be distinguished from the study of neural mechanisms that determine autonomic nervous system activity. The purpose of research on neural mechanisms is to discover which parts of the brain control autonomic activity and to identify the pathways over which this control is exerted. The study of neural mechanisms is discussed in Chapter 2 of the present volume, which summarizes what is presently known about the neural control of cardiovascular responses in several species. Structures of the brain that regulate cardiovascular activity, however, perform other behavioral functions as well. Research on the functional organization of the autonomic nervous system asks, what are these other functions? For example, are diencephalic centers that control cardiovascular responding imbedded within a neural system that modulates sensory input, as some theories of cardiovascular organization propose (Sokolov

The author's research is supported by grants from the Ontario Mental Health Foundation (345) and the National Research Council of Canada (APA-132).

1963)? Or, are they part of a neural system which is responsible for the initiation and execution of consummatory activities, or of previously learned instrumental responses (Black and de Toledo 1972)? Although the problems of functional organization and neural mechanism are separable, both are basic to an understanding of how cardiovascular and other autonomic adjustments are achieved in the behaving animal.

The present chapter provides an interpretative review of some recent research on the functional organization of two autonomic systems, the electrodermal and the cardiac.[1] Attention is focused primarily upon the study of these systems during conditioned emotional response (CER) training, in which aversive classical conditioning is superimposed upon an appetitive operant base line (Estes and Skinner 1941). It should be stressed, however, that the model of functional organization suggested by the CER studies may not properly describe the organization of behavior in other experimental situations, where performance may be mediated by different neural systems. This possibility will be considered briefly at the conclusion of the chapter, where some research on electrodermal correlates of instructed movement is discussed.

Two themes will be apparent as the chapter unfolds. The first is that experiments that compare the relationship of different autonomic responses to behavior provide much more information about functional organization than do experiments that consider each autonomic response separately. A growing awareness of this fact is one of the reasons comparative studies are, as they should be, a contemporary trend in the psychophysiological analysis of the cardiovascular and other autonomic systems. The second and more specific theme of the chapter is that there appear to be important differences between the electrodermal and cardiac systems regarding the extent to which they are regulated by movement control processes and attentional or motivational mechanisms. An analysis of these differences can be expected to contribute substantially to our understanding of the functional organization of these systems, and to suggest new approaches to the study of the functional significance of other autonomic responses.

THEORIES OF THE FUNCTIONAL ORGANIZATION OF THE ELECTRODERMAL AND CARDIAC CONTROL SYSTEMS

We begin with a description of three processes that have been suggested by many investigators to determine electrodermal and heart rate responses in various behavioral situations, and that might account for the organization of responding during CER training as well. Although these processes do not exhaust the list that has been proposed, most of the suggestions which are not discussed may be interpreted as variations of one of the following theories of the organization of the electrodermal and cardiac systems.

Movement Theories

Many investigators have suggested that electrodermal and heart rate responses are determined by neural processes that control the initiation and execution of movement. According to this hypothesis, autonomic responses may be excited· directly by central motor outflow, or by proprioceptive feedback over pathways that connect with the electrodermal and cardiac control systems in the brain or spinal cord. Both possibilities were suggested by Wang (1930), who provided what is perhaps the most explicit statement of a movement or somatic theory of electrodermal responding.

> The galvanic skin reaction is also closely linked up with muscular activity. This is strongly suggested by the fact that the sweat center is closely associated with the motor center in the cerebral cortex and the tuber cinereum, and also by the nature of the stimuli which induce the galvanic skin reaction. Painful and emotional stimuli all excite a man to violent muscular movement, while the galvanic skin responses caused by deep breathing and loud recitation of multiplication tables are evidently due to the stimulation of proprioceptors in muscles . . . The adequate stimuli of this reflex may therefore be assumed to be either excitants for violent muscular activity, or ones produced by muscular activity itself. [Wang 1930, p. 25]

Because his contributions were cited by Carney Landis in a widely read review in the 1930s (Landis 1932), it is possible that Wang's remarks had a considerable influence on investigators who later espoused movement theories of electrodermal functioning (Freeman 1948; Smith 1967). One of these described the galvanic skin response (GSR) as "probably the best general index of total neural muscular activity that we have today" (Freeman 1948, p. 13). More recently, somatic-motor arousal has been emphasized as a determinant of both electrodermal and heart rate responses by somatic theories of classical and operant autonomic conditioning (e.g., Black 1971a; Smith 1967). These theories view classically and operantly conditioned electrodermal and heart rate responses as secondary to an effect of conditioning on skeletal-motor behavior.

Movement theories of functional organization make two general predictions that have attracted a good deal of experimental attention. The first of these is that autonomic and somatic responses ought to be positively correlated with one another in a variety of experimental situations. The nature of this relationship is that changes in autonomic responding should be observed whenever changes in somatic responding take place. The second prediction is that any experimental manipulation that affects somatic responding, such as the operant conditioning of specific skeletal movements or the prevention of skeletal responses by physical restraint, brain lesions, or pharmacological blockade, should affect autonomic responding as well. Some experiments comparing electrodermal and heart rate responses with respect to these predictions in the CER situation will be reviewed later in the chapter.

Motivational Theories

A second class of theories proposes control of the electrodermal and cardiac systems by neural processes that set the occasion for overt responding and facilitate subsequent performance when it occurs. Since these are among the several functions normally ascribed to motivational processes, I shall call theories of this sort "motivational" theories of electrodermal and heart rate responding.

Motivational theories of functional organization have many historical roots. Cannon (1936) was the first to document many of the autonomic changes that accompany behavioral expressions of fear, anger, and other emotional or motivational states, and to point out the adaptive utility of these in meeting the metabolic requirements of sustained muscular and other activities. More recently, the motivational significance of autonomic arousal and its assumed tendency to anticipate overt behavioral responding have been stressed by two-process theories of learning (Rescorla and Solomon 1967). Proponents of activation theory have also ascribed the control of autonomic responding to motivational rather than to movement control mechanisms, although their view of the relationship between these two neural systems is somewhat more complex than that proposed by two-process or Hullian theories of learning (Malmo 1962). Heart rate has been studied most intensively among autonomic responses as a possible measure of motivational processes by both activation and learning theorists (e.g., Malmo and Belanger 1967; Overmier 1966). However, some attention has been paid to skin conductance and potential as well (Pinneo 1961; Roberts and Young 1971).

Although all motivational theories appear to distinguish between processes that set the occasion for performance, on one hand, and processes which are responsible for response execution, on the other, there is little agreement regarding the specific function of the former, motivational process. In the present chapter, motivation will be viewed as a response selection and potentiation process that is aroused by punishment or by depriving the subject of needed substances, or by presenting reward-related or punishment-related cues. According to this interpretation, motivational processes are responsible, not for the initiation and execution of overt responses, but merely for their selection and potentiation. After selection and potentiation has occurred, response elicitation and execution is carried out by movement control processes whose excitation requires appropriate movement cues. The effect of motivational arousal on movement control processes may be viewed as highly selective and precise, in that some instrumental responses and innate behaviors may be facilitated while others are inhibited, depending upon the motivational process that is excited and upon the subject's previous learning experience. There may, of course, be several distinguishable motivational systems, these differing with respect to the class of reinforcing object or deprivation manipulation that excites them, with respect to the specific pattern of response biases that is imposed upon movement control mechanisms, and possibly also with respect to which autonomic systems are excited when the motivational process is aroused.

The relationship between autonomic responses and overt behavior expected on the basis of motivational theories such as the one just described differs greatly from that predicted by movement theories of functional organization. Movement theories such as those proposed by Smith (1967) and Wang (1930) regard increased somatic activity as sufficient and perhaps necessary for excitation of various autonomic systems. Motivational theories, on the other hand, hold that autonomic responding may anticipate skeletal-motor behavior by a considerable period of time, or that autonomic arousal may occur in the absence of somatic activity, if appropriate movement cues are not present. Motivational theories predict further that autonomic responses are sensitive to drive manipulations and to presentation of reinforcement or reinforcement-related cues, and that the effects of these variables on autonomic responding are independent of their effects on skeletal-motor behavior. Several experiments comparing electrodermal responses and heart rate with respect to these predictions during CER training will be reviewed later in the chapter.

Attentional Theories

Both movement and motivational theories of functional organization attribute control of autonomic responding to what might be called efferent processes of the brain (i.e., movement control processes or neural systems that modulate these). A third class of theories, on the other hand, proposes control of autonomic responding by afferent processes of the central nervous system. These theories, which I shall call "attentional" theories of functional organization, attribute changes in autonomic responding to neural mechanisms that regulate sensory perception.

Two very popular attentional models have been described by the Laceys (1970) and by Sokolov (1963). Although there are substantial differences between these models with respect to their scope and the specific mechanisms involved, both propose the regulation of autonomic arousal by attentional processes, and suggest that feedback arising from visceral responding has a modulating effect on the flow of sensory information into the central nervous system. A fuller description of these attentional theories may be found in Chapters 3 and 26 of the present volume.

Experimental evaluation of attentional theories appears to have followed one of two general approaches. In the first approach, an attempt is made to determine whether cardiovascular and electrodermal responses are related to stimulus parameters or to the attentional requirements of various tasks as the theories require. Experiments following this approach have typically examined the direction, amplitude, and other features of cardiovascular and electrodermal responses as a function of stimulus quality and intensity (Weisbard and Graham 1971), stimulus repetition (Maltzman et al. 1971), temporal uncertainty (Bowers 1971a), and so on. Experiments following the second approach have attempted to relate autonomic manifestations of orienting or attention to behaviors which are believed to be strongly influenced by attentional processes. Among the behaviors that have been studied in relation to autonomic responding are electroencephalographic indices of stimulus detection such as alpha-blocking (Sokolov 1963), response latency in reaction time experiments (Obrist et al. 1970a), slow cortical potentials or the "contingent negative variation" (CNV) (Lacey and Lacey 1970), and verbal reports indicating whether a particular stimulus change was noticed (Bernstein 1969). Much of this work has been summarized elsewhere in this book (see Chapter 3, Cook; Chapter 25, Elliott; Chapter 26, Lacey and Lacey) and will not be considered here. However, findings that appear particularly important for understanding the functional organization of the cardiac and electrodermal systems will be discussed when appropriate.

Summary

Each of the theories reviewed above attributes control of autonomic responding to neural processes that perform specific functions in behavior. These theories differ, however, with respect to the specific functions proposed. Movement theories of functional organization suggest the regulation of cardiovascular and electrodermal activity by neural systems which are responsible for the initiation and execution of movement. Alternatively, motivational theories hypothesize the regulation of autonomic arousal by response selection and potentiation or similar processes, rather than by movement control systems. Attentional theories suggest that the function of processes which regulate autonomic responding involves the modulation of sensory input. Each theory specifies different variables as determinants of autonomic responding, and, in some cases, different classes of behavior as correlates of autonomic nervous system activity.

The task for the remainder of the chapter will be to determine which of the foregoing models provides the most satisfactory account of the organization of electrodermal, cardiac, and skeletal-motor responding during CER training. Particular attention will be paid to experiments that have compared the relationship of electrodermal and heart rate responses to overt behavior during CER training, since the results of these appear to be especially important for understanding the organization of the electrodermal and cardiac control systems.

ELECTRODERMAL AND CARDIOVASCULAR CORRELATES OF THE CER

Motivational theories of functional organization accept repeated pairing of a conditioned stimulus (CS) with shock as one procedure that establishes stimulus control of motivational arousal (Mowrer 1947). Consequently, if motivational theories are correct, presentation of an aversive CS would be expected to provoke widespread changes in autonomic responding that can be shown to be independent of the effects the CS may have upon striatemuscular activity. Movement theories of functional organization, on the other hand, maintain that autonomic responding will occur to an aversive CS only if skeletal-motor responding takes place as well. An analysis of dependencies among autonomic and somatic responses to· conditioned aversive stimuli during CER training is a major concern of the present section.

We begin with a discussion of our published work on electrodermal and cardiac correlates of the CER in rats (Roberts and Young 1971). Then, several other CER studies will be reviewed.

The Roberts and Young Studies

The preparation we have used for studying electrodermal and heart-rate responses during CER training may be described briefly, as follows. Rats were restrained on a Lucite platform that contained openings for the hind legs and scrotum. The method of restraint allowed the rat to move its body and head freely, and to manipulate a lever made available to the forepaws. Reinforcement for lever-pressing was a drop of chocolate Metrecal dispensed through a hypodermic needle situated just in front of the rat's head. Electrodermal responses were measured by means of silver-chloride electrodes attached to the plantar surfaces of the rear feet and referred to reference electrodes on the tail. Subdermal EKG electrodes were implanted on each side of the rib cage to measure heart rate and were connected to an electrode assembly cemented to the rat's skull. Changes in skeletal-motor behavior during conditioning were assessed by recording lever-pressing and gross body movement. The latter variable was measured by a capacitative system that detected virtually every movement the rat made, including respiratory maneuvers. In all of our experiments, the unconditioned stimulus (UCS) was a brief shock applied to the tail. Conditioned stimuli were a clicker and a tone. The interstimulus interval was 3 minutes.

Our first experiment examined the relationship of changes in skin conductance (SC) to changes in lever-pressing during CER training. Rats were first given five days of preliminary training during which a movement baseline was established by rewarding lever-pressing on a VI-20-second schedule of reinforcement. Discriminative classical conditioning was then superimposed upon the operant schedule and continued for an additional eight days. The main findings are summarized in Figure 9.1, where response patterns on the fourth and eighth days of conditioning are shown. Presentation of the stimulus that was paired with shock (CS+) elicited a substantial increase in SC that was sustained and amplified throughout the conditioning trial. The effect of CS+ on skeletal-motor activity, on the other hand, was opposed, with little lever-pressing occurring during CS+ on the fourth conditioning day and only slightly more on the eighth. These results are clearly inconsistent with theories that attribute increased electrodermal arousal primarily or exclusively to increased somatic activity, as Smith (1967) and Wang (1930) appear to have proposed.

It is possible, however, to defend a movement theory in several ways. For example, one might argue that changes in lever-pressing did not reveal the true course of somatic outflow during the conditioning trial, or that lever-pressing was correlated with somatic activities that did not have a significant impact on autonomic function. How can these interpretations be ruled out?

We attempted to evaluate them by determining whether classically-conditioned electrodermal responses would be found independent of a somatic variable (gross body movement) that appeared to determine a second autonomic response. Heart rate was chosen as the second autonomic response, since many investigators have found it to be closely related to somatic activity in other behavioral situations (Black 1971a; Obrist et al. 1970b). In order for this strategy to be convincing, heart rate must be shown to depend upon movement, rather than upon motivational or attentional effects that may accompany the movement response.

The procedure for conditioning was similar to that of the previous study, with the following exceptions. First, measures of skin potential (SP), heart rate, and overt movement were added to those of SC and lever-pressing taken previously. Second, shock intensity was increased from 3.2 to 5.8 ma. The purpose of this was to suppress the movement baseline, in order to provide greater opportunity to examine autonomic responses that occurred when movement increased, decreased, or did not change following the presentation of CS+. A third difference between the present study and the previous one was that conditioning was extended from 8 to 11 days, to provide sufficient data for an analysis of steady-state behavior patterns.

The main results are summarized in Figure 9.2. Autonomic responses were computed by subtracting measurements taken 10 seconds before CS onset from measurements recorded 10 seconds before termination of the CS. Changes in movement and lever-pressing, on the other hand, are portrayed by means of "suppression ratios" which rep-

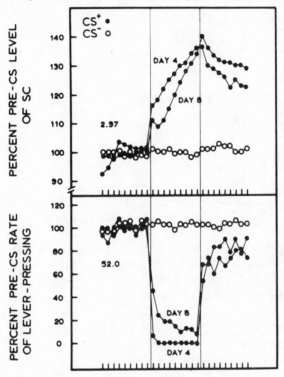

CONSECUTIVE 20 SEC. INTERVALS

FIGURE 9.1. *Skin conductance and lever pressing during positive and negative trials on the fourth and eighth conditioning days. Responses on negative trials were combined across conditioning days, since there was no difference between them. The first vertical line denotes onset of the CS; the second indicates CS termination and, on positive trials, the delivery of shock. The numbers to the left of the first vertical line are pre-CS means. (SC in micromhos, lever pressing in responses/minute. From Roberts and Young 1971).*

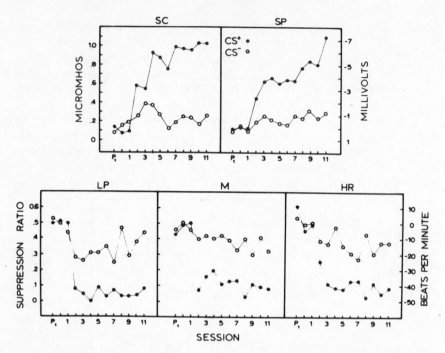

FIGURE 9.2. *Effect of CER training on skin conductance (SC), skin potential (SP), lever pressing (LP), movement (M), and heart rate (HR). The letter P on the abscissa denotes a pretest day on which the conditioned stimuli were presented without shock. (From Roberts and Young 1971).*

resent responding during the last 20 seconds of the CS as a proportion of the total observed during this interval and a comparable interval 20 seconds before CS onset. Thus, a ratio of 0 indicates complete suppression of lever-pressing or movement by the CS, whereas a ratio of .5 indicates that the CS had no effect. Inspection of the figure reveals that lever-pressing and movement decreased during positive trials, while the electrodermal response was an increase in SC and the negativity of SP. This outcome is consistent with the results of Figure 1, and, like those findings, is incompatible with theories that attribute electrodermal arousal primarily or exclusively to excitation of movement control processes. However, in striking contrast to the electrodermal responses, the direction of the heart rate response was the same as the changes in movement and lever pressing. This finding suggests a principle of cardio-somatic coupling and is consistent with the results of many earlier studies of classical heart-rate conditioning (Obrist et al. 1970b).

While the results of Figure 9.2 indicate that the relationship of electrodermal and heart rate responses to movement is different, the most compelling evidence for differential organization of these two auto-nomic systems was provided by detailed analyses of the response pat-terns that occurred on various types of conditioning trial. We turn to these analyses next. Since elucidation of the mechanisms that control electrodermal activity requires an understanding of the processes that control heart rate, our first effort will be devoted to an analysis of the heart rate response.

Mechanism of the Heart Rate Response. The results of Figure 9.2 are compatible with several interpretations of the decelerative heart rate response. Obviously, the fact that heart rate and somatic responses were of the same direction is consistent with theories that attribute reg-ulation of heart rate to movement control processes. However, presen-tation of CS+ may be assumed to have provoked motivational and attentional arousal as well, and the decelerative heart rate response may have been due to one of these processes. Or, the decrease in heart rate may have been secondary to an effect of sympathetic activation that was correlated with, but causally independent of, overt movement. Two such effects might have been the release of norepinephrine from the adrenal medulla (Wenger et al. 1960), or an increase in blood pres-sure with subsequent initiation of the baroreceptor reflexes (Scher 1966).

These interpretations were evaluated by comparing autonomic responses that occurred on trials on which movement increased, decreased, or did not change following presentation of CS+. The autonomic patterns associated with each type of movement response are shown in Figure 9.3. Each pattern represents the mean of 15 trials sampled randomly from those displaying the appropriate movement response, with the single restriction that the average number of CS-UCS pairings (trials) for each pattern had to be approximately the same. Because the facilitation of movement by CS+ was confined largely to the first 30 seconds of the interstimulus interval, only the 30 seconds immediately prior to and following presentation of CS+ were analyzed. The results portrayed in Figure 9.3 may be interpreted in the following way. Since the number of CS-UCS pairings was com-parable for each response pattern (M = 19.6), classically-conditioned motivational effects of the CS+ should have been similar on each type of conditioning trial. The fact that very little lever-pressing occurred during CS+, even when movement increased, is consistent with the view that the subjects were in a state of fear. Comparison of the pat-terns also shows that electrodermal responses of comparable amplitude accompanied each type of movement change. This suggests that the subjects attended to the onset of CS+ on each trial, and that sympa-thetic activation was approximately the same. Therefore, if the decel-

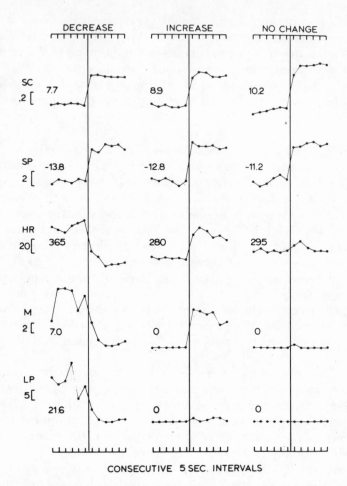

FIGURE 9.3. *Autonomic responses attending a decrease in movement (left panel), an increase in movement (middle panel), and little change in movement (right panel). The average number of CS-UCS pairings for each pattern was 20.4, 20.5, and 17.7 respectively. The vertical line denotes onset of CS+. The numbers to the left of the vertical line are pre-CS means. (SC in micromhos, SP in millivolts, heart rate in beats/minute, movement in inches/minute, and lever pressing in responses/minute. From Roberts and Young 1971).*

erative heart rate response was determined primarily by motivational or attentional arousal or by sympathetic activation, a decrease in rate should have been elicited by CS+ on each type of conditioning trial. If, on the other hand, heart rate was regulated by somatic control processes, the direction of the heart rate responses should have been the same as the movement responses.

The results were very clear. Heart rate decreased by 49 bpm when movement was suppressed by CS+ (p < .01), but increased by 36 bpm when movement was elicited by CS+ (p < .025). Heart rate was unchanged when movement remained constant, although an increase of 6 bpm (t < 1) accompanied small, phasic movement responses that frequently occurred on this type of trial. These findings clearly implicate somatic arousal as one process controlling the heart rate response.

A complementary analysis examined the effect of nonsomatic processes on heart rate, and evaluated the importance of these relative to somatic events. For this purpose, a multiple regression model was employed to partition predictable variability in the heart rate responses into additive components that reflected the contribution of different processes to cardiac change. The first predictor variable, movement, was chosen to reflect neural activity in somatic control processes that appear to have affected heart rate. The second predictor, trials, was viewed as a determinant of classically-conditioned motivational or attentional processes that may have affected the heart rate response. The third predictor was the SC response, which was chosen to examine the effect of sympathetic activation on cardiac change. Multiple regression analyses were applied to the responses of positive trials and were computed separately for each rat.

The results are summarized in the left hand panel of Table 9.1. Since

TABLE 9.1 *Partitioning the variability of heart rate and skin potential responses*

	Heart rate				Skin potential			
Rat	R	βM	βT	βSC	R	βM	βT	βSC
98	.76	−.10	−.72	−.17	.86	.09	.61	.26
110	.62	.50	−.15	.04	.62	−.06	.27	.43
111	.74	.60	−.32	.13	.89	.02	.62	.31
122	.82	.67	−.20	.01	.59	.07	.07	.35
134	.70	.55	−.31	.05	.79	−.07	.77	.01
141	.80	.64	−.11	−.24	.63	.00	.27	.49
144	.75	.42	−.05	−.39	.60	.10	.51	.04
155	.62	.25	−.07	.20	.49	−.18	.39	.19
159	.73	.66	.14	−.23	.50	.00	.12	.42
168	.67	.51	−.15	−.12	.45	.22	.12	.18
M	.73	.49	−.22	−.08	.68	.02	.41	.27
t	20.11	6.05	−2.44	−1.23	7.90	.55	4.30	5.03
p	<.01	<.01	<.05	ns	<.01	ns	<.01	<.01

NOTE — Means and t-tests were computed after an r to z transformation had been applied. Probabilities are two-tailed. Abbreviations: M = movement; T = trials; SC = skin conductance; R = multiple correlation between heart rate or skin potential responses and M, T, and SC.

the β-coefficients for a given predictor are independent, the contribution of each predictor may be evaluated statistically by means of a sign or t-test. Inspection of the t-statistics provided in Table 9.1 reveals that movement contributed substantially to variability in the heart rate responses (M $\beta = .49$), but that SC did not (M $\beta = -.08$). This outcome, of course, corroborates the results presented earlier in Figure 9.3. However, trials also made a statistically reliable contribution to variability in the heart rate responses (M $\beta = -.22$) when the effects of movement and sympathetic activation were partialed out. This contribution was small compared to movement for most subjects, although a notable exception was provided by one rat (#98) that displayed decelerative heart rate responses approximating 20 bpm on several trials on which movement did not change. Analyses of the pooled data revealed that 65% of the predictable variability in heart rate responding could be attributed exclusively to the movement response, whereas the proportion attributable to trials was 2%. These findings suggest that the heart rate responses of the Roberts and Young study were determined by nonsomatic processes as well as by movement control mechanisms. However, for most rats, movement appeared to be a far more important determinant of cardiac change than did nonsomatic factors.

Mechanism of the Electrodermal Responses. The results regarding the electrodermal responses were very different. The response patterns of Figure 9.3 show that electrodermal responses of comparable amplitude occurred on trials on which movement either increased, decreased, or did not change when CS+ was presented. This outcome is clearly incompatible with a somatic interpretation of the control of electrodermal responding, but is generally consistent with motivational or attentional theories. Moreover, the apparent independence of electrodermal and somatic activity cannot be attributed to insensitive measures of somatic involvement or to the study of overt behaviors that failed to affect autonomic function, since movement appeared to be an important determinant of heart rate.

The contribution of nonsomatic processes to the electrodermal responses, and their importance relative to somatic factors, were evaluated by multiple regression analyses, as was done for heart rate. Inspection of the right hand panel of Table 9.1 shows that trials contributed significantly to predictable variability in the SP responses (M $\beta = .41$), but that movement did not (M $\beta = .02$). The same result was obtained when the SC responses were examined, although these data are not reported in Table 9.1. Analyses of the pooled data indicated that up to 73% of the predictable variability in SP was attributable to conditioning trials, while the corresponding value for SC was 77% (Roberts and Young 1971). The contribution of movement to SC and SP, on the other hand, was not significantly different from zero.

The significance of the present findings for somatic theories of the control of electrodermal responding may be illustrated further by considering how a somatic theory might be defended. For example, one might argue that the electrodermal responses were secondary to an increase in generalized muscle tension that was not detected by measuring overt movement (cf. Smith 1967). This possibility seems unlikely, however, since the hypothesized increase in muscle tension would have been expected to accelerate the heart on each conditioning trial, or at least when overt movement remained constant, but this did not happen. An alternative interpretation attributes the electrodermal response to the tensing of particular muscles, rather than to a general increase in somatic activation (Smith 1967). However, this possibility is rendered unlikely by the response patterns of Figure 9.3, which show that electrodermal responses were nearly identical even when overt movement changed in different directions, or not at all, when CS+ was presented. If the electrodermal responses were due to the tensing of particular muscles, the pattern of muscle contractions that occurred would have to have been compatible with all three of the observed movement changes.

A final form of somatic theory attributes electrodermal arousal to respiratory maneuvers that may have been elicited by CS+. However, measurements of respiratory frequency taken on trials on which movement did not change following presentation of CS+, indicated that respiratory frequency remained constant as well (M = 1.70 and 1.76 breaths per second for pre−CS+ and CS+ intervals, respectively, t < 1). Yet electrodermal responses on this type of trial were substantial, as Figure 9.3 shows. Also, heart rate on these trials remained substantially unchanged. Had the electrodermal responses been secondary to a sustained and undetected respiratory maneuver such as hyperpnea or reduced respiratory frequency and amplitude, cardiac sinus arrhythmia or perhaps a substantial bradycardia would have been expected (Obrist et al. 1970b), but neither of these occurred. These findings suggest that the electrodermal responses of the present study were not elicited by altered patterns of respiratory activity.

We appear, therefore, to be left with the following question. If the electrodermal responses of the present study were not due to movement control mechanisms, how were they determined? The apparent dependence of electrodermal responses upon CS-UCS pairings rather than upon movement is clearly consistent with a motivational theory of the organization of the electrodermal system, but is compatible with an attentional theory as well. Can a choice between these models be made?

Some data bearing upon this question were provided by an analysis of the results of our first CER study, which showed that phasic electrodermal responding failed to occur to the onset of CS+ on only 2% of positive trials beyond the second conditioning day. Responses to the onset of CS−, on the other hand, failed to occur on more than 40% of the trials on these days. In view of the intensity of the CSs (a 70 db tone or clicker) and the potential significance of auditory cues in the experimental situation, it seems highly unlikely that the subjects failed to detect CS− on these trials. Rather, it seems more plausible to attribute the absence of electrodermal responding to a failure of CS− to have a motivational effect. Of course, this analysis rules out only those attentional theories that treat electrodermal arousal as an indicant of stimulus detection.

To summarize, the main implications of the Roberts and Young studies are twofold. First, the results appear fatal to any theory that proposes control of the electrodermal system primarily or exclusively by somatic events, at least in the CER situation. Second, the mechanisms of classical electrodermal and heart rate conditioning are clearly different. The nature of this difference is that the electrodermal system appears more closely coupled with motivational or possibly attentional processes than with mechanisms that control movement, while the reverse is true for heart rate.[2] In the next section, we consider whether further support for these conclusions can be found in other studies of relationships among electrodermal, heart-rate, and overt behavioral responses during CER training.

Other CER Studies

One way to test the hypothesis that the electrodermal and cardiac systems are organized differently with respect to movement control mechanisms is to hold movement control processes constant during conditioning, and see whether electrodermal and heart rate responses are affected differently. Autonomic responses may be examined once again when movement is permitted to occur, to determine whether manipulation of the movement response alters some components of the response pattern and not others. An unpublished experiment by Muzzin (1970) in our laboratory followed this approach.

Briefly, the experimental procedure involved superimposing aversive classical conditioning upon two types of movement baseline: On some days, classical conditioning trials were given while restrained rats pressed a lever for food reward (movement days). On other days, classical conditioning was carried out while the subjects were rewarded for holding still (no-movement days). A within-subject design was used, in which the lever was removed on no-movement days in order to indicate which operant contingency was in effect. Movement and no-movement days were given in a predetermined order, so that within each block of four conditioning days the average number of cumulated trials (CS-UCS pairings) for movement and no-movement sessions was the same. Therefore, classically-conditioned effects of the CS+ on motivational or attentional processes would have been comparable on the two types of day. The operant contingencies employed on the two types of day, however, ensured that the movement responses would be very different.

The results are summarized in Figure 9.4, where the amplitude of autonomic and somatic responses on no-movement days is plotted as a proportion of response amplitude on movement days. As in our previous work, the prevailing response to CS+ on both days was a decrease in movement and heart rate, and an increase in SC and SP. However, the movement response was greatly attenuated on no-movement days, as was the heart rate response, but the electrodermal responses were enhanced. The differential effect of manipulating the movement baseline on electrodermal and heart rate responses was observed for each of the four rats in the experiment and was statistically reliable for the group as a whole. Moreover, reinforcement for holding still lowered the movement baseline and heart rate in all rats, but had no consistent effect on the tonic level of SC or SP. Although we cannot explain why the electrodermal responses were enhanced, these results are obviously consistent with the view that the electrodermal and cardiac systems are organized differently with respect to movement control processes.

Unfortunately, the experiments by Roberts and Young (1971) and Muzzin (1970) are the only ones presently available that have studied the relationship between electrodermal responses and movement during CER training, or that have compared the relationship of electrodermal and heart rate responses to movement in the CER situation. However, the relationship between cardiovascular responses and skeletal-motor behavior during CER conditioning has been the object of study by many investigators. These experiments will be given careful attention since, although many of them support a principle of cardiosomatic coupling, some have been interpreted as providing strong evidence for the independence of cardiovascular and movement control systems (Brady 1971).

One of the most comprehensive analyses of the relationship between heart rate and skeletal-motor activity during CER training was carried out by Sutterer (Sutterer 1970; Sutterer and Obrist 1972) who, like Muzzin (1970), examined the effect of superimposing an aversive CS+

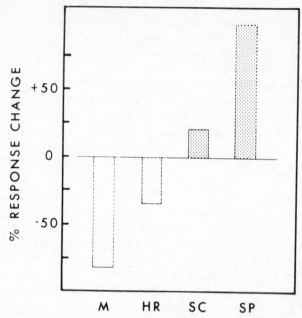

FIGURE 9.4. *CER training superimposed on movement and no-move-ment base lines. Responses on no-movement days are represented as a pro-portion of response amplitude on movement days. Results from the last four days of conditioning are shown. (From Muzzin 1970).*

upon different operant baselines. Sutterer's experimental procedure may be described by referring to Figure 9.5, which presents the results obtained from subjects that completed all segments of training. Briefly, hungry dogs were first trained to press a panel for food reward. Several sessions of discriminative classical conditioning were then car-ried out, while the manipulandum was removed. Each conditioning session consisted of 15 positive and 15 negative trials of 15-second duration, with electric shock as the UCS. The results from this stage of training are portrayed in the first row of Figure 9.5 (the "classical" procedure). Next, the manipulandum was reintroduced and classical conditioning continued for several sessions while the subject worked for food reward on a VI-30-second schedule (the VI-30 procedure of Figure 9.5). Subjects were then switched to a DRL-8 second schedule of reinforcement (differential reinforcement of low rates) for several sessions during which the CSs employed previously were presented several times without shock. Following this, classical conditioning was begun again, first employing a weak shock (DRL + low UCS in Figure 9.5) and later a strong shock (DRL + high UCS) as the UCS. Heart rate and panel-pressing were recorded continuously throughout each session. In addition, general activity was measured by means of a tamber-mounted floor in the subject's experimental chamber.

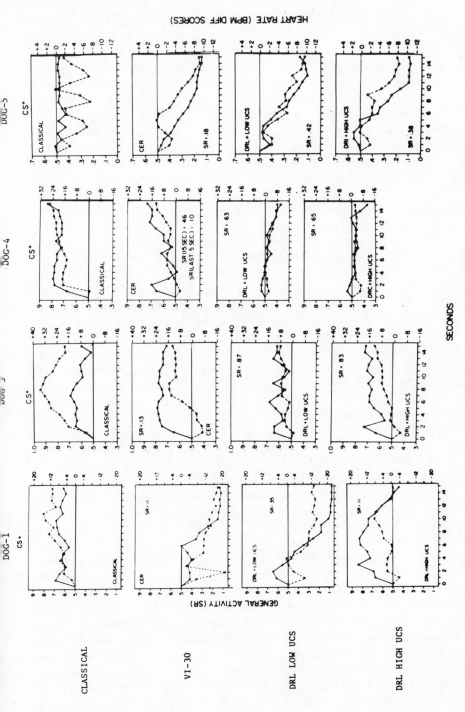

FIGURE 9.5. *Cardiac and movement responses to an aversive CS superimposed upon different types of operant base line. (Broken line = heart rate; solid line = movement. From Sutterer and Obrist 1972).*

Figure 9.5 portrays the changes in heart rate and general activity that occurred on positive trials for each dog during the various stages of training. The heart rate responses shown here were computed by subtracting the pre-CS+ rate from the rate that occurred during each second of the trial. Second-by-second changes in general activity are portrayed by means of suppression ratios computed as described earlier. In addition to these measures, the effect of CS+ on operant behavior for the trial as a whole is reported as a suppression ratio, placed in most cases in the upper right corner of the last three panels for each dog. Inspection of the figure shows that although the direction of responding varied substantially from animal to animal and from procedure to procedure, the direction of the prevailing movement and heart rate responses was always the same. Dog 1, for example, displayed increased heart rate and somatic activity in the presence of CS+ during classical conditioning and when the CS+ was followed by strong shock on a DRL schedule. However, the direction of both heart rate and movement responses was reversed when the CS+ was presented on a VI schedule or on a DRL schedule when a weak UCS was employed. On the other hand, the direction of the heart rate and somatic responses for Dogs 3 and 5 was the same in all conditions, but for Dog 3 the pattern was an acceleration of movement and heart rate, while for Dog 5 a decelerative response prevailed throughout all segments of training. On the whole, the degree of relationship between heart rate and movement apparent in these data is quite remarkable and clearly consistent with theories that attribute control of heart rate primarily to somatic processes.

The response patterns of Figure 9.5 also provide major difficulties for attentional and motivational theories of the control of cardiac activity. These theories would have predicted considerable consistency in the direction of the heart rate response to CS+ across the various conditions, since the same CS+ was utilized during all phases of the experiment. There was, however, little consistency in the direction of responding either within subjects or within conditions in Sutterer's study. It is difficult to understand why the subject would attend to the CS+ under one condition and not another, or why motivational processes should be excited under some circumstances and inhibited under others, when the CS+ that was presented in each case was the same. Of course, one might defend an attentional or motivational theory by arguing that the effect of CS+ on attentional or motivational processes depends upon UCS intensity and the number of prior conditioning trials, or upon the movement baseline. A defense of this sort is possible since there are large differences among experimental conditions with respect to these variables in Sutterer's experiment. However, there are no differences among the response patterns of Figure 9.3 with respect to the number of conditioning trials or UCS intensity, nor with respect to the movement baseline in 2 of the 3 patterns portrayed. Nevertheless, the form of the heart rate response on each trial is different and is the same as the movement response. Taken together, the results of Figures 9.3 and 9.5 provide grave difficulties for theories that contribute control of the heart to attentional or motivational processes. They are, however, highly consistent with movement theories of functional organization.

Further consideration of Sutterer's data reveals an additional finding of considerable importance. Although, for the most part, heart rate and movement changed in the same direction, heart rate and panel pressing often did not. For example, heart rate and movement increased significantly when CS+ was superimposed upon a VI schedule in Dog 3, but panel-pressing during the CS was greatly reduced (suppression ratio = .13). On the other hand, Dog 4 decreased its heart rate and movement significantly when CS+ and weak shock were superimposed upon a DRL baseline, although panel-pressing increased (suppression ratio = .63). A more detailed analysis of response relationships reported by Sutterer revealed that heart rate and movement responses were very highly correlated with respect to response direction across experimental conditions, but that the directional relationship of both of these variables to changes in panel-pressing was not significantly different from zero (Sutterer and Obrist 1972). Why should heart rate be related to general activity, but not to panel-pressing?

The answer to this question is probably that measures of operant behavior are not related to total somatic outflow as closely as are measures of gross body movement. If this interpretation is correct, and if heart rate is strongly determined by total somatic outflow, one would expect the correlation between heart rate responses and changes in operant behavior ($r$hr−ob) to increase with the magnitude of the correlation between changes in operant behavior and gross body movement ($r$ob−m). The expected trend is apparent in Figure 9.6, which plots $r$hr−ob as a function of $r$ob−m, using individual rats from the Roberts and Young study as the unit of observation. Figure 9.6 also shows that $r$hr−ob was quite substantial in the Roberts and Young study ($M\ r$ = .75), presumably because $r$ob−m was also ($M\ r$ = .88). In contrast, changes in heart rate and operant behavior were unrelated across experimental conditions in Sutterer's study, presumably because operant responding and general activity were unrelated as well. A stronger prediction that can be derived from the present interpretation is that when gross body movement and operant behavior are imperfectly correlated, heart rate should be more closely related to changes in movement than to changes in operant responding. This, of course, is what

Sutterer found. However, further corroborative evidence is provided by de Toledo (Black and de Toledo 1972), who compared the relationship of heart rate responses to changes in general activity and lever-pressing during CER training in rats. She found that heart rate responses were consistently more closely related to changes in general activity than to changes in lever pressing.

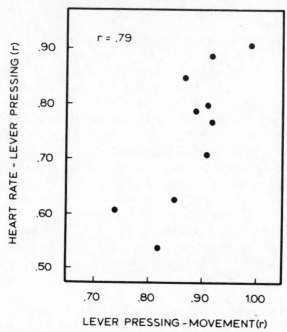

FIGURE 9.6. *Correlation between heart rate and lever-pressing responses (rhr-ob) plotted as a function of the correlation between lever-pressing and movement responses (rob-m). Individual rats from Roberts and Young (1971) are the unit of observation.*

The failure of operant responding to accurately portray total somatic outflow may explain the results of several recent studies which have reported clear dissociations between heart rate responses and the suppression of operant behavior during CER conditioning. De Toledo (1971), for example, compared the rate at which cardiac responses and the suppression of lever-pressing were acquired when independent groups of rats received CER training with different types of CS (white noise interrupted either 3 or 15 times per second), and various shock intensities (.8, 1.3, or 3.0 ma). She found that when white noise interrupted at a low frequency was used as CS+, suppression of lever-pressing and decelerative heart rate responses were acquired at the same rate at each shock level. However, when white noise interrupted at a high frequency was used as CS+, increasing shock intensity seriously retarded the acquisition of the decelerative heart rate response but did not affect the rate at which suppression was learned. De Toledo suggested that dissociation of the heart rate and suppression responses may have been due to a failure of changes in lever-pressing to accurately reflect changes in general activity during the CS+. In her words, "when changes in bar-pressing form the major component of changes in general activity, the correlation between changes in heart rate and in bar-pressing will be high; when changes in bar-pressing form only a minor component of changes in general activity, and the two are controlled by different independent variables, the correlation between changes in heart rate and in bar-pressing rate will be low" (de Toledo 1971, p. 536). The results portrayed in Figure 9.6, of course, support this prediction.

Another series of experiments reporting dissociations between changes in heart rate and operant behavior during CER training has been carried out by Brady and his co-workers (Brady 1971; Brady, Kelly, and Plumlee 1969). Unlike the studies reviewed above, which employed either rats or dogs as subjects, the experiments reported by Brady were performed on the monkey. As is true in the rat and dog, the effect of CS+ upon operant responding in the monkey is usually a decrease in response rate. However, Brady found that the cardiac response is frequently a decrease early in training and an increase later on, even though lever-pressing is suppressed by CS+ at all conditioning stages. He suggested that decelerative heart rate responses which develop early in CER training are largely secondary to a suppression of lever-pressing and other skeletal-motor activities by CS+, but that acceleratory heart rate responses which prevail later in training are determined by some other, nonsomatic process (Brady, Kelley and Plumlee 1969).[3]

Unfortunately, the data presently available on CER training in the monkey do not permit a thorough evaluation of Brady's hypothesis. There are, however, two reasons for interpreting his findings cautiously. First, it is quite possible that the changes in operant behavior which occurred in Brady's experiments failed to portray changes in general activity that took place during conditioning trials. This suggestion is supported by two recent studies in which general activity was measured during CER training in the monkey (Nathan and Smith 1971; Zeiner, Nathan, and Smith 1969). Like Brady, these investigators reported that the prevailing effect of CS+ upon operant behavior during the terminal stages of training was a suppression of lever pressing. However, general activity increased during CS+, as did heart rate.

The second reason for interpreting Brady's findings cautiously is that increases or decreases in heart rate which occurred during CER training in the monkey were usually accompanied by corresponding changes in systolic blood pressure, and to a lesser extent in diastolic blood pressure as well. Correlation coefficients computed among these responses from data provided in various Brady publications are reported in Table 9.2. The correlations shown here are independent in the sense that no overlapping sets of data were used in the computation, although in several cases the data were taken from the same animal during different stages of experimentation. Inspection of Table 9.2 reveals a strong correlation between heart rate and systolic blood pressure (median $r = .75$), and a similar but somewhat weaker relationship between heart rate and diastolic pressure as well (median $r = .47$). Interestingly, increments in heart rate and systolic blood pressure, and less consistently in diastolic pressure, are highly characteristic of the cardiovascular response to exercise (Rushmer 1970). One wonders, therefore, whether the cardiovascular responses recorded in Brady's experiments might have been associated with movement responses that were not detected by measuring lever-pressing.

TABLE 9.2   *Correlations derived from Brady data*

Source	Monkey	Correlation			
		HR-SBP	HR-DBP	SBP-DBP	HR-OB
1	A	.92	.89	.93	−.13
2	B	.81	.47	.74	.22
3	B	.69	.29	.50	.15
4	B	.79	.51	.72	.38
5	C	.92	.45	.63	.58
6	C	.71	.43	.52	−.34
7	D	.02	−.14	.19	−.05
8	E	−.45	−.46	.86	.47
9	1	.68	.89	.59	
10	S-300	.93	.93	.98	−.10
Median		.75	.47	.68	.22

NOTE: HR = heart rate; SBP = systolic blood pressure; DBP = diastolic blood pressure; OB = operant behavior. Sources: 1 = Brady et al. (1969) Fig. 1; 2 = Brady et al. (1969) Fig. 2; 3 = Brady et al. (1969) Fig. 7; 4 = Brady et al. (1969) Fig. 8; 5 = Brady et al. (1969) Fig. 9; 6 = Brady et al. (1969) Fig. 6; 9 = Brady (1971) Fig. 9, conditioning only (operant behavior not available); 10 = Brady (1971), Fig. 10.

While the results of Table 9.2 suggest the possibility of cardio-somatic coupling in Brady's data, there are some exceptions. Perhaps the most striking of these was provided by one animal (Monkey D) that displayed large acceleratory heart rate responses of up to 75 bpm without apparent changes in either systolic or diastolic pressure during conditioning trials. In another animal (Monkey E), decelerative heart rate responses of up to 40 bpm occurred without attending blood pressure changes. Unfortunately, the reasons for these exceptions are unclear. However, like Rat 98 in the Roberts and Young studies, they suggest that integration of cardiovascular and somatic activity may be fragmented for a minority of subjects during CER training.

Summary

The experiments reviewed in this section have been concerned with an analysis of dependencies among electrodermal, heart rate, and skeletal-motor responses in the CER situation. The major conclusions to emerge are twofold. First, changes in heart rate that occur during CER training are highly correlated with changes in gross body movement, and with changes in operant responding as well, when these are closely related to fluctuations in gross body movement. The magnitude of the relationship between cardiac and somatic activity is such that classical conditioning appears to have only a small effect on heart rate when the contribution of movement is partialed out. The second conclusion is that, unlike heart rate, electrodermal responses appear to be independent of movement during CER training. These findings indicate that the electrodermal and cardiac control systems are organized very differently with respect to neural mechanisms that determine striate muscular activity and motivational or attentional arousal. Unlike heart rate, which appears to be regulated primarily by movement control mechanisms, electrodermal activity appears to be determined mainly by motivational or attentional arousal, or by some other nonsomatic process.

Although the evidence for cardio-somatic coupling during CER training is undeniable, there are also repeated indications that dissociation of cardiovascular and somatic arousal is possible, at least under some circumstances. Continued study of apparent dissociations and the conditions under which they occur seems desirable, particularly in view of the implications such study may hold for our understanding of the origin of cardiovascular pathology. However, future studies would undoubtedly profit from a comparative analysis of the relationship of different measures of somatic activity to one another as well as to various indices of cardiovascular function. If independence of several highly intercorrelated measures of somatic arousal from cardiovascular activity can be demonstrated, the conclusion that cardiovascular and movement control systems function independently under some conditions would have to be accepted. Unfortunately, the studies of cardiovascular concomitants of the CER presently available have not provided a demonstration of this sort.

CONCLUSION

The research reviewed in the present chapter has attempted to characterize the behavioral function of neural processes that control electrodermal and heart rate responding during CER training. In concluding, we consider briefly whether the model of functional organization suggested by the CER studies properly describes the organization of behavior in other situations, where performance may be mediated by different neural systems.

As other chapters in this volume testify, a remarkably close relationship between heart rate and somatic activity has been documented in a variety of situations in addition to CER training. What is perhaps more significant, however, is that attempts to demonstrate control of heart rate by motivational or other nonsomatic processes have met with only limited success. To date, the only convincing demonstration of changes in heart rate independent of somatic activity has been described by Obrist et al. in Chapter 8 of this book. The nonsomatic effects observed by these investigators were confined to the early trials of a stressful reaction-time task, and, like the electrodermal responses described in the present chapter, were sympathetically mediated. This demonstration notwithstanding, the weight of the evidence suggests that movement control mechanisms are the major determinant of heart rate variability in most experimental situations.

The results regarding electrodermal responding are more complex. Although there is little evidence for an effect of somatic processes on electrodermal arousal during CER training, an effect of somatic events on electrodermal responding does appear to be demonstrable under other, apparently less aversive, circumstances. For example, Culp and Edelberg (1966) found that instructing human subjects to flex the toes of the right foot produced an electrodermal response in the ipsilateral hand that was larger, relative to a homologous contralateral palmar site, than responses produced by flexing the toes of the left foot. Segmental patterning of electrodermal responses with respect to movement was also apparent. These effects do not appear attributable to motivational or attentional processes that may have been excited when subjects were instructed to perform a particular movement, since these processes as elaborated in the present chapter would have been expected to affect electrodermal responding in all limbs equally. Rather, it seems more plausible to attribute electrodermal asymmetry to movement control mechanisms. An effect of somatic events on electrodermal arousal is also suggested by recent studies which have compared electrodermal reactions to cues that require either the performance of a specific movement or merely an attentional response. These studies typically report larger electrodermal responses to stimuli that require movement, although substantial responding invariably occurs to attentional cues as well (e.g., Harding and Punzo 1971).

Demonstrations of somatic control of electrodermal responding lead one to ask whether any general conclusions can be drawn about the relative importance of motivational and movement control processes as determinants of electrodermal responding in various behavioral situations. The following conclusions seem possible. Clearly, the extent to which electrodermal arousal is determined by motivational or movement processes will depend upon the degree to which these systems are engaged by the task the subject is required to perform. However, whenever both systems are engaged to a substantial degree, as undoubtedly happened during CER training, motivational arousal will be a more important determinant of electrodermal responding than will motor activity. Motor activity, however, will be a more important determinant of heart rate than of electrodermal responding.

NOTES

1. In this chapter, I shall use the term electrodermal control system to refer to those brain structures and nerve pathways that determine skin conductance and skin potential. The cardiac control system, on the other hand, refers to structures and pathways that determine heart rate. A more precise definition of these systems is offered by Roberts (1972).

2. This model of the organization of the cardiac control system makes sense in view of the importance of heart rate in adjusting cardiac output to meet the metabolic requirements of striate muscular activity. Obviously, the functional organization of the electrodermal control system would be clearer if the adaptive utility of palmar and plantar sweating were known (see Roberts and Young 1971).

3. Brady (1971) and de Toledo (1971) also recorded electromyographic activity during CER training (the former in one subject only). Electromyographic activity (EMG) was not significantly related to changes in lever pressing or heart rate. On the other hand, Obrist et al. (1970b) reported strong relationships between heart rate and EMG in studies of classical conditioning and reaction time, but in their experiments EMG and general activity were also correlated. Like lever pressing, EMG may be related to heart rate only when it is correlated with general activity.

10

NEIL SCHNEIDERMAN

The Relationship Between Learned and Unlearned Cardiovascular Responses

INTRODUCTION

Major physiological interventions have traditionally been used to study the mechanisms involved in cardiovascular regulation. These interventions have included peripheral electric shock, electrical stimulation of the brain, hypoxia, exsanguination, or transection of neural structures. Peiss has pointed out that: "To a large degree these procedures represent major crises to the organism and involve massive activation of homeostatic mechanisms. In this light many investigations have dealt with central control mechanisms which operate in emergency states of the organism" (Peiss 1965, p. 180).

Many experiments studying the integration of cardiovascular responses have additionally used acute procedures upon anesthetized animals. Unfortunately, the cardiovascular responses of anesthetized animals cannot be expected to reflect normal, dynamic cardiovascular control mechanisms. General anesthetic agents, for example, have direct actions upon the central nervous system, the heart, and the blood vessels, and markedly alter cardiovascular responses to stimuli (e.g., Herd 1970; Korner, Langford, and Starr 1968; Korner, Uther, and White 1968).

Whereas physiologists interested in the cardiovascular system tradi-

The research from my laboratory described in this chapter was primarily supported by research grants from the National Science Foundation and by the cooperative funds of the Florida Heart Association and its chapters.

190

tionally worked with acutely prepared, anesthetized subjects, some cardiovascular- and neurophysiologists have in recent years begun to study the integration of cardiovascular responses in chronically prepared, unanesthetized animals. This has increasingly led to an overlap of interests with psychophysiologists studying the influence of behavioral manipulations upon autonomic responses in unanesthetized individuals. Due to this convergence of interests, questions are now being raised about the mechanisms of cardiovascular regulation that are operative in the behaving organism. In this context, the classical- (Pavlovian) conditioning paradigm—because of its simplicity, exact control over stimulus events, and feasibility for use in restrained animals —offers one of the most appropriate vehicles for studying mechanisms of cardiovascular regulation in the unanesthetized behaving organism.

In my own laboratory, the classical-conditioning procedure has allowed my co-workers and me to compare unlearned cardiovascular responses elicited by massive interventions such as noxious electric shock with learned cardiovascular responses to initially innocuous stimuli (e.g., lights or tones). The present chapter examines the relationship of these unlearned (unconditioned) and learned (conditioned) cardiovascular responses to one another. These relationships between unconditioned responses (UR) and conditioned responses (CR) have important implications for our understanding of both cardiovascular regulation and behavior.

Most of the research in my laboratory has been performed upon rabbits; some has been conducted upon rats and rhesus monkeys. In one series of experiments we examined aversive classical-conditioning of heart rate (HR), using peripheral electric shock as the unconditioned stimulus (UCS). In another series of experiments we used chemical or electrical stimulation of the brain (ESB) as the UCS. The present chapter first reviews our research findings concerning the relationships between cardiovascular CRs and URs. This exposition is followed by a more general discussion about the role of cardiovascular CRs as adaptive adjustments of the organism.

PERIPHERAL ELECTRIC SHOCK AS THE UCS

The cardiovascular URs to peripheral electric shock in the loosely restrained rabbit include a change in HR and an increase in blood pressure (BP); whereas, the CRs usually include a change in HR, but no change in BP.

If the rabbit does not move in response to peripheral shock, the HR UR consists of a monophasic decrease in rate; whereas, if the rabbit moves, the HR change includes an increase in rate. Both monophasic decreases in HR and biphasic HR changes in which the initial component is an increase in rate have been observed using essentially the same experimental procedures (Kazis and Powell 1971; Schneiderman 1972; Schneiderman et al. 1969; Yehle, Dauth, and Schneiderman 1967).

We (Powell et al. 1971) have provided evidence that characteristics of the conditioned stimulus (CS) as well as the UCS can also influence the direction of HR responses in rabbits. In this experiment, in which peripheral shock was the UCS, the HR CRs were decelerative for a group having tone as the CS, but were accelerative for a group in which a change in ambient illumination was the CS. Conditioning began earlier in training with the auditory than with the visual CS. Our data suggested that the direction of the HR CR was related to the activity of our animals at the time when conditioning first occurred. The HR decrease to the tone CS appeared to be related to behavioral freezing (i.e., somatic motor inhibition), which occurred early in training. In contrast, the HR increase to the visual CS occurred later in training after behavioral freezing was reduced. Our data, as well as those of other investigators, indicate that theories relating HR CRs and URs must be able to elucidate (a) relationships between HR responses and movement; and (b) circumstances under which the same UCS can induce different HR URs.

When tone is the CS and peripheral electric shock is the UCS, the cardiovascular CRs in rabbits and rhesus monkeys are very different from one another. In the rabbit, the CR includes bradycardia which is usually unaccompanied by a change in BP. In contrast, both the CRs and URs of rhesus monkeys include concomitant increases in HR and BP. A theory describing the role of cardiovascular CRs as adaptive adjustments needs to take these species differences into account.

ELECTRICAL STIMULATION OF THE BRAIN AS THE UCS

In several of our experiments conducted on rabbits we have used ESB as the US. For our purposes the procedure has offered us several advantages over peripheral electric shock. First, because the cardio-vascular URs to hypothalamic or septal region ESB do not readily habituate, whereas the URs to peripheral shock do, responses to ESB following injection of various drugs can be studied over the course of several sessions. Second, by merely adjusting the current intensity of ESB, the relationship between the direction of HR changes, and so-matic activity can be separated easily, conveniently, and reliably into two distinct classes (i.e., HR increases accompanied by overt movement; HR decreases unaccompanied by obvious movement). Third, by using UCS electrode placements that are empirically determined to be either appetitive or aversive, HR CRs and URs can be related to the motivational properties of the UCS. Fourth, by using long pulse-trains of ESB as the UCS, various patterns of cardiovascular URs can be elicited by stimulating different brain locations.

Coupling Between Cardiac and Somatic Responses

The use of short pulse-train ESB has provided us with an experimental preparation characterized by extremely stable cardiovascular responses. When electrical stimulation of the midbrain or hypothalamus is presented at current intensities eliciting pronounced movement, the HR UR consists of an increase in rate. Conversely, when stimulation via the same electrodes is presented at current intensities below the threshold for eliciting gross movement, the HR UR consists of a decrease in rate. This dichotomy permitted Elster, VanDercar, and Schneiderman (1970) to examine the relationship between movement on the one hand and the topography of HR URs and CRs on the other.

In this experiment we used a differential conditioning procedure with intracranial stimulation as both the CSs and the UCS. Our UCS consisted of a 1-second train of 200 pulse per second (pps) stimulation of the midbrain, subthalamus or hypothalamus. The CS+ was immediately followed by a UCS, whereas the CS− was not. Duration of the CS was 6 seconds as was the CS-UCS interval. In some rabbits the CS+ consisted of electrical stimulation of one medial geniculate nucleus, and the CS− consisted of stimulation of the contralateral medial geniculate nucleus. In other animals, stimulation of one lateral geniculate nucleus was CS+ and stimulation of the contralateral lateral geniculate nucleus was CS−. In all instances the CS consisted of low-frequency (i.e., 9 pps) stimulation.

Our major findings were as follows: (1) Differential HR conditioning was induced by midbrain, subthalamic, or hypothalamic UCSs. (2) Greater differential conditioning was induced by diencephalic (subthalamic, hypothalamic) than by midbrain stimulation as the UCS. (3) In both the midbrain and diencephalon, UCS electrode placements were found that elicited accelerative HR conditioning. (4) Particularly in the diencephalon, a strong positive relationship existed between diffuse movement and accelerative HR CRs and URs.

In summary, decelerative HR CRs were obtained in subthalamic and hypothalamic placements in which the UCS elicited a decrease in HR and an absence or inhibition of pronounced movements. In contrast, when stimulation of UCS placements in the diencephalon elicited diffuse somatic movements, accelerative HR CRs and URs were concomitantly elicited. These findings suggest the presence of a firm cardiac-somatic response linkage when electrical stimulation of the diencephalon is used as the UCS. Kaada (1960) previously implicated various limbic structures in the concomitant inhibition of cardiac and somatic URs. Conversely, Eliasson, Lindgren, and Uvnäs (1952) implicated various hypothalamic structures in the concomitant regulation of cardiovascular responses and muscular activation. The nature of the cardiac-somatic linkage has also been examined with regard to exercise (e.g., Rushmer 1962; Rushmer and Smith 1959; Rushmer, Smith, and Franklin 1959), and to conditioning (e.g., Obrist 1965; Obrist and Webb 1967; Obrist, Sutterer, and Howard 1972a).

The Elster et al. (1970) experiment demonstrated a strong positive relationship between HR increases and movement. Consequently, in order to examine the bases of HR conditioning in the absence of gross movement, the UCS intensity of our subsequent experiments was always kept below the threshold for eliciting gross somatic activity.

Autonomic Relationships

The absence of concomitant cardiovascular measures in the Elster et al. (1970) experiment precluded an analysis of any autonomic relationships involved in HR classical conditioning. Therefore, in our next experiment, VanDercar, Elster, and Schneiderman (1970) concomitantly examined HR and BP changes during differential classical conditioning induced by UCS stimulation of the hypothalamus or septal region. In this study, electrical stimulation of one lateral geniculate nucleus (CS+) in rabbits was paired with septal or hypothalamic stimulation as the UCS, whereas stimulation of the contralateral lateral geniculate nucleus was the CS−. The CS duration and CS-UCS interval were 2 seconds.

We found that HR differential conditioning developed between the CS+ and CS−. However, no conditioned BP changes of any kind were observed. The HR CRs and URs in this experiment consisted of decreases in rate. The BP URs consisted of increases in systolic and diastolic pressures. Latencies of the BP URs were invariably shorter than the latencies of the HR URs.

The results obtained by using septal region or hypothalamic ESB as the UCS agreed with our previous findings in which peripheral electric shock served as the UCS (Schneiderman et al. 1969; Yehle, Dauth, and Scheiderman 1967). In these earlier studies we suggested that bradycardia as a UR might be a compensatory reflex response to a sympathetically-induced increase in BP.

The possibility that the HR UR in the VanDercar et al. (1970) study was a reflexive response to a BP increase is of particular interest, because the HR CR, which also was a decrease in rate, typically occurred in the absence of a BP CR. This indicates that the HR CR is not a reflexive response to a change in arterial pressure. Consequently, the CR and UR may be controlled by very different central nervous system mechanisms.

In order to investigate the nature of these relationships we conducted a series of experiments in which cardiovascular URs and/or CRs were selectively abolished by various adrenergic and cholinergic blockades. The overall strategy was one in which we blocked a particular cardiovascular response in order to examine the effect upon another cardiovascular change. This permitted us to determine the relationship between (a) HR and BP changes following short pulse-train stimulation of the hypothalamus or septal region; and, (b) HR URs and CRs induced by this stimulation.

In the drug experiments we used the alpha-adrenergic blocking agent, phentolamine, to antagonize sympathetic vascular tone. The beta-adrenergic blocking agent, propranolol, and the cholinergic blocking agent, atropine, were used respectively, to antagonize sympathetic and parasympathetic influences upon the heart. Since atropine (sulfate) is known to have marked central nervous system effects, methyl atropine was also studied because it does not readily pass the blood-brain barrier into the central nervous system and, consequently, has primarily peripheral effects when injected systemically (e.g., Carlton 1962; Giarman and Pepeu 1964). We have also shown that atropine sulfate, but not methyl atropine, abolishes classically conditioned somatic CRs in rabbits (Downs et al. 1972).

In our initial study—examining the effects of autonomic blockades on cardiovascular responses to ESB—we (Powell et al. 1972) assessed the effects of pharmacological blockade on URs. Unanesthetized rabbits received high frequency (200 pps), short pulse-train duration (1 second) electrical stimulation of the septal region or hypothalamus at current intensities not producing obvious gross movements. Dose-response and time-response effects were obtained for the HR and BP changes following intracranial stimulation under the alpha-adrenergic (phentolamine), beta-adrenergic (propranolol), and cholinergic (methyl atropine, atropine sulfate) blocking agents.

Stimulation at all 42 of our electrode placements elicited an increase in arterial BP. In 40 or 42 of these placements the HR response was either a monophasic HR decrease or a brief acceleration followed by a much larger and longer duration HR decrease. In one septal region and in one subthalamic location, stimulation resulted in a unidirectional increase in HR. In the drug portion of the experiment we found that appropriate doses of the alpha-adrenergic blocking agent, phentolamine, abolished the BP increase and HR decrease seen after ESB. The HR and BP changes to stimulation of a representative rabbit, DS-5, before and 10 to 45 minutes after injection of phentolamine are shown in Figure 10.1. The changes in systolic and diastolic BP (not shown) following stimulation were comparable to those shown for mean BP in Figure 10.1.

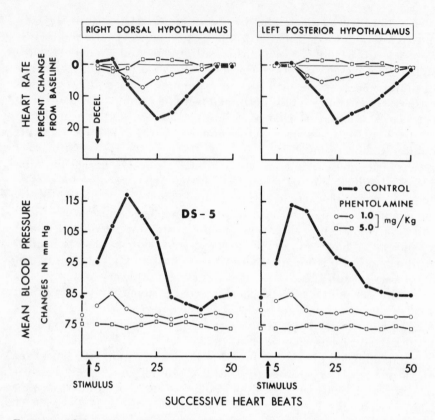

FIGURE 10.1.   *Heart rate and blood pressure changes occurring during the 50 heart beats following stimulation of the right dorsal hypothalamus (left) frames or the left posterior hypothalamus (right frames) in rabbit DS-5. Changes are shown following injection of saline (control) or 1.0 mg/kg or 5.0 mg/kg of phentolamine. (From Powell, Goldberg, Dauth, Schneiderman, and Schneiderman 1972).*

The HR and BP changes to ESB in the Powell et al. (1972) experiment were abolished or markedly reduced following systemic injection of phentolamine. Since phentolamine blocks the innervation of the arterioles rather than the heart, it would appear that the decelerative HR change normally occurring after stimulation was a compensatory baroreceptor response that was secondary to the BP increase. The additional finding that the HR decrease to ESB was converted to cardioacceleration following injection of phentolamine (see Figure 10.1) suggests that the HR decrease to stimulation in the nondrugged animal masked a sympathetic cardiac response.

Although HR decreases are generally considered to be primarily parasympathetic responses mediated by the vagus nerves, the magnitude and form of the HR decrease may be influenced by the interaction at the heart of sympathetic and parasympathetic innervations. The Powell et al. (1972) experiment provided important information about the relationship between parasympathetic and sympathetic influences upon the heart in determining the form and magnitude of the HR decrease following ESB. The principal aspects of these relationships can be seen in the performance of rabbit DS-6 in Figure 10.2.

Figure 10.2 presents percent changes from baseline for the 60 heart beats following the onset of ESB. The dashed line (with open circles) in each frame represents the HR change to stimulation prior to drug administration. The solid line (with open circles) represents the HR change to stimulation approximately 15 minutes after injection of the drug specified in each frame. The thin solid line (with open triangles) shown in the upper right hand frame shows the HR change to ESB following injection of both propranolol (5 mg/kg) and methylatropine (20 mg/kg).

Figure 10.2 indicates that injection of propranolol (5 mg/kg) increased the magnitude of the HR decrease. Since propranolol is a beta-blocking agent that blocks the sympathetic input to the heart, the augmentation of the HR decrease under propranolol appears to largely reflect the full influence of the parasympathetic innervation of the heart. (The propranolol induced displacement of the curve towards ESB onset merely reflects a drug-induced slowing of the HR baseline.)

The augmentation of bradycardia under propranolol and the change from cardiodeceleration to cardioacceleration under phentolamine indicate that in the normal, nonblockaded animal, the parasympathetic and sympathetic inputs to the heart actively oppose one another, but that the parasympathetic activity predominates. This view is further confirmed in the frames on the right hand side of Figure 10.2. These show that the atropine blockades unmasked the sympathetic, cardioaccelerative influence upon the HR change.

The atropine frames of Figure 10.2 also indicate that from beat 40 onward the HR response to ESB showed a small deceleration under atropine. This HR deceleration, although quite small, showed up reliably in almost all of the electrode placements tested, and even occurred after bilateral vagotomy. Note in the top right hand frame, however, that the combination of propranolol and methyl atropine abolished the small HR decrease. Thus, the small HR deceleration at the end of the HR response to ESB seems to reflect a sympathetic inhibitory process.

In the Powell et al. (1972) experiment we examined the effects of pharmacological blockades upon cardiovascular responses to subcortical ESB in unanesthetized rabbits. By means of drug interventions we were able to show that following ESB the HR decrease that was typically observed is (a) a compensatory response to an increase in BP,

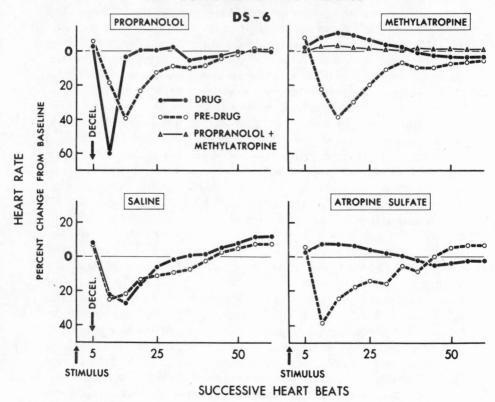

FIGURE 10.2.   *Heart rate percentage changes from baseline occurring during the 60 beats following stimulation of the left dorsomedial hypothalamus in rabbit DS-6. Solid lines and closed circles represent heart rate changes occurring before saline or drug administration. Dashed lines and open circles represent heart rate changes occurring during the same session after injection of saline, propranolol (5 mg/kg), methylatropine (20 mg/kg), or atropine sulfate (20 mg/kg). (From Powell, Goldberg, Dauth, Schneiderman, and Schneiderman 1972).*

and, (b) a complex response involving synergistic and antagonistic relations between the sympathetic and parasympathetic innervations of the heart. In a subsequent experiment Fredericks, Moore, Metcalf, and I used similar pharmacological methods to compare the physiological bases of HR CRs and URs in unanesthetized rabbits.

We differentially classically conditioned rabbits using electrical stimulation of one lateral geniculate nucleus as CS+, and stimulation of the contralateral lateral geniculate nucleus as CS−. The UCS consisted of a short pulse-train of ESB in the hypothalamus or septal region. The UCS parameter values were the same as those used by Powell et al.

(1972). Once differential conditioning was established, we compared the effects of selective autonomic blockades upon HR CRs and URs by including UCS alone as well as CS+ and CS− trials.

The changes in baseline HR and the changes in HR URs to intracranial stimulation after systemic injections of the blocking agents were consistent with those observed by Powell et al. (1972). As in the previous study, HR responses to the ESB UCS included an abolition of bradycardia under phentolamine, and a reversal or the bradycardia to tachycardia under atropine sulfate and methylatropine. Whereas phentolamine severely attenuated the HR UR, its influence on the HR CR and on HR differential conditioning were considerably less (see Figure 10.3). In some instances the HR UR was totally abolished, by alpha-adrenergic blockade, but on temporally adjacent trials HR CRs continued to occur. Since the baselines were similar on the CS+ and UCS alone trials, this indicates that the diminution of the HR UR was not merely due to a change in the HR baseline. The results emphasize that while the HR UR to high frequency, short pulse-train ESB in unanesthetized rabbits is a response to a sympathetically-induced change in BP, the HR CR is not.

In another experiment, Sampson, Francis, and Schneiderman (in press) used the conditioned emotional response (CER) paradigm to examine the effects of various autonomic blockades upon the differential classical-conditioning of bar-pressing, HR, and BP in rabbits. Although the parameter values of the intracranial UCS remained the same as in the experiment by Fredericks, Moore, Metcalf, and myself, our study using the CER paradigm differed from it in several important respects. Thus, in the experiment with Sampson et al. (in press) our CS-UCS interval was 1 minute instead of 2 seconds, there were many fewer trials per day, and during acquisition sessions the classical conditioning procedure was superimposed upon a situation in which the rabbits bar-pressed for water on a variable interval schedule.

We observed differential conditioning of bar-press and HR, but not BP responses. The bar-press CRs to the CS+ consisted of a decrease in rate; the HR CR consisted of bradycardia. Both occurred in the absence of obvious BP changes. Alpha adrenergic blockade abolished the HR and BP URs, but only slightly attenuated HR and bar-press suppression CRs. The results are consistent with our other findings that the UR to short pulse-train ESB is a compensatory response to a sympathetically-induced change in BP, but that the HR CR is not.

In the experiment conducted by Sampson et al. (in press) the rabbits were also studied after injections of propranolol, atropine sulfate, and methyl atropine. Propranolol had little effect upon HR, BP, or bar-press responses. Following the administration of atropine sulfate, however, bar-press responses (including those during baseline periods) as

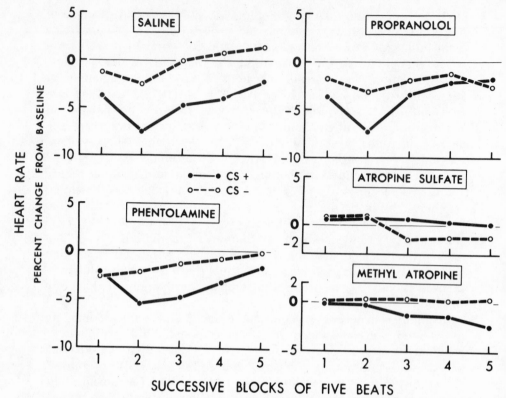

FIGURE 10.3.   *Heart rate changes from baseline for the 25 heart beats occurring after onset of CS+ (solid line and closed circle) and after onset of CS− (dashed line and open circles) following systemic injection of saline, phentolamine (5-10 mg/kg), propranolol (5 mg/kg), methylatropine (20 mg/kg), and atropine sulfate (20 mg/kg).*

well as HR CRs and URs were abolished. In contrast, at appropriate doses, methyl atropine abolished neither the bar-press baseline nor the bar-press suppression CR, but did abolish HR CRs and URs. Our findings therefore suggest that: (a) HR URs to short pulse-train stimulation of the septal region or hypothalamus consist of compensatory responses to sympathetically-induced increases in BP, and, (b) HR CRs produced in these experiments represent primary parasympathetic responses mediated via the vagus nerves.

Motivational Properties of the US

Several theorists (e.g., Malmo and Belanger 1967; Overmier 1966) have related cardiovascular changes to motivational processes. Typically, motivational theories have treated motivation as a response selection process that is influenced by depriving the organism of a needed substance (e.g., food or water), or by presenting the organism with an aversive or appetitive stimulus. In our experiments using peripheral electric shock, the UCS was obviously noxious (e.g., Schneiderman et al. 1969; Yehle, Dauth and Schneiderman 1967). In the case of our ESB experiments the motivational properties of the UCS were less self-evident. Since motivational properties have been alleged to be involved in the organism's selection of cardiovascular responses, and since our research interest includes discovering the variables influencing the form of cardiovascular CRs and URs, Sideroff, Elster, and Schneiderman (1972) examined cardiovascular classical conditioning using appetitive or aversive hypothalamic stimulation as the UCS. As in our previous studies using ESB, and UCS consisted of short pulse-trains of stimulation.

Twelve rabbits were implanted with stimulating electrodes in either the lateral (n = 6) or medial (n = 6) hypothalamus. Upon recovery each animal was tested to determine if it would bar-press to receive ESB in the lateral or medial hypothalamus. A day later each rabbit was tested in a shuttle-box preference situation in which the subject received or did not receive stimulation by being on the appropriate side of the box. During the final stage of the experiment each animal received differential classical conditioning in which stimulation of one lateral geniculate nucleus was CS+, and stimulation of the contralateral lateral geniculate nucleus was CS−. The UCS consisted of the medial or lateral hypothalamic stimulation received during the previous operant conditioning tests. Current intensity and other parameter values within the pulse-train of the UCS were identical with those used in the operant conditioning tests.

We found that the rabbits having access to lateral hypothalamic stimulation, bar-pressed to receive stimulation and made approach responses in the shuttle-box. The rabbits having access to medial hypothalamic stimulation did not bar-press and made escape responses in the shuttle-box. The cardiovascular URs of all rabbits consisted of a BP increase and bradycardia; CRs consisted of bradycardia. Thus, while medial and lateral hypothalamic stimulation had different motivational properties, both provided effective UCSs for eliciting similar HR CRs. The data, therefore, indicate that at least in our experimental situation the directionality and topography of HR and BP responses are not directly influenced by whether the US is appetitive or aversive.

Although the sign of the motivational stimulus may not be important, it is possible that an arousing UCS (i.e., either appetitive or aversive) is required to elicit HR conditioning. An experiment conducted by Sideroff, Schneiderman, and Powell (1971) suggests that this is actually the case. We used operant and classical conditioning procedures similar to those used by Sideroff and his co-workers (1972) to evaluate septal region ESB as the UCS. We found that HR classical conditioning occurred at high but not at low intensities of septal region ESB, even though the low and high intensities of ESB both elicited reliable URs.

Cardiovascular Responses Elicited by Long Pulse-Trains

In contrast to the uniform response pattern elicited in our experiments using 1-second trains of ESB, we (Francis et al. 1973) observed several different patterns of cardiovascular responses after stimulating various areas of the hypothalamus or septal region with 10-second pulse-trains. These patterns, which to some extent were specific to particular areas stimulated, consisted of: (1) a concomitant decrease in HR and BP; (2) a concomitant increase in HR and BP; (3) an increase in HR and decrease in BP; and, (4) a decrease in HR accompanied by an increase in BP. In a subsequent experiment, still in progress, we have been using 10-second pulse-trains of ESB as the UCS for inducing classical conditioning. Thus far, we have ascertained that long pulse-train stimulation of the medial septal region can induce decreases in BP as both CRs and URs. Further use of the long pulse-train UCS should provide us with opportunities for examining important relationships among a variety of cardiovascular CRs and URs.

CHEMICAL STIMULATION OF THE BRAIN AS A UCS

In addition to using ESB as the UCS to study cardiovascular conditioning in situations in which UR patterns are different, Elster, Sideroff, and I have used intracranial microinjections of acetylcholine (ACh) or norepinephrine (NE) as the UCS. Besides allowing us to study the relationships between different patterns of CRs and URs, our experiment provides the first demonstration that intracranial microinjections can be used as a UCS to induce classical-conditioning.

Initially, we examined HR changes in unanesthetized rabbits receiving several different intracranially administered dosages each of NE bitartrate monohydrate and ACh chloride, as well as separate control microinjections of saline and sodium bitartrate. Control solutions were adjusted with hydrochloric acid to match the pH of experimental drugs. The various drug and drug dosages were delivered through the same cannula on different days in a random order. The cannulae were aimed at the septal region, lateral ventricles, hypothalamus, or third ventricle.

We found that the control substances did not elicit cardiovascular responses. In contrast, intracranial microinjection of ACh elicited a pronounced decrease in BP with a concomitant increase in HR. Conversely, intracranial microinjections of NE elicited a marked increase in BP accompanied by a decrease in HR. Onset of the BP increase to NE occurred significantly earlier in time than the recorded HR decrease.

The HR and BP changes to intracranial microinjections of NE were examined following separate systemic injections of methylatropine, phentolamine, propranolol, and saline. We found that systemic injections of the autonomic blocking agents modified the cardiovascular responses to intracranial microinjections of NE in the same way that they influenced cardiovascular responses to short pulse-train ESB. Thus, phentolamine eliminated the BP increase and HR decrease that followed microinjection of NE, and methylatropine abolished the decelerative HR UR. Our findings suggest that, as was the case for ESB, the bradycardia following intracranial microinjection of NE is mainly a reflexive response to a sympathetically-induced increase in BP. In contrast to the cardiovascular changes elicited by NE, intracranial microinjection of ACh elicited tachycardia accompanied by a BP decrease. Our findings did not distinguish whether the HR or the BP changes occurring after intracranial microinjection of ACh were reflexively related to one another.

The major differences in cardiovascular changes between those elicited by electrical or chemical intracranial stimulation were in terms of latency and temporal duration. Following short pulse-train ESB, latencies of HR and BP changes in our experiments were less than 1 second, and response durations were typically under 10 seconds (e.g., Powell et al. 1972; VanDercar, Elster, and Schneiderman 1970). In contrast, for the rabbits in the study using intracranial chemical stimulation mean latencies of the HR changes to NE and ACh were generally more than 20 seconds and mean peak latency usually exceeded 30 seconds.

Having demonstrated that cardiovascular URs to central injection of NE resembled those elicited by high frequency, short pulse-train ESB, we set out to determine whether intracranial administration of NE could serve as the UCS to induce differential classical conditioning and whether the HR—if it occurred—would consist of an HR decrease.. We also tested whether intracranial administration of ACh could serve as a UCS to induce differential classical conditioning.

In the conditioning phase of the study, we differentially classically conditioned rabbits using a microinjection of either NE or ACh into the lateral hypothalamus as the US. Because of the relatively long latencies of the BP and HR changes elicited by the microinjections, we used a backward conditioning procedure in which a 10-second injection of drug (ACh or NE) or saline was followed by a 30-second train of 8 pps ESB. A differential conditioning procedure was used in which stimulation of one lateral geniculate nucleus (CS+) was preceded by an injection of drug, and stimulation of the contralateral geniculate nucleus (CS−) was preceded by an injection of saline. On test trials, stimulation of each lateral geniculate nucleus was preceded by an injection of saline. Differential conditioning occurred using either NE or

ACh as the UCS. The CR consisted of cardiodeceleration for rabbits in which NE was the UCS, and cardioacceleration for rabbits in which ACh was the UCS. Neither HR CR was accompanied by a BP CR.

Our study indicated that intracranial microinjection of NE or ACh can be used to induce cardiovascular URs and that either drug can be used as a UCS to induce HR classical conditioning. When NE was the UCS, the cardiovascular CRs and URs resembled responses previously seen when short pulse-trains of hypothalamic or septal region stimulation was the UCS. Thus, the decelerative HR URs to both short pulse-train ESB and NE appeared to be reflexive responses to sympathetically-induced increases in BP, whereas the conditioned HR decreases were not related to conditioned changes in BP.

For the purposes of the present chapter the primary significance of our findings based upon intracranial chemical stimulation is that it demonstrated that HR increases and HR decreases in rabbits can each be classically conditioned. The HR CRs in each case occurred in the absence of concomitant BP changes. In the next section we shall discuss in detail the implications of these as well as our other findings.

THE CR AS PREPARATORY RESPONSE

At one time many conditioning theorists advocated a "stimulus substitution" interpretation of conditioning. The stimulus substitution hypothesis held that the responses made to the CS following conditioning are the same as the responses evoked by the UCS. Once investigators began to compare the topographies of CRs and URs and began to look at a number of response systems concomitantly, the stimulus substitution formulation became untenable.

An important difference between the CR and UR has been documented in HR classical conditioning studies conducted upon rats or humans. Several investigators have noted that in these species the UR is almost invariably an increase in HR, but the CR is frequently a decrease in HR (e.g., de Toledo and Black 1966; Obrist, Wood, and Perez-Reyes 1965; Parrish 1967; Zeaman and Smith 1965). Sideroff, Schneiderman, and Powell (1971) have additionally indicated that when ESB is used as the UCS in HR classical conditioning of rabbits, the topographies of the HR URs and CRs are often different. We observed, for instance, that electrical stimulation of the medial septal region elicited a biphasic UR, consisting of a brief HR increase accompanied by a larger and longer lasting HR decrease. In contrast, the CR consisted of a monophasic HR decrease.

The VanDercar et al. (1970) experiment indicated that the CR constellation is not a replica of the UR constellation. Whereas, the cardiovascular URs consisted of changes in both BP and HR, the CRs included a change in HR unaccompanied by any visible changes in BP. Moreover, our subsequent ESB studies (e.g., Powell et al. 1972; Sampson, Francis, and Schneiderman (in press)) indicated that the HR UR to short pulse-train ESB is a compensatory response to a sympathetically-induced increase in BP, whereas the HR CR is a parasympathetic response that is unrelated to any change in BP. Several converging lines of evidence, therefore, have clearly shown that the stimulus substitution hypothesis is untenable.

An alternative view of the relationship between the CR and the UR is that the CR is a fractional component of the UR. Since the HR CRs and URs in the VanDercar et al. (1970) experiment both consisted of decreases in rate, the HR CR could be looked upon as a fractional component of the response constellation evoked by the UR. A difficult question for advocates of this position to answer, however, is why the HR rather than the BP response invariably becomes conditioned. A serious objection to the fractional component hypothesis is raised by instances in which the CR consists of a decrease in HR, but the UR consists of an increase (e.g., deToledo and Black 1966; Obrist, Wood, and Perez-Reyes 1965; Zeaman and Smith 1965).

Another hypothesis about the form of the CR is that it is determined by the UCS. According to this view, the CR may not be related to the UR at all. Instead, each UCS is said to have associated with it a set of CRs that becomes conditioned. If, indeed, the UCS determines the form or direction of the CR, as the hypothesis proposes, then the CRs for any given UCS ought to be the same. In our studies using peripheral electric shock as the UCS in the rabbit, however, the same UCS led either to an increase or a decrease in HR depending upon the sensory modality or characteristics of the CS (Powell et al. 1971). Moreover, even in experiments in which tone is the CS, peripheral shock is the US, and other parameter values (e.g., CS-UCS interval) are kept constant, a few rabbits will consistently show accelerative rather than decelerative CRs (e.g., Downs et al. 1972). Another issue that is difficult for the hypothesis to deal with concerns the reason why peripheral shock as a US leads to decelerative HR CRs in rabbits, but accelerative HR CRs in monkeys.

Motivational theories, too, tend to relate the form of the CR to properties of the UCS. The experiment by Sideroff and his co-workers (Sideroff et al. 1972) in which the form and direction of the HR CR were the same to both an appetitive and an aversive US, however, indicates that differences in the directionality of HR CRs cannot be due solely to differences in the motivational properties of the UCS.

Cardiovascular psychophysiologists have consistently observed that the directionality of both HR CRs and URs are related to movement. Thus, it has commonly been observed that HR increases accompany somatic movements, whereas HR decreases accompany the inhibition or absence of somatic movements. Convincing demonstrations of cardiac-somatic coupling have been provided for exercise (e.g., Rushmer, Smith, and Franklin 1959; Rushmer and Smith 1959), and for conditioning (e.g., Elster, VanDercar, and Schneiderman 1970; Obrist 1965; Obrist and Webb 1967; Osbrist, Sutterer, and Howard 1972a). Although HR changes during conditioning are usually related to gross somatic activity, this is not always the case. Several classical conditioning studies have found that the HR CR is qualitatively the same whether animals are run under a paralyzing drug or in the normal state (e.g., Black 1965; Yehle, Dauth, and Schneiderman 1967). The experiments using paralyzing drugs indicate that the direction of HR changes is related to the integration of movement processes within the brain rather than to actual somatic movements.

Some evidence indicates that HR increases may actually precede overt signs of movement. When movement of a treadmill was used as a UCS, dogs showed increases of HR and BP in the presence of the CS (Bolme and Novotny 1969). In the experiment by Elster, Sideroff, and Schneiderman, in which we infused chemicals into the brain and recorded cardiovascular activity, we concomitantly monitored somatic activity using a phonograph cartridge. We found that somatic activity occurred much more often during or after infusion of ACh than during or after infusion of NE. Whereas movement only occurred on some trials during ACh injections, HR increases occurred on every trial. Moreover, in the instances in which movement was observed, somatic activity followed rather than preceded increases in HR.

The research investigating cardiac-somatic coupling suggests that there is an important relationship between HR and movement, but that HR is not merely a passive concomitant of overt somatic activity. Even if it was, however, we would still have to ask what determines whether a CR will consist of an increase or a decrease in somatic activity. Thus far, we have ruled out explanations contending that the CR is either a replica or a fractional component of the UR, but have not provided an alternative hypothesis.

Some theorists have emphasized the role of the CR as part of an attentional process (e.g., Sokolov 1963; Graham and Clifton 1966; Lacey and Lacey 1970). Sokolov has related the elicitation of autonomic CRs to neural mechanisms that facilitate or inhibit the reception of sensory input. According to Sokolov, low-to-moderate intensities of stimulation elicit autonomic and somatic responses (i.e., the orienting reflex) that facilitate afferent input; whereas, very intense stimulation elicits a different constellation of responses (i.e., the defensive reflex) that protects the organism from over-stimulation by inhibiting sensory input. Sokolov suggested that sympathetic responses such as HR increases are characteristic of the orienting reflex, but Graham and Clifton, as well as Lacey and Lacey, have contended that HR decreases rather than increases are indicative of orienting.

While various constellations of CRs may or may not differentially influence sensory input, the directionality of HR CRs does not appear to be directly related to attentional processes. None of the attention theories, for example, account for our findings that when a broad range of peripheral shock intensities are used as the UCS; rhesus monkeys show cardioacceleration, but rabbits show cardiodeceleration as the CR. It would also be difficult for Sokolov's theory to explain how tone and changes in visual illumination, which are both innocuous CSs, could produce different HR CRs with the same parameter values of peripheral electric shock as the UCS (Powell et al. 1971). The findings of Sideroff and his colleagues (Sideroff, Schneiderman, and Powell 1971; Sideroff, Elster, and Schneiderman 1972) raise additional problems for the Sokolov formulation that the directionality of autonomic responses is related to the intensive properties of stimulation. Thus, the HR CRs in our rabbits maintained the same directionality across a broad range of US current intensities. The HR CRs also maintained the same directionality across a spectrum of UCS motivational properties, including very pleasant, mildly pleasant, mildly aversive, and very aversive stimulation.

My own working hypothesis (speculation) about CRs is that they are related both to the UCS and to URs. The CR is conceptualized as an adaptive response that prepares the organism to either augment or cope with the effects of the UCS. This depends upon the constellation of URs that is elicited. If, for example, the UCS leads to prolonged movement with a concomitant demand for increased energy expenditure, then the cardiovascular CRs will augment the cardiovascular URs, thereby increasing cardiac output. Similarly, if the US leads to a general quieting of the organism with decreased energy expenditures, the cardiovascular CRs and URs may both include concomitant decreases in HR and/or BP. If on the other hand, the UCS leads to an increase in BP, but also to behavioral freezing or an absence of movement (e.g., VanDercar, Elster, and Schneiderman 1970), then the cardiovascular CRs will consist of compensatory responses. In this instance, a decelerative HR CR would decrease the stress placed upon the cardiovascular system by the UR constellation.

The cardiovascular CRs and URs obtained in our experiment using intracranial microinjections of ACh, can also be interpreted within the framework of the compensatory adjustment hypothesis. The URs to intracranial injection of ACh included an increase in HR and a decrease in BP, but the CR consisted of an increase in HR unaccompanied by a change in BP. According to the present interpretation, the cardioaccelerative CR could be conceived of as a preparatory response, which helped to compensate for the decrease in BP elicited by the UCS. When decreases in arterial BP—such as those resulting from pronounced vasodilation and venous pooling in muscle—are not countered by compensatory mechanisms, reduced blood flow to the brain may occur with resulting syncope (fainting).

The notion that CRs may have compensatory functions was suggested by Subkov and Zilov (1937). At the outset of their experiment, dogs injected with Ringer solution did not produce HR changes. The injection procedure can thus be conceived of as a neutral CS. After the original injection of Ringer solution, the dogs were subsequently given systemic injections of adrenaline. These injections of adrenaline were given every two or three days for several weeks. Each of these injections produced an increase in HR. After several of the adrenaline injections were given, Subkov and Zilov again injected the dogs with Ringer solution. This time the injection elicited a decrease in HR. Pairing of the injection procedure (CS) with the administration of adrenaline (UCS) apparently elicited a compensatory, decelerative HR CR. Subsequent injection of adrenaline, again elicited an increase in HR.

Siegel (1972) has also conducted an experiment which supports the view that CRs can serve a preparatory, compensatory function. Rats were first injected with physiological saline. This did not lead to a change in the level of blood glucose. The rats were subsequently injected with insulin every other day for several sessions. Each injection elicited a decrease in blood glucose (hypoglycemia) as the UR. After receiving several sessions of insulin injection, the animals were given a test session in which they were injected with physiological saline. This induced an increase in blood glucose (hyperglycemia) as the CR. Thus, the CR and the UR in Siegel's study consisted of opposite glycemic responses.

Since it is essential for an animal to maintain an adequate glucose level, an insulin injection given to a normal animal could dangerously reduce this level. A hypoglycemic CR would therefore be maladaptive. In contrast, a hyperglycemic CR could be viewed as a preparatory response by the organism in anticipation of a reduction of blood glucose by the insulin US. Siegel's (1972) finding of conditioned hyperglycemia in rats therefore supports the view that the CR is a preparatory adaptive response.

The present formulation seems plausible. But how well does it stand up to the objections raised to other theories? In the Powell et al. (1971) experiment, for example, the same UCS led to an increase or a decrease in the HR CR depending on whether the CS consisted of a tone or a change in illumination. The present formulation has little difficulty handling these results, if we merely assume that the directionality of the HR CR is determined at the time when conditioning first occurs. The decelerative HR CR to tone occurred while the rabbit showed behavioral freezing; whereas, the accelerative HR CR to the visual CS first occurred after behavioral freezing was diminished. These findings, therefore, are consistent with the hypothesis that the directionality of HR CRs are jointly influenced by the BP and somatic motor characteristics of the UR.

Our present hypothesis also has little difficulty handling the differences in the direction of the HR CRs which have been observed between monkeys and rabbits conditioned with a peripheral shock UCS. Thus, the first few times that the UCS is presented, monkeys typically struggle; whereas, rabbits move very briefly, if at all, and then tend to freeze.

The present formulation encounters its greatest difficulty in attempting to explain how in humans and rats the HR CR can be decelerative, whereas the HR UR is accelerative. Actually, the difficulty may be only that a comprehensive analysis of the temporal relationships among HR, BP, and movement URs has not yet been conducted on humans or rats. Such an analysis would be most cogent for the trials immediately preceding the onset of conditioning. While sometimes described as accelerative, the HR UR is often really biphasic, consisting of an HR increase followed by a subsequent decrease (e.g., Zeaman and Smith 1965). The HR UR is dynamic and its response topography often changes over the first few trials. It would thus appear, that the discrepancy between the direction of HR CRs and URs in rats and humans has considerable theoretical significance and deserves further study.

With the one exception just discussed, the available data support the hypothesis that the CR is an adaptive response that prepares the organism to either augment or cope with the effects of the UCS. Since the hypothesis is based upon post hoc analysis, however, its credibility will ultimately depend upon whether it successfully predicts behavioral outcomes in new experimental situations. The finding by Francis et al. (1973) that various patterns of cardiovascular URs can be elicited by long pulse-trains of ESB should provide us with an opportunity for examining new relationships between cardiovascular CRs and URs. Many of the techniques described in the present chapter (e.g., pharmacological blockades; concomitant recording of HR, BP, and movement) will be useful in this analysis.

The present formulation has emphasized the relationship among HR, BP, and movement. Study of additional parameters such as cardiac output and regional blood flow would provide valuable information and more rigorous tests of our hypothesis. Our speculation about the relationship of CRs and URs in the rhesus monkey, for instance, was based upon information about HR and BP. Since increases in HR and

BP can be accompanied by either an increase or a decrease in cardiac output, knowledge of this variable would be useful in distinguishing whether the HR and BP CRs are augmenting or compensatory responses. Similarly, information about cardiac output as well as HR, BP, and movement would help us to understand the relationship between decelerative HR CRs and accelerative HR URs in the rat.

In experiments based upon classical conditioning, our information about the relationship existing among HR, BP, and movement is correlational. Our knowledge about the relationship between CRs and URs is also correlational. One useful strategy for assessing whether relationships exist between URs and CRs (i.e., the constellation of URs determines the CR) would be to selectively manipulate aspects of the UR situation, and assess the effects upon the CR.

Suppose, for example, we construct an experimental situation in which one group of rhesus monkeys is presented with a green light immediately followed by the presentation of a yellow light. If we now train these monkeys (e.g., through shock avoidance or by positively reinforcing ESB) to increase their BP and not to move when the yellow light goes on, we can assess the effects of this manipulation upon cardiovascular response during presentation of the green light. A second group of monkeys could be trained to move when the yellow light goes on, and we could similarly assess the cardiovascular changes occurring to the green light preceding it. According to our formulation the first group of monkeys should reveal HR decreases to the green light; whereas, the second group of monkeys should show elevations in BP during illumination of both the green and yellow lights. These and similar experiments manipulating movement and cardiovascular URs could be used to rigorously test the hypothesis that the HR CR is an adaptive response that prepares the organism to either augment or cope with URs.

11

J. A. HERD, R. T. KELLEHER,
W. H. MORSE, AND S. A. GROSE

Sympathetic and Parasympathetic Activity During Behavioral Hypertension in the Squirrel Monkey

INTRODUCTION

Recent studies in the squirrel monkey have shown that persistent as well as transient elevations of systemic arterial blood pressure can be induced by schedule-controlled behavior (Grose, Herd, Morse, and Kelleher, 1971). However, the cardiovascular mechanisms underlying behavioral hypertension are not known at the present time. Because sympathetic and parasympathetic influences have been implicated in other well characterized states of arterial hypertension (Frohlich, Tarazi & Dustan, 1969; Frohlich, Ulrych, Tarazi, Dustan & Page, 1967; Julius & Conway, 1968), the role of the autonomic nervous system in regulating cardiovascular function has been investigated in normal squirrel monkeys and monkeys with behavioral hypertension. The objective of the present study was to determine how drugs that have relatively specific effects on the cardiovascular system would affect schedule-controlled behavior and behaviorally induced changes in heart rate and systemic arterial blood pressure in the squirrel monkey (Kelleher, Morse & Herd, 1972). Phentolamine, propranolol, methyl atropine, and atropine were studied as prototypes of drugs with antagonistic actions on neurotransmitters involved in cardiovascular regulation.

METHODS

The subjects were adult male squirrel monkeys weighing between 750 and 1050 gm. Under sterile conditions, while the animals were anesthetized with mixtures of halothane and oxygen, one end of a small polyvinyl chloride catheter (id 0.38 mm and od 0.76 mm or id 0.64 mm and od 1.04 mm) was implanted into the aorta of each animal

211

through the right internal iliac artery, and was threaded in a retro-grade direction to a position with the intravascular end of the catheter below the renal arteries (Herd, Morse, Kelleher & Jones, 1969). The other end of the catheter was passed through the skin in the middle of the back. The catheter was filled with heparin solution and sealed with a stainless steel obturator. For measurement of right atrial pres-sure and intravenous administration of drugs, another catheter was implanted by way of the right internal iliac vein through the inferior vena cava into the right atrium. Each day, the catheters were flushed with saline solution, filled with heparin solution, and sealed with stain-less steel obturators.

Arterial blood pressure was measured while each animal sat in a restraining chair in a sound-attenuating isolation chamber. The im-planted arterial catheter of each monkey was connected by Teflon tub-ing to the fluid-filled chamber of a Statham P23 Db strain gauge pres-sure transducer, which in turn was connected to a constant infusion syringe pump. A heparin and saline solution was infused continuously through the gauge and the tubing at a rate of 0.01 ml/min to prevent blood from clotting in the tubing. The hydrostatic pressure attributable to the continuous flow of fluid through the gauge, the connecting tub-ing, and the small polyvinyl chloride catheter was found to be less than 2 mmHg at 0.01 ml/min (Herd, et al., 1969). The Wheatstone bridge connections of the pressure transducer were attached to a polygraph recorder. Because of the distensibility of the chronically implanted catheter, no attempt was made to measure systolic or diastolic blood pressure. Patency of the arterial catheters was verified by the free flow of blood out of the open end before each experimental session, and was assessed during sessions by the amplitude of pressure oscillations synchronous with each beat of the heart. Average daily mean arterial blood pressures were calculated using horizontal lines of best fit drawn through polygraph records. Heart rate was measured by a car-diotachometer triggered by the amplified undamped output of the arterial pressure transducer. The heart rate was recorded simultane-ously with the blood pressure on the polygraph. The system used for measuring right atrial pressure was identical to that used for measuring arterial pressure, except that a Statham P23 Bb gauge was used. Car-diac output was measured by indicator dilution technique using indocyanine green (Drazen & Herd, 1972). A known amount of dye was injected into the right atrium through the catheter implanted for pressure measurements. Aortic blood was drawn by a motor-driven syr-inge through a modified low volume cuvette densitometer from the catheter implanted for aortic pressure measurements. Approximately 3 ml of blood were withdrawn for each determination and returned to the animal on detection of recirculation. Blood was withdrawn from the animal for calibration and linearity checks of the cuvette-recorder system 20 minutes after the final determination. Cardiac output was determined from the polygraph record by the technique of exponential replot.

During the two-week period following surgery, several control measurements of mean blood pressure and heart rate were made for periods of 1 to 4 hours, during which the isolation chamber was illuminated by a 25 watt overhead light. After control measurements had been made, experimental sessions of 1- to 3-hour duration were conducted daily with each animal. Between experimental sessions the monkeys were kept in individual cages. During all sessions, each monkey was restrained in the seated position by a waist lock, and its tail was held motionless by a small stock. Electric current could be delivered through the tail by two hinged brass plates which rested lightly on a shaved portion of the tail. A noncorrosive electrode paste ensured a low resistance electric contact between the plates and the tail. The electric stimulus was 650 volts alternating current 60 Hz delivered through a series resistance to give currents of 1 to 10 ma for 200 msec. A response key was mounted on the right side of a transparent Lucite wall in front of the monkey. When the key was pressed with a force of 28 gm or more, a response was recorded, accompanied by the audible click of a relay. Green and white 6 watt lights mounted above the front of the chair were used as visual stimuli.

Each monkey was studied under a procedure in which noxious electric stimuli were scheduled to occur periodically in the presence of a green light (Morse & Kelleher, 1966). Pressing the key a fixed minimum number of times (10, 30, or 100) turned off the stimulus-shock complex for a 1-minute time-out period ("fixed-ratio" schedule). For example, under the 30-response fixed-ratio schedule, electric shocks were scheduled every 30 seconds. During the time-out period, the experimental chamber was dark, electric shocks were never delivered, and key-pressing had no programmed consequences. When the time-out period ended, the green light came on again and the cycle repeated.

Propranolol hydrochloride, phentolamine methanesulfonate, atropine methyl nitrate, and atropine sulfate were dissolved in saline (0.9% NaCl). Doses refer to the salt of each drug. The drugs were injected intramuscularly just before the experimental session in a volume that never exceeded 1 ml. Various doses of the different drugs were studied in an irregular order. Drug sessions were conducted only after a control session in which the animal's blood pressure, heart rate, and rates of key-pressing were generally consistent with the values of these measures in immediately preceding sessions. Differences between the average values for the individual animals in successive control and drug sessions were computed for each dose. Summary dose-effect curves of the mean differences are presented.

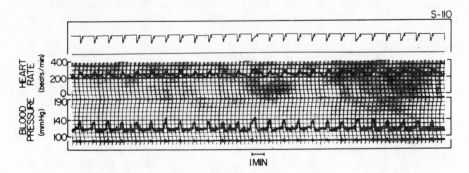

FIGURE 11.1. *Characteristic patterns of lever-pressing and changes in heart rate and mean arterial blood pressure in* monkey S-110 *under a schedule in which noxious stimuli were scheduled to occur every 30 sec in the presence of a panel light and in which the 30th response turned off the light. Top record shows cumulative recordings of lever-pressing responses. Slope of cumulative record is directly related to rate of lever-pressing. Recording pen reset to bottom of record when light was turned on automatically. Short diagonal strokes show where the light was turned off and 1-min time-out period began. Top polygraph record is heart rate and bottom polygraph record is blood pressure.*

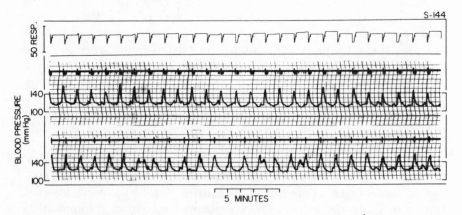

FIGURE 11.2. *Mean arterial blood pressure in* monkey S-144 *during behavioral experiments in which noxious stimuli were scheduled to occur in the presence of a panel light. Top polygraph record is blood pressure measured under the same behavioral schedule described in Figure 11.1. Bottom polygraph record is blood pressure measured in the absence of a lever under a schedule in which a panel light occasionally associated with noxious electric stimuli was turned off 1-4 sec after blood pressure had risen 5-10 mm Hg above the level recorded during time-out periods.*

RESULTS

Systematic studies of blood pressure conducted with monkeys before they were trained revealed that average mean arterial blood pressure was 121 mmHg (SD 11.1), during repeated 1 to 4 hour sessions in which the animals sat in the isolation chamber with no behavioral schedule in effect (Herd, et al., 1969). Average mean arterial blood pressure measured continuously 24 hours a day in the home cage was 125 mmHg (SD 8.1) (Grose, et al., 1971). In 12 monkeys trained under the fixed-ratio schedule, mean arterial blood pressure during control (non-drug) sessions was 149 mmHg (SD 11.0), and mean heart rate was 270 bpm (SD 3.0) (Kelleher, et al., 1972).

During preliminary training under the fixed-ratio schedule, noxious stimuli were delivered frequently to each monkey. Each noxious stimulus usually caused a momentary increase in mean blood pressure followed by a transient decrease. As rates of key-pressing increased, all monkeys had elevated mean arterial blood pressures in the presence of the green light. Results of a typical experimental session are illustrated in Figure 11.1. When the panel light came on, the monkey pressed the key rapidly, while its blood pressure and heart rate increased. When the required number of responses had been made, the light automatically was turned off, the animal stopped responding, and blood pressure and heart rate decreased. For all monkeys, mean blood pressure and heart rate were highest when the green light was on.

Elevations of arterial blood pressure in the presence of a panel light were not merely the effects of physical activity associated with pressing a lever, because elevations of blood pressure continued even after the lever had been removed from the chair (Benson, Herd, Morse & Kelleher, 1969). In Figure 11.2, the top half of the polygraph record shows the changes in arterial blood pressure observed when an animal pressed the lever in the presence of a panel light. The bottom half shows changes observed in the same animal in the presence of a panel light presented periodically while the animal sat motionless in the chair after the lever had been removed.

Other animals were continued in daily sessions, in which they were required to press a lever to turn off a light. After many daily sessions, blood pressure was elevated throughout each session, not only during periods of responding but also during time-out periods (Grose, et al., 1971; Herd, et al., 1969). In Figure 11.3, records A and B were obtained 126 days after training began, and C and D were obtained 162 days after. In both sessions, the monkey pressed the lever at a high rate and no noxious stimuli were delivered during the time these data were recorded. Blood pressure was markedly elevated on day 162.

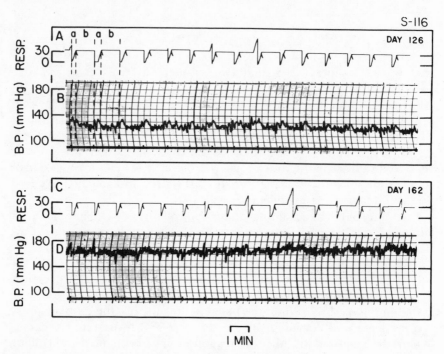

FIGURE 11.3. *Mean arterial blood pressure in* monkey S-116 *on* day 126 *(A and B) and* day 162 *(C and D) under the same behavioral schedule described in Figure 11.1. Light was turned on automatically at beginning of period* a *and turned off during period* b.

Continuous measurements of blood pressure recorded 24 hours a day revealed that elevations of arterial blood pressure induced by behavioral techniques persisted between experimental sessions. Control animals maintained in the same way as animals subjected to behavioral procedures, including daily flushing of the intravascular catheter, had no significant elevations of mean arterial blood pressure (Grose, et al., 1971).

The average resting cardiac output of five normal untrained squirrel monkeys was 319 ml/min (SD 65) (Drazen, et al. [in press]). The average resting heart rate and blood pressure of these same monkeys was 283 bpm and 123 mmHg, respectively. The average calculated stroke volume was 1.2 ml/beat and the average calculated peripheral resistance was 31,900 dynes•sec/cm^5.

Effects of propranolol

The most marked effect of propranolol was to decrease heart rate at doses of 0.1 mg/kg and higher (Figure 11.4). In individual monkeys, the magnitude of this decrease was directly related to the heart rate

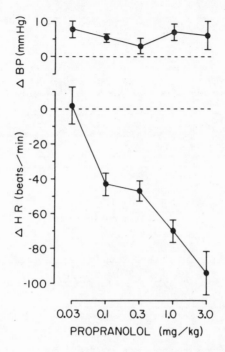

FIGURE 11.4.   *Effects of propranolol on mean blood pressure and heart rate of squirrel monkeys during 2-hour experimental sessions. The drug was given intramuscularly immediately before the start of the session. Summary dose-effect curves were obtained by computing the mean change from control to drug sessions. Dashed lines at zero indicate mean control values; vertical lines, standard errors of the means. The number of monkeys studied at each successive dose was 3, 5, 6, 9, and 4, respectively. Propranolol produced dose-dependent decreases in heart rate, whereas blood pressure was slightly increased.*

in control sessions, and was similar in subjects with normal pressures and those with behavioral hypertension. Propranolol had little or no effect on mean changes in systemic arterial blood pressure and no consistent effect on average rates of key-pressing. After 3.0 mg/kg of propranolol, episodic changes in heart rate were almost completely eliminated, whereas episodic changes in blood pressure were not affected (Figure 11.5).

Similar changes were seen in three animals in which the effects of propranolol on cardiac output were studied. In these animals, at 3.0 mg/kg there was an average decrease of 92 ml/min in cardiac output. Heart rate decreased by an average of 72 bpm at this dose. No significant change was observed in mean systemic arterial or mean right atrial pressure after propranolol. Peripheral vascular resistance was increased after propranolol and stroke volume was unchanged.

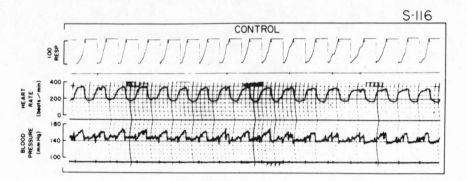

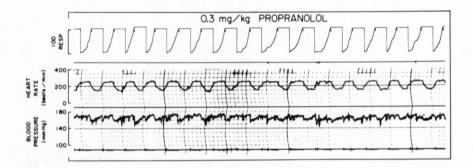

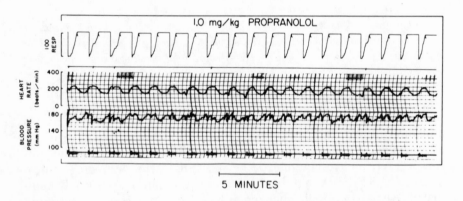

5 MINUTES

FIGURE 11.5. *Effects of propranolol on marked episodic changes in heart rate associated with key-pressing under a 100-response fixed-ratio schedule in monkey S-116. The upper record in each frame is a cumulative record of key-pressing responses. Polygraph recordings as in Figure 11.1. In this monkey, propranolol increased the mean blood pressure. Note the decrease in mean heart rate and the decrease in the magnitude of episodic heart rate changes after propranolol.*

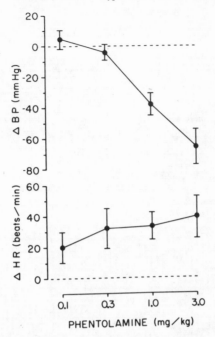

FIGURE 11.6. *Effects of phentolamine on mean blood pressure and heart rate of squirrel monkeys during 2-hour experimental sessions. The drug was given immediately before the start of the session. Summary dose-effect curves were obtained by computing the mean change from control to drug sessions. Dashed lines at zero indicate mean control values; vertical lines, standard errors of the means. The number of monkeys studied at each successive dose was 2, 5, 5, and 3, respectively.*

Effects of phentolamine

Mean blood pressure was decreased and heart rate was increased after doses of 1.0 or 3.0 mg/kg of phentolamine (Figure 11.6). This drug decreased the episodic changes in heart rate, but not the episodic changes in blood pressure. In monkeys whose blood pressure fell to a minimum value at the beginning of the time-out period and then slowly rose to a maximum value in the presence of the green light, the magnitude of the rise was often larger after phentolamine. During the first 45 minutes after the injection of phentolamine, the blood pressure gradually increased in the time-out period, and then rose to a maximum and fell during the fixed-ratio schedule (Figure 11.7). In the second hour after injection of phentolamine, the patterns of episodic changes were similar to those observed in control sessions, as mean blood pressure increased toward control values.

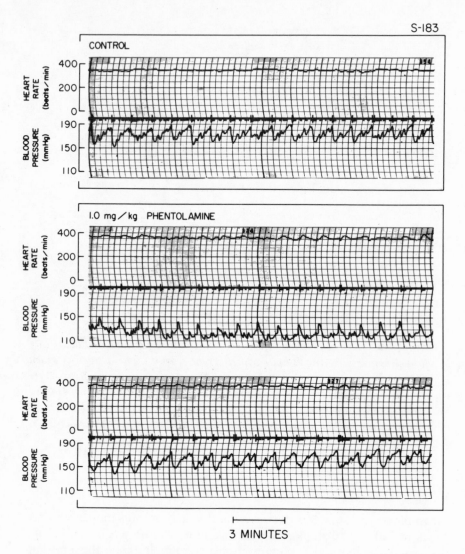

FIGURE 11.7. *Modification of the pattern of episodic blood pressure changes after phentolamine* (monkey S-183, fixed-ratio 30). *Recording as in Figure 11.1. The drug was injected about 5 minutes before the start of the records shown in the middle frame; the records shown in the bottom frame were taken about 60 minutes later, as the blood pressure was returning to control levels.*

Effects of methyl atropine and atropine

Doses of 0.1, 0.3, and 1.0 mg/kg of methyl atropine resulted in mean heart rate increases of approximately 37 bpm with no consistent change in mean arterial blood pressure. In individual subjects, the magnitude

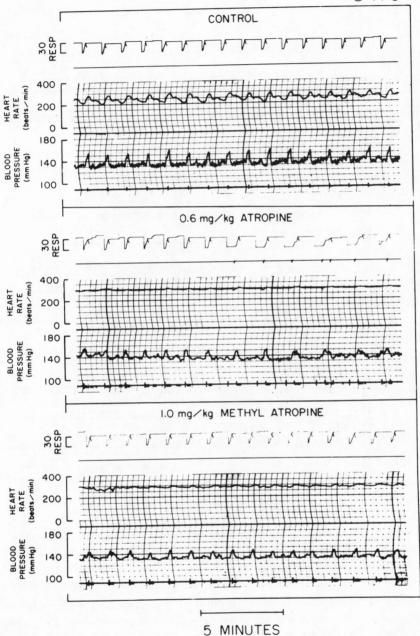

S-110

FIGURE 11.8. *Comparison of the effects of atropine and methyl atropine on key-pressing, heart rate, and blood pressure* (monkey S-110, fixed-ratio 30). *Recording as in Figure 11.1. Note that both drugs had comparable effects on heart rate, but only atropine decreased rates of key pressing.*

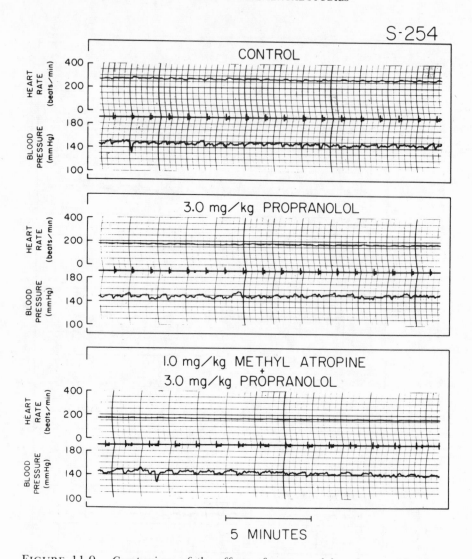

FIGURE 11.9. *Comparison of the effects of propranolol and a combination of propranolol and methyl atropine on heart rate and blood pressure* (monkey S-254, fixed-ratio 10). *Recording as in Figure 11.1. Note that the combination of drugs decreased heart rate to about the same level as propranolol alone.*

of the heart rate increase after methyl atropine was inversely related to the heart rate in control sessions. Episodic changes in blood pressure were not affected by methyl atropine, whereas episodic changes in heart rate were markedly diminished (Figure 11.8). A few experiments with atropine produced changes similar to those of methyl atropine, but atropine markedly decreased rates of key-pressing in the presence of the green light.

Effects of combinations of drugs

In some experiments, both methyl atropine (0.3 or 1.0 mg/kg) and propranolol (0.3, 1.0, or 3.0 mg/kg) were injected immediately before the experimental session. The results were generally similar to those obtained with propranolol alone (Figure 11.9). The mean heart rate change was an increase of 36 bpm after methyl atropine alone, a decrease of 90 bpm after propranolol alone, and a decrease of 77 bpm after the combination. Neither the individual drugs nor the combination produced consistent changes in mean systemic arterial blood pressure.

DISCUSSION

The fixed-ratio schedules used in this study engendered high rates of responding, and both episodic and sustained increases in mean systemic arterial blood pressure. In most animals, blood pressure generally increased gradually during the time-out period, rose abruptly to a maximum during the fixed-ratio schedule, and then decreased again at the start of the time-out period. Episodic changes in heart rate, which differed in magnitude in different monkeys, usually occurred in phase with the increases in blood pressure. Therefore, under the circumstances of these behavioral experiments, the baroreceptor or moderator reflexes were apparently overshadowed. For example, increases in blood pressure of up to 30 mmHg were accompanied by increased heart rates. Such increases in both blood pressure and heart rate, as observed in the present study in association with schedule-controlled behavior, have been frequently reported in association with behavioral events in unanesthetized individuals (MacDonald, Sapru, Taylor & Donald, 1966; Nicotero, Beamer, Moutsos & Shapiro, 1968; Ulrych, 1969).

The behaviorally induced blood pressure increases in the present experiments were little affected by doses of propranolol that decreased cardiac output in the squirrel monkey. Previous studies with anesthetized animals (cats, rats, dogs) have shown that doses of propranolol that decreased heart rate and cardiac output and antagonized the cardiovascular effects of isoproterenol had little or no effect on systemic arterial blood pressure (Black, Duncan & Shanks, 1965; Nakano & Kusakari, 1966; Farmer & Levy, 1968; Dunlop & Shanks, 1969). Studies of unanesthetized human subjects also indicate that propranolol consistently decreases heart rate and cardiac output, whereas its effects on arterial blood pressure in normotensive and hypertensive subjects are relatively small (MacDonald, et al., 1966; Nicotero, et al., 1968; Epstein, Robinson, Kahler & Braunwald, 1965; Shinebourne, Fleming & Hamer, 1967; Ulrych, Frohlich, Dustan & Page, 1968).

The effect of phentolamine in decreasing mean blood pressure and increasing mean heart rate is similar to results reported in both anesthetized and unanesthetized subjects (Drill, 1965). The tachycardia that characteristically occurs after the injection of phentolamine is usually attributed both to the baroreceptor reflexes in response to the decrease in blood pressure, and to a direct stimulant effect of phentolamine on the heart. The hypotensive effect of phentolamine has been attributed both to its direct effects as a vasodilator and to its indirect effects as an alpha-adrenergic antagonist. In the present experiments, the magnitude of the behaviorally induced episodic increases in blood pressure was enhanced even with relatively large doses of phentolamine.

Propranolol and methyl atropine are specific antagonists of cardiac responses to direct or reflex stimulation of sympathetic and parasympathetic nerves, respectively. Comparisons of the independent and combined effects of these drugs on heart rate provide an indication of the relative opposing sympathetic and parasympathetic influences. Methyl atropine (1.0 mg/kg) alone increased the mean heart rate from approximately 270 bpm to approximately 300 bpm, and markedly diminished the episodic changes in heart rate. After methyl atropine, heart rate should be minimally affected by changes in parasympathetic tone, but changes in sympathetic activity could alter the heart rate. That episodic heart rate changes were minimal after methyl atropine suggests that parasympathetic influences play an important role in the behaviorally induced changes in heart rate. In individual monkeys, the heart rate after methyl atropine was similar to the maximum heart rate recorded during the fixed-ratio period under control conditions. This suggests that the episodic increases in heart rate resulted from a decrease in parasympathetic activity. After propranolol (3.0 mg/kg) alone, the mean heart rate was decreased to approximately 180 bpm, and episodic heart rate changes were slight. The combination of these relatively large doses of methyl atropine and propranolol had an effect on heart rate similar to propranolol alone.

Combinations of atropine and propranolol that minimize neurogenic and neurohumoral control of the heart have been used to estimate the intrinsic heart rate (i.e., the rate after block of sympathetic and parasympathetic influences). Thus, a mean heart rate of approximately 180 bpm can be considered as the intrinsic heart rate of the squirrel monkey. As compared with other species, the intrinsic heart rate of the unanesthetized squirrel monkey is quite low relative to its control heart rate. In man (Jose, 1966; Robinson, Epstein, Beiser & Braunwald, 1966; Cumming & Carr, 1967; Jose & Taylor, 1969), in the rhesus monkey or baboon (unpublished observations), and in the dog (Donald & Samueloff, 1966), the control heart rate is characteristically lower than the intrinsic heart rate. These species all have control heart rates that are much lower than that of the squirrel monkey. The present results indicate a relatively high degree of sympathetic tone that is only slightly damped by parasympathetic tone in the control of heart rate in the squirrel monkey. Perhaps it is because of this continual high degree of tone of the sympathetic nervous system that behaviorally induced hypertension can be developed and sustained in the squirrel monkey.

III

Animal Operant Conditioning

This section contains six chapters on the operant conditioning of autonomic responses, and one chapter on the side effects of curare. They consider two main issues. The first concerns the changes in effector systems that are produced when one operantly conditions an autonomic response. Does one produce changes only in the autonomic effector system that controls the reinforced response? Or, does one produce changes in other effector systems that precede or are correlated with change in the reinforced response? If changes in other effector systems are involved, are they necessary for the change in the reinforced autonomic response (or perhaps vice versa)? The issue is usually discussed under the heading of "mediation" or the "cardiac-somatic relationship." It is dealt with at length in the chapter by Black, and more briefly in the chapter by Brener, Eissenberg, and Middaugh.

A second issue concerns operant autonomic conditioning in the curarized subject. This issue is considered by all of the authors in this section, and is the primary interest of the authors of the last five chapters—DiCara, Hahn, Miller and Dworkin, Roberts et al., and Howard et al. Conditioning under curare seems to be a narrow problem on which to focus so much attention, and one is naturally led to ask about the reasons for this effort. One obvious purpose of the curarized preparation is to rule out skeletal mediation. It is true that this preparation does rule out *peripheral* skeletal mediation of autonomic changes; it does not, however, rule out the possibility of mediation by central nervous system events, particularly central components of those effector circuits that control skeletal responses. The use of the curarized preparation for studying mediation is very limited, and, therefore, does not

227

explain the great interest in the preparation. The main source of interest is the failure by Miller and his colleagues to replicate their earlier
unexpected and exciting findings on operant autonomic conditioning
in the curarized rat. It is the attempt to replicate these results—or to
find out why they cannot be replicated—that motivates this great interest in the curarized preparation at present.

All of the chapters in this section discuss the various sources of possible error in working with the curarized preparation. Particular
emphasis is given to the ganglionic blocking effects of curare by Black,
Hahn, and Howard. Whereas Brener, Eissenberg, and Middaugh and
DiCara discuss respiratory factors in some detail. The chapter by Miller
and Dworkin summarizes their attempts to isolate the factors associated
with the current and prevalent difficulties reported in the experimental
replication of operant cardiovascular phenomena.

The implications of these chapters for our understanding the
cardiac-somatic relationship, and the meaning and consequences of the
failure to replicate earlier results in the curarized rat are discussed in
the Summary.

12

A. H. BLACK

Operant Autonomic Conditioning: The Analysis of Response Mechanisms

The purpose of this chapter is to discuss the neural and behavioral mechanisms that must be activated for the performance of operantly conditioned autonomic responses. I shall discuss the value of research on response mechanisms, as well as research strategies for studying them. The discussion will be illustrated by data from research on the operant conditioning of heart rate.

SIGNIFICANCE OF RESEARCH ON RESPONSE MECHANISMS

The first goal of research on operant autonomic conditioning is, of course, to demonstrate that one has successfully changed some autonomic response by means of operant conditioning rather than by some other experimental manipulation (for example, classical conditioning or the noncontingent presentation of a reinforcer). I won't deal with this issue, since I've already made my contribution to the interminable discussions of the meaning of the statement, "Operant conditioning produced an autonomic change," and of the procedures (bidirectional control groups, yoked control groups, etc.) for ruling out possible alternative causes of the autonomic change (Black 1967a,b; 1971a).

The preparation of this paper and the research described in it were supported by research grant APA-0042 from the National Research Council of Canada, research grant 258 from the Ontario Mental Health Foundation, and research grant 7-476 from the Foundations' Fund for Research in Psychiatry. The research described in the paper was carried out in collaboration with Mr. G. Young and F. Brandemark. I would also like to thank C. Batenchuk and D. Berry for their assistance in carrying out this research.

Once this first goal has been achieved, a number of other goals are open to the experimenter. One could take on the lifestyle of the game hunter or collector, search for new autonomic responses whose operant conditioning has not been demonstrated before, and attempt to operantly condition them. One could attempt to determine the optimum procedures for rapid and stable conditioning. One could study the factors that limit or constrain the degree to which one can change a particular autonomic response by operant conditioning. One could apply operant autonomic conditioning procedures therapeutically. Or, one could attempt to determine the neural mechanisms that are involved in operant autonomic conditioning. In this paper, I would like to concentrate on the last of these goals.

There are all sorts of "mechanisms of operant conditioning" to which one might direct his attention: for example, mechanisms which function to process information from discriminative stimuli (S^Ds); mechanisms by means of which reinforcers (S^Rs) have their effect; and mechanisms involved in the performance of particular operant responses. The latter are what I have called "response mechanisms."

One can consider these response mechanisms in two ways. First, one can attempt to identify the particular neurobehavioral systems of which the operantly conditioned response might be a component. Heart rate, to take an obvious example, is a part of the cardiovascular system; therefore, the response mechanism for a heart rate change would involve a particular pattern of activity in this system. Second, one can attempt to identify other neurobehavioral systems to which the operantly conditioned response might be uniquely related. For example, the system controlling somatic movement might be intimately related to the cardiovascular system; in this case, the response mechanism would involve a particular pattern of activation in the systems controlling somatic movement as well as in the cardiovascular system.

Of the various mechanisms of operant conditioning that one could study, the response mechanism has captured the attention of researchers on operant autonomic conditioning. The reason for this is obvious. Interest has focused on the response mechanism because of concern with the problem of mediation. (Black 1971a; Crider, Schwartz, and Shnidman 1969; Katkin and Murray 1968; Katkin, Murray, and Lachman 1969.) According to the mediation hypothesis, when one thinks that one has operantly conditioned an autonomic change, one has actually operantly conditioned some other response inadvertently, and feedback from this other response elicits the autonomic change. There are a number of different types of mediating responses. The most obvious is peripheral mediation by skeletal responding. One can also consider two types of central mediation. The first type involves the activation of the central components of neural circuits that control skeletal movement directly. The second involves the activation of other types of central circuits, e.g., associative, motivational, information processing, etc.

Why should one be concerned about the occurrence of mediation? A possible reason is the belief that one hasn't operantly conditioned an autonomic response when mediation occurs (Lynch and Paskewitz 1971). I would like to suggest that this belief is incorrect. When we say that a change in some response was operantly conditioned, what we usually mean is that the change in the response was produced by the pairing of, or contingency between, response and reinforcer. If we accept this position, then a change in an autonomic response can be produced by operant conditioning whether mediation occurs or not, as long as the response-reinforcer contingency produced the change. When there is no mediation, the operant conditioning procedure changes the autonomic response directly. When there is mediation, the operant conditioning procedure changes the mediating response which in turn changes the autonomic response: That is, the operant conditioning procedure changes the autonomic response indirectly. One might be tempted to argue that the operant conditioning procedure really affected only the mediating response. But as long as the mediating and mediated responses are positively correlated, it seems more correct to say that it affected both.

Is there any other reason for being concerned about the occurrence of mediation? One possibility is this. If the mediating response is skeletal, the odds are that it has been operantly conditioned in the past. Therefore, one could argue that we really haven't done anything "new" when we have operantly conditioned some autonomic response that is skeletally mediated. It is important to note that this argument about a lack of "novelty" applies only to skeletal mediation. It does not apply to central mediation, especially central mediation of the second type (i.e., mediation by attentional processes, motivational processes, etc.). When central mediation occurs, one has directly conditioned processes at least one step back from the periphery. In such cases, one has done something quite novel as far as operant conditioning is concerned.[1]

While one can understand this reason for being upset about skeletal mediation, one must ask whether the fear that operant autonomic conditioning is old hat is sufficient rationale for research on the response mechanisms in operant conditioning. I think not. As a number of others have pointed out recently (Brener, 1970a; Engel 1972; Obrist 1970), research on response mechanisms may address some very significant issues regardless of whether we have conditioned a novel response.

1. *System Analysis:* As I stated earlier, research on response mechanisms provides data on the neurobehavioral systems of which the

reinforced autonomic response might be a component, and on the systems to which it might be related—in particular, the changes that must take place in these systems for the performance of the reinforced response. This infommation is particularly important in therapeutic situations, especially those in which a given autonomic change could be produced by different response mechanisms.

2. *Specificity:* Research on the neurobehavioral systems that are activated when an operantly conditioned autonomic response is performed could inform us about the specificity of autonomic conditioning (Miller 1969). The performance of some autonomic responses may be correlated with activity in a number of neurobehavioral systems or it may occur in relative isolation. If, for example, heart rate changes are related to attentional and motivational systems, the performance of an operantly conditioned heart rate response would be correlated with widespread changes in psychological functioning. If heart rate changes are relatively independent of attentional and motivational systems, the performance of the operantly conditioned heart rate response would not be correlated with changes in psychological functioning. This analysis suggests that the more specific the response, the less its performance would be related to psychological functioning, and the less interesting it might be from a psychotherapeutic point of view.

3. *Constraints:* Research on such systems may demonstrate contraints or limitations on operant autonomic conditioning. Suppose that a response is related to a neurobehavioral system, such that the response can be changed only if other components of the system are permitted to change at the same time. In this case, one could prevent the conditioning of that response by holding the system in a steady state. For example, suppose that heart rate was linked to the system controlling skeletal movement, so that heart rate increases could not occur unless skeletal movement occurred. We could then prevent the conditioning of heart rate responses by requiring the subject to hold still during training, and so establish a constraint on the operant conditioning of heart rate. Again, this would be very important information for therapeutic applications.

4. *System Reorganization:* Finally, such research may provide information on the changes in the organization of response systems that might be produced by operant autonomic conditioning. Heart rate changes, for example, may be intimately related to changes in motor control systems before conditioning, but may be broken free from that relationship as a consequence of some special form of operant conditioning. One might say that the conditioning procedure broke the constraints of skeletal activity on heart rate. If this happened, the operant conditioning of autonomic activity would be a very powerful technique indeed.

Research on response mechanisms is not incompatible with the attempt to demonstrate that we have done something novel when we have operantly conditioned an autonomic response. In practice, however, the two approaches could take us in very different directions. Consider, for example, correlations between the operantly conditioned autonomic response and other responses that are measured during conditioning. When we are trying to understand response mechanisms, we are happy to find that skeletal responses are correlated with heart rate responses, because such correlations provide us with clues about the neurobehavioral systems to which heart rate changes might be related. When we are trying to demonstrate that we have done something novel, on the other hand, we are unhappy to find such correlations with skeletal responses, because they open the possibility of mediation. I'm not suggesting that our expectations concerning our future happiness will determine our results. But these expectations could determine the research strategies that we employ. An exclusive concern with "pure" unmediated examples of operant control may lead us to give up when we find correlations between the reinforced response and other responses. As a consequence, we may be diverted from the task of analyzing these correlations in order to find out more about response mechanisms. Such a diversion would, I think, be harmful.

RESEARCH STRATEGIES

In this section I shall discuss strategies for carrying out research on response mechanisms in operant autonomic conditioning. Again, I shall employ data on the operant conditioning of heart rate to illustrate the discussion.

The point has been made at this conference and elsewhere that a single measure of cardiovascular function, such as heart rate, can only be understood if it is considered in the context of the functioning of the cardiovascular system as a whole. From this point of view, operant conditioning of heart rate should be treated as a psychological manipulation that influences functioning of the cardiovascular system. The first step in studying response mechanisms should be to analyze the changes in the cardiovascular system that are required for the performance of a conditioned change in heart rate (see Chapter 7, Cohen). One might subsequently attempt to relate these cardiovascular changes to changes in other neurobehavioral systems; for example, in respiratory or skeletal response systems, in order to determine their role in the response mechanism.

This seems to be a reasonable approach. The trouble is that many of us have not followed it; we have omitted the middle step. We have attempted to relate changes in a single index of cardiovascular activity to changes in the functioning of other neurobehavioral systems, without relating these changes to the activity of the cardiovascular system. In my own research, for example, we have attempted to relate operantly conditioned heart rate changes to central and peripheral changes in the systems controlling skeletal movement.

I must admit, in retrospect, that I agree with the view that this approach is inadequate. There are, however, two points that could be made in its support. First, the data on the relationship between heart rate and skeletal activity can be incorporated into a more complete picture when other measures of cardiovascular function are taken. The data, then, are not useless; they are incomplete. Second, the research strategy that has been developed for studying the role of skeletal activity in the response mechanism for operantly conditioned heart rate changes is much the same as that which would be employed in studying the role of other indices of cardiovascular activity in this response mechanism. Therefore, a consideration of the successes and failures of the research strategy should be instructive from a methodological point of view, even though the data may give us an incomplete picture.

Correlational Procedures

One approach to finding out which neurobehavioral systems must be activated for the performance of an operantly conditioned autonomic response is based on correlational analyses.[2] One begins by measuring a variety of different responses during the performance of the operantly conditioned heart rate response. Then one determines which of these concomitantly measured responses are correlated with changes in the reinforced response.

One caution must be mentioned at this point. In correlational experiments, one must employ a bidirectional design at least. For example, in heart rate conditioning experiments, one should train one group of subjects to accelerate and another to decelerate heart rate. Without this bidirectional procedure, one would not be able to distinguish between measures that were correlated with the reinforced responses, and those which were correlated with some other aspect of the conditioning procedure. Suppose that one operantly conditioned only heart rate accelerations and found that an increase in general activity was correlated with the occurrence of the conditioned response. One would not know whether this increase in activity was related to the processing of information from the S^D to a motivational change, to central integrating processes, or to the neurobehavioral system controlling the response. Suppose, however, that one conditioned heart rate accelerations in one group of subjects and decelerations in another group, employing the same S^D, S^R, and training procedure, and found that the increase in general activity occurred only during accelerations. It is unlikely that the increase in activity would be related to processing information from the S^D or central integrating processes, since these would probably be the same for both groups. It is more likely that it would be related to the heart rate response, since it is the only factor that differs between the two groups.

This approach is illustrated by an experiment in which we employed a bidirectional design to study the relationship between operantly conditioned heart rate changes and skeletal movement. This experiment has been described in more detail elsewhere (Black 1967b; Black 1971a): Therefore, it will be described only briefly here. The subjects were 15 mongrel dogs. Nine were operantly conditioned to increase heart rate, and six to decrease heart rate to avoid shock. In addition, six of the dogs that were operantly conditioned to increase heart rate, and three of the dogs that were operantly conditioned to decrease heart rate, were trained to pedal-press before operant heart rate conditioning. The remaining six dogs were given no pedal-press pretraining.

The dogs were curarized (employing d-tubocurarine chloride) during operant heart rate conditioning. A medium level of curarization was employed. At this level of curarization little or no movement was observed, but electromyographic activity (EMG) was recorded.

During the avoidance conditioning procedure for increases, the maximum heart rate during 20 seconds of the intertrial interval was determined just prior to the onset of the S^D. This rate was employed as the criterion level. After S^D onset, the dogs were reinforced by S^D termination and avoidance of shock for maintaining heart rate above the criterion level for 6 seconds. If no avoidance occurred after S^D onset, the dogs were given a series of brief pulsed shocks which continued until the appropriate response occurred. Each dog was trained to a criterion of 20 consecutive avoidances. If the dog did not reach this criterion of 20 consecutive avoidances within 150 trials, the conditioning session was terminated. A similar procedure was employed in training decelerations; shaping was employed during the early stages of training.

The results of this experiment are straightforward. First, there was a significant increase in the number of avoidances during training in both groups. Second, 8 of 9 dogs that were operantly conditioned to increase heart rate met the criterion; only 2 of 6 dogs that were operantly conditioned to decrease heart rate met the criterion. It would seem, therefore, that the operant conditioning of heart rate occurs, and that it is easier to operantly condition heart rate accelerations than decelerations with the experimental procedure that we employed.

Our main interest is in the relationship between heart rate and EMG activity. Again the results are quite clear. On 532 of 588 trials, operantly conditioned heart rate accelerations were accompanied by an increase in EMG activity. The remaining heart rate accelerations, which were of small magnitude, were not accompanied by EMG.[3] All successful operantly conditioned heart rate decelerations followed a brief burst of EMG activity.

The pattern of responding in the two cases was quite different. During heart rate accelerations, the dogs produced EMG at S^D onset and continued to do so until the S^D was turned off. During heart rate decelerations, the dogs produced a brief burst of EMG activity at the beginning of, or before the onset of, S^D, and then stopped producing EMG activity during the remaining portion of the S^D presentation. The brief burst of EMG activity was correlated with an increase in heart rate, and the cessation of EMG activity was correlated with a heart rate deceleration.

One obvious interpretation of these results is that the response mechanism employed by the dogs was to produce two different patterns of skeletal activity, which in turn led to different patterns of heart rate change. This conclusion is not completely compelling, however, because the dogs may have been changing some internal process which affected both movement and heart rate. It might be, for example, that heart rate changes and changes in skeletal activity are related to certain types of motivational changes. Perhaps the dogs in the acceleration group increased motivational level throughout the S^D, and the dogs in the deceleration group learned to increase motivation briefly at S^D onset.

There are a number of approaches one might take in order to deal with such alternative interpretations. For the example given above, one could measure motivational level in one way or another, and could determine whether it is correlated with the reinforced response. If it is not, then one can reject the hypothesis that the heart rate changes were related to motivational level. If it is, then one has to determine whether motivational level or general activity, or both, are necessary for operantly conditioned heart rate changes. A procedure that has been commonly employed to accomplish this task is the intervention procedure that is so familiar in physiological psychology. One blocks or holds constant the concomitantly measured event that is correlated with the reinforced response, and studies conditioning or performance of the response that has been previously conditioned. These intervention procedures will be discussed in the next section.

Intervention Procedures

As was pointed out above, the main purpose of intervention procedures is to study the relationship between correlated events. It provides a method for determining whether a change in one event is necessary for the operant conditioning of another. The basic feature of the method is to hold constant or block a given response system. This can be accomplished in a variety of ways. Consider skeletal movement. One can block skeletal responses peripherally by curarelike drugs, or centrally by lesions, or by requiring the subject to hold still. We have employed the first and third approaches in research on operant heart rate conditioning. I shall discuss each separately.

Curarization One of the most popular intervention procedures in research on the relationship between skeletal and operantly conditioned heart rate changes employs d-tubocurarine chloride to block transmission at the neuromuscular junction. This procedure blocks peripheral activity in motor control systems, but leaves the central components of these systems relatively intact. Therefore, if curarized subjects can be operantly conditioned to change heart rate, one can conclude that peripheral activity in motor control systems (i.e., the contraction and relaxation of skeletal muscles, and feedback from this muscular activity) is not necessary for such conditioning.

There is, however, a problem with *d*-tubocurarine. In large doses, it blocks transmission in peripheral autonomic ganglia, as well as at the skeletal neuromuscular junction (Miner 1951). One must ask, therefore, whether the dose that is required to block skeletal musculature is less than the dose that is required to block autonomic ganglia.

In order to answer this question, we first studied the effects of electrical stimulation of the distal portion of the cut vagus nerve using different doses of *d*-tubocurarine under acute conditions in anesthetized dogs, and of electrical stimulation of the vagus and sympathetic nerves to the heart under chronic conditions in awake dogs (Black 1967b, 1971a). Data on three dogs were obtained under acute conditions. As is shown in Figure 12.1, *d*-tubocurarine interfered with the decelerative response to vagal stimulation. In one case, neostigmine was injected and counteracted the effects of *d*-tubocurarine. Stimulation was carried out under chronic conditions on two dogs—one vagal and one sympathetic. The *d*-tubocurarine interfered with the effects of both vagal and sympathetic stimulation.

In the chronic preparations, we also studied the effects of presenting an S^D for a previously operantly conditioned heart rate acceleration in six dogs. The dogs were operantly conditioned under a medium level of *d*-tubocurarine chloride paralysis. Then, the rate of infusion of *d*-tubocurarine was increased, and the S^D for heart rate acceleration was presented periodically. The S^D was presented during recovery from curarization after infusion was terminated.

Data on the effects of S^D presentations on heart rate and EMG activ-

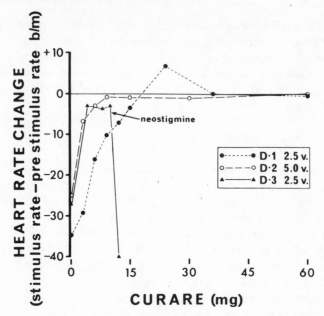

FIGURE 12.1   *Responses to stimulation of the vagus in three dogs after vary-ing doses of* d*-tubocurarine chloride. In one case, neostigmine was injected at the point shown by the arrow.*

ity for two dogs are shown in Figures 12.2 and 12.3. Both dogs showed a decrease in the magnitude of the cardiac acceleration to the S^D as the level of curarization became deeper, and then showed an increase in the magnitude of heart rate acceleration during recovery. In one case, the heart rate response was blocked before complete disappear-ance of EMG activity, while in the other case, the opposite occurred. Also, responding to the S^D became variable, and a number of failures to avoid occurred under deep paralysis.

The answer to our question concerning the dose levels that are required to block movement is ambiguous. In some cases, the dose that was required to block skeletal activity was less than that which blocked autonomic ganglia, but in other cases, the opposite seemed to be true. Such individual differences will obviously increase the variability among groups of dogs trained at levels of curarization great enough to block all EMG activity.

The results of this work on the effects of large doses of *d*-tubo-curarine made us hesitant about attempting the operant conditioning of heart rate under deep curarization in dogs. We did, however, carry out one study in which three dogs were trained to increase heart rate, and three to decrease heart rate under deep *d*-tubocurarine chloride paralysis. As in our previous experiments, *d*-tubocurarine was adminis-

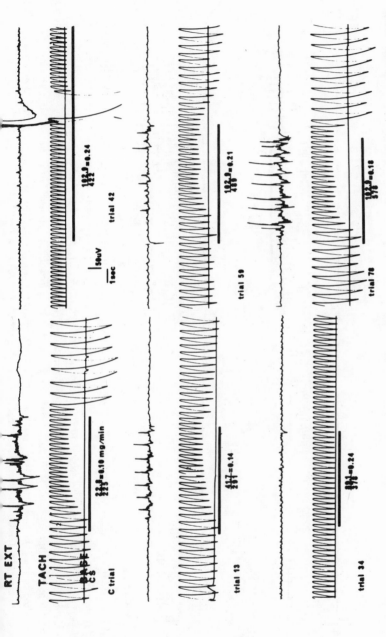

FIGURE 12.2 EMG and heart rate responses in a single dog to the presentation of an S^D shock was avoided. C trial-control trial at the end of training under a medium level of curarization. At this point the rate of injection of curare was increased, and the S^D was presented periodically during the transition to deep curarization (trials 13, 34, and 42). At this point, curare injections were terminated, and the S^D presented during recovery from curarization (trials 59 and 78). The total amount of curare, the total time from the first injection and the ratio of the two are shown for each trial. The solid horizontal bar indicates the duration of S^D. The interference during trial 42 indicates the presentation of a shock when the cardiac avoidance response failed to occur. RT EXT: shows EMG from right forelimb extensor. TACH: shows a tachographic recording of heart rate.

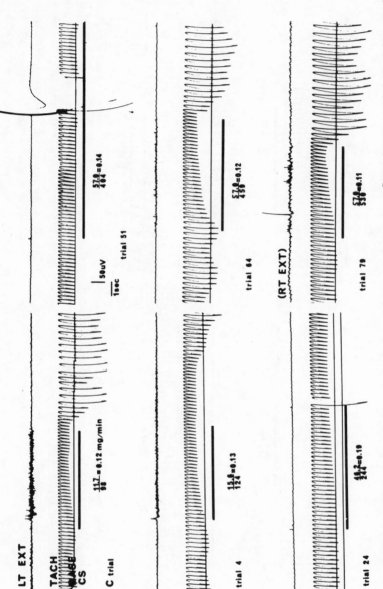

FIGURE 12.3 *EMG and heart rate responses in a single dog to the presentation of an S^D shock was avoided. C trial–control trial at the end of training under a medium level of curarization. At this point the rate of injection of curare was increased, and the S^D was presented periodically during the transition to deep curarization (trials 4, 24, and 51). At this point, curare injections were terminated, and the S^D presented during recovery from curarization (trials 64 and 79). The total amount of curare, the total time from the first injection, and the ratio of the two are shown for each trial. The solid horizontal bar indicates the duration of S^D. The interference during trial 51 indicates the presentation of a shock when the cardiac avoidance response failed to occur. RT EXT: shows EMG from right forelimb extensor. TACH: shows a tachographic recording of heart rate.*

tered via an intravenous catheter. Dose levels were chosen to maintain complete paralysis. EMG was monitored.

The conditioning procedure was similar to that described by Miller and DiCara (1967). Approximately 15 minutes after curarization, the dogs were exposed to a series of 5-second presentations of an auditory S^D (preconditioning trials). Then, during a period in which no S^Ds were presented, a BRS logic circuit determined whether heart rate during approximately 1 second was above or below a criterion level. The criterion level was set such that 12 responses per minute (20%) would have been reinforced, had reinforcement been administered. Then conditioning began. On each trial, the S^D was presented. If a correct response occurred within 10 seconds, the S^D was terminated and shock avoided. If the correct response did not occur, a series of brief shocks was presented once every 3 seconds until a correct response occurred. Shocks were delayed, however, when the heart rate was changing in the correct direction. Every tenth trial was a test trial. On the test trials, the S^D was presented for a fixed 5-second period, and then continued as a regular trial. Shaping was carried out as follows. If the median latency of response was less than 5 seconds on each block of 10 trials, the criterion was made approximately 2% more difficult. If it was greater than 10 seconds, the criterion was made approximately 2% less difficult.

The dogs received 200 conditioning trials during the first training session. They received preconditioning trials (during which the S^D alone was presented), and 40 additional conditioning trials during a second training session which occurred either one or two days after the first session.

Because curare blocks circuits that control skeletal movement peripherally but not centrally, we were curious about the activity of central components of circuits controlling movement. One possible measure of activity in central components of movement control circuits is provided by hippocampal electroencephalographic activity (EEG). Vanderwolf (1969, 1971) has proposed that hippocampal theta waves (regular sinusoidal waves between 4 and 7 Hz in the dog) accompany voluntary phasic skeletal movements such as running, walking, head turning, etc. Our data has generally supported this hypothesis (Black 1971; Black and Young 1972a,b). Therefore, we measured hippocampal theta activity during heart rate conditioning in the hope that it would provide some index of activity in central movement control circuits.

Data on heart rate for the dogs trained to accelerate and decelerate heart rate are presented in Figure 12.4. Heart rate during the first 5 seconds of the S^D on test trials, and heart rate during a 5-second period of the intertrial interval (blank trials) before the test trial are shown. Data are presented for preconditioning trials, and for the first and last four trials of the first training session. Also, data are shown for the four training trials of the second training session for four of the six dogs. Data are omitted for the other two dogs because for these dogs (one in each group), heart rate was unresponsive even to shock at the end of the first training session, the acceleration to shock being less than 10 bpm. These dogs were not continued in the experiment after the first day.

Data on the number of theta waves for the same period are shown in Figure 12.5.

I would like to make three points about these results. First, we were not successful in operantly conditioning increases and decreases in heart rate. All dogs showed an increase in baseline heart rate. There were no significant differences in heart rate between blank and S^D trials during the first training session.[4] The obvious explanation of our failure to demonstrate bidirectional heart rate conditioning in this experiment is some inadequacy in our procedure. We must await a resolution of the problem concerning the replicability of the results of operant heart rate conditioning in curarized rats that was reported by Miller at this conference in order to determine whether this explanation is correct (see Chapter 8).

The second point is this. Although there were no significant changes in heart rate to the S^D, there was a significant interaction between type of trial (blank versus S^D) and stage of training for theta responding ($F=7.97$, $df=2,8$, $p<0.05$). Dogs in *both* groups showed an increase over trials in the number of theta waves to the S^D as compared to blank trials. (This resembles a classical conditioning effect.) The fact that we found significant theta conditioning to the S^D but no significant heart rate conditioning *to the same S^D in the same dog* is important for our attempts to determine how d-tubocurarine interferes with heart rate conditioning. Two rough types of interference can be identified. One is that d-tubocurarine has a central effect which incapacitates the subject generally so that he cannot learn. The second is that d-tubocurarine has a specific effect on the cardiovascular system (probably peripheral) which interferes with the performance of heart rate responses. Our data support the second of these possibilities, since the dogs did display a conditioned EEG response to the S^D at the same time that the heart rate response to the S^D was not significant.

The third point that I would like to make about these results is that there was a significant correlation between changes in heart rate to the S^D and changes in the number of hippocampal theta waves to the S^D. The correlation of the difference between S^D and blank trials for heart rate and theta was $+0.69$ ($p<.01$). (This correlation indicates that the dogs did demonstrate heart rate accelerations to the S^D. The failure to find a significant difference in heart rate between blank and S^D trials

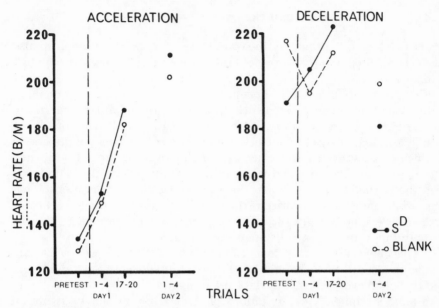

FIGURE 12.4 *Heart rate data for three dogs trained to accelerate heart rate under deep curarization, and three dogs trained to decelerate heart rate under deep curarization. Data are shown for the heart rate response during the first 5 seconds of the S^D on the test trials and for 5 seconds during the intertrial period (blank).*

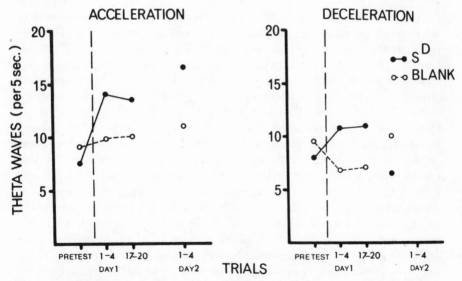

FIGURE 12.5 *Data on the number of hippocampal theta waves for three dogs trained to accelerate heart rate under deep curarization, and three dogs trained to decelerate heart rate under deep curarization. Data are shown for the heart rate response during the first 5 seconds of the S^D on the test trials and for 5 seconds during the intertrial period (blank).*

was produced, I think, by the variability of the heart rate response which resulted from the peripheral autonomic blocking action of *d*-tubocurarine.)

The correlation between theta and heart rate responses suggests that the heart rate accelerations which occurred to the S^D during heart rate conditioning were accompanied by changes in central components of the neural circuits that control skeletal movement. This tempts one to conclude that the response mechanism employed by the subjects when they were deeply curarized was the same as that which they employed in the partially curarized state to produce cardiac accelerations. That is, while they were curarized, they tried to move in the presence of the S^D. Peripheral signs of this attempt to move did not occur, but the central movement control system was activated.

The generality of this conclusion is limited because we aren't sure that the heart rate changes in this experiment were operantly conditioned. Nevertheless, the data does suggest that the use of curare to block peripheral manifestations of skeletal motor activity is not an adequate procedure for studying response mechanisms in the operant conditioning of heart rate, because it is the activation of central not peripheral aspects of movement control circuits that is important.[5] Techniques for dealing with these central components of movement control circuits are discussed in the next section.

Dissociative Conditioning.   It is clear from the previous section that we must understand the relationship of central components of movement control circuits to heart rate changes if we are to understand the response mechanism in operant heart rate conditioning. The usual technique for attempting to achieve such understanding is, as I pointed out above, to block or hold constant these central components of movement control circuits. To do so either by lesions or pharmacological techniques is an extremely difficult task, since we know so little about these circuits. A simple alternative approach that we employed is based on the assumption that holding still keeps central components of the neural systems that control skeletal movement in a steady state. Therefore, if we study the operant conditioning of heart rate in subjects who are required to hold still, we should be able to provide information on the role of central components of the neural systems that control movement. We called the procedure in which we attempted to operantly condition rats to accelerate heart rate while simultaneously holding still "dissociative conditioning" because it requires the subject to dissociate two related responses by performing one, while holding the other in a steady state.[6]

Operant conditioning was carried out in a running wheel. Movement in the running wheel was measured by an Electrocraft Movement

Transducer. The output of the activity detector was fed into an integrator and then to a Schmitt trigger which provided dichotomous measures of movement and nonmovement. In addition, videotape records were made in order to provide a continuous check on the movement detector. Heart rate was recorded by a BRS Foringer logic circuit which measured the interval between ORS complexes. A reinforceable "heart rate acceleration" was arbitrarily defined as three consecutive interbeat intervals, the rate of each of which was higher than a preset criterion level.

The reinforcement was brain stimulation. Before heart rate conditioning, bar-pressing was reinforced with brain stimulation to the lateral hypothalamus in order to make sure that the reinforcer was effective.

In order to obtain a reinforcement for holding still and accelerating heart rate, the rat had to hold still for 2 seconds; then it had to continue to hold still and simultaneously produce a heart rate response. No additional reinforcement could be obtained for 3 seconds after each reinforcement had been presented.

A shaping procedure was employed in order to train the rats to accelerate heart rate. Each rat was trained for a series of 10 to 12 trials per day. Each trial terminated after 50 seconds of holding still. During the 30-second intertrial period a tone was turned on. Also, the number of reinforced responses during the previous trial was counted. If this number was greater than 15, the heart rate criterion level (measured in beats per second) was increased by 0.4 Hz; if it was greater than 12, by 0.2 Hz; if it was greater than 10, by 0.1 Hz. If it was less than 6, the heart rate criterion level was dropped by 0.1 Hz; if it was less than 4, by 0.2 Hz. At the beginning of the first operant conditioning session, the lower limit of the interbeat interval range was set at a level that would have produced 10 reinforceable responses in 50 seconds on the basis of the data obtained during the preconditioning session. At the beginning of each subsequent day's session, the rat began at 0.2 Hz below the point at which it had ended on the previous day.

This experiment is still in progress. The rats that we have trained so far, however, did learn to increase heart rate while holding still. Data for two rats are shown in Figure 12.6. Cumulative distributions of the average number of heart rate responses (three consecutive interbeat intervals between 4 and 10 Hz) during holding still for the first 40 seconds of each trial are plotted. One distribution is shown for the first four trials of training, and another for the last four trials of training. In addition, a cumulative distribution of heart rate responses for selected 40-second periods during movement is also plotted. For one rat, the average number of responses per trial was greater on the last four trials of training than on the first four; for the other rat, it was

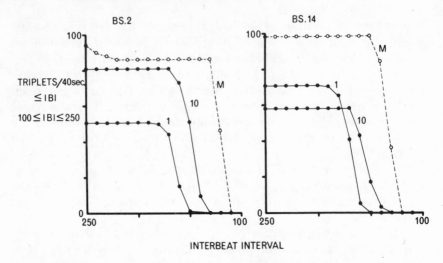

FIGURE 12.6 *Data are shown on heart rate conditioning for two rats who were trained to accelerate heart rate while holding still in the normal state. Cumulative distributions of the number of heart rate responses are shown. A heart rate response was arbitrarily defined as three consecutive interbeat intervals between 250 and 100 msec. Cumulative distributions were shown for the first four trials of training (1), for the last four trials of training (10), and for the period during which the rats were moving (M).*

less. Also, both rats showed more high-rate responses after training than before. Finally, neither number nor rate of responses was as high during holding still as during movement.

It would seem that the training procedure produced an increase in high heart rate responses during holding still. The question that is of primary interest, of course, is how the rats accomplished this. That is, what response strategy did the rats employ to accelerate heart rate while simultaneously holding still at the end of training? In order to deal with this issue, I shall have to digress for a moment. The procedure that we employed in this experiment was actually developed in earlier work on the operant conditioning of hippocampal EEG activity. In this experiment, rats were required to hold still and simultaneously produce three consecutive hippocampal theta waves, each of which had a frequency that was above a criterion level. In addition, the rat had to hold still for 0.5 seconds before the recording circuits would operate. We began heart rate conditioning with an identical procedure. We had been training the first rat for only a few minutes before we realized that it was developing a strategy to produce high heart rates while holding still, which could best be described as "a pumping response." The rat would be active for a brief period of time, and then stop suddenly.

When this happened, the heart rate gradually decelerated during the period following movement. By simply moving and stopping, the rat could meet the criterion for reinforcement while holding still. The rats that were being trained to produce EEG waves did not employ this strategy, because higher frequency hippocampal theta waves terminate within a fraction of a second after a rat stops moving. It is as though heart rate and hippocampal EEG had decay functions following the cessation of skeletal movement which differed in terms of the time constant; the EEG rate decayed rapidly, but heart rate decayed slowly.

One solution to this problem is obvious. It is to increase the amount of time that the rat is required to hold still before the reinforcement circuits become operative, so that heart rates that occur immediately after a movement are not counted. Therefore, we required the rat to hold still for 2 seconds (rather than 0.5 seconds) following cessation of movement before it could obtain reinforcement. The data that were shown in Figure 12.6 were obtained with this procedure. The rat whose data are shown on the right section of Figure 12.6 did not employ the pumping strategy; unfortunately the other rat did, even with the 2-second delay. An analysis of the videotapes indicate that the latter rat, in fact, employed a variety of strategies. In some cases, the correct heart rate response was produced by pumping. In others, the rat held still and the heart rate acceleration anticipated a sudden movement. Finally, in other cases, the heart rate acceleration occurred while the rat was holding still; no large amplitude movements preceded or followed the reinforced response.

These latter examples which occurred in both rats indicate that a shift in the distribution of heart rate to higher levels can be produced by operant conditioning in rats that are holding still, even though the rats do not reach the high levels of heart rate when they are holding still that they reach while moving. This suggests that rats can learn to accelerate heart rate independently of skeletal movement to some extent. But before we can be sure of this conclusion, we need to measure isometric muscle activity and respiration in order to assess their roles in producing heart rate changes in the nonmoving rat. In addition, we require control groups that are given random reinforcements, and groups in which heart rate decelerations are operantly conditioned while the rats are holding still in order to achieve a proper understanding of the response mechanism in this situation.

Even though we have not carried this research too far, it is apparent, I think, that the dissociative conditioning procedure is a useful technique. It is useful because it permits us to deal with central components of the neurobehavioral circuits to which heart rate accelerations may be related, and because it provides some data on the strategies employed by the subject in performing the reinforced response.

Summary

The examples given in this section illustrate, I hope, that the correlational and the intervention procedures can provide useful information on the response mechanism in operant autonomic conditioning.

One is naturally led to compare the two intervention procedures that I have described, the curarization procedure and dissociative conditioning. While the curarization procedure has provided information on peripheral components of the response mechanism, and perhaps on other issues (see Footnote 5), it has, I think, been overworked. It doesn't provide information on central components of the response mechanism; in fact, it may have adverse effects if we conclude that these central components are inactive just because we fail to see the normal peripheral manifestations of central activity in the curarized subject. In addition, certain curare-like drugs block peripheral responses that we don't want blocked. At this stage, therefore, we might be wise to employ other intervention procedures, such as dissociative conditioning, more extensively, especially since the available data indicate that some of the more important linkages between neural systems that control different types of behaviour are central.

CONCLUSION

The purpose of this paper was to suggest that the attempt to understand response mechanisms in operant autonomic conditioning is worthwhile, and to discuss some research procedures for doing so. Data on heart rate conditioning was presented to illustrate this discussion. Most of our data indicated that heart rate is correlated with the activity of central circuits that control skeletal movement, and that the activation of neural systems that control skeletal movement plays an important role in the response mechanism for operantly conditioned heart rate changes. Additional data that are consistent with these results are described in Chapters 8 and 13. This, of course, does not imply that the relationship between heart rate and the activity of central circuits controlling movement is simple, nor that the two occur together in every situation. This was made clear by data in Chapter 8 by Obrist et al., and by the last experiment described in this paper, in which there is a tentative indication that one can train subjects to increase heart rate without the involvement of the central components of movement control systems when a dissociative conditioning procedure is employed. It is important to note, however, that even with dissociative conditioning, holding still acts as a constraint on the heart rate because when the rats were holding still they were not able to produce heart rates that were as high as those that they produced when moving.

I shall not discuss the evidence for and against the cardiac-somatic relationship since it is treated extensively in chapters 8, 9, 13 and 25. The only point that I want to make is that research on the response mechanism in operant autonomic conditioning is necessary if we are to understand this relationship. If a subject can employ different strategies to accelerate and decelerate heart rate, as seems to be the case, we need research on response mechanisms to identify the different strategies, to identify the conditions which lead to the use of one strategy as opposed to another, to determine the limits on the magnitude of change that can be produced by a given strategy with a given training procedure, and to determine whether special training procedures can change these limits. In other words, in order to deal with the somatic-cardiac relationship in operant cardiac conditioning, we need more information on response mechanisms (especially on the issues mentioned earlier in this chapter—on systems analyses, specificity, constraints, and system reorganization), and this information will be provided in large part by research of the type outlined under "Research Strategies" in this chapter (especially dissociative conditioning techniques). The same, I think, holds true for other autonomic responses.

This information on response mechanisms will be of use not only to those interested in basic mechanisms, but also to those interested in therapeutic applications of operant autonomic conditioning. Research on constraints on operant autonomic conditioning that are produced by properties of the response mechanism will be especially useful, at present, when so many overblown claims are being made for "biofeedback" and "operant autonomic conditioning." As has been pointed out in other chapters in this volume, if these claims are not fulfilled, we may be exposed to a "backlash" which could lead to the rejection of some potentially useful procedures. We can take some small comfort about these exaggerated claims, however, by noting that hyperbole in this field is not a novel phenomenon, as is demonstrated by the following observation which I quoted in another paper recently, and which I'll quote again (Black 1972b).

It may be of interest to you to know that some years since a gentleman—Colonel Townsend, lived who possessed the power of controlling the actions of his heart and lungs. You will tell me this is quite simple—you can do it yourself. Not so fast. It is quite impossible, at all events improbable, that you have any such ability. Draw in your breath now, and you are, bloated like the frog in the fable, undergoing your torture with heroic fortitude. The gallant gentleman I have mentioned, however, could really influence his heart in much the same way as you can control the action of your forefinger, which I fancy I see elevated in an attitude of scepticism; as the Ingoldsby legend goes:

"The sacristan, he says no word, to indicate a doubt,

But he puts his thumb unto his nose, and draws his fingers out."

Colonel Townsend performed the experiment once in the presence of his physician, who cautioned him strongly against its repetition. Nevertheless, he did again exhibit the control he had over his circulatory organs, and this time more triumphantly than ever, for he so completely suppressed the heart's action that it never throbbed again. The unlucky individual added another name to the list of scientific martyrs . . . (H. Lawson 1873, p. 64).

NOTES

1. One could also argue that these techniques are novel in that they extend the range of our voluntary control. I don't want to discuss voluntary control, however, except to point out that I do not consider "voluntary" control to be equivalent to "operant" control. The operational criteria for deciding whether one has established "voluntary" control over behavior are more complex than those for deciding whether one has established "operant" control over behavior.

2. There are a variety of other procedures that are employed for this purpose. One is what might be called a "transfer procedure." In this case, one determines the effects of the occurrence of the operantly conditioned heart rate response on behavioral processes with which it is not apparently correlated. For example, one might operantly condition subjects to change heart rate, and then study the effects of such training on subsequent shuttle-box operant conditioning (DiCara and Weiss 1969). One could also carry out the opposite procedure in which one first trains animals to perform some specific skeletal response, and studies the effects of such training on subsequent operant heart rate conditioning (Goesling 1969).

3. Other data on non-curarized dogs (Black 1971) suggest that small EMG changes were occurring during these small magnitude cardiac accelerations but were masked by the action of curare.

4. On the second day of the experiment, two dogs in each group displayed the appropriate heart rate and theta responses, i.e., higher heart rates and number of theta waves to the S^D in the acceleration group, and lower heart rates and theta to the S^D in the deceleration group. Why there was a shift from increased heart rates to the S^D at the end of Day 1 to decreased heart rates at the beginning of Day 2 in the deceleration group is not clear.

5. I do not want to give the implication that I think that the occurrence of peripheral movement is completely irrelevant to cardiovascular functioning. There will be differences between those cases in which only central components of movement control circuits are activated, and those cases in which both the central components are activated and movement occurs simultaneously. For example, the initial increase in heart rate when an instruction to move goes out may be the same in both cases, but differences may arise if the instructions are maintained, because maintained changes in heart rate depend on feedback from movement. In order to describe such differences accurately, we need a paralytic agent that does not produce ganglionic blocking.

6. Schwartz (1971b) has referred to this process as "differentiation." Data obtained by this dissociative or differentiation procedure is relevant to another issue. Operant heart rate conditioning has been reported to be better in curarized rats than in normal rats (Miller et al. 1970). One hypothesis that has been suggested to account for these results is that the curarized rat is prevented from receiving a great deal of extraneous information as compared to the normal rat. If this hypothesis is correct, rats who are required to hold still during operant heart rate conditioning should do better than rats who can move, since the noise is reduced during holding still.

13

JASPER BRENER, ETHEL EISSENBERG,
AND SUSAN MIDDAUGH

Respiratory and Somatomotor Factors Associated with Operant Conditioning of Cardiovascular Responses in Curarized Rats

INTRODUCTION

When research on learned control of the viscera first began to appear in the literature, the Zeitgeist, reflecting centuries of prejudice against the voluntary status of visceral responses, demanded evidence that the reported autonomic changes were not an artifact of "true voluntary" somatomotor activity. Since the characteristics of such true voluntary responses have not been made explicit, the difficulty of proving that cardiovascular responses are members of this class is insurmountable. Nevertheless a response was and is still often thought to be voluntary only if it is not "mediated" by some other response (Katkin and Murray 1968). Although it is doubtful that the issue of mediation is resolvable at an empirical level (Brener 1970a), experiments involving curarized rats were initiated to bolster the case for operant and voluntary visceral phenomena. Thus Miller and his colleagues (Miller et al. 1970) provide the following rationale for the long series of experiments emanating from his laboratory: "In order to prevent the rats from affecting their heart rates indirectly by changes in breathing and muscular activity, the skeletal muscles were completely paralyzed by curare and the rats were maintained on artificial respiration." (Miller et al. 1970, p. 1-4) That the curare literature served to establish the scientific respectability of these phenomena contains a double irony. In the first instance, the rationale provided for performing these experiments is open to a

This research was supported by NIMH Grant 17061.

number of substantial criticisms. Secondly, the magnitude and reliability of the phenomena reported in the initial publications of DiCara and Miller (Miller and Dworkin, Chapter 16) are open to question.

We have tended towards the view expounded by Obrist et al. (1970b) which regards somatomotor and cardiovascular activities as outputs of a single control system. Within this theoretical framework the interpretation of operant conditioning of cardiovascular responses in the curarized animal is of special interest. The major implication drawn from these studies appears to have been that the control of cardiovascular and somatomotor activities is autonomous. In reality, the curare evidence demonstrates only that cardiovascular control may be achieved in the absence of peripheral feedback from the striate muscle effectors which are immobilized by the drug. Such a demonstration, although interesting, is not particularly relevant to the specification of the mechanisms involved in operant cardiovascular change. Neither does it speak with any clarity on the issue of somatomotor involvement in cardiovascular change. Any somatomotor process proximal to the myoneural junction may retain an influence over cardiovascular activity in the curarized subject. This possibility cannot be overlooked since it has been well-established that following acquisition, the role of peripheral feedback in the maintenance of somatomotor activities is of a vastly diminished importance. The possibilities exist that feedback of a central nature may dominate in the control of well-learned skills, or that the control of such skills may be organized as a purely efferent sequence (Festinger and Cannon 1965).

In view of these considerations, we inaugurated a series of studies directed ultimately at resolving these issues but initially at replicating operant cardiovascular effects of the type and magnitude reported by Miller and DiCara and their colleagues. Although we (Hothersall and Brener 1969; Middaugh 1971) succeeded in replicating the basic phenomenon reported by those investigators, it was not without considerable tribulation. The primary problem encountered in our attempts to condition cardiovascular responses in the curarized rat involved maintaining subjects in a healthy condition for periods long enough to execute the procedures. In these studies we have consistently found it impossible to maintain curarized rats by employing the techniques of artificial respiration described by those authors. Whereas DiCara and Miller and their associates employ the same pre-specified parameters of artificial respiration for all of their subjects, we have found it necessary to set the parameters separately for each subject. This methodology is clearly not as powerful as that employed by DiCara and Miller et al. since it is well known that very subtle differences in artificial respiration can produce profound alterations in the cardiovascular activity of curarized rats. As a result of the foregoing, we embarked on a series of experiments designed specifically to investigate the influence of various respiratory manipulations on the cardiovascular activity of curarized rats. A description of these experiments forms the first part of this chapter. The second part is comprised of a description of experiments relating to the issue of mediation as it pertains to this area of research.

ARTIFICIAL RESPIRATION, CURARE, AND THE CARDIOVASCULAR SYSTEM

It is difficult to overemphasize the importance of respiratory variables in determining the cardiovascular activity of the curarized preparation. Not only must the normal intimate linkage between the activities of the respiratory and cardiovascular systems be taken into account, but, in addition, one must consider the pharmacological effects of curare together with the physiological abnormalities introduced by the procedure selected to artificially ventilate the lungs of the curarized subject. Almost universally, investigators have ventilated the curarized preparation employing a positive pressure system to deliver room air to the subject through a face mask. Three critical parameters are involved in this method of artificial respiration: the respiratory rate (RR), the ratio of time during each cycle spent in inspiration and expiration (I:E ratio), and the peak inspiration pressure (PIP). The differences between normal and positive pressure respiration are described in detail by Mushin et al. (1969). Particularly relevant to procedures currently employed by investigators in the area of operant cardiovascular conditions are the following factors:

1. During normal respiration, the alveolar pressure falls to 1 to 2 cm H_2O below atmospheric pressure during inspiration, and increases to 1 to 2 cm H_2O above atmospheric pressure during expiration. In contrast, during positive respiration, the alveolar pressure approximates the PIP employed during inspiration and is approximately equal to atmospheric pressure during expiration. The pulmonary pressure differences are therefore not only greatly exaggerated during positive pressure respiration, but are also out of phase with those produced by normal respiration. These pressure differences almost certainly result in out-of-phase baroceptive feedback to the respiratory and cardiovascular centers.

2. The drop in intrathoracic pressure contingent upon normal inspiration produces an increased "downhill" pressure gradient, augmenting venous return to the heart by drawing blood into the great thoracic veins. Because the intrathoracic pressure during inspiration in positive pressure respiration is greatly in-

creased, this important mechanism is disturbed and venous return to the heart is attenuated.

3. Given the relationship between intrathoracic pressure and venous return, it follows that if the inspiration phase is unduly prolonged, the cardiac output will be severely diminished. In this connection Mushin et al. (1969, p. 13) note: "The higher the peak pressure and the longer the time during which it acts, the greater is the cardiac tamponade and the interference with cardiac output." Thus, intrathoracic pressure decreases cardiac output by decreasing venous return and also by a direct mechanical compression of the heart. It is reported by Morgan et al. (1966) that when an I:E ratio of 1:1 is used with a PIP of 20 cmH$_2$O, the cardiac output is decreased by 22%. The values assigned to these parameters in most of the experiments reported by DiCara and Miller and their colleagues were: I:E ratio=1:1; PIP=20 cm H$_2$O; and RR=70 cpm.

The influences on cardiovascular activity contingent upon positive pressure ventilation of the lungs are further compounded when this method is employed with subjects that have been immobilized with d-tubocurarine chloride. Curare in and of itself is a source of considerable influence on cardiovascular activity. Goodman and Gillman (1970) report these influences in great detail and refer to the autonomic ganglionic blockade which has been investigated and somewhat substantiated in three species by Hahn (Chapter 15); Howard et al. (Chapter 18); and Black (1967b). Of more general relevance is the fact that the loss of skeletal muscle tone with motor paralysis interrupts an important circulatory mechanism eventuating in blood pooling and the attenuation of venous return. When and if sympathetic pathways are also interrupted, the attendant loss of vasomotor control prevents peripheral vasoconstriction and thereby provides yet another mechanism for diminished blood flow back to the heart. The histamine release which accompanies curare injection and initiates tracheobronchial and salivary secretion frequently and differentially causes airway constriction and congestion. The resulting diminished and/or variable air flow remains undetected in the absence of proper measuring devices, and the secondary changes in heart rate may be misinterpreted as a desirable "variable heart rate."

These issues are further complicated if a constant value of positive pressure is maintained to ventilate the lungs of curarized subjects. Massion (1957), among others, has demonstrated that curare leads to substantial changes in the elastic properties of the thorax. In particular, it was noted by that investigator that an intravenous injection of curare led to a 42.2% decrease in lung compliance and a 5.9% decrease in the compliance of the chest cage. Since the lungs become progressively more rigid under curare, if the animal is maintained by constant pressure respiration, the actual alveolar gas turnover will decrease successively. Massion concludes that if the ventilating device does not correct for this change in lung elasticity by an increase in pressure, serious hypoventilation may occur with time. These problems appear to demand an investigation of the influences of various respiratory parameters on the cardiovascular activity of curarized subjects. To this end the following series of studies was undertaken.

Only two papers reporting methods for respirating curarized rats have appeared in the literature. Hahn (1970) determined his respiratory parameters on the basis of heart rate data. This method of assessing the adequacy of respiration has obvious deficits if the experimental goal is the manipulation of cardiovascular variables. Ideally, respiration should be evaluated on the basis of gas transport within the curarized preparation. DiCara (1970a) employed arterial blood gas analyses to validate the respiratory parameters employed by him and his colleagues for the maintenance of curarized rats. That investigator obtained P_{CO2} and P_{O2} values of 25.4 mmHg and 75.1 mmHg, respectively, for the arterial blood of normal noncurarized rats. He further observed that these blood gas values were achieved in curarized subjects weighing between 400 to 500 gm by using an RR of 70 cpm, an I:E ratio of 1:1, and PIPs between 17 to 19 cm H_2O. Previous to this investigation, however, DiCara reported that he employed a peak inspiration pressure of 20 cm H_2O.[1]

Our experience in employing these parameters led us to conclude that they result in hyperventilation of the curarized rat. Rats respirated by this technique display profound invariant tachycardia at the inception of the session, show a systematic decrease in heart rate throughout the session, and are unresponsive to peripheral stimulation. In order to resolve this discrepancy between our observations and those of DiCara and his associates, an investigation of the influence of two critical respiratory variables on cardiovascular activity was undertaken.

EFFECTS OF PEAK INSPIRATION PRESSURE AND
RESPIRATORY RATE ON HEART RATE
AND MEAN BLOOD PRESSURE

The subjects in this experiment were 24 male albino rats of the Sprague-Dawley strain divided into four equal groups according to the weight ranges 200 ± 25gm, 300 ± 25gm, 400 ± 25gm, and 500 ± 25gm. The carotid arteries of four subjects in each group were cannulated to permit blood pressure measurement. All subjects were curarized with an intraperitoneally injection of 3.6 mg/kg tubocurarine chloride, and connected to a respirator via a moulded nylon face mask. In this experiment, respiratory rate and pressure were varied but the I:E ratio was held constant at 1:1 for all animals. Three subjects in each weight range were respirated according to Schedule A and three subjects were respirated according to Schedule B.

Schedule A: During the first 20 minutes each rat was respirated at a PIP of 20 cmH_2O, and at a RR of 70 cpm (written 20/70). This period was followed by successive 10-minute exposures to each of the following pressure/rate combinations: 20/70, 16/70, 12/70, 8/70, 20/70, 20/50, 16/50, 12/50, 8/50, 20/50.

Schedule B: During the first 20 minutes each subject was respirated at 20/50, followed by 10-minute exposures to 20/50, 16/50, 12/50, 8/50, 20/50, 20/70, 16/70, 12/70, 8/70, 20/70.

The difference between Schedules A and B was simply that the order in which the two respiratory rates were presented was reversed. The 20 cmH_2O pressure was repeated under each rate setting in order to determine whether the 10-minute periods employed were indeed sufficient for obtaining accurate assessments of the influence of each pressure/rate setting, regardless of the immediately preceding setting. The data analyzed in this experiment were derived from the last 5 minutes under each pressure/rate setting.

The reliability with which a given respiratory setting produced a given heart rate and/or blood pressure was ascertained by comparing the heart rates and blood pressures recorded during the final 5 minutes of the first and second 20 cmH_2O pressure setting separately for each respiratory rate. It was found that at a RR of 70 cpm, neither heart rate nor blood pressure differed significantly between the first and second presentations of the 20 cmH_2O pressure setting. At 50 cpm, the blood pressure did not differ significantly between the first and second presentations of this pressure setting, although the heart rate was observed to be significantly lower on the second presentation (t = 2.24, df = 23, p < .05). Despite the statistical significance of this difference, it should be noted that the mean difference in heart rate was only about 12 bpm, which is small compared to the differences induced by the different pressure settings.

Heart Rate: Analysis of variance indicated that respiratory pressure alone contributed significantly (F = 60, df = 4/80, p < .01) to the observed heart rate variability. The influence of respiratory rate was virtually nondiscriminable. Although between-subject variability led to a nonsignificant body weight effect, this effect is nevertheless worthy of scrutiny and is illustrated in Figure 13.1. As can be seen, in all weight groups, heart rate is a function of peak inspiration pressure.

The 200, 300, and 400 gm groups display graduated mean heart rate differences, but the 500 gm group displays a somewhat anomalous effect, especially at the intermediate pressures. Of particular significance here is the observation that peak respiratory pressures of above 16 cmH$_2$O produce abnormally high heart rates (greater than 450 bpm) in all groups.

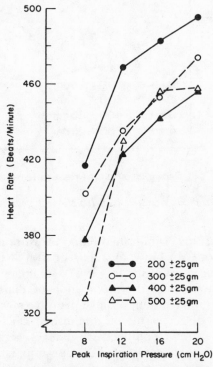

FIGURE 13.1. *Mean heart rate as a function of peak inspiration pressure in four groups of curarized rats.*

Blood Pressure: The only significant effect indicated by the analysis of variance performed on the blood pressure data was due to body weight (F = 5.18, df = 3/12, p < .05). Reference to Figure 13.2 which illustrates this effect will, however, indicate that it is not readily amenable to explanation. Although statistically insignificant, it was observed that the mean blood pressures recorded during respiration at 50 cpm were higher at all pressures than those recorded at 70 cpm.

We have concluded, on the basis of this research, that respiratory rate does not greatly influence heart rate or blood pressure within the range investigated. On the other hand, it is true that heart rate is significantly influenced by changes in peak inspiration pressure.

The absence of blood pressure changes even in the presence of pres-

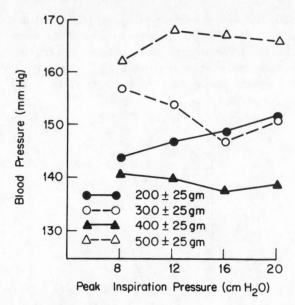

FIGURE 13.2.   *Mean blood pressure as a function of peak inspiration pressure in four groups of curarized rats.*

sure extremes is baffling. Diminished blood pressure is to be predicted with hyperventilation (Mushin et al. 1969), or with tachycardia on pressure cycled ventilators (Rawitscher 1967). Maloney and Handford (1954) clearly demonstrated the attenuation of diastolic and systolic blood pressure with intermittent positive pressure machines which they explained to be a direct result of diminished cardiac output. It is possible that in this study blood pressure changes were immediate with respiratory pressure change and of short duration, i.e., within the first 5 minutes, and therefore were not apparent during the interval selected for the determination of significant change. Restoration of blood pressure level, accomplished by cardiovascular autoregulation, may have led to our failure to detect significant blood pressure changes.

Since the rate of change in heart rate with pressure manipulation is greatest at the extreme ends of the pressure continuum employed, a pressure range of 12 to 16 cmH_2O appears to be optimal for the maintenance of the curarized rat. Weight factors associated with heart rate and blood pressure point to the advisability of grouping subjects within a narrow weight range and of avoiding extreme weights.

ARTERIAL BLOOD GAS COMPOSITION
OF THE NONCURARIZED RAT

The data of primary interest to us in this experiment were those indicating that peak inspiration pressures of 16 to 20 cmH_2O produced tachycardia in the curarized rat. Although the observed tachycardia could be attributed to a variety of causes secondary to the peak respiratory pressure, at the time it seemed most likely to us that this response was due to hyperventilation. DiCara employed analysis of arterial blood from normal and curarized rats to validate his respiration parameters. Since in our experiments these parameters led to apparent hyperventilation, it was decided to investigate further the blood gas composition of the normal noncurarized subject. In addition, our decision to undertake this experiment was based on the fact that we could find no corroborative evidence in support of that investigator's contention that the arterial P_{CO2} of normal rats was 25.4 mmHg. In the light of available evidence (Blood, Elliott, and D'Armour 1946; King and Bell 1966; Jones, MacGrath, and Aculthorpe 1950), this value appears abnormally low. Given that DiCara's respiratory technique produced such values in the curarized subject, it seemed likely that this technique would lead to hyperventilation.

Seven rats ranging in weight from 326 to 422 gm ($\overline{X}$ = 370.86, SD = 36.98) had cannulae chronically implanted in the external iliac artery. Two days following surgery, blood samples were withdrawn from these cannulae and their gas composition analyzed. These analyses provided a mean pH of 7.48 (SD = .01), a mean P_{O2} of 81.66 (SD = 10.09) and a mean P_{CO2} of 33.32 (SD = 1.12). It is clear that the mean P_{CO2} value obtained in these analyses is significantly higher than that reported by DiCara. This observation lends support to our suggestion that the artificial respiration parameters suggested by that investigator lead to hyperventilation.

Having ascertained to our satisfaction that the standard procedures reported for maintaining curarized rats in a healthy condition were inadequate, we set about specifying alternative procedures. In the development of these procedures we attended to two factors not previously investigated in this preparation, viz: the decreased lung compliance evidenced in curarized animals, and the influence of the I:E ratio on cardiovascular activity.

CONSTANT PRESSURE RESPIRATION AND DECREASE IN LUNG COMPLIANCE

It has been mentioned that curare induces a substantial loss of lung compliance. In view of this and because investigators using curarized preparations in cardiovascular conditioning experiments have consistently employed a constant pressure setting throughout their procedures, it might be expected that the subjects in these procedures become successively more hypoventilated as a function of time. In order to investigate this possibility, we measured heart rate, circumferential chest movements, and body temperature in two groups, each comprised of eight curarized rats.

One group of subjects was respirated at a constant pressure of 18 cm H_2O, and the other group at a constant pressure of 14 cmH_2O. The RRs and I:E ratios for both groups were set at 70 cpm and 1:1, respectively. Measurements of mean heart rate, circumferential chest movements (1 mm change in gage circumference=pen deflection of 15.7 mm), and rectal temperature were made at regular 10-minute intervals for 90 minutes following curarization. All subjects were curarized with an i.p. injection of 3.6 mg/kg of d-tubocurarine chloride, and were connected to the respirator via a moulded nylon face mask following the first signs of respiratory difficulty.

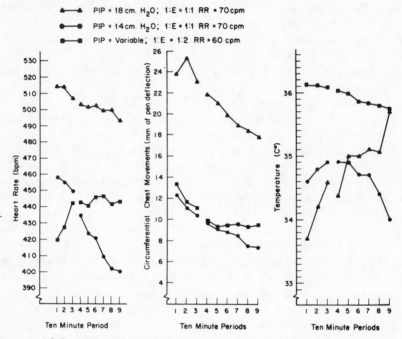

FIGURE 13.3.   *The effects of constant pressure artificial respiration at two peak inspiration pressures (14 & 18 cm H_2O) on mean heart rates, circumferential chest movements, and rectal temperature compared to the effects of a variable pressure procedure (see text).*

The 10-minute averages of each measure for each of the groups are presented in Figure 13.3. For purposes of comparison, parallel data derived from a third group of eight curarized rats respirated by what we believe to be an optimal procedure are also presented in this figure. The comparison group was respirated at a rate of 60 cpm at an I:E ratio of 1:2. The PIP for this group was adjusted from the 40th through the 90th minute of the session to maintain constant circumferential chest movements in each of the subjects.

In both groups respirated at constant pressures, it will be observed that heart rate declines systematically as a function of time, as do chest movements. We attribute the decline in the latter measure, which serves as an index of tidal volume, to the loss of lung compliance contingent upon the administration of curare. Since subjects in the 18 cmH_2O group were obviously hyperventilated—judging from their profound tachycardia—the reduction in gas turnover secondary to the curare-induced loss of lung compliance did not lead to hypoventilation in these subjects. The same cannot, however, be said of the 14 cmH_2O group. By the 180th minute of curarization, all but two of the animals in this group had died. Thus a respiratory pressure that was sufficient to maintain these animals in a healthy condition at the inception of the procedure had, by the 180th minute of the session, led to fatal hypoventilation in all but two of the subjects. The data from the variable pressure group clearly differ from those of the other two groups. It will be seen that the chest movements of this group were maintained relatively stable from the 40th through the 90th minute of the session. During this period it will be observed that the heart rate measure remains relatively stable and does not display the same decrement as is evidenced in the constant pressure groups. It is important to note that during this period pressure was adjusted to maintain constant chest movements, rather than a constant heart rate. The procedure employed to determine the appropriate chest movements will be described in the next section.

The temperature data are worthy of careful consideration. Unlike the other two groups, the 18 cmH_2O subjects display successive increments in body temperature throughout the session. It is suggested that this trend is attributable to a steady reduction in thoracic pressure, as tidal volume is diminished due to decreased lung compliance. Cardiac output is essentially disinhibited as cardiac tamponade and pressure on the great thoracic veins is attenuated, with the result that temperatures rise with improved circulation. Although the temperatures of all groups of subjects are somewhat subnormal, our experience with curarized rats has led us to consider rectal temperatures lower than 34.5° C as indicative of serious physiological stress. The 14 cmH_2O subjects display an initial increment in temperature followed by a more pronounced decrement, reaching 34°C by the 90th minute of the session. We attribute the latter trend in temperature to the hypoventilation discussed above. Of particular note are the temperature recordings of the variable pressure group which, although displaying a slight decrement over the session,[2] are at a considerably higher level than the other groups represented. The higher temperature displayed by this group is attributed primarily to the lower I:E ratio (1:2) employed with these subjects. As was mentioned earlier, diminished cardiac output is a joint function of the level of PIP and the time during which it acts. Cardiac output in this group was then less attenuated, because the intrathoracic pressure was elevated for a proportionately shorter period of time than in the other two groups.

It is evident from these data that the selection of appropriate respiration parameters poses a very considerable problem. With respect to pressure alone, a balance must be struck between increasing pulmonary pressures to the degree that they interfere with cardiac output, and maintaining settings so low that the subjects become hypoventilated. Because the duration of increases in intrathoracic pressure acts jointly with the peak inspiration pressure to attenuate cardiac output, it remained to investigate the effects of varying I:E ratio on the variables, heart rate and temperature.

EFFECTS OF MANIPULATING THE I:E RATIO

Since the reduction in cardiac output that is associated with positive pressure respiration varies as a direct function of the time during which the lungs are inflated, it follows that the inspiration phase of the respiration cycle should be kept as short as possible. In other words the I:E ratio should be reduced to the smallest value which, at the same time, will permit adequate pulmonary turnover in the animal. The present experiment investigated the influence of different I:E ratios on heart rate and body temperature in curarized rats. In all cases PIP was adjusted so as to maintain constant circumferential chest movements in each subject, and the respiratory rate was maintained at 60 cpm.

Eight rats in the weight range of 400 to 500 gm were run under each of the following I:E ratios: 1:1, 1:1.5, 1:2, and 1:3. All subjects were immobilized with an i.p. injection of 3.6 mg/kg of d-tubocurarine chloride, and following the first signs of respiratory difficulty (usually within 5 seconds) were attached to the respirator via a moulded nylon face mask. During the first 30 minutes of each session, respiratory pressure was adjusted until the subject's heart rate fell within normal limits.[3] When this was achieved, the circumferential chest movements of the subject were noted, and, throughout the remainder of the session, the pressure was adjusted so as to maintain these movements at the same level. Continuous recordings of rectal temperature, chest movements, pressure, and heart rate were made throughout the session, which lasted until the subject displayed evidence of recovering from curare. The data reported here and illustrated in Figure 13.4 were derived from recordings made during the 110 minutes immediately following curarization.

Although attempts were made to maintain constant chest movements

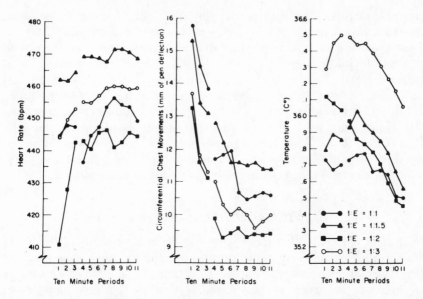

FIGURE 13.4.   *The effects of variations in the I:E ratio on the mean heart rates, circumferential chest movements, and rectal temperatures of curarized rats. In all cases subjects were respirated at a rate of 60 cpm, and peak inspiration pressure was varied so as to maintain constant chest movements following the first 30 minutes of curarization.*

during the last 80 minutes it will be noted that this index does vary during this period with a range of approximately 1.5 mm pen deflection in the 1:1 group to approximately .65 mm pen deflection in the 1:2 group. Although the heart rate means do show a tendency to increase over the last 80 minutes, with this tendency being most marked in the 1:1 group, the trend is not invariant and apart from the 1:1 group, the magnitude of the increment is not substantial.

During the initial 30 minutes of the procedure, it will be seen that body temperature is an inverse function of the I:E ratio, suggesting again that the lower this ratio, the smaller the inhibition of cardiac output. Although the temperatures of all groups display a systematic decline during the last 80 minutes of the session, it will be noted that the total decrement in temperature does not amount to more than .5°C in any group. Comparison of these data with those described in Figure 13.3 will indicate that all groups display consistently higher body temperatures than subjects respirated at a constant pressure setting, with an I:E ratio of 1:1.

In view of the stability of the heart rates of subjects respirated at a 1:2-1:E ratio and also because of the relative ease with which a constant respiratory volume may be maintained with this setting, it is suggested that this procedure is the most efficient of those investigated by us for maintaining curarized rats in a healthy condition.

Of great importance is the fact that we have found these results to be reproducible, i.e., there are extremely small differences in temperature and heart rate curves obtained from groups of subjects maintained on the same ratio with this variable pressure technique. On the other hand, initial mean pressures for such groups differ even though they fall within the range which we have found to be desirable, namely, 12 to 16 cmH$_2$O. This finding only substantiates our belief that individual variations in resistance to air flow, both mechanical and physiological, demand that pressure settings be individualized as well.

IMPLICATIONS OF THE CURARE LITERATURE

In spite of the difficulties experienced in replicating many of the operant cardiovascular phenomena reported in the literature (see Chapter 16, Miller and Dworkin; Chapter 15, Hahn; Chapter 17, Roberts et al.) it must nevertheless be conceded that such phenomena exist. Numerous evidences have emanated from the laboratories of Miller and DiCara, and independent replications of the basic phenomena have been reported by Hothersall and Brener (1969) and Slaughter, Hahn, and Rinaldi (1970). In our laboratory, Hothersall (1968) successfully conditioned either heart rate increases or decreases in 13 curarized rats. All the subjects employed in his experiments displayed the desired effect, although in certain cases it did not emerge until the third or fourth sessions of conditioning. Middaugh (1971), although unable to produce operant heart rate conditioning effects employing the methods reported by Miller and DiCara (1967), did obtain positive evidence of this phenomenon (a change in the reinforced direction during conditioning and a reversal of this direction during extinction) in 12 of 20 curarized rats when she adjusted respiratory parameters. Apart from the Hothersall study which employed multiple conditioning sessions, we have been unable to obtain results as reliable as those reported by Miller and DiCara. Certain subjects provide convincing evidence, while others do not despite the use of equivalent procedures. Possibly, the standardization of respiration procedures as suggested above may facilitate the reproducibility of these phenomena. Thus we do not question the existence of such phenomena, but rather the reliability and magnitude of the reported effects.

Given that operant cardiovascular phenomena are demonstrable, the question of the significance of these phenomena still awaits clarification. It will be recognized that curare operates primarily at the myoneural junction to prevent motor impulses from producing striate muscle activity. The observation that profound alterations in cardiovascular activity may be produced in curarized animals establishes only that such changes are independent of afferent feedback from the striate musculature. Such a conclusion is not surprising—a voluminous literature indicates that cardiovascular and somatomotor responses are integrated at a central level (Hoff, Kell, and Carroll 1963). Since any somatomotor process proximal to the myoneural junction may exert an influence on the cardiovascular activity of the curarized rat, the question remains open as to whether cardiovascular conditioning in this preparation is specific to the cardiovascular system or whether it involves a modification of the somato-cardiovascular Gestalt.

The purpose of the experiments described in this section is to demonstrate that, even under curare, somatomotor processes continue to exhibit their effects through cardiovascular performance. Our interest in this problem was prompted by the initial experiments with curarized rats (Trowill 1967; Miller and DiCara 1967). In these experiments, subjects were first trained to press a bar for brain stimulation. Given the integral relationship between somatomotor and cardiovascular processes, it could be proposed that this pretraining involved not only the conditioning of bar-presses in the subjects, but also the conditioning of a response complex involving cardiovascular components which were subsequently manifested in the curarized state. This hypothesis can be questioned in the light of more recent work (DiCara and Miller 1969a; Slaughter, Hahn and Rinaldi, 1970) in which it has been shown that cardiovascular responses may be conditioned without any pretraining in the noncurarized state, and that the amount of pretraining does not influence the magnitude of the response conditioned under curare. However, the evidences to be described below indicate that there is a kernel of truth in the proposition that somatomotor processes continue to exert an influence on cardiovascular activity in the curarized animal.

SOMATOMOTOR-CARDIOVASCULAR RELATIONS DURING CONDITIONING

That cardiovascular and somatomotor activities are related in a lawful manner is not a speculative issue, but a fact that may be validated by simple observation. The nature of coupling between these two systems is, however, of critical significance to the analysis of learned cardiovascular activity. It has been suggested by DiCara and Miller and their associates that the neural control circuits involved in cardiovascular adjustment are demonstrably independent of the circuits involved in somatomotor control. On the other hand, Obrist and Webb (1967), Black (1967b), and Brener and Goesling (1968) have suggested that

cardiovascular and somatomotor processes are the peripheral manifestations of a common neural control center. Much of this discussion has
centered about data derived from experiments involving curarized
subjects.

Certainly in the noncurarized animal, somatomotor and cardiovascular activities occur in concert and are highly correlated in a variety
of learning situations (Obrist et al. 1970b). Obrist et al. (see Chapter
8) have also recently reported that the magnitude of operantly conditioned heart rate responses in noncurarized human subjects is inversely related to the degree of somatomotor restraint employed during conditioning. Black (1967b) has similarly observed that heart rate
and somatomotor responsiveness in dogs decrease as a function of level
of curarization. That investigator entertains the possibility that the reduction in heart rate responsiveness under curare is due to a vagal
blocking effect exhibited by this drug in large doses. Autonomic blockade by curare has also been demonstrated by a number of other investigators in this area of research (see Chapter 15, Hahn; Chapter 18,
Howard et al.). Despite this autonomic effect of curare, however, a considerable body of literature indicates that profound changes in cardiovascular activity may be produced in deeply curarized animals. The
focal question here is whether such changes are independent of the
somatomotor activities they accompany in the normal state. Since curare prevents the experimenter from observing the overt manifestations of somatomotor activity, the empirical answer to this question
must be sought by employing a transfer design.

Some of the strongest evidence in support of the integration of somatomotor processes in the operant cardiovascular effects observed in
curarized rats comes from the studies by DiCara and Miller and their
associates. Following conditioning of heart rate increases in one group
of curarized rats and heart rate decreases in another group, DiCara
and Miller (1969b) tested for retention of the conditioned response in
the noncurarized state. In this test, subjects that had previously been
reinforced for heart rate increases under curare displayed substantially
higher respiratory rates and general activity levels than subjects that
had been reinforced for heart rate decreases under curare. Since in
the pretest conditioning procedure, there was no possibility of fortuitous reinforcement of activity and respiratory changes, it must be concluded that the conditioned response was not specifically cardiovascular
in nature, but involved a constellation of biologically-related activities.

Surprisingly, these transfer data are directly contradicted by data reported in the same year by DiCara and Weiss (1969). Although the
conditioning and transfer procedures employed in this experiment
were very similar to those reported by DiCara and Miller (1969b), it
was found that subjects that had been reinforced for heart rate incre-

ments under curare displayed lower respiration rates and activity levels in the noncurarized test than subjects previously reinforced for heart rate decrements. Despite the contradictory nature of these results, it must still be concluded that, in both cases, conditioning was not specific to the cardiovascular system. Of the two sets of transfer data, those provided by DiCara and Miller (1969b) fit better with other reported evidence of somato-cardiovascular integration, including data derived from noncurarized rats by DiCara and Miller (1969a). In this experiment, heart rate responses were operantly conditioned in two groups of noncurarized rats. It was observed that subjects reinforced for heart rate increases displayed higher activity levels than and similar respiratory rates to subjects reinforced for heart rate decreases.

Our initial attempt to investigate the influence of somatomotor learning on the cardiovascular activity of curarized rats involved shuttle-box training prior to heart rate conditioning under curare (Brener 1970b). Following extended avoidance training in the shuttle-box, rats were curarized and submitted to a conditioning procedure in which they could avoid electric shock either by increasing or decreasing their heart rates. Rats that had learned to avoid in the shuttle-box displayed heart rate changes during the curare conditioning phase of the experiment that were consonant with the Law of Effect. However, rats that had not learned to avoid the shock in the shuttle-box (escapers) displayed substantial heart rate changes in a direction opposite to that predicted by the Law of Effect during the curare phase of the experiment. Although these data lent some support to the assertion that somatomotor learning continues to exert an influence on cardiovascular activity in the curarized animal, they were also subject to alternative interpretations. For example, the relationship between shuttle-box and heart rate avoidance may have been based upon a difference between the two groups of animals in general learning ability. This possibility cannot be overlooked in the present case since the nonavoiders failed to develop a shuttle-box avoidance response in over 600 training trials.

A similar experiment which tends to favor a transfer of training interpretation has been reported by Black (1967b). That investigator trained dogs to avoid an electric shock by pressing a pedal in the non-curarized state. Thereafter, these subjects were compared in heart rate avoidance under curare to dogs that had not been similarly pretrained. It was found that the pretrained subjects displayed slightly but not significantly better heart rate conditioning under curare than did the subjects that had not been pretrained.

In order to more adequately assess the transfer of learning from the noncurarized to the curarized state it was decided to examine the effects of conditioning mutually antagonistic somatomotor-cardiovascular responses in two groups of subjects prior to heart rate conditioning under curare (Goesling and Brener 1972). The responses of choice were the broad classes "activity" and "immobility." Given the integrated nature of the somatomotor and cardiovascular systems, we assumed that increased activity would be associated with heart rate increases and immobility with heart rate decreases. We reasoned that if curare simply blocked one component of the general response set, then subjects that had been conditioned to be immobile would display better conditioning of heart rate decrements under curare than subjects that had been conditioned to be active, and vice versa.

In summary, the plan of the experiment was as follows: Ten experimental and 10 yoked-control rats served as subjects in an immobility conditioning experiment. An additional 20 rats were arbitrarily divided into equal experimental and yoked-control groups in an activity conditioning experiment.

Activity was conditioned in a running wheel under an S^D/S procedure and was implemented for 10 40-minute sessions. During S^D, the house lights were on and the experimental subjects had to rotate a wheel whenever a tone came on in order to avoid shock. The tone was presented whenever a subject failed to rotate the wheel for 5 seconds. The stimuli that were contingent upon the experimental subject's activity were also presented to its yoked-control subject. During S , the house lights were off and no experimental stimuli occurred.

Immobility was conditioned in a small open field. An S^D/S procedure was employed here as well and all rats were run for 10 40-minute sessions. During S^D, the house lights came on and if the experimental subject moved (as sensed by an ultrasonic motion detector) a tone came on; if it continued to move when the tone was on, it received a shock on each recorded activity unit. The yoked-control subjects received the same stimuli as those controlled by the experimental subjects' activity. During S , the house lights were off and no stimuli were presented.

In both procedures, activity responses were recorded throughout each session and heart rate was measured on the final (10th) session. The results derived from the 10th session of this phase of the experiment are summarized below in Table 13.1.

TABLE 13.1 *Group mean heart rate and activity scores recorded during the final day of conditioning.*

		S		S^D	
		Activity	HR	Activity	HR
Immobile	Experimental Ss	32.85	428	2.60	404
	Yoked-control Ss	34.30	424	15.50	415
Active	Experimental Ss	47.20	386	600.50	461
	Yoked-control Ss	159.00	396	202.10	409

It will be seen that experimental and yoked-control immobile subjects displayed lower heart rates and activity levels in S^D than in S . This overall difference was significant for both measures at the .05 level. The difference between experimental and control subjects, although in the predicted direction, was not of sufficient magnitude to satisfy statistical criteria of significance. Statistical analyses of the data derived from the active subjects, on the other hand, indicated that both measures were significantly higher in S^D than in S (p<.01) *and* that the experimental subjects displayed a significantly greater increment in both heart rate and activity from S to S^D than did their yoked controls (p<.01).

It is clear from these data that heart rate reflects the level of somatomotor activity. The lower the activity, the lower the heart rate. Since similar aversive contingencies were employed to condition both activity and immobility, it also seems fair to suggest that the heart rate does not reflect the emotional substrate of the behavior which was presumably similar in the two procedures.

Following these pretraining procedures, all subjects were curarized and submitted to a procedure in which they could avoid an electric shock by altering their heart rates. Half the subjects in each experimental and yoked-control group could avoid the aversive stimulus by increasing their heart rates, and the other half could avoid the aversive stimulus by decreasing their heart rates. All subjects were immobilized with an i.p. injection of 16 units/kg of d-tubocurarine chloride and respirated at55 cpm at pressures ranging between 12 and 18 cmH^2O. Heart rates were stabilized during the first 20 minutes of the curare session, and the conditioning procedures were implemented during the subsequent 40 minutes. Heart rate avoidance criteria were established separately for each subject during the initial 20 minutes and were selected to approximate the median heart rate displayed by the subject during this period. During conditioning, whenever the subject's heart rate failed to meet criterion for five successive heart beats, a warning stimulus (tone) came on. If the subject continued to display non-criterion heart rates for an additional 20 heart beats, it received a brief shock (0.75 ma for 0.1 seconds) following which there was a 6-second time out, and the procedure was recycled. If the subject failed to avoid for six consecutive 30-second periods, the criterion was made less stringent, and if it succeeded in avoiding for six consecutive 30-second periods, the criterion was made more stringent.

Heart rate measures were recorded every 30 seconds throughout the procedure. Eight-minute averages were then computed for each subject and the mean preconditioning heart rate (recorded during the last 8 minutes of adaptation) was subtracted from each of these averages to provide five consecutive heart rate change measures for each subject.

These measures were then averaged for each group and are described for rats that served as experimental subjects in the pretraining procedure (see Figure 13.5) and for rats that served as yoked-control subjects in the pretraining procedure (see Figure 13.6). Attending first of all to Figure 13.5, it will be observed that subjects which were trained to be active prior to curarization display heart rate increments under curare regardless of the reinforcement contingencies imposed during this latter procedure. Subjects which were trained to be immobile prior to curarization display decrements in heart rate under curare regardless of the reinforcement contingencies. Although it is true that within both the active and immobile groups there are slight differences in heart rate in a direction predictable by the Law of Effect, these differences are not statistically significant and are trivial in comparison to the effect attributable to the pretraining procedure. Analysis of variance indicated that the pretraining effect (Active versus Immobile) was significant at the .05 level. Consideration of Figure 13.6 indicates that all subjects serving as yoked controls in the pretraining procedure displayed decrements in heart rate under curare regardless of contingencies imposed. Differences in the reactions of the experimental and yoked-control subjects to the curare procedure are reflected in a significant Pretraining (Active versus Immobile) by Groups (Experimental versus Control) interaction ($p < .01$). Active experimental subjects displayed greater increments under curare than did their controls, whereas immobile experimental subjects displayed greater decrements than did their controls. Neither the curare contingency effect (high heart rates avoid versus low heart rates avoid) nor any of its interactions were significant. We are forced to conclude therefore that the dominant influence over heart rate in these curarized rats was the pre-curare training received by subjects in the normal nondrugged state.

DISCUSSION AND CONCLUSIONS

The experiments reported in this chapter have centered about two issues, both associated with the conditioning of cardiovascular responses in curarized rats. The first section attended to a methodological aspect of the curare literature, namely, the influence of respiratory procedures employed in the maintenance of curarized rats. The second section has dealt with an interpretive aspect of these phenomena: in particular, the extent to which curare provides a method for eliminating somatomotor influences on cardiovascular activity.

Two conclusions appear to be warranted by the data presented. First, it must be conceded that the cardiovascular activity of curarized rats maintained on positive pressure artificial respiration is subject to a mul-

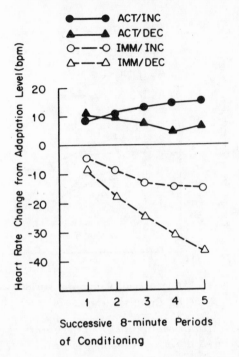

FIGURE 13.5. *Heart rate changes in groups of curarized rats that were previously trained to be either active (ACT/) or immobile (IMM/) while being reinforced for heart rate increases (INC) or decreases (DEC).*

titude of abnormal influences. These influences go far beyond achieving striate muscle paralysis, the empirical goal of this procedure. Consequently the generality of principles derived from the study of such preparations is limited. Second, data have been provided which suggest that curare does not achieve its primary purpose: Somatomotor influences on cardiovascular activity may be observed even in the curarized rat. As was suggested earlier, the principal effect of this drug is to prevent experimenters from observing the integrated behavioral processes in which cardiovascular responses are imbedded. Despite these negative conclusions, the curare literature is considered here to have served several important functions although these were tangential to its intended function.

As was mentioned in the introduction to this chapter, the demonstration of operant cardiovascular effects in paralyzed animals appears to have established the scientific respectability of these phenomena. In so doing, the curare literature has contributed to a major reconceptualization regarding the structural boundaries within which different learning principles are effective. Cardiovascular activities are clearly not

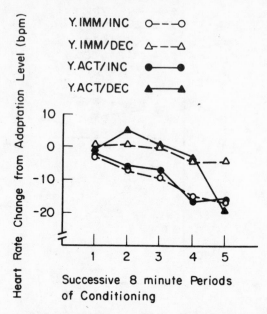

FIGURE 13.6.   *Heart rate changes in groups of curarized rats that previously served as yoked-controls during conditioning of activity (ACTl) and immobility (IMMl) while being reinforced for heart rate increases (INC) or decreases (DEC).*

immune to the influences of response-contingent reinforcement. Although operant cardiovascular responses have not been demonstrated to be independent of somatomotor processes, the demonstration of such responses in curarized animals does delimit the possible mechanisms linking the activities of these response systems.

Four models of somato-cardiovascular linkage are illustrated in Figure 13.7. Implicit in these models is the assumption that operant control rests upon the availability of response feedback to the cortical centers involved in the regulation of the responses in question (see Chapter 19, Brener).

The most conservative model of the relationship between somatomotor and cardiovascular processes is described in diagram (a) of this figure. This model, erroneously ascribed to Smith (1954) and implicated in a previous controversy in which curare figured prominently (Smith 1964; Smith 1964; Black and Lang 1964), assumes that the cardiovascular system responds to the peripheral demands of the striate musculature. Clearly this model cannot assimilate the cardiovascular phenomena reported for animals immobilized by curare.

Smith (1967) proposed that somatomotor activity is primary with respect to somato-cardiovascular adjustments only insofar as the feedback

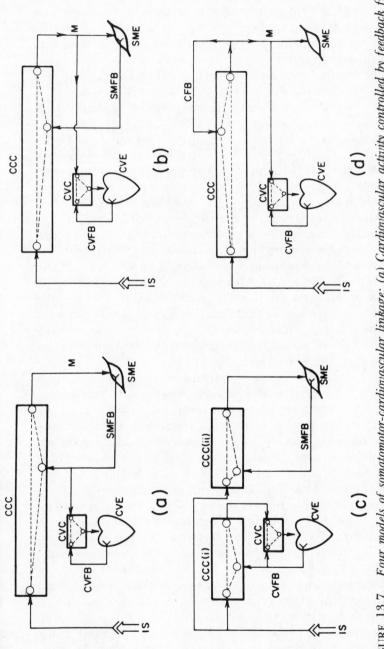

FIGURE 13.7. *Four models of somatomotor-cardiovascular linkage: (a) Cardiovascular activity controlled by feedback from somatomotor effectors. (b) Cardiovascular and somatomotor activities controlled in parallel by same neural center. Parallel outputs of the center regulated via feedback from somatomotor effectors. (c) Independent control of somatomotor and cardiovascular activities with each regulated via its own intrinsic feedback. (d) Parallel control of somatomotor and cardiovascular activities with parallel output regulated via central feedback from motor control center.*

ABBREVIATIONS:

CCC = Cortical control center	SME = Somatomotor effectors	CVE = Cardiovascular effectors
M = Efferent motor pathway	SMFB = Somatomotor feedback pathways	CVFB = Cardiovascular feedback pathways
	CVC = Cardiovascular control center	IS = Initiating stimulus

from this system serves to regulate the output of the common neural control center serving both response systems. Although this model, illustrated in Figure 13.7 (b) is also unable to account for cardiovascular change in the immobilized animal, it is inherently attractive and consonant with a considerable body of experimental literature dealing with behavioral regulation in intact, free-moving animals.

If we assume that operant cardiovascular learning is a cortical phenomenon (DiCara, Braun, and Pappas 1970) and that it relies upon the availability of feedback from the effector system being conditioned, we may accommodate the operant cardiovascular phenomena reported for curarized animals in terms of the model illustrated in Figure 13.7(c). This model which seems to be implicit in the theoretical approaches of Miller and DiCara et al. assumes autonomy in the circuits responsible for the control of cardiovascular and somatomotor activities. While such a mechanism can accommodate evidences of learning effects that are specific to the cardiovascular system, it does not easily accord with the wealth of evidence indicating the commonality of somato-cardiovascular regulation. In assessing the nature of the somato-cardiovascular relationship it is important to take into account not only the behavioral evidence (Obrist et al. 1970b), which indicates a close correlation between the effector processes of the two systems, but also the neurophysiological evidence (Hoff et al. 1963; Germana 1969) which indicates considerable overlap in the neural circuits involved in the control of somatomotor activities and the cardiovascular adjustments that are observed to accompany them.

In view of these considerations it is proposed that the model presented in Figure 13.7 (d) can most readily describe the relationship between somatomotor and cardiovascular control observed in the curarized animal. It is assumed here that the regulation of the somato-cardiovascular response is achieved via central feedback or "efferent monitoring" in the normal adult organism. It is well established that feedback from the periphery is essential only during the initial development of motor control. In well-practiced skills such peripheral feedback becomes redundant (Kimble and Perlmuter 1970). Particularly relevant to the current topic is an observation recorded by Campbell, Sanderson, and Laverty (1964). These investigators observed that human subjects who were pharmacologically immobilized reported executing vigorous movements although, objectively, the movements were very small or nonexistent. In this case it must be assumed that subjects assessed the vigor of their movements not on the basis of peripheral feedback but rather in terms of efferent monitoring or central feedback. Whether or not such central motor circuits are involved in the production of operant cardiovascular changes would seem to be easily amenable to an empirical answer.

Despite the strong evidence in favor of somatomotor involvement in operant cardiovascular change, it is generally conceded that dissociation between these activities may occur under certain circumstances. Specification of the conditions under which decoupling of these activities is facilitated may well have important clinical ramifications. Essential hypertension, for example, may be thought of as the result of such a dissociative process. Early in this disease the only manifest symptom is that the levels of cardiovascular activity observed are inappropriate to the somatomotor context in which they occur.

The experiments of DiCara and Miller (1969b) and DiCara and Weiss (1969) referred to earlier in support of somatomotor involvement in operant cardiovascular effects observed in curarized rats also provide evidence of decoupling of the two systems. With further testing and training in the noncurarized state, these investigators report a convergence of somatic activities between groups reinforced for heart rate increases and decreases and a divergence of heart rate. A similar effect was not observed by DiCara and Miller (1969b) during heart rate conditioning in the noncurarized state. This disparity suggests that the implementation of reinforcement contingencies that are specific to heart rate when somatomotor responses are blocked may predispose the organism towards acquiring a dissociation of the two activities. Possibly, in such cases, cardiovascular activity becomes more reliant on its intrinsic self-regulatory capacity and less subject to the influences of cortical motor processes. Within the context of the views presented here such dissociation of normally coupled activities is seen as a functional aberration rather than as indicative of the normal processes of behavioral regulation. For this reason, the use of immobilizing agents, such as curare, may well be limited where the interest is in understanding the general principles of cardiovascular learning.

NOTES

1. An explanation of these apparent discrepancies may be obtained by reference to Chapter 14 by DiCara.

2. Use of nonrecirculating respirators will inevitably lead to a gradual reduction of body temperature over the period of artificial respiration. This is due simply to nonrecoverable heat transferred to the expired air and vented to atmosphere.

3. We consider a normal heart rate in the curarized rat weighing between 400 to 500 gm to have a mean value somewhere between 360 and 460 bpm. Species differences contribute significantly to this wide variation. More important than the absolute heart rate, however, is the heart rate variability. Invariant heart rates generally indicate hyperventilation, and profound sinus arrhythmias indicate hypoventilation. Ideally, the subject should display 10 to 30 bpm bidirectional variations that have time course unrelated to respiration rate. Systematic unidirectional trends in mean heart rate generally indicate inadequate respiration, and, therefore, assessment of the heart rate should be made employing a sample of at least 10 minutes in duration.

14

LEO V. DiCARA

Some Critical Methodological Variables Involved in Visceral Learning

INTRODUCTION

For the past several years a number of students and colleagues associated with Neal Miller and me have published the results of experiments which clearly indicated that visceral responses can be trained by operant learning techniques (Miller 1969; DiCara 1970b). During these years, despite confirmation and extension of the basic phenomena in some laboratories (Hothersall and Brener 1969; Slaughter, Hahn, and Rinaldi 1970), it was equally clear that some investigators including Brener, Hahn, and Black were having difficulty in working with curarized animals. Consequently, one of the goals of this conference was to bring together the major investigators in this field to exchange ideas and information.

The results of this conference have been quite profound. The conference has clearly identified three different types of problems in the area of visceral learning. The first type has to do with the reliability of the basic learning phenomena itself. As Miller has pointed out (Chapter 16) the size of the learned heart rate obtained in different heart rate learning experiments has declined progressively over the past five years. To illustrate, in my last reported experiment on the heart rate learning of neodecorticate rats (DiCara, Braun, and Pappas 1970) I obtained an average learned effect of only 4.5% in normal Ss

The preparation of this paper and the unpublished research described within was supported by Research Grant MH21403 from the USPHS; and by Research Grant 71-774 from the American Heart Association to Leo V. DiCara.

DiCARA: *Techniques in Visceral Learning*   277

as compared to 20% in 1967 (Miller and DiCara 1967). To add to the confusion of this matter, during the past year, Miller has reported no success whatsoever in obtaining learned heart rate changes in curarized rats using electric shock. Unfortunately, at the present time, I cannot speak definitively to this issue since my recent relocation and development of a laboratory at the University of Michigan has slowed my research program to a temporary crawl.

The second type of problem is far more subtle; it has to do with an examination, and, insofar as it is possible, a comparison of current techniques with those used several years ago. The third problem pertains to the theoretical argument for and against the use of curare.

I would like to address myself, in the main, to a discussion of past and present techniques for working with curarized animals, especially those used to demonstrate heart rate learning with electric shock as a reinforcer. Insofar as they do not markedly divert me, I will try to answer explicit, as well as implicit, questions and to discuss the current activities of my laboratory relevant to them.

In keeping with the spirit of this conference, my paper will be relatively informal. In many ways, it exemplifies the growth pains of a new area of research and its methodological and conceptual difficulties. However, it is my hope that resolving the current problems will bring us that much closer to an understanding of the basic phenomena of learning, and its relationship to the autonomic nervous system.

PERSPECTIVES

There are numerous autonomic responses and at least two well known methods of reinforcement—delivery of rewarding intracranial brain stimulation, and avoidance and/or escape from mild electric shock. For example, if we exclude heart rate, the list of other responses which have been instrumentally modified in curarized rats by electric shock is impressive: blood pressure (DiCara and Miller 1968c), the PR and PP intervals of the heart beat cycle (Fields 1970b), intestinal motility (Banuazizi, 1972), uterine motility (Pappas, DiCara and Miller 1972c unpublished results), vasomotor tone in the stomach wall (Carmona, Demierre, and Miller 1972, unpublished results), and gastric pH (Carmona 1971). I think that it would be wise to remember the number of positive and different demonstrations of successful learning of visceral responses when discussing the general validity of the basic phenomena of visceral learning.

At this point, I would like to make some comments regarding the graph that Miller has presented in this volume (see Chapter 16). I think that the graph in its present form is somewhat misleading. I believe that the 1967 intracranial brain stimulation, and 1968 electric shock experiments that Miller and I reported (Miller and DiCara 1967; DiCara and Miller 1968a), were unusually successful ones; they should not be used as contemporary targets to shoot for. If we continue to expect such large changes in learned heart rate responses, it is easy to fall prey to the error of equating smaller, but significant learned heart rate changes, with failure to demonstrate the basic phenomena. For example: Pappas, Miller, and I have just submitted for publication an experiment in which we report on the significant learning of heart rate increases and decreases in infant rats, as well as their subsequent relearning of heart rate, as adults, to avoid noxious electric tail shock (Pappas, DiCara, and Miller 1972a). However, the heart rate changes obtained in this experiment averaged about 7%, not 20%.

Having the advantage of several years of hindsight and being acutely aware of how difficult it is, under the best conditions, to work with curarized preparations, I believe that the replication difficulties being encountered now will turn out to be due, in part, to one or more of the following variables: (1) precurarization treatment of the subject; (2) procedures for curarization; and, (3) respiration techniques.

One can curarize and try to train an unlimited number of animals without obtaining evidence of instrumental learning if any one of the preceding variables is ignored. It is unfortunate—but true—that, although there are a million ways that things can be done wrong, there is only one correct way.

Before embarking on a discussion of each of the above variables, I would like to confess how obvious it has become to me just how incomplete and, sometimes, incorrect my previous reports of my techniques and procedures have been. Looking back, I can see how some investigators could have ended up with curarized rats suffering from hyperventilation, as evidenced by invariant and unresponsive tachycardia, conditions obviously incompatible with learning, instrumental or classical. If only I had had the foresight to know how critical it was to have detailed the things I had taken for granted; unfortunately, I didn't. Let me give you an example: Until recently I have measured the amount of electric shock delivered to each S by needle deflection on an ammeter as shown during the shock pulses. In view of the physics of momentum, this procedure constitutes a serious error in experimental design, since the amount of shock can be grossly underestimated depending upon the amount of inertia of the needle, the coefficient of friction of moving parts, the lubrication, and so forth. Obviously, this procedure could easily lead to other investigators either overshocking or undershocking the S, depending on how they measured the intensity of the shock.

Precurarization Treatment of S

During 1965 and 1966, I used to house my animals in colony cages. I abandoned this practice soon after I discovered that it was the more emotional animal that was apt to be chosen last. That is, since I opened the cage only a few inches and picked up the animal closest to the front, the highly emotional S would more likely be in the back of the cage during my early selections. I also noted that animals curarized toward the end of an experiment (i.e., more emotional or frightened ones) appeared to be subject to greater cardiac arrhythmias and to sudden death if rewarded for decreases in heart rate, than animals rewarded for decreases who were curarized and trained early in the experiment (i.e., the animals near the front of the cage). The more emotional animals also seemed to take longer to recover from the effects of curare. It was these observations which led us to investigate the behavioral (DiCara and Weiss 1969) and biochemical consequences of heart rate learning (DiCara and Stone 1970). Unfortunately, it is just these types of observations which most journal editors will tend to discourage; sad to think that some years passed between the time that these observations were made and the time that experiments based on them were designed, executed, and reported.

The above effect, that is, the differential effect of curarized heart rate training on rats of differing emotionality is an extremely important one, which, if not controlled for, can confound an experiment before it gets off the ground. For example, it is apparent to me that rats handled daily will behave differently than Ss who have not been handled. Consequently, accurate reporting of handling techniques are very important. Handling is very important since it affects emotionality which, in turn, has an effect on a rat's physiological response under curare. For example, Stone (unpublished Ph.D. thesis 1970) has found that more emotional rats show a greater lowering of body temperature during the initial 30 minutes under curare compared to normal animals. However, the drop was not accompanied by metabolic changes, i.e., oxygen consumption.

Emotional animals also tend to have their core temperature move in the direction of the ambient temperature faster and to a greater extent than do normal Ss. This latter effect is presumably due to metabolic factors and to changes in cutaneous blood flow which reduce the insulation of the skin and thereby increase heat transfer. However, here also, Stone found nonmetabolic effects of emotionality on thermoregulation. Stone also found it more difficult for highly emotional rats to maintain normal body temperature in either a normal, warmer-than-normal, or cooler-than-normal, ambient environment. In view of the high correlations between body temperature, oxygen consumption, and heart rate these results might help to explain drifts in heart rate first in one direction and then in the opposite direction during the adaptation or pretraining phase of curarization.

The particular method of curarization, as well as the precurare handling of the rat, can have profound effects on heart rate behavior under curare. Since adult, as well as infantile, handling of the rat reduces emotionality, I recommend that each investigator look carefully at his housing conditions, and check whether the animal attendant and graduate students play with some Ss and not others, tease the Ss, etc.

It is my conviction that highly emotional or animals overly frightened during the process of curarization have little if any chance of learning cardiac responses under curare. In the successful report of operant conditioning of heart rate in curarized rats using intracranial brain stimulation, Hothersall and Brener (1969) used the gentling technique of Weininger, Mcleeland, and Arima (1954) which has been shown to decrease activity in the sympathetic nervous system. Their animals were also deprived of food for 12 hours prior to the experiment. These facts are reported in Hothersall's dissertation (1968). It would be very interesting to know if Brener is experiencing his current difficulties with or without gentling. With hungry or satiated animals?

Because of the complex interaction of core and ambient temperature with heart rate and the role of emotionality on the thermostability of the preparation, as well as its interaction with the training procedures, I have conducted my experiments under conditions of a controlled environment. This is not the case with many of the investigators in the field. I suggest that they look into this matter very carefully, especially in view of the fact that they often report Ss dying within 30 minutes of curarization.

Precurarization treatment of the S does not only include physical parameters such as housing, ambient temperature, noise, and light, but also the behavioral experience of the animal up to the time the experimenter closes the experimental chamber door. In this regard, Goesling and Brener's experiments (1972) aimed at investigating the somatic-visceral question can be viewed as precurarized treatment of the S. In one of these experiments, the effects of prior shuttle-box training on avoidance conditioning of heart rate under curare was investigated. Animals were trained to learn a two-way shuttle, and then were curarized and required to learn heart rate increases and decreases under curare. The results of this experiment indicated that Ss that acquired the shuttle-box response displayed significantly better heart rate learning of both increases and decreases under curare, than did Ss that had not acquired the shuttle-box response. The animals learned approximately 10% changes in baseline heart rate. This is quite impressive, since the reinforcer used in this experiment was avoidance of electric shock. In many ways, this experiment was a mirror image of the DiCara and Weiss experiment (1969).

Procedures for Curarization

Since several participants have presented excellent papers on the factors, dangers, and intricacies involved in curarizing an animal, it would not be very productive for me to repeat the technical and pharmacological aspects of curarization. Instead, I would like to address myself to simpler matters. For instance, even with as simple a procedure as injecting a neuromuscular blocking agent, different investigators have different techniques, not to mention the use of different dosages. For example, Carmona successfully used dosages as high as 4.5 mg/kg to operantly train cortical electroencephalographic (EEG) activity (Carmona unpublished Ph.D. thesis 1967).

I think I can be most helpful by describing certain habits I have developed over the years which have never been described elsewhere. One of these regards the handling of the animal; and, the other, the timing of the different steps involved in curarization.

Before handling the rat, I have always let my hand run over that rat's home cage and gridfloor in order to get some of the rat's body odor on my hand before picking the animal up. I found this does not frighten the animals as much as a "naive" hand. Some facts which may be of interest include the following: I never let any technician carry out the curarization. In addition, I do not smoke nor does anyone in my laboratory when we curarize rats. I never use gloves and try wherever possible to minimize discomfort to the S by gentle handling and blowing quickly on the rat's snout, to distract it, at the instant of injection entry. I do not, as some experimenters do, push the animal's hind limbs against a table to expose its abdomen, or have another person help by eagle-spreading the animal. Both procedures are extremely stressful to the rat. In these regards, it is interesting to note Hahn's observation that: "a S that had received nembutal was extremely easy to curarize and respirate without complications while animals which had not received nembutal invariably were difficult to stabilize following curare injection" (Chapter 15).

An experiment is in progress in my laboratory with very interesting results. The experiment consists of comparing animals receiving nembutal with those receiving a saline injection prior to curare. The saline control Ss are placed in the face mask either according to my procedures or those of other investigators (see Chapter 15, Hahn); i.e., after the S has ceased struggling from the curare injection. Initial results indicate that normal conscious animals placed in the face mask rapidly after curare injection behave physiologically like the animals "protected" from the stress by nembutal; they have normal heart rate and variability, condition in a classical situation, and show few abnormalities of rhythm. Conversely, Ss that receive control saline injections and are placed in the mask after they have ceased struggling from curare, show abnormalities of heart rate and rhythm and condition very poorly, if at all.

One way to try and describe what is essentially an art or interaction between man and animal, such as the process of curarization, is to give a description of events over time. In regard to timing, the entire process of reaching for a S to curarize it and place it into the face mask should take place in less than 45 seconds; certainly, it should not take as long as 2 or 3 minutes as some investigators have reported. In the sense that I always was able to achieve this in the time specified, my procedure could, in the hands of an investigator with less success, be used as a criteria to screen subjects. The possibility that I may have inadvertantly screened subjects has been raised by Hahn (Chapter 15) and Middaugh (unpublished Ph.D. thesis 1971, p. 4). Middaugh also has recognized that the "site of injection and speed of onset of paralysis in the rat has an important bearing on the stability of the S's heart rate under curare (ibid., p. 107).

I have found that, if injected correctly, the S will cease struggling immediately after being placed in the face mask. However, it will be necessary to hold the S in the mask for another 1 or 2 minutes until it is totally paralyzed. One can determine that the S is not completely paralyzed by momentarily moving it so that it is not being respirated. It will start to struggle immediately. This procedure of placing the S in the mask very quickly will minimize bronchoconstriction, laryngospasm, obstruction of the glottis, and other defensive pulmonary reflexes. In addition, this procedure lowers intrathoracic pressure. Conversely, waiting for the rat to become totally paralyzed, as many investigators do (see Chapter 15, Hahn), before applying the face mask results in great trauma and an increased intrathoracic pressure which interferes with the venous return.

In summary of this and the preceding section on the precurarized treatment of the S, I would like to say that the most important thing that an investigator can do to obtain good curarized preparations is to design the procedures to allow the animal to keep as much of its composure as it possibly can while undergoing curarization. In order to achieve this, the individual handling the animals must be experienced. Too often, principal investigators utilize minimally trained technicians, or two-week volunteer students to carry out this very critical work—this is a deadly trap. Unless the experimenter has had extensive experience with animals, knows how to handle them without gloves, and is clearly not afraid of being bitten, the experiment may be sabotaged before it begins.

Respiration Techniques

Before starting out I would like to state that, for those who may not have already experienced it, proper curarization and artificial respiration constitute, at best, very fragile preparations. Over the years, I have discovered certain procedures which have helped me with these exceedingly difficult preparations. In view of this, I believe that I can be most helpful if I direct my comments to those seemingly unimportant things I did which missed getting into print. That is, metaphorically speaking, I will, in the main, stay "outside" of the organism. In some instances, I will even do without the organism. For example, concentrate on comparing and calibrating the small animal respirator pumps used for the artificial respiration of curarized rats. (Model V5KG, Narco-Biosystems Inc., Houston, Texas).

Prior to my arrival at Yale in 1965, two graduate students of Miller's, Drs. Jay Trowill and Eric Stone, had developed a relatively simple technique for the artificial respiration of curarized rats, the face mask. I inherited this apparatus, and, as is the case when things are going well, did not change a thing—not even the tubing or the respirator. In addition, because of differences in elasticity, I went as far as to try and use the same balloon for the mask as long as possible. For example, all things being equal, an elastic balloon effectively increases the dead air space, a very important variable. In addition, in our laboratory we have found that, all other things being equal, decreasing compliance of the balloon is equivalent to increasing the pressure in the system. These results are especially important in view of the fact that some investigators change the balloon for each experimental session.

To help me accomplish my goal, that is, to use one balloon as long as I could, I initially put a tiny swab of cotton over the rat's top incisors to avoid puncturing the balloon. Somewhere along the way, I think in 1967, I instituted two changes. They did not get into print. I do not know why. I probably thought that they were unimportant; obviously, they were not. One change was instituted in order to avoid the necessity for using Xylocaine which has effects on the central nervous system. This involved the construction of a plastic "sling" so that the rat could be placed on its belly and its entire snout forced into the mask, held by special rubber tipped braces as shown elsewhere (DiCara 1970a). This change accomplished its aim; that is, it eliminated the need for a Xylocaine injection since I no longer had to pinch the upper portion of the balloon and nose skin with a hemostat, in order to insure a tight fit. However, the side effects of this change meant that the rat's mouth would be kept closed and the animal placed on its belly. Prior to use of the sling, the S lay on its side on a towel in the experimental chamber. These changes are important because the air entering the animal's lungs now had to raise, as well as expand, the animal's lungs and thorax. This in turn, resulted in less air entering the animal's lungs at any given pressure. In addition, the change in position had differential effects on the passive expiration phase of the inspiration-expiration cycle.

In order to discuss artificial respiration of small animals using the small animal respirator it is necessary to consider the respirator with and without a S. That is to consider: (a) respiration of a curarized rat using the respirator; and, (b) the respirator's design, performance, and operating characteristics without a S attached to it. As we shall see, the respirators have independent and unique operating characteristics. In view of the difference between respirators, I recommend that nothing be taken at face value. Instead, each investigator should obtain a direct measure of tidal volume. Other useful controls are to obtain pneumograms based on a strain guage around both the chest and abdomen of the S. However, we have found that a pneumogram based on chest measurements alone can be misleading, depending on the amount of air which is entering the animal's stomach and the body weight of the rat, as well as such obvious variables as lung compliance and true tidal volume.

Respiration of a Curarized Rat.   In every experiment prior to 1970, Miller and I used the same parameters—a 1-to-1 inspiration-expiration ratio, 70 cpm and a peak pressure reading of 20 cm of water. From 1967 to the present, the mouth of the S was closed. Many investigators do not close the S's mouth. These parameters when used with a 500 gm rat, in my laboratory, resulted in a tidal volume of approximately 4 ml and a viable physiological preparation as evidenced by heart rate of approximately 420 bpm, normal body temperature, and steady peripheral vasomotor tone. These values agree with independent measurements made by Stone (unpublished Ph.D. thesis 1970) on tracheotomized rats.

Certain arguments have been made questioning the possibility of heart rate learning in curarized rats on the basis that curarization results in a massive vagal blockade. The work of Hahn (Chapter 15) on the external stimulation of the vagus nerve of curarized rats, and that of Vertes and Ball in Miller's laboratory, in stimulating a central structure, the nucleus ambiguous, an outflow of the vagus nerve clearly indicate that curarization does not result in a total vagal blockade. In addition, Fields' (unpublished Ph.D. thesis 1970a) report of independent PR and PP learning constitutes evidence of reasonable vagal function since the PR interval, as well as the amplitude of the P-wave, is primarily, if not wholly, under vagal control.

In early 1970, I undertook to analyze arterial blood PO_2 and PCO_2 of rats respirated as described above (DiCara 1970a). The results of this experiment indicated that, compared to the control noncurarized rats in the experiment, I was respirating them properly; however, compared to the results of other investigators using normal noncurarized rats, I was hyperventilating them. Confusing? Yes! Let me explain. Brener's data on normal rats are accurate and, as he correctly points (see Chapter 13), the PCO_2 values I obtained for the control group of noncurarized rats in my experiment (25.4 mm) was low. When Brener brought this to my attention, I was puzzled and dismayed with this discrepancy until I remembered that most Ss used in my experiment on blood gases had been previously trained in the noncurarized state to increase or decrease systolic blood pressure, in order to avoid noxious electric shock (Pappas, DiCara, and Miller 1970). These animals were extremely frightened at my approach, and they exhibited abnormal patterns of respiration at the time of blood withdrawal. Incidentally, I got bit several times. In contrast, Brener's animals had been previously prehandled and had adapted to a restraint apparatus prior to blood withdrawal (personal communication).

Why did I use non-naive Ss? I used them in order to save the time and effort that the catherization of 48 animals would consume. I also assumed, erroneously, that the respiration procedures under curare were simply a matter of gas exchanges and that participation in a previous behavioral experiment could not possibly affect the outcome. Consequently, when the experimental group of rats in this experiment were respirated at the usual parameters and showed a PCO_2 of approximately 25 mmHg, I was delighted. I wrote the experiment up, omitting the now apparent critical issue of the Ss' prior behavioral experience. The reader may, at this point, arrive at the conclusion that I was, since 1965, hyperventilating my curarized rats. This does not turn out to be the case. I had, indeed, been correctly respirating them using the 1-to-1, 70 cycle, 20 cmH_2O parameters. However, the reasons that they were correctly ventilated were not the same ones I thought at the time I was writing the blood gas paper. To explain, it will be necessary for me to describe the physical setup of the face mask, the inspiration and expiration tubes, the respirator, the position of the rat, and so on.

The small animal respirator consists of two parts, the respirator proper and a poorly ventilated housing unit with ventilation slits to the ambient environment which start approximately 1½ inches from the base. The expiration tube also empties into the housing cabinet so that expired CO_2 has a tendency to collect on the floor of the housing assembly, since it is heavier than air. In the blood gas experiment, I used a respirator placed in the middle and on top of a table; and, since there was no need for placing the rat in a special environment, the inspiration and expiration tubes from the respirator to the rat were kept very short, under 1 foot. The use of short tubes resulted in a relatively low total dead air space. In addition, the respirator was itself well ventilated. The combination of these factors resulted in little, if any, rebreathing of expired air, or air loaded with CO_2. The result of this, in turn, was a hyperventilated rat which I concluded was properly respirated despite unusually high heart rates, close to 480 bpm, because of my error in design which permitted rats with prior shock avoidance training to be used as subjects.

To explain the situation in the visceral learning experiments it will be necessary for me to describe the geometry and location of the respirator in regard to the walls and the other equipment in the room. In the past years, the respirators, sometimes two or three of them, were stacked on top of one another with one side of the respirator's housing cabinet propped up against a side of the experimental chamber, and the other side just some 3 to 4 inches away from a wall. This lack of ventilation and blockage of the slits in the housing cabinets of the respirators often resulted in overheating of the respirator. In addition, we used to run the inspiration and expiration tubes through special apertures to get them to the subject. The total distance of the tubes often reached 4 feet. Obviously, the longer the inspiration tube the greater the pressure necessary to push the air along.

In summary, during visceral learning experiments in the past, the necessity to keep the S in a soundproof and temperature controlled environment, coupled with our ignorance, resulted in our running the inspiration and expiration tubes some 4 feet from the respirator into the experimental chamber. This resulted in an enormous amount of dead air space, and, coupled with the physical location of the respirator and the respirator's intake valve and operating characteristics, permitted a great deal of rebreathing of expelled air loaded with CO_2. I believe that I can put forth the hypothesis that the heart rates of the same rat strain vary in different laboratories as a function of that laboratory's policy regarding the geometry and length of tubing connecting animal and respirator. In this context, it is important to note that the addition of approximately 5% CO_2 will bring a rat's heart rate into normal ranges of rate and variability (see Chapter 16, Miller and Dworkin).

Although it is impossible to use the same respirators I did in 1966, I currently possess two respirators of that vintage, serial numbers 110 and 111. By respirating a rat under standard conditions and measuring the CO_2 content in the fáce mask, I have found a buildup of CO_2 in the face mask to a maximum of 2 to 3%. In addition, the buildup is significantly correlated with the rat's level of heart rate and heart rate variability. It is also interesting to note that an inspiration-expiration ratio of 1-to-2 or 3 is more effective in producing a homeostatic cardiovascular response under curare, as is using 60 cpm instead of 70 cpm. These observations are both interesting and consistent with my previous observations, since both of these procedures facilitate the removal of expired air from the face mask. Furthermore, other things being equal, the lower the inspiration:expiration (I:E) ratio and cpm, the greater the volume of air delivered to the S per stroke. In this regard it should be called to attention that some investigators utilize different experimental parameters while attempting a replication. To be sure, a parametric study of respiration variables is needed very badly; however, what is not very illuminating during the present confusion is the varying of parameters while attempting replications. For example, in Goesling's dissertation (1969), a 1-to-1 and 40 cpm is used. In another series of experiments, Brener reports using 55 cpm (personal communication), and, yet in another report, Hothersall and Brener (1969) report that 70 cpm were employed.

I would now like to consider the importance of the position of the respirator with respect to the S's lungs. If the respirator is higher than the S, the CO_2 in the tube containing the passively expelled air will flow back into the face mask and be rebreathed for quite awhile. (CO_2 is heavier than air.) If the respirator is lower than the S's lungs, and the expiration tube is bent sharply downwards, the passively expelled air will flow more readily through the tube and there will be less chance of its being found in the face mask. Unfortunately, as I mentioned earlier, the expiration tube ends inside the housing cabinet of the respirator where the expelled air will tend to collect on the floor, especially if the respirator is located against a wall, in a corner, or in an area with poor ventilation and/or air currents. Furthermore, since the housing unit does not have forced ventilation and has its first row of ventilation slits approximately 1½ inches from the floor, there is a high probability that residual CO_2 in the housing unit will be swept up through the intake valve during the inspiration phase and delivered to the S.

I would like to conclude this section by illustrating how critical it is to respirate curarized animals properly, and how easy it is to conclude incorrectly that instrumental learning has not been secured instead of correctly concluding that one has been respiring the animals improperly. Cohen (personal communication) has stated that if one respirates curarized pigeons such that there is 5% of CO_2 in the expired end tidal volume of air, one can demonstrate excellent evidence of classical cardiac conditioning. However, let the expired and tidal volume of CO_2 vary but 1%, that is to 4% or 6%, and it will be impossible to obtain evidence of classical conditioning.

Respirator Operating Characteristics: Old and New. A set of variables, perhaps as important as any other and more important if ignored, concerns the performance characteristics of the Narco-Biosystems respirator. I was somewhat superstitious in my early research; I always used the same respirators, serial numbers 160, 192, and 246. Although I no longer have these respirators in my laboratory, I am currently in the process of comparing the operating characteristics of old and new respirators. I have been told that the old and new respirators perform exactly the same and that the changes in the valves in 1966 and other aspects of the pumps design did not affect their operating characteristics. I wish to state that I have data which conflicts with that claim. Perhaps the differences I have obtained are peculiar to the respirators I have and are not general ones. At any rate, at the present time, I am examining respirators which are pre- and post-1966. Our results indicate that there are functional differences between pre- and post-1966 respirators in several areas. Some of the comparisons I have made between old and new respirators include: determination of maximum rate, internal resistance, volume output, internal and external operating temperatures; determination of passive and volume output stability over a 12-hour period; comparison of output of old and new respirators against an identical resistance, stroke to stroke variability, and needle hysteresis. Perhaps some of the current confusion in results from different laboratories are due to the use of different respirators which have been assumed to be equivalent!

I believe that the experiments Brener reported at the present convention utilized respirator serial number 322, received in 1967 (personal communication). Another one of his respirators, 293, was received in 1966. Which pump did he use in the experiments in which he successfully trained rats to increase or decrease heart rate (Hothersall and Brener 1969)? Has he ever compared the functioning of pump number 322 against 293? Which of these or other pumps did he use for each of his other reported experiments?

What I would like to do in this section is to state the functional differences between the old and new respirators, point out their significance and conclude with relevant results regarding the issue in question.

There were leakage problems in the old pumps. Presumably, this would not affect respiration of the rat if the leakage occurred before passing through the pressure sensing system; however, if leakage occurred afterward, one might be respirating the *S* while reading a higher false pressure. Since I no longer have the original respirators in my possession I cannot state what was likely the case in 1965. In any case, I doubt that those old respirators are still in action or that they have been updated or repaired.

Prolonged use of a single pump, operation of several pumps in close proximity and/or poor ventilation, all contribute to an abnormal build-up of operating temperature in the pumps. This is a very important factor since the housing cabinet does not have any forced ventilation; consequently, at a higher temperature the percent of oxygen per unit volume of inspired air is decreased. This physical factor is significant at the levels of temperature reached by the respirators. For example, we have observed, under the preceding conditions, a buildup of temperature up to 125°F in an ambient temperature of 76°F. I was told by the company that this was not an unusual temperature for the pumps to reach!

Internal resistance of the pump, as indicated by a needle deflection even when the respirator's inspiration and expiration valves are left completely open, is rather critical since internal resistance would have to be subtracted from the peak pressure reading in the old respirators in order to obtain a corrected value. With the volume output set on maximum we have observed internal resistance readings as high as $7 cmH_2O$ in the old pumps. New pumps do not have this error. Consequently, it is possible, although I do not believe highly likely, that in past years, although I was respirating rats at what I read as $20 cmH_2O$ water pressure, it was in fact 13 to 15. I would like to note here that when using the older pumps it was often necessary to set the volume adjustment to maximum.

Needle hysteresis, especially over prolonged usage, can amount to 5 to 10% of full scale, depending on when the system was lubricated and the rate at which the pump is operated. Incidentally, in all these years, no investigator has ever mentioned lubricating the system. In general, hysteresis is a relatively negligible error amounting to no more than 1 or 2 cm of water pressure. However, during the period 1965 to 1969, each respirator saw an enormous amount of activity. Combined with other errors, hysteresis could contribute to misinformation. We have experimentally determined the extent of hysteresis in our pumps using the respirator needle to break different photoelectric beams set at different pressure levels, while direct pressure readings were recorded simultaneously. We did not use a rat, but used a clamp on the inspiration tube to obtain a constant resistance. We then left the pump on for several hours (up to 12 hours).

Perhaps the most critical difference between the old and new respirators is their volume output per cycle against a given resistance. Figure 14.1 presents a polygraph record comparing one old and three new respirators. The system was calibrated so that all four channels had the same amplification. All of the pumps were run at $15 cmH_2O$

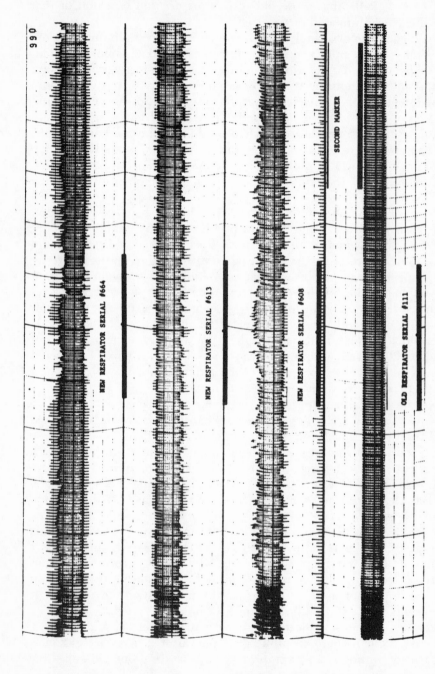

990

NEW RESPIRATOR SERIAL #664

NEW RESPIRATOR SERIAL #613

NEW RESPIRATOR SERIAL #608

SECOND MARKER

OLD RESPIRATOR SERIAL #111

FIGURE 14.1 Stroke-by-stroke variability of output of old and new respirators against a fixed resistance at equal amplification.

pressure. It is apparent that the old respirators were more reliable. In addition, it is equally clear, from the recorded excursions, that the old respirator when set at 15 cmH_2O pressure delivered less output per stroke. To systematically investigate this operating characteristic, we calibrated the polygraph so that an excursion of 15 mm of deflection represented 15cm of water pressure. This was done using a new respirator; and, we then substituted an old respirator in its place. We have observed that the stroke-to-stroke variability of the new respirators we have can vary as much as 50%. For example, we found that when we adjusted the pump to deliver 15 cm of water pressure, the deflection on the polygraph was only 10 or 11 mm.

The importance of an accurate and reliable stroke volume is critical. A variable output may average what you set the pump for; however, its variability would make instrumental learning very difficult, if not impossible. Discriminative learning would be especially difficult. For example, imagine an animal trying to increase its heart rate on a particular trial when the respirator is delivering 50% less tidal volume per stroke.

I am currently in the process of replicating my original study (Miller and DiCara 1967), using a permanently indwelling tracheal tube to assure each animal of exactly the same volume of air per stroke. We have also abandoned the old respirators; we now use a fixed volume small animal pump that has a higher ceiling than 70 cpm as well as more flexibility in regard to adding pure O_2 or CO_2 to inspired air.

In addition to each of the above variables, both old and new respirators have poorly ventilated housing cabinets, with rather narrow ventilation slits communicating to the ambient atmosphere. As was mentioned earlier, this is especially important since the expiration valve empties into the housing chamber, and there is no forced ventilation in these models. Consequently, the location of the respirator with respect to air currents in the room, walls, other heat producing equipment, and distance from the subject can all have effects on the buildup of temperature and carbon dioxide in the housing cabinet. There is little doubt in my mind that many of the difficulties encountered are due to uncontrolled differential rebreathing of previously expired air loaded with CO_2. If this is true, it could help explain the continued discrepancy between laboratories regarding initial heart rate in the otherwise undisturbed curarized rat. For that matter, it might also help explain the discrepancy between the heart rates of rats obtained in earlier experiments conducted in this laboratory with ones obtained in recent years—415 (Miller and DiCara 1967) versus 460 (Pappas, DiCara, and Miller 1972b).

Before moving on, I would like to comment on Hahn's suggestion to reexamine previous heart rate learning experiments in the light of the hypothesis that "uncontrolled variables were artifactually enhancing the results" (see Chapter 15). In order to comment on this position, I have to backtrack a bit. In our early experiments, we found and were amazed at the stability of the curarized rat's heart rate. In 1967, Miller and I reported that: "At the beginning of training the standard deviation of the heart rates of individual S's measured over 5 minutes, averaged only 2 bpm (or only 0.5%) for both groups" (Miller and DiCara 1967).

In these experiments, heart rate was determined by measuring heart rate over five consecutive 1-minute periods. Although the mean and standard deviation of heart rate during this 5-minute period was highly regular, during any 5-second period within this 5-minute period large deviations were obvious. Indeed, if this were not the case, it would be almost impossible to train heart rate increases or decreases, since the criterion steps were in 2% jumps. Although heart rate as measured in this manner was very stable, it most certainly was not "locked in" in the sense that Brener, Black, and Hahn (see Chapters 12, 13 and 15) use the term; that is, an invariant unresponsive tachycardia. Furthermore, it cannot be taken as evidence of a non-homeostatic preparation since temperature and peripheral vasomotor tone remained normal throughout the curarization period, responses which would clearly indicate an atypical physiologic condition.

In continuing his line of reasoning, Hahn states that the death of three S's in our experiment is "a fact which speaks for itself as regards the physiological condition of the animal" (see Chapter 15). However, contrary to the clinical profile of death from hypoventilation, the rats died of what is termed "sudden death," presumably due to massive vagal inhibition. In fact, it was impossible to duplicate the symptoms of these rats' last few minutes of life even by direct manipulation of respiration parameters for an hour.

CONCLUDING REMARKS

In view of space limitations, I have not addressed myself to a host of extremely important topics which deserve intensive discussion such as: (1) The somatic-visceral, specifity and mediation issues which clearly are unresolved; for example, heart rate learning is independent of intestinal learning (Miller and Banuazizi 1968); and, although the p-r interval can be singled out for training (Fields 1970b), the results of heart rate training have been shown to have profound effects on the animal's behavior and physiology (DiCara and Weiss 1969; DiCara and Stone 1970). Just how can visceral training be so highly specific yet be shown to have such diffuse effects? (2) The importance and value of the curarized preparation, despite its shortcomings, to investigate what Black (Chapter 12) has termed "response strategies," as well as to help us understand in just what ways the organism can "uncouple" the normally coordinated somatic-visceral mechanisms, (3) The use of cardiovascular responses as indices of psychological function; for example, Hahn and his associates have shown that stimulation of the vagal nerve during conditioned emotional response (CER) training inhibits the interference of fear conditioning on subsequent avoidance learning—that is, vagal stimulation is incompatible with the development of fear. (4) The role of visceral learning in investigating critical periods. Although our working definition of a critical period is overly simplistic, the results of a recent experiment (Pappas, DiCara, and Miller 1972b) clearly indicate that if a critical period does exist, it is certainly not at the 30-day mark for rats. (5) The role that visceral learning may play in the etiology of psychosomatic symptoms. We may find that individuals with certain autonomic profiles are more or less susceptible to certain diseases. (6) The evidence of human visceral learning while under curare, i.e., the experiment reported by Lapides, Sweet, and Lewis (1957). In general, see Miller (Chapter 16) for his excellent presentation of this work, as well as a discussion of placebo effects, interceptive perception, and the possible role of hypnosis in visceral learning. (7) The use of instrumental learning techniques to study the effect of higher central mechanisms on visceral functions. Despite little direct cortical representation of the viscera, neodecorticate rats cannot learn visceral responses (DiCara, Braun, and Pappas 1970). These results have obvious implications for the concept of the unity of the learning process, since the same rats could be classically conditioned. (8) The application of operant conditioning techniques to the treatment and, possibly, prevention of certain psychosomatic symptoms.

The preceding list is not exhaustive. Many other important issues could be listed. However, before it is possible to make efficient headway in any of the above areas, it will be necessary to demonstrate visceral learning, consistently and under a wide variety of conditions. I hope that this conference has served as a stimulus and that—in the ensuing solution of the difficulties that Brener (Chapter 13), Hahn (Chapter 15), and Miller and Dworkin (Chapter 16) have discussed—we will all advance toward the goal of being able to obtain learned visceral changes, and will understand the conditions that are essential for obtaining them.

In regard to the future, there is no doubt that clarification of the mechanisms of visceral learning and the sequential factors of how one learns to control his heart rate will help the therapeutic work. This area seems to have attracted the most interest and in some ways presents the most problems. The current inability to replicate the animal work has had a significant negative effect on the human work. Just why this is so is unclear; perhaps it is a crutch phenomena. That is, the scientists working in the human area are leaning on the animal work for encouragement until they can develop their own techniques and procedures. While this attitude is understandable, especially when working in a new field, there is no a priori reason why investigators interested in the potential of the therapeutic and preventative aspects of visceral learning should wait until the animal work has been totally spelled out. Indeed, many clinicians appear to be moving ahead, in parallel with the animal experimenters and with considerable success (see Chapter 23, Engel).

My own work, up to the present, has been conducted exclusively with rats. It is quite possible that the best procedures for rats are not the best ones for humans. The differences in specie go beyond obvious differences; they extend to the very nature of the innervation, central representation, and control of the cardiovascular system itself.

As one might imagine, I encourage research on normal humans, as well as "autonomic athletes." I believe that this would, so to speak, put the human research on its own feet, and perhaps would tend to mellow the refractory stance that some medical scientists and clinicians have assumed in regard to the area—often equating it with faith healing, parapsychology, and so forth. Finally, sick people are, by definition, different; it may turn out that they are so different we may eventually have to take therapeutic "measurements" and fit each individual with a procedure, much as a tailor does a customer for a suit.

As has been pointed out by several participants, the need for accurate publicity cannot be overemphasized. Unfortunately, if one looks back in time, these warnings are always made after the fact. Science is a human activity, and, as humans, we all seek recognition for our work. However, in this instance, heartbreaking letters testify to the false hope that has been aroused. In addition, this unwarranted publicity tends to encourage poorly trained and unqualified individuals to submit grant proposals in the hope of getting some easy money. This behavior tends to lend credence to the belief of certain medical authorities that biofeedback is populated by basically incompetent researchers. Because of each of these reasons, I think that, to the extent to which it is humanly possible, we should continually endeavor to correct the erroneous and gross over-publicity that this work has received.

15

WILLIAM W. HAHN

The Learning of Autonomic Responses by Curarized Animals

Since Trowill's (1967) innovative study and the dramatic impact of the more impressive sequelae (Miller and DiCara 1967; DiCara and Miller 1968a-d; Miller and Banuazizi 1968), the phenomenon of autonomic instrumental conditioning has been recognized as an event of major theoretical and practical significance. Most of these studies were carried out with curarized rats as subjects (Ss) and Heart Rate (HR) was the response manipulated. Despite the fact that we were able to replicate the principal results of the HR conditioning study in one instance using positive brain stimulation (+ESB) (Slaughter, Hahn, and Rinaldi 1970), we had no success whatsoever in a 12-month attempt to condition HR in curarized animals using avoidance conditioning with tail shock, and we have learned at this conference that others have also experienced considerable difficulty in attempting to establish instrumentally conditioned HR changes in curarized animals. Because of the potential usefulness of such conditioning and because of the flurry of experimental attempts to demonstrate and extend these findings it is important to carefully reassess the studies that have been conducted. This reassessment will examine two principal factors involved in this issue: the effects of curare on the HR response to vagal stimulation, and the possible contamination of previously published results by factors other than operant contingencies.

Throughout the course of our investigations with curare we have

These studies reported here were supported in part by NIMH research grant MH 20180-01.

observed anomalous unconditioned HR reactions in curarized Ss (Hahn, Slaughter, and Rinaldi 1969). We first cautioned against the inadvertent attainment of excessively stable HR which appeared to be "locked in" and unresponsive to stimuli in a technical note (Hahn 1970), and reported on paradoxical HR changes which we hypothesized were due to altered cardiac reactivity produced by curare in a study on the classical conditioning of HR in curarized rats (Hahn and Slaughter 1970). We became even more concerned about the effects of curare upon learning that in dogs it was capable of producing a blocking of the vagus at relatively low dosages, and a blocking of sympathetic accelerator nerves at higher dosages (Black 1967b; Guyton and Reeder 1950); and that it had been found to produce a large decrease in lung compliance (Safar and Bachman 1956; Maisson 1957), and to elicite a considerable release of histamine upon injection (Koelle 1970).

It became apparent to us at this point that it would be useful to systematically examine the unconditional HR reactions of curarized rats to several stimuli, in order to know what the "baseline" reactivity was for the various conditioned stimuli (CSs) and unconditioned stimuli (UCSs) employed in instrumental and classical conditioning studies, and to explore various physiological parameters that might elucidate the sources of the altered HR reactivity. A major problem faced in interpreting available data was the conflict between the reports of "complete" vagal block produced by moderate dosages of curare, and the repeated reports of "successful" conditioning of HR decreases in deeply curarized animals. Although it might be possible that an organism with a nonfunctional vagus could produce some HR deceleration through decrease in sympathetic tone, it is difficult to conceive of decelerations specific to a discriminative stimulus, total decelerations of as much as 80 bpm, and "superior" HR conditioning occurring without the participation of the vagus nerve.

If there were a significant degree of vagal blocking occurring, one might expect the increased HR to be larger than decreases in studies using bidirectional shaping. One might also expect studies in which higher dosages were used to show more of this effect as the amount of vagal blocking was reported to increase with increasing dosages of curare (Black 1967b). To attempt to assess those possibilities, and also, in an effort to compare the results using different species and routes of administration of curare, we assembled the summary of studies shown in Table 15.1. It can be seen that not only are decreases in HR readily obtained in curarized animals, but that in a number of studies it appears to be easier to obtain a HR decrease than an increase. It is very difficult to assess pharmacological effects across different species and routes of administration; however, it can be seen that in most of the work using rats as Ss the dosage has been an initial intraperitoneal injection of 2.0 to 3.6 mg/kg of body weight often followed by additional injections of .5 to 1.0 mg/kg every hour. The levels used for intravenous (i.v.) administration of larger animals is about .6 mg/kg per hour. One crude way to compare the relative strength of these is by noting the length of time needed for the return of voluntary muscular activity and unassisted respiration. For adult humans, when curare is used as an adjunct to general anesthesia, a usual recommended dose of .3 mg/kg wears off in approximately 20 minutes. Recovery rates are not reported in detail in the studies using i.v. injections in dogs, but in albino rats an initial i.p. injection of 1.2 mg/kg will cause muscular relaxation to a level that requires artificial respiration with recovery in 1 to 2 hours. An injection of 3.0 mg/kg will keep an animal in very deep relaxation for 2 to 4 hours, and, if additional supplementary injections of 1.0 mg/kg every hour are given, the animal can be maintained in a deeply curarized condition for 3 to 4 hours and will require an additional 2 hours for recovery after termination of the injections. Thus, if one accepts these rough comparisons, the animals used in most of the autonomic conditioning work are definitely deeply curarized, and it would seem that they must be in at least as deeply curarized a state as cats that received approximately .6 mg/kg i.v. and were reported to show "100% blocking" of vagal activity at this dosage (Guyton and Reeder 1950).

We undertook a study to determine the presence of vagal blocking in rats injected with 3.0 mg/kg curare. If a large degree of blocking were found in a high percentage of animals, then some alternative explanations must be sought for the "successful" operantly conditioned HR decreases which were vagally produced, according to one report in which a cardiovascular specialist examined the EKGs (Miller and DiCara 1967). If vagal blocking does not occur to the degree expected from previous studies then we may be faced with a species difference or other methodological differences between our studies and those of previous investigators.

Our initial studies were run with animals implanted with a chronic electrode for stimulation of the vagus. After obtaining a baseline response of at least −60 bpm we injected with 3.0 mg/kg curare. One-half hour was allowed for respiratory adjustments and stabilization of HR and then 36 trials were administered at preset intervals of 30, 120, or 150 seconds. Of the eight animals stimulated under these conditions, an increase of stimulating voltage was needed for each S in order to obtain the same level of HR response that had been obtained prior to curarization; the average increase for the group was 3.27 times the pre-curare voltage. We concluded at the time that this was evidence for the occurrence of partial vagal blocking induced by curare. However, this conclusion was tentatively accepted. We were aware that

TABLE 15.1 *Survey of Some Studies in Which Changes in Heart Rate are Produced in Curarized Subjects*

Study	Dosage	Route	Species	Type of Study	Results
Trowill 1967	1.2 mg/kg/hr	IP	Rat	Instrumental conditioning of HR changes with +ESB	15 of 19 increased HR average of 18 bpm 15 of 17 decreased HR average of 19 bpm
Miller & DiCara 1967	Initial Dose of 3.6 mg/kg	IP	Rat	Instrumental conditioning of HR changes with ESB	12 Ss increased HR average of 88 bpm 11 Ss decreased HR average of 84 bpm
Miller & Banuazizi 1968	Initial Dose 3.0 mg/kg 1 mg/kg each hr thereafter	IP	Rat	Instrumental conditioning of HR changes with ESB	3 Ss increased HR average of about 35 bpm 3 Ss decreased HR average of about 50 bpm
DiCara & Miller 1969	Initial Dose 3 mg/kg & 1 mg/kg/hr infusion subsequently	IP	Rat	Instrumental conditioning of HR changes with ESB	7 Ss transferred from noncurarized training a decrease average of 37 bpm and 7 Ss transferred increase of 33 bpm (failure to get "additional learning" of HR response under curare)
DiCara & Miller 1968d		IP	Rat	Avoidance condition of HR	Transfer from curarized to noncurarized state of 5% increase & 16% decrease, change enhanced to 11% increase & 22% decrease with additional training in noncurarized state.
DiCara & Weiss 1970	3 mg/kg	IP	Rat	Instrumental avoid condit. of HR	Decrease of 31 bpm 100% retained after 2 wks.; increase of 35 bpm declined to 13 bpm after 2 weeks

TABLE 15.1 Continued

Study	Dosage	Route	Species	Type of Study	Results
Hothersall & Brener 1969	1.8 mg/kg	IP	Rat	Instrumental changes of HR using ESB	Approximately a 25 bpm change in each direction in total of 12 Ss after 4 sessions of training.
Slaughter, Hahn, & Rinaldi 1971	3.0 mg/kg	IP	Rat	Instrumental changes of HR using ESB	15 of 15 Ss increased average of 58 bpm; 12 of 15 Ss decreased average of -37 bpm
Pappas, DiCara, & Miller 1972	3.0 mg/Kg plus 1.0 mg/kg/hr infused	IP	Rat	Fear retention of classically conditioned HR changes in normal & sympathectomized rats	No consistent conditioned HR changes observed, but reliable blood-pressure changes conditioned.
Safar & Bachman 1956	Different doses up to "many times" paralyzing dosage	Presumably IV	Dog	Study of distensibility of lungs & thorax after inject. of several muscle relaxants	Distensibility of lungs reduced 50-86% in 80% of subjects injected with curare.
Maisson 1957	1.2 mg/Kg	Femoral vein injection	Dog chest	Changes in elastic properties of Lung compliance evaluated	Lung compliance decreases of 42-61% obtained in 15 dogs. Similar results produced by Histamine. After Pyribenzamine curare failed to produce this effect.
Guyton & Reeder 1950	.6 to 3.8 mg/Kg	Presumably IV	Dog	Effect on muscle & cardiac innervation	.3 mg/Kg produced total paralysis of gastrocnemius muscle; .4 mg/Kg paralysis respiratory muscles; .3-.6 mg/Kg produces blocking of vagus (100%) at .6; 3-7 mg/Kg needed to produce 90% inhib. of cardiac symp-accelerator nerves

TABLE 15.1 Continued

Study	Dosage	Route	Species	Type of Study	Results
Church, LoLordo, Overmier, Solomon, & Turner 1966	12 mg administered to 7-13 Kg dogs (about .9 mg/Kg)	Inj. into recurrent Tarsal vein in 2.6 mg injections	Dog	Study of conditioned effects of shock on HR	HR increased in response to shock and fell below baseline after shock response. Both responses were a function of duration and intensity of shock. HR deceleration was positively correlated with base rate.
Black 1967	.8 mg/Kg over 1½ hrs	Presumably IV ("inj. thru catheter")	Dog curare	Better increase HR conditioning under	Vagal block occurred in 3 out of 3 Ss at this dosage. Sympathetic block more variable.
Howard (Chap 18)	Rate of infusion "gradually increased" until complete muscular blockade obtained	Infusion into Femoral vein	Cat	Effects of curare in HR response to stimulation of the vagus	Large degree of vagal blocking obtained in 4 cats.
Smith, Brown, Toman, & Goodman 1947	500 units or about 744 mg administered	IV	Man	Large dosage of curare administered to Smith	No "cerebral effects"—i.e., no interference with pain reception, auditory reception, memory, etc., according to subjective report of Smith.

NOTE: To construct this Table it was at times necessary to estimate HR changes from graphs; data on the number of Ss showing changes in each direction were not always available; dosage has been translated from units to mg/Kg wherever possible; although in some studies total amount of curare injected is not reported.

generally damped HR responses can occur under curare due to some problems associated with the setting of respiratory parameters, and we were concerned that alterations in the effective voltage delivered by the chronic electrode might have occurred due to changes in the position of the subject. It seemed possible that placement of the subject in the curarization apparatus—where the head is elevated and stretched slightly forward—might have resulted in minimal contact between the electrode and the nerve. To reduce these doubts we determined to repeat the study using acute stimulation of the vagus and to take more detailed records of the physiological state of the organism.

For the acute stimulation studies we injected animals with 50 mg/kg Nembutal, exposed the cervical vagus, and administered a standard stimulus of 1 volt, 20 pps, 2 msec per pulse for 3 seconds. After obtaining three baseline responses to this stimulus the S was injected with 3.0 mg/kg curare, and an additional 10 trials at 1 per minute were administered 10 minutes following curare injection. The results of this study indicated that no vagal blocking occurred in a group of eight animals subjected to these procedures!

Baffled by these contradictory results we attempted to analyze the differences between the two studies. One of the most obvious differences was that Nembutal had been used in the second, but not in the first. A second relevant point was that a minimum of ½ hour delay was allowed between the injection of curare and the first stimulation in Study No. 1, while trials began almost immediately after curare injection in Study No. 2. At this point we began to entertain the hypothesis that an aberrant physiological state caused by improper setting of respiratory parameters might explain much of the "damped" HR responsiveness, which was interpreted as vagal blocking in our first study. We observed that a S that had received Nembutal was extremely easy to curarize and respirate without complications, while animals that had not received Nembutal invariably were difficult to stabilize following curare injection. In both studies we had rejected some animals because of unacceptable HR levels or responsiveness, and we had not kept careful record of this selection factor.

We conducted a third and final study with more rigidly standardized procedures and collection of data on baselevel HR, HR variability, and body temperature. Test stimuli were presented continuously for 1 hour after total curarization. The procedure and results of this study will be presented in some detail here, since it is our belief that these data reflect some basic and reliable characteristics of the HR response of curarized rats to acute vagal stimulation. Furthermore, some of the current confusion in this field may stem partly from incomplete reporting of certain facets of each study, and it might be useful if all investigators would present data on selection of Ss, baselevel HR, and variability and

body temperature of the animals used in curare studies since this information can serve as a check on the adequacy of the preparation.

THE RESPONSE OF CURARIZED RATS
TO ACUTE VAGAL STIMULATION

The animals used were Sprague-Dawley derived Simonsen albino male
rats all weighing between 400 and 500 gm. (We have indications that
the respiratory settings used in these studies may not be sufficient for
animals outside this weight range.) After injection with 50 mg/kg of
sodium pentothal (Nembutal), the cervical vagus was exposed and
placed carefully in the loop of two insulated stainless steel electrodes
placed 1.5 cm apart. The nerve and cavity were covered with mineral
oil, an insulating sheath of Silastic was placed around the nerve and
electrodes, and the animal was released from all restraints so that it
assumed a natural supine position with its ventral aspect exposed.
Several test stimuli were given to determine the Ss response to a 1 volt
20 pps 20 msec per pulse stimulus. As soon as baseline responses were
obtained each S was injected with an initial dose of 3.0 mg/kg curare.
Experimenter (E) waited until respiration had ceased and then placed
the respirator mask on the animal. Respiration was begun at a 1 to
1 inspiration:expiration (I:E) ratio, 70 breaths per minute, and a peak
pressure reading of 12 cmH_2O. The peak pressure was readjusted
whenever it varied by more than 1 cmH_2O from the preset level. The
S was then allowed to rest for 10 minutes to provide time for the curare
to be thoroughly absorbed; then the stimuli were presented again at
1-minute intervals for the next 60 minutes. Animals were given maintenance dosages of .10 cc of 50 mg/ml solution of Nembutal as needed
and .05 cc of a 3 mg/ml solution of curare 20 minutes and 40 minutes
after the initial curare injection. Throughout this phase, body temperature was recorded every 5 minutes, HR base level and response to
stimulation were recorded on every trial, and, on a few animals, a 1
ml sample of blood was drawn from the carotid artery at the end of
the series of trials.

Because some problems may have resulted from inadvertent selection of Ss in previous work, we kept a careful record of every animal
on which we even attempted to gather data. There were a total of 19
Ss attempted. Of these, one failed to achieve an adequate level of
anesthetization with the Nembutal, one was discarded because of a very
abnormal EKG, two had respiratory infections and developed mucus
blocking and had to be artifically respirated before curarization, two
did not produce an adequate baseline response to vagal stimulation,
two were discarded due to equipment problems, and one developed
respiratory problems about 50 minutes after curarization. Thus, of the

total of 19 animals attempted, 10 yielded unstable records. However, of the nine rejects, only one was given test trials under curare and then discarded. The results of this S for the first 40 trials differed in no substantial way from the averaged curves shown.

The results are shown in Figures 15.1 to 15.4. It can be seen in Figures 15.1 to 15.3 that body temperature, HR level, and HR variability do not show major changes in the post-curare period when compared to the pre-curare periods, although there is a steady decrease in the basal HR level and a slight decrease in body temperature which are probably the result of the problems associated with curare and positive pressure respiration detailed elsewhere (see Chapter 13, Brener, Eissenberg, and Middaugh). However, HR variability of 7 to 15 bpm is maintained throughout the session, and HR level and body temperature remain within a nominal range. The response to vagal stimulation remains at an average of 94.8 bpm over the entire 60 trials of the experiment (Figure 15.4). Heart rate response to vagal stimulation is evaluated by taking the lowest HR recorded during or immediately after the stimulus is applied if it is maintained for at least two beats; ordinarily this response slowly returns to baseline or slightly above baseline in 5 to 10 seconds following stimulation.

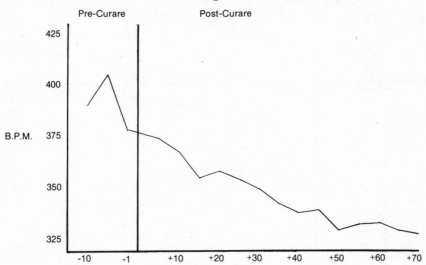

FIGURE 15.1. *Resting heart rate level prior to curare injection and for 70 minutes after curarization.*

While this is a decrease in response from the pre-curare baseline of −147 bpm, it still represents a marked and consistent response to vagal stimulation. It is important to know if this decrease represents a slight

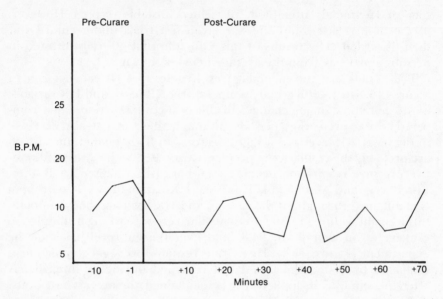

FIGURE 15.2. *Heart rate variability prior to curare injection and for 70 minutes after curarization.*

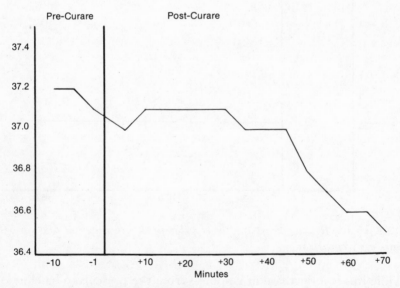

FIGURE 15.3. *Body temperature prior to curare injection and for 70 minutes after curarization.*

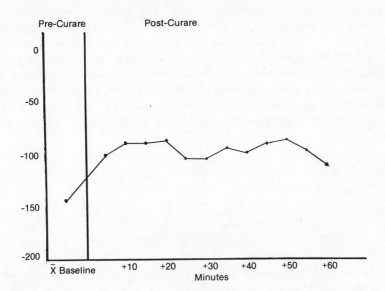

FIGURE 15.4. *Average response to vagal stimulation prior to curare injection and for 60 trials at 1-minute intervals beginning 10 minutes after curarization.*

damping of vagal response in all Ss or if a few Ss are showing marked vagal blocking, while the response of others is unaffected by the administration of curare. The data in Table 15.2 are presented to show the range of responses to vagal stimulation in the pre- and post-curare phases, and the relationship of this response to other potentially relevant measures. The "vagal blocking score" was obtained by taking the average cardiac deceleration of every fifth post-curare trial and dividing that figure by the average pre-curare response for each S. The scores are then arranged in increasing order of magnitude, thus ranking Ss in order of the degree of inhibition of vagal response (a score of .1 indicates a 90% loss of vagal response post-curare, etc.). For each S there is listed the average post-curare HR level and body temperature and the number of adjustments of peak pressure needed to maintain a peak inspiratory pressure of 12 cmH$_2$O. These data are presented in order to determine if these indices of adjustment of the animal might reflect systematic differences between high and low blockers that might, in part, explain the differences in vagal responding.

As can be seen from Table 15.2 there were no systematic differences in any of these scores, and, on the basis of these limited response measures, we would conclude that the demonstration in some Ss of a high degree of vagal inhibition is not simply due to a debilitated physiological state of those Ss. As a further check on this we computed correlation coefficients between the vagal blocking score and initial, average, and terminal temperature and HR measures for the group and found that none of these six correlations approached a significance level of P < .05. Only 3 of the 10 experimental animals showed a marked degree of vagal blocking—defined here as a 50% or larger decrease in response—and these Ss account for the 50 bpm difference in the total group's post-curare HR response. When the HR responses of the remaining seven animals are averaged, the post-curare response level is equal to slightly more than 100% of the pre-curare response level.

TABLE 15.2 *A comparison of vagal inhibition and other indices of physiological adjustment*

S#	*Vagal Blocking Score	Average Post-Curare HR Level (bpm)	Average Post-Curare Temperature (°c)	Total Number Peak Pressure Respiration Adjustments Needed
17	.1	325	37.6	4
10	.3	357	36.4	3
18	.3	377	37.8	12
6	.6	335	37.3	7
3	.7	367	36.8	8
2	.8	368	37.5	4
16	.9	351	36.6	4
1	1.2	326	35.6	10
5	1.3	355	36.5	3
19	1.8	304	36.9	3
X =	.80	346.5	36.9	5.8

*Average Post-curare HR response to stimulation divided by average Pre-curare HR response.

There is clear evidence that vagal blocking is not a universal phenomenon in albino rats given large i.p. dosages of curare and adequately respirated. Three out of 10 Ss demonstrated a substantial degree of vagal blocking, while the remaining seven animals demonstrated a post-curare response level that was comparable to the pre-curare level.

In the second pilot study, when we began to get indications that vagal responding was continuing under curarization, we became concerned that our stimulus was too intense or too prolonged to enable the blocking to be demonstrated. To test for this we used lower levels of stimulation (.5 volts) for .5 seconds and still obtained responses. We injected atropine into three experimental Ss and in these animals the response was either eliminated or markedly reduced.

It is clear from Figures 15.1 and 15.3 that these Ss are not in an ideal physiological state. However, the lowest average body temperature is well above the danger level of 34°C cited by Brener, et al., Chapter 13, HR remains between 325 and 375 bpm, and HR variability is maintained at about 12 bpm throughout the session. The fact that continued vagal responding is obtained in spite of a condition of slight hypoventilation only strengthens the conclusion that vagal block is not a necessary concomitant of curarization. There is little doubt that we are dealing with a specific response to the stimulus; onset is immediate and dramatic—a 50 to 150 bpm decrease occurring within 1 second of onset of stimulation and returning to baseline within 5 to 10 seconds in nearly all cases. We are clearly not dealing with any sort of tonic decrease, or increased variability or other artifacts of that nature.

The question has been raised as to whether the Ss might be incompletely curarized. We did not obtain electromyogram (EMG) or electroencephalogram (EEG) recordings on these Ss as all are anesthetized with Nembutal, and, therefore, such recordings would not be terribly useful as an index of curarization. We know from extensive past experience that an i.p. injection of 3.0 mg/kg effectively and completely paralyzes a subject for periods of time considerably longer than those used in this study. The injections were all done by an experienced laboratory technician and—to guard against the possibility of a misplaced injection and the inadvertent running of a noncurarized S—E always waited until the S ceased all respiration movements before initially placing the face mask on the S. Again, at the end of the session, the face mask was removed and a check made for any reflexive respiratory movements to be certain that the effects of curare had not worn off. By these indicators, at least, Ss were completely curarized; whether they were as deeply curarized as the Ss in the Black (1967b) and Howard et al. studies (see Chapter 18) is another matter.

It is possible that our stimulation of the intact vagus produced central effects through vagal afferent influences which affected the HR decrease by some nonvagal means. This seems unlikely but we are in the process of stimulating the severed vagus to check on this possibility.

If we add together the results of all animals receiving acute vagal stimulation under 3.0 mg/kg of curare we have a total of 18 animals run for a total of 680 trials and showing an average decrease in HR of more than 100 bpm. We believe the conclusion that vagal block is not a ubiquitous phenomenon in rats run under these conditions is justified. Blocking of the vagus *may* occur in some animals; but, if so, a substantial degree of blocking apparently occurs in less than 50% of an unselected population of rats given this amount of intraperitoneally administered d-tubocurarine chloride.

To some extent these results are in contradiction to previous reports in the literature. Reports of vagal blocking in cat and dog may be found in Koelle (1970); Grob (1967); Black (1967b); Guyton and Reeder (1950); and Howard (see Chapter 18). The most obvious explanation for these differences is that there is a species difference; the rat showing less susceptibility to d-tubocurarine-produced ganglionic blocking than either cat or dog. However, it is also possible that differences in technique and level of curarization may account for the discrepant results. Perhaps i.v. administration of curare to the point of complete absence of EMG response will result in substantial vagal block in rat also. Nevertheless, the results of this report are important because of the demonstration that Ss receiving curarization procedures *like those used in the previous autonomic conditioning studies* do retain some degree of vagal control over HR.

STUDIES USING THE CURARIZED RAT

Reexamination of Some Published Studies

To demonstrate that vagal control of HR may be retained in curarized rats is only one small step in attempting to clarify the current paradoxical state of affairs. An alternative to the slow process of gathering new data on the complex issues surrounding curare is to scrutinize the published studies available, in an attempt to find some pattern or clue to help explain the highly variable results obtained. Table 15.1 was constructed to achieve an overview and to look at possible relationships among the major independent variables and the results obtained. One can also examine each study in detail, and, from the present perspective of slightly increased knowledge about the curarized rat, try to guess what factors may have been operating in these studies.

Space limitations do not permit an analysis of even a portion of the studies listed in Table 15.1. As an example of the kind of analysis that can be done, we can examine the first report of Miller and DiCara (1967) as a prototype of the studies in this area. In that investigation there are several indications that the Ss were in an atypical and non-homeostatic cardiovascular state. The authors state: "throughout this experiment the heart rates were remarkably regular. At the beginning of training the standard deviations of the heart rates of individual Ss measured over 5 minutes averaged 2 bpm (or only .5%) for both groups." (Miller and DiCara 1967, p. 15) As we have pointed out (Hahn 1970), this can be regarded as a sign of hyperventilation and is usually associated with an unreactive cardiac system—a phenomenon we referred to as a "locked in" HR pattern. This also undoubtedly reflects the same phenomenon that Brener refers to as "profound invariant tachycardia" which he observed when using the same respiratory parameters and which resulted in animals that were "unresponsive to peripheral stimulation" (see Chapter 13). There is further corroborative evidence that these animals were in this pathophysiological state of hyporeactivity, since the authors note that a strong (3 ma) shock to the tail elicited less than a 10% increase in HR in the curarized rat (Miller and DiCara 1967, p. 17). It was also noted in the Miller and DiCara study that three animals in the group rewarded for slow HRs died during the experiment—a fact which speaks for itself regarding the physiological condition of the animals. It is common in our experience to observe decreases in HR as the time under curare progresses. Unless respiratory parameters are changed to correct this baseline shift, the S will expire in 30 to 60 minutes following this decline. One final difficulty is the fact that Ss in the group to be shaped to a HR increase had a mean resting HR prior to training of 422 bpm, while those shaped to have lower HR started trials at 400 bpm. Despite the authors' attempt to control for biased assignment of Ss, this rather large difference suggests that Ss assigned to an increase group may already have been tending toward tachycardia, while those in the decrease group may have been progressing in the opposite direction.

At this point it is impossible to say just exactly how the large and reliable differences were obtained, but it can be seen that most of these subjects were probably in very poor condition regarding their cardiovascular and general physiological state. If this is true, then either the autonomic shaping procedures are so potent that they were effective in spite of the existing conditions, or the results reflect "chance" and other uncontrolled variables that somehow systematically influenced the results.

Through most of the studies in this series on autonomic conditioning the same respiratory parameters and techniques were used, and the problems generated by the condition this induces in the animal apply also to these subsequent studies. In one recent study curarized animals have a mean HR level of about 460 bpm and an absence of significant conditioned HR responses (Pappas, DiCara, and Miller 1972a). The hypothesis that uncontrolled variables were artifactually enhancing the results is further strengthened by reports that "superior" HR conditioning occurs in curarized as compared to noncurarized rats (DiCara and Miller 1968d); by much smaller changes found by other experimenters even when virtually identical methodology is used (Hothersall and Brener 1969; Slaughter, Hahn, and Rinaldi 1970); and by recent difficulties in replicating the original results (Miller and Dworkin, Chapter 16).

Further analysis of existing literature reveals some additional perplexing problems; for example, both Trowill (1967) and Brener and his colleagues (Chapter 13) have reported changes in control Ss that are in a direction opposite to that produced in an experimental group or that predicted by the "law of effect." Brener and his co-workers appear to have demonstrated that prior activity or immobility training can facilitate later HR shaping under curare. But it is intriguing that animals that failed to learn the previous avoidance task showed HR changes nearly as large and in a direction opposite to that which would be produced by the operant contingencies.

In Trowill's study, rats rewarded for an increase in HR increased only about 6 bpm, while their yoked-controls showed a decrease of −20.4 bpm. It seems quite possible that such results reflect, in part, an unconditional HR response to the stimuli used. In Brener's study, where tail shock was used, the predominant response was a HR increase (nearly 50 bpm compared to a decrease of only 12 bpm), while in Trowill's study, where +ESB was used, the predominant trend was a decrease in HR. *If* there are systematic and reliable changes produced in yoked-control animals, the investigation of the source of these changes may shed considerable light on the "instrumentally learned" HR responses produced in other *S*s.[1] Brener's demonstration of a link between previously learned skeletal muscle responses and direction of the HR response conditionable under curare provides an interesting lead for subsequent studies in this area. Perhaps an unravelling of the complexities of curarization and investigations of the interactions between unconditional HR response and centrally-linked coping attempts will help resolve some of these perplexities.

The Control Group Problem

When the series of studies on autonomic conditioning began, it was generally thought that the use of curare was a considerable, even critical, asset in answering the "muscular mediation" problem, and the use of bidirectional shaping and a discriminative stimulus (in some cases) were thought to be adequate control for the most obvious noncontingent factors. It now would seem that curare may have introduced more problems than it solved, and part of its contribution is to weaken our confidence in the adequacy of the controls used.

To be more specific, we now know of a variety of factors associated with the curarization procedures (artificial respiration, etc.) which can cause HR to regularly increase or decrease; and there are evidently a number of important systemic physiological changes which occur as a result of curare injection which can also produce HR increases and decreases. Perhaps, had we known what a delicate preparation it is, there would have been even greater care taken to demonstrate that the reward contingency was the major determinant of response change.

To increase our confidence in this phenomenon we now need to learn more about the unconditional effects of the stimuli used on HR of the curarized rat and to find out how this interacts with increase or decrease shaping. We need to find out if a learned response will vary with the schedule of rewards and if it will demonstrate extinction, and we need to use yoked-control groups to illustrate that it is not merely the effects of curarization and unconditional HR responses which are producing the effects observed.[2] Although some studies have attempted some of these procedures, the majority of these issues have not been systematically studied, and, as noted above, some attempts at greater precision—such as the use of yoked-controls—have yielded data that are not very convincing.

The criticisms which have been indicated here, and to whatever extent the reader chooses to generalize them to other studies, are intended to apply *only* to instrumental HR conditioning studies using curarized rats. This writer has no expertise or experience in some of the other autonomic responses that have been conditioned and, in the absence of such experience, does not wish to appraise studies involving intestinal contractions or vascular responses, or those experiments which have used animals other than albino rats as the experimental subjects of study.

SUMMARY

The effects that have been attributed to operant conditioning of HR responses in the curarized rat *may* not be due strictly to operant conditioning effects. The phenomenon may well be a valid one: Some success has been obtained by many different investigators and in several different laboratories. There are no convincing logical reasons why it should not be possible to obtain operant control over autonomic responses and the data presented above indicate that vagal control of HR responsiveness *is* retained in deeply curarized rats. What appears to be needed is further investigation of the physiological effects of curare, especially on cardiovascular responsiveness, and additional control procedures which will demonstrate that the operant contingency is the primary factor responsible for the changes produced. Now that we are gaining some much needed information about the problems of curarization perhaps we can return to the operant conditioning attempts, exercise the needed controls, and determine in a more convincing fashion the strength and specificity of the operant control over autonomic processes.

NOTES

1. The author is indebted to Dr. Jay Trowill for pointing out the potential significance of these responses.

2. The author's awareness of this problem was enhanced by the remarks of Dr. Neil Schneiderman who emphasized the importance of this issue at the conference.

16

NEAL E. MILLER and BARRY R. DWORKIN

Visceral Learning: Recent Difficulties with Curarized Rats and Significant Problems for Human Research

First let me say that I can join the ranks of those of you who are having problems with the technique of respirating rats paralyzed by curare and difficulties in replicating earlier results from my laboratory. Then I want to make some brief comments on a variety of topics: some neglected evidence for human visceral learning, the danger of over-optimistic publicity, the need to control for placebo effects in studies aimed at therapeutic use of visceral learning, interactions between the skeletal and autonomic nervous systems, and a number of different high-priority problems in the area of visceral learning.

You will remember that my earlier attempts to secure instrumental learning of visceral responses encountered a considerable variety of difficulties (Miller 1966a). Eventually, Carmona and I succeeded in teaching one group of thirsty dogs, during 40 days of training, to salivate more to get water and another group to salivate less to get it (Miller and Carmona 1967). The dogs trained to increase salivation tended to have an aroused, fast, low-voltage electroencephalogram (EEG), while those trained to decrease tended to have a nonaroused, slow, high-voltage EEG. Carmona (1967) also found that the EEG or normal

This paper is written in the first person singular, the style in which it was presented by the senior author at the symposium. The junior author has been added to give recognition to his ideas and to the enormous amount of hard and frustrating work involved in the attempts to replicate the earlier work on cardiac learning by curarized rats and to improve the technique. The unpublished work described here as performed in the author's laboratory was supported by USPHS grants MH 13189, MH 19183, and GM 01789.

cats and curarized rats could be changed by instrumental learning (Miller 1966b, 1969). Concurrently, Trowill (1967) trained highly reliable increases or decreases in the heart rate of rats paralyzed by curare, but these changes were relatively small, averaging only 5%. Subsequently, by using the procedure of shaping to reward progressively larger changes, both DiCara and Banuazizi were able to produce considerably greater increases and decreases in heart rate (Miller and DiCara 1967; Miller and Banuazizi 1968). Everything was going very smoothly and Dr. Leo DiCara and other colleagues with me forged ahead with a considerable variety of studies (Miller 1969).

DIFFICULTIES IN REPLICATION

But more recently, in trying to extend some of these studies in a new direction, Barry Dworkin and I have run into difficulties in getting any learned changes in heart rate. At first we thought that these difficulties were a function of the new problem we were studying, but eventually we decided to check our technique by trying to replicate an earlier study in which changes in heart rate were rewarded by avoiding or escaping electric shocks (DiCara and Miller 1968a). After considerable time without success in this venture, Dworkin looked back at other studies of heart rate in our laboratory and noticed the progressive downward trend illustrated in Figure 16.1. We were and are hovering near the zero mark to be predicted from the extrapolation of this trend. It was encouraging, however, to note that two studies from other laboratories represented here had reported effects that statistically were highly reliable and of the same general magnitude secured in our laboratory at the same period of time.

Although greatly puzzled and disappointed, we thought that in learning what was wrong and how to correct it we might discover something that would help us to improve human visceral learning and perhaps would even have therapeutic value. Thus, our difficulties could turn out to be a disguised opportunity if we only had the wit to comprehend what they were telling us.

Along with the failure to repeat our earlier results was the fact that the initial heart rate of rats respirated under apparently comparable conditions was from 10 to 20% higher and apparently much less variable, seeming to be "locked in" at the higher rate. If rats were simply anesthetized, their heart rates seemed nearer the initial baseline rates of those in the earlier experiments. Artificial respiration produced an increase in heart rate, and the curare a second increase. Finally, the rats seemed to go under curare faster than they had and to stay under less long.

While we were discovering these difficulties, DiCara was deeply

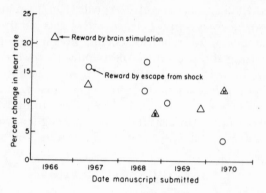

FIGURE 16.1. *Progressive decline in learned heart rate changes during five years. Experiments were performed under approximately similar conditions in the senior author's laboratory, except for point B from data by Hothersall and Brener (1969) and point H from data by Slaughter, Hahn, and Rinaldi (1970). For each experiment, increases and decreases were converted into percent changes and then averaged. (From Miller, Seminars in Psychiatry, 1972, 4, p. 247; by permission of Grune & Stratton, Inc.)*

involved in his move to Michigan. He had been giving us considerable advice, and we finally got him in to give a demonstration during one of his trips back to New York. To his amazement, he found that both of the rats that he tried had far too fast and unvarying initial heart rates under curare. The recording was so different from what he had been used to that he did not think it was worthwhile to train either of them. As we were sitting around puzzling about what possibly could be different, the thought finally occurred that the injections of Xylocaine that he had used earlier to relieve possible pain at the site of the electrodes had been omitted in the rush of the occasion. When these injections were given, the heart rate came down to a more reasonable level. The problem seemed to be solved, but there was not enough time to train the rat before DiCara was scheduled to leave. Subsequent tests showed that the reduction in the heart rate was from a general pharmacological effect of the Xylocaine rather than from a relief in any pain. For a brief time we had delightful thoughts that we might have discovered a relatively innocuous drug that might greatly facilitate both animal and human visceral learning. But we soon found that Xylocaine was not the answer we were looking for. In fact, the gradual wearing off of its effect seemed to produce an undesirable upward drift in the baseline heart rate, so we abandoned it as a distraction.

After varying many other parameters without success, we thought that perhaps something peculiar had happened to the strain of rats

(Charles River Sprague-Dawley) that we were using. So we tried a large, calm, old Hormone Assay rat that happened to be available; he seemed to learn. Excitedly, we sent in an order for more Hormone Assay rats. They were somewhat smaller, more excitable, had higher heart rates under curare, and did not learn. So we thought of the calmest rats that we know about: hypophysectomized ones. In order to avoid any unconscious bias, we always made all of the respirator adjustments first, then flipped a coin to see whether the rat was going to be trained to increase or decrease, and did not touch any adjustment after that. The first two hypophysectomized rats happened to be rewarded for decreases. Their unconditioned response to electric shock was a slight increase in heart rate. In spite of this, both of them acquired beautiful decreases in heart rate quite specific to the positive stimulus. But when subsequent tosses of the coin dictated rewarding increases, the rats showed exactly the same decreases. Apparently, hypophysectomy greatly facilitates either pseudo-conditioning or a decreased heart rate to classically conditioned fear—a problem we hope to investigate subsequently.

We have explored many other possibilities. The problem is that, whereas there often are millions of ways of doing something wrong, there may be only one or two ways of doing it right. Thus, one positive result can yield vastly more information than many negative ones. But, if one does not understand exactly what the right combination of circumstances was that led to the positive result, there may be a distressingly large number of parameters to canvass before one gets back on the right track again. Furthermore, when one has an effect, it is easy to see whether varying a given parameter—for example, increasing the rate of respiration—increases the desired effect, decreases it, or leaves it unchanged. But when one is not getting any effect, one does not have such guidance; one does not know whether one is not varying the parameter enough in the right direction, or is varying it in the wrong direction, or whether the parameter is a relatively irrelevant one. I have fervently wished that, when things were going well, we had taken much more time to specify all of the conditions in more accurate detail. But then, of course, one does not necessarily know which of the myriad details are crucial until something goes wrong. I also have wished that I had spent much more time watching and participating in each experiment, as had been my custom when I was younger. If I had done this then, I might possibly have acquired some better clues as to what might be wrong now.

Faced with the foregoing situation, one searches for strategies that will reduce the enormous amount of slow trial-and-error. Since one of the changes that occurred along with the disappearance of visceral learning was an increase in the initial heart rate, a considerable amount

316 ANIMAL OPERANT CONDITIONING

of our work has been directed to avoiding this increase in the curarized rat. While we cannot be certain that this increase is the cause of the difficulty, at least we can tell whether a specific change in our procedures is changing the initial heart rate in the correct direction.

Another of our strategies has been to try to produce normal blood gases in the rat—another effect that we can measure. Of course, this strategy will be wrong if it turns out that some abnormal condition of blood gases is essential to produce an anti-homeostatic effect favorable to visceral learning.

Back when I originally started this work, Dr. John Lacey told me that I must monitor the pCO_2 of the expired air during artificial respiration. So I scraped up the funds to buy a Beckman gas analyzer, only to find that I could not make it work reliably with the small volume of air from rats respirated with a mask. I am encouraged at this meeting to learn that I am not alone in failing to solve that difficulty. Highly motivated to find out what is happening to respiration, we recently bought an apparatus for analyzing blood gas. We used rats with a chronic catheter into the abdominal aorta to get arterial blood. Respirating at our previously standard level of 20 cm water, the pCO_2 seemed to be somewhat on the low side, ranging from 15 to 25 (instead of the normal 35 to 45), and the pO_2 about right, ranging from 50 to 75—perhaps a little on the low side of the ideal which probably is 75 to 100. If we respirated at lower pressures, we could bring the pCO_2 more into line, but the pO_2 became too low. Finally we tried respirating with 5% CO_2. This brought both the pCO_2 and the heart rate to a more reasonable level, and restored the reactivity of the heart to various stimuli, such as opening the box or touching the rat. Eight of the next 8 rats changed in the rewarded direction and most of the changes were quite large. Such a proportion would be expected by chance only one time in 240. Happy days were here again!

But then some rats began showing changes that were also quite large in the opposite direction. The more we ran, the less reliable the overall effects became. In looking back over the series of results, we noted a tendency for rats respirated under our conditions to show an upward drift in their baseline. We also noted that the flips of the coin had determined that 5 of our 8 good rats were rewarded for increases and only 3 for decreases. Furthermore, perhaps the first two good rats should not really be counted, because it was their performance that caused us to decide to continue with this procedure. In any event, it became painfully clear that we had not solved our problem.

By this time we were carefully monitoring not only pneumograph/chest expansion, but also air flow. Under constant settings of respirator pressure, strange changes sometimes occurred in these measures, accompanied by changes in heart rate or temperature. At other times, the temperature of the rat would unaccountably start to drift without changes in respiration. This was usually accompanied by a drift in the level of heart rate. Occasionally the heart rate of rats run without any training would show large shifts, first in one direction and then in another. To make a long story short, we began to feel as though we were wandering at midnight through a haunted forest with strange, unknown things rustling past us in the dark.

If this story of difficulties and false leads seems somewhat long-winded, I can assure you that it is greatly abbreviated. We have explored many possibilities.

Faced with this extraordinarily perplexing dilemma, I even explored the possibility that we were the victims of some mass hallucination in my laboratory. This does not seem probable because of the number of people involved—Trowill, Carmona, DiCara, Banuazizi, Fields, and Pappas. Although the fact of stubborn failure to replicate can eventually drive one to doubt one's own memory, I can be certain of some vivid details—such as standing with DiCara and watching a rat that was scheduled to turn off shock respond to the shock by an unconditioned increase, which consistently kept him too fast to meet the criterion. We stood until we could not bear watching any longer and then walked out of the room to get a Coke, returning to find that the rat had finally come down to meet the criterion and now was proceeding to learn the demanded decreases.

I also can remember Banuazizi's initial resistance to trying the first experiment on intestinal contractions, and our shared excitement when his first rat learned the changes that are illustrated in the published record (Miller and Banuazizi 1968). The next experiment in the same paper was on intestinal contraction versus heart rate and 12 out of 12 rats learned sizable changes. Both of these experiments happened to be performed in a room in Professor Allan Wagner's laboratory. After having been told about our present difficulties, he has authorized me to say that, since he was highly skeptical at first, he watched these experiments especially carefully and, of course, he also watched carefully the later dissertation performed under his supervision (Banuazizi 1972). Although he says that he cannot be as confident of spotting some subtle artifact in these experiments as he could in one on eyelid conditioning with which he has had much more experience, he is certain that the procedures were followed conscientiously and that the results occurred exactly as they are reported. He cannot think of any possible artifacts or alternative interpretations.

Recently, I have had a naturally skeptical and ingenious postdoctoral student, Dr. David VanDercar, try to see if, remaining roughly within the general ground rules of the procedures of these experiments,[1] he can produce similarly appearing results as any sort of an artifact—such as an accumulative unconditioned effect of the reinforcement—or an unusual—possibly biphasic—type of classical conditioning. Mr. Robert Vertes and Dr. Gordon Ball have been encouraged to try a similar venture. In my present state of intense perplexity and vexation, having lost many hours of sleep puzzling about the problem, I would welcome anything, even a plausible artifact, that would reproduce the original effects.

To illustrate how far we were pushed in trying to find an explanation, I remembered that there had been an epidemic of bedbugs in the Yale animal room, located near my laboratories. Therefore, the rooms and cages were heavily sprayed with a Chlordane and pyrethrin mixture. On the extremely long chance that the wearing off of the chloridane residue could be responsible for the decline in the effects, I had Dworkin try giving rats minute injections of it. Larger ones made them sick but did not seem to interact with curare to affect heart rate or to induce learning. I have not yet had the courage to suggest introducing an epidemic of bedbugs into the Rockefeller University, although I consider that it is just possible that they and other parasites to which rats used to be subjected might toughen them up to resist histaminic or other effects of curare.

Since I have been referring to these difficulties in public lectures, I have learned about similar ones encountered by other investigators. Pribram (1970, pp. 53-66) has called my attention to the fact that for several years he was unable to replicate one of his earlier findings on the effects of central stimulation on electrophysiological indices of reactions to visual cues. He reports: "Successive groups of graduate and postdoctoral students came to the laboratory fired with enthusiasm by our finding. But alas, as so often occurs when a really new result is obtained, we could not replicate" (Pribram 1970, p. 53). Happily, the problem was solved when it was found that the phenomenon in question depended on the monkey being sufficiently bored so that attention was not already near its asymptote.

Baxter, Tewari, and Raeburn report that:

> From 1966 through 1969, the stimulatory effect of GABA upon protein synthesis was observed quite consistently in hundreds of experiments. Early in 1970, however, when we were studying the time relationship of the GABA effect with respect to a variety of parameters, the stimulatory action of GABA in the *in vitro* system disappeared. . . . Several other characteristics of the system which had been observed consistently and repeatedly for 3½ years previously were found to have changed. Something had happened that either affected the experimental animals, the *in vitro* system, or the methodology of the experimental procedures (Baxter, Tewari, and Raeburn 1972, p. 211).

Finally, lending credence to the possibility that supplies of rats may have changed, Gorski tells me that in the last dozen years the dose of testosterone required to sterilize neonatal female rats has greatly increased. This phenomenon is briefly mentioned in Gorski and Shryne (1972). I shall be interested in hearing of other recent cases in which the responses of rats have changed. Perhaps they will give us some clue as to what has happened.

On my first inquiry, our chief rat supplier claimed that nothing at all had changed in their procedures of producing rats but added that "our rats are much better now than ever." After thinking over this remark, I submitted a list of very specific questions and found that some things had changed. During the period of time in question, they had changed their shipment from rail to air express, adopted a superior canned food during shipping, and changed to a more absorbent bedding material which enabled them to reduce the handling of preweaned rats during changes to clean cages from two times to one time. Since somewhat before this time they had been deriving their foundation stock by Caesarean operation in absolutely sterile environments and inoculating them with pathogen-free cultures of the intestinal flora required for normal gastrointestinal functioning. It is conceivable that the wide adoption of such procedures by the rat industry is preventing infant rats from being subjected to the kinds of stresses that could be necessary for the development of capacities for visceral learning.

We have tried securing rats from a few different suppliers and subjecting our adult rats to the experience and stress of active avoidance learning, followed by a reversal to passive avoidance learning. So far, I have not met any marked success along these lines. We may have to investigate much more thoroughly strain differences and the effects of early experience. I am currently trying habituating rats to increasing periods of severe restraint, and also to other sources of stress.

Most recently, we have concentrated our efforts on further attempts to control the parameters of respiration. Dworkin has found that it really is quite easy to tracheotomize rats[2] and that it may even be possible to recover such rats by cementing the trachea together with Eastman 910 cement. The procedure eliminates changes of resistance in the nasal passages, and changes in the position of the glottis which may allow some of the air to be forced down into the stomach or to escape by the mouth.

By changing from a constant pressure to the Harvard respirator, we thought we were changing to a constant volume system which would be good, since moderate changes in volume probably are more important than moderate changes in pressure. But we have found, to our horror, that the slide valve on the Harvard respirator is designed so that there is an appreciable period when the inhale and exhale ports are simultaneously open, allowing a leakage which makes the system a compromise between constant pressure and constant volume. We are hoping to correct this. Even so, we seem to be on our way to removing a number of hobgoblins from the haunted forest and thus materially increasing the stability of our baseline. Figure 16.2 shows the record of one of the mercifully atypical rats in which a buildup in pressure during "constant volume" respiration must have been due to blockage of the air passages—for example, by mucus, since it was corrected by briefly inserting a fine flexible tubing down the trachea and aspirating. I illustrate this to show that changes in respiratory function may not necessarily be due to changes in the compliance of the lungs. Fortunately, the vast majority of our rats are like those recorded in Figure 16.3, where the respiratory flow and pressure and also the heart rate are the same after 3 hours of curarization as they were at the beginning of it.

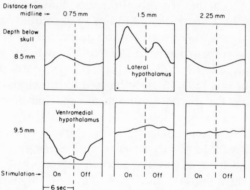

FIGURE 16.2. *Effect of apparent mucus block on respiratory pressure of curarized rat maintained on "constant volume" respiration with 5% CO_2, 95% air. Initial pressure is 15 cmH_2O.*

Still more recently (actually as a result of a suggestion at the conference), we have added a recording of blood pressure from an acute catheter inserted via the femoral artery. Samples of blood are obtained also via such a catheter, since it is our opinion that animals prepared in this way often are in better condition than those which have had the more severe operation of implanting a chronic catheter into the abdominal aorta. Throughout the period of maintenance on 5% CO_2, the blood pressure remains quite stable except for transient fluctuations. That the tracheotomy plus curarization has not produced such a state of pain, shock, or terror that nothing else matters to the rats is indicated by the fact that they show blood pressure changes to

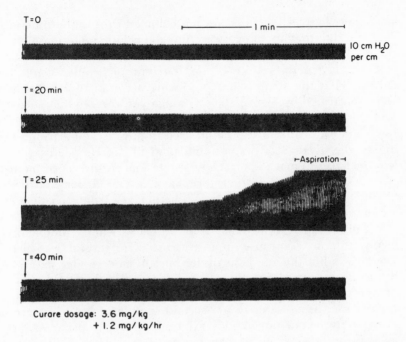

FIGURE 16.3. *Constancy of respiratory parameters during a session of 2 hours and 40 minutes. In each pair of records the top tracing is of pressure, the bottom one of flow. The tracheotomized and curarized rat is respirated by a relatively constant volume respirator on 5% CO_2, 95% air. Throughout the 2-hour-and-40-minute period, the volume remains constant at 2 cm^3 and the pressure at 14 cmH_2.*

stimuli, such as 0.3 ma shocks to the tail, opening the door to the sound-deadened compartment in which they are reclining, or bringing the hand near enough the head to touch the whiskers.

On the chance that our difficulties might be specific to the cardiovascular system, we have tried to replicate the avoidance conditioning of intestinal motility that Banuazizi (1968 1972) performed as his dissertation in Wagner's laboratory at Yale University but have been unsuccessful.

The fact that half a dozen different investigators in my laboratory were able to produce such large and consistent changes by visceral learning makes it seem unlikely that the phenomenon required a hairline precision adjustment of any specific parameter, such as respiration. Conversely, it seems highly probable that whatever is producing our present difficulties must be some quite general change that produces a large effect. Thus we have tried to investigate such factors. One of these could be the diet that is fed to the animals, but the food companies swear that their diet has not changed during the time in question and that they monitor it carefully to exclude pollution by sex hormones or antibiotics.

Another general source of our current difficulties could be the curare. That this drug is not producing a complete ganglionic block is demonstrated by Figure 16.4, in which you can see that Dr. Gordon Ball finds that with 3.6 mg/kg d-tubocurarine and maintained on the same kind of artificial respiration used in our visceral learning experiments, the average effect of stimulation in the lateral hypothalamus is to increase stomach contractions while that in the ventromedial nucleus is to stop them. Furthermore, back in 1968, I started Mr. Robert Vertes on the problem of seeing whether rewarding changes in the activity of the nucleus ambiguus, a source of the vagal nerve, would affect heart rate. He was able to locate places where stimulation at or below 10 μamp will cause the heart to stop for several beats, irrespective of whether the animal is under anesthesia or under paralysis produced by various doses of curare. Even at the threshold stimulation of approximately 5 μamp, which will cause the heart to be approximately one beat slower in a 2-second sample, doses of curare up to 7 mg/kg (twice our normal dose) did not appear to make any appreciable difference. We believe that tests of the effects of the drug on responses elicited by central stimulation probably are more physiological than those involving the direct stimulation of an isolated nerve. On the other hand, although the results by Ball and by Vertes show that the curare is not completely blocking the vagal nerve, it is conceivable that it is blocking just those components that are involved in learned changes. Since Vertes did not get clear-cut evidence for learning of changes in the nucleus ambiguus that in turn affected heart rate, we are going to try the effects of dimethyl tubocurarine iodide and other agents suggested at this conference. We have in the past given succinylcholine some brief trials without any obvious great improvement in heart rate learning.

One of the early things we did was to inquire of the drug company that supplied our d-tubocurarine. The first expert I contacted in this company assured me that curare is a USP product that has not changed at all within the time during which results from my laboratory have been declining.

After I began to refer to our difficulties in public lectures, however, Dr. Russell C. Leaf got in touch with me and said that he knows that curare is an imperfectly purified drug and, hence, varies with the source of the raw material, even with the year in which it is collected—much as wine varies from vintage to vintage. He put me in touch with Dr. Zola Horovitz, Director of Pharmacology at E. R. Squibb and Sons, who confirmed this fact and set about looking back into their

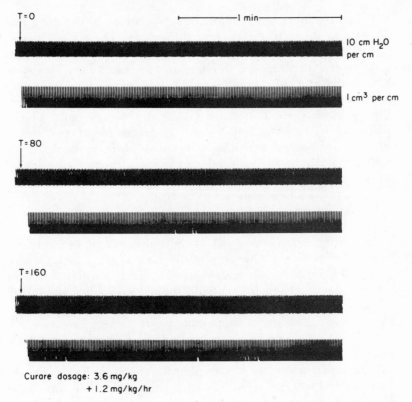

FIGURE 16.4. *Effects on pressure in a stomach balloon of 50 μa electrical stimulation of various points in the brain. Each curve is a computer average of eight stimulations. Stimulation in the lateral hypothalamus produces an increase in pressure, and in the ventromedial nucleus a decrease. Other points are relatively ineffective. From unpublished data by Dr. Gordon Ball in the senior author's laboratory.*

records concerning curare. Unfortunately, since we had purchased the drug (rather than securing it free from the company) and had not bothered to note the serial numbers on the labels of the bottles, it was impossible to be certain exactly when our drug was manufactured. But Miss Barbara Stearns, who was doing the investigation, eventually discovered that Squibb had stopped manufacturing their own curare in 1969 and started purchasing it from another firm. This change opens up additional possibilities that the curare (which I am beginning to view as a witch's brew) has changed. Fortunately Miss Stearns was able to secure for us some samples that had been set aside approximately seven years ago, and we are proceeding to test the effect of this older version of the drug.

There are three possibilities. First, variations in the drug may have nothing to do with our current difficulties. The second possibility is that the new drug contains some potent contaminant that interferes with visceral learning and also increases the heart rate. The third possibility is that the older samples may have contained an anti-homeostatic agent which greatly aided the learning, but which is now absent. This third possibility would in many ways be the most favorable one because, when isolated, such an anti-homeostatic agent might conceivably speed up human visceral learning without producing paralysis. You will remember that, once acquired, our animal learning transferred from the curarized to the normal condition. It will be interesting to see which of these possibilities turns out to be true.

We have been forced by our difficulties to consider the admittedly remote possibility that during the time when our experiments were successful, the curare contained an anti-homeostatic agent that helped learning to get started by temporarily loosening up the tight servo controls. This consideration has led us to institute a wider search for such possible agents. If such agents do indeed exist, they should manifest themselves by an increased variability in one or more functions and/or by a decreased ability to compensate for disturbing factors.

For most purposes, such effects would be highly undesirable, so compounds showing them would be likely to be discarded very early in the screening processes of the pharmaceutical industry. But I would be delighted to hear about any such compounds that any of you may know about.

SOME NEGLECTED HUMAN EVIDENCE

Some of the strongest evidence for human visceral learning has been available for some time but has been overlooked because of disciplinary compartmentalization. Although the urethral sphincters are innervated exclusively by the autonomic nervous system, I trust that all of you have learned to control urination under the favorable conditions of strong motivation and immediate knowledge of results. In the past, there has been controversy about whether skeletal musculature, for example, tensing the abdominal muscles and increasing pressure on the bladder, is involved in such control. That the overt action of such muscles is not necessary for performing voluntary control has been shown by an experiment in which Lapides, Sweet, and Lewis (1957) paralyzed 16 human subjects—some by curare and some by succinylcholine—so completely that they had to be maintained on artificial respiration. These subjects did not become incontinent, a finding in line with observations of clinicians who have used curare for treating tetanus. The new finding was that these paralyzed subjects could initiate urination on command about as fast as ever and could stop it in about twice the time required before paralysis. Catheterization showed that a large amount of fluid still remained in the bladder. These people could exercise their learned voluntary control over urination when all effects of overt contraction of the skeletal musculature were ruled out.

Furthermore, other, less heroic human experiments are continuing to provide evidence for human visceral learning that is becoming cumulatively more impressive (Barber et al. 1971a,b).

DANGER OF OVER-OPTIMISTIC PUBLICITY

When I began work on visceral learning, the general climate was so skeptical that it was difficult to get students to try any experiments. Now the climate has completely changed; there is a great deal of interest in this kind of work. But I deplore the exaggerated publicity in the popular press about this and other kinds of work commonly called biofeedback. I fear that such exaggerated articles are raising impossible hopes which will inevitably result in a premature disillusionment that may interfere with the hard work that is necessary and desirable to explore this new area of research.

NEED TO CONTROL FOR PLACEBO EFFECTS

In investigating the possible therapeutic applications of visceral learning, most investigators, including myself, have adopted the strategy of concentrating first on trying to produce a significantly large and permanent effect, deferring the time-consuming effort of running suitable control tests until we are sure that we have a phenomenon to control for. Scientifically, it is very important to know whether we are dealing with classical conditioning or instrumental learning, and to know whether the effects are produced by the direct learning of autonomic control or are indirectly mediated by learned skeletal responses. As far as therapy is concerned, these questions are not necessarily crucial. But it is important to determine that the results are from the specific training procedures used, rather than from the hope raised by the impressive apparatus and personal attention.

With the one case of hypertension with which we have had the greatest success (Miller 1972a), we have attempted to control for placebo effects by rewarding the patient first for producing small decreases and then, as soon as she appeared to be reaching an asymptote, for producing increases, but never above the original baseline level. From the point of view of training, this increase gives the subject a better opportunity to succeed in practicing a subsequent decrease and provides a sense of movement that prevents the hypertensive patient from becoming so frustrated that his pressure goes only up. The immediate contrast between down and up and down again may also be of value. In any event, during a period of three months this patient improved from only a few mmHg as the range of her voluntary control to the point where the average diastolic pressure during a minute of trying to bring pressure down would be approximately 30 mmHg below the average of a minute of effort to raise blood pressure. Such an increase in voluntary control does not seem likely to have been a mere placebo effect.

Interestingly enough, this increase in voluntary control was accompanied by therapeutically significant decreases in overall blood pressure. However, when a series of extremely difficult circumstances seemed to overwhelm her, she lost her ability for voluntary control. Her hypertension returned and she had to be restored to drugs (Miller 1972b).

I mention this single case not as a proof of therapy, but to illustrate what I believe to be a profitable type of training that contains some immediate control for placebo effects. I would be much happier about various claims for therapeutic success with biofeedback techniques if the investigators would train patients to change first in one direction and then in the opposite one, without any suggestion about which type of change will be beneficial. Then consistent reports of benefit following reward for one direction of change and exacerbation following reward for the opposite one would be especially convincing.

AUTONOMIC-SKELETAL INTERACTIONS

The whole thrust of my work in the area of visceral learning has been to emphasize that there is nothing uniquely different about the autonomic nervous system. From this point of view, one would expect autonomically mediated responses to be integrated with skeletal ones in the same way that different skeletal responses are combined into various integrated patterns, such as swinging the arms while walking. And, indeed, such patterns of autonomic and skeletal responses are well known. But, just as specific training can select the performance of a more specific skeletal pattern, such as swinging only one arm or wiggling one finger, I find it to be able to select the performance of a more specific autonomic one.

At first curare was used as a control for the effects of gross overt skeletal responses. Such overt responses can result in a greater production of heat and carbon dioxide, and in other effects that place greater demands on the cardiovascular system. But in our initial paper, DiCara and I realized that subjects may learn to send out from the motor cortex central impulses for skeletal responses, such as struggling, and that these impulses might elicit innate or classically conditioned changes in heart rate (Miller and DiCara 1967, p. 17). In that paper we present various arguments against such an interpretation—for example, the fact that a very strong, 3-ma, electric shock that would be expected to elicit maximal struggling produced only a 10% increase in heart rate, whereas instrumental learning produced an average increase of 20%. The strongest argument against explaining all visceral learning as mediation comes, however, from the fact that with appropriate training such responses can be made quite specific (Miller 1969). As the possibility for learning specificity is demonstrated with an increasing number of visceral responses, it becomes harder to imagine enough different patterns of skeletal responses to account for such specificity. For example, it is hard to imagine any skeletal response, or even emotional thought, that would cause the rat to blush in one ear but not in the other (Miller 1969).

SOME URGENTLY NEEDED, HIGHLY SIGNIFICANT STUDIES

In spite of the difficulties that have become all too obvious to me recently, I still believe that the new area of visceral learning is an extremely important one to investigate. I believe that it is likely to make at least several, and perhaps all, of the following significant contributions: (1) provide a powerful tool for investigating the functions of the autonomic nervous system and the mechanisms involved in cardiovascular and other visceral responses; (2) increase our understanding of what we mean by voluntary control and improve our methods for teaching such control over both visceral and skeletal responses;[3] (3) increase our understanding of mechanisms of normal homeostatic control; (4) contribute to our understanding of the etiology of psychosomatic symptoms and, hence, perhaps to techniques of preventive medicine with respect to such symptoms; (5) provide, perhaps, an improved type of therapy for certain psychosomatic, and conceivably even certain organic, symptoms; and, (6) provide a technique for screening drugs for the counteraction of specific psychosomatic symptoms. Therefore, I am continuing to invest a major portion of my time and energy in this area.

One of the most important steps in achieving any of the foregoing goals is to improve our techniques of producing sizable learned changes in visceral responses. My concluding comments will briefly summarize my views in this area.

In spite of our difficulties in replicating them now, I am impressed with the fact that in our earlier experiments the animals paralyzed by curare learned so much more rapidly than those that were not curarized. Was this effect primarily produced by the paralysis or was it some other pharmacological effect of the drug or physiological effect of the procedure? Was some unusual set of circumstances crucial, or are our current difficulties the results of a failure to produce normal enough physiological states in the curarized rat?

A number of similarities to the practice of yoga make me believe that the paralysis induced by the curare may be a key variable (Miller et al. 1970).[4] The yogis practice absolutely regular breathing, maintain a constant posture, and further rule out stimulus variability by monotonously concentrating their attention on a single point. My curarized rats have absolutely regular breathing, a constant posture, and a monotonous constancy of the environmental cues, because of both the paralysis and the sound-deadened box.

A possible rationale for the utility of paralyzing skeletal muscle runs as follows. If, for any reason, it is initially easier for the subject to produce rewarded visceral changes indirectly via skeletal responses, such as changes in breathing, then the subject should learn to produce more and more of such mediating responses. Unless there is a considerable transfer of training from the mediated visceral responses to the directly elicited ones, a smaller and smaller part of the variance will be produced by the latter so that it will rapidly become difficult to reward any of the direct responses. Paralysis of skeletal muscle movements may tend, at least partially, to correct such a source of difficulty. On the hypothesis that paralysis may play such a role, I have initiated work with patients who are severely paralyzed by polio, muscular dystrophy, or some other cause that affects the skeletal musculature while sparing the autonomically mediated visceral responses. Yet another possibility is to record undesirable skeletal responses responsible for most of the interference and to have changes in them turn off the reward circuit (Miller 1972a, p. 249; 1972b).

On the other hand, the opposite possibility should be investigated, namely, that there may be enough transfer of training from the visceral response mediated as a part of a pattern to the autonomic component of that pattern so that deliberately encouraging and rewarding appropriate skeletal responses, which if necessary could be phased out later, might be a good way to achieve visceral control. In some therapeutic instances, it might not even be necessary to phase out the skeletal response. For example, a certain patient reports to me that he can abort an attack of paroxysmal tachycardia by taking a sudden deep breath. If he is correct, this is a useful skeletal maneuver. I am pleased that some of Brener's work reported here (see Chapters 13 and 19) seems to be headed along this second and opposite track.

Many other aspects of the problem of maximizing visceral learning deserve intensive investigation. Is a highly sophisticated type of reward which depends on a strongly motivated subject identifying a certain feedback signal as a signal of success the most effective one? Or would it be better to use some more direct physiological reward that does not depend upon such elaborate conscious mediation? What level of motivation is most effective, at what stage of training, for what type of subject? Certainly there is some indication that trying too hard may prevent a hypertensive patient from lowering his blood pressure. What is the optimal choice between the strategies of rewarding very frequent minute changes and much less frequent larger ones? How long should the periods of training be? What type of feedback is most efficient for what type of response? Some of these problems are being investigated in laboratories across the country, but we are only beginning to scratch the surface.

We have talked about the mediation of visceral responses via overt or covert skeletal ones. What about mediation via thoughts or imagery? There is one kind of thought that might cause the rat to blush in one ear but not the other—namely, a vivid image that one ear was exposed to the hot sun and the other to an icy blast. After a discussion of this experiment on the rat's ears, Maslach, Marshall, and Zimbardo (1972) demonstrated that self-hypnotized subjects can produce a difference averaging approximately 4°C in the temperature of the two hands. They apparently do this by imagery—for example, by thinking of one hand in hot and the other in cold water. Similarly, Luria (1968) reports on a mnemonic expert with unusually vivid imagery. By imagining that he was chasing a train, he could increase his heart rate from a normal 70-72 to 80-96, and finally to 100 bpm.

Autogenic training (Schultz and Luthe 1959) seems to be another example of using imagery to acquire control over autonomic functions. In a preliminary test of this approach, Dr. David Blizard, Miss Patricia Cowings, and I have used the bidirectional type of control for placebo and other spurious effects recommended earlier in this paper. On alternate periods we had subjects practice the autogenic procedure of imagining that their hands are warm and heavy, and the anti-autogenic procedure of imagining that their hands are cool and light. The first procedure did, indeed, produce a reduction in heart rate and apparently also blood pressure, while the second had the opposite effect of definitely increasing both heart rate and blood pressure.

Although visceral changes induced by imagery may depend on classical conditioning, they are encouraging indications of a possible route to voluntary control. We need much more work on the use of imagery as a route to voluntary control over the viscera. The use of specific imagery of thoughts of this kind should not be considered incompatible with the idea that visceral and skeletal responses follow the same laws. As I have pointed out: "And if one assumes a more direct, specific connection between different thoughts and different visceral responses, the notion becomes indistinguishable from the ideomotor hypothesis (W. James, 1950 edition) of the voluntary movement of skeletal muscles" (Miller 1969, p. 445).

Closely related to the use of imagery is the idea of training subjects to improve their perception of visceral changes. Extensive work in Eastern European countries (Ádàm, 1967) has shown that animals and people can be trained to discriminate a considerable variety of visceral stimuli that once were considered to be entirely unconscious. As Brener has pointed out at this conference (see Chapters 13 and 19), the ideomotor hypothesis would lead one to expect such training to be directly conducive to better visceral control; and, as I have pointed out in a discussion of such training (Miller 1972a), it would enable the subject to substitute his own direct perceptions for feedback from elaborate instrumentation. Various means of giving such training should be investigated; for example, starting with large changes first and then working down to smaller ones, or using the anticipation method (Miller 1972b). A patient who, by such training, has learned to perceive changes in blood pressure might then proceed to learn to control his blood pressure by being rewarded for success in producing changes in the correct direction, much as a bicycle rider is rewarded for moving the handlebars in the direction that restores his balance. With sufficient practice it seems quite possible that such corrections could be performed relatively automatically, like those of the skilled bicycle rider. Finally, if there are situations that are so disturbing that voluntary control over blood pressure is impossible, the patient who is aware of his blood pressure might learn to remove himself from those situations.

In conclusion, it should be clear that there are many exciting, significant, and difficult problems to be investigated in the new area of visceral learning.

NOTES

1. Trowill early became aware of the possibility of what he called "trapping," namely, that if there was a slowing of heart rate as an unconditioned aftereffect of brain stimulation, when an animal being rewarded for a decrease finally fluctuated downward far enough to be rewarded the aftereffect of that reward could force his rate further down so that he would continue to meet the criterion, be rewarded, and held at the lower rate. Similarly, with a biphasic fluctuation, first in one direction and then another, it would be conceivable that meeting the criterion on a free operant schedule would space stimulation closer together for one group to produce trapping in one direction, and slightly further apart for the other group to produce trapping in the opposite direction. That is why he introduced an 8-second time-out after each reward. In order to be absolutely safe, DiCara extended this period to 20 seconds. Furthermore, both Trowill (1966) and Banuazizi (1968) ruled out the possibility that the unconditioned effect of the reinforcement when the response is high is to drive it still higher, but when the response is low is in the opposite direction of driving it still lower. Such level-dependent, opposite, unconditioned effects (which neither Trowill nor Banuazizi found any evidence

of in their experiments), if they had been present, could have been classically conditioned to the time-in stimulus and/or the entire experimental apparatus and thus have given a false impression of instrumental learning. On the other hand, the Law of Effect might produce an immediate strengthening of whatever change is occurring as a part of true instrumental learning. See the discussion of a hypothetical go-mechanism (Miller 1963).

2. For the tracheotomy, the rat is first anesthetized in an 8-liter jar containing 1 ml of Metofane. Additional anesthetic may be administered, if necessary, throughout the procedure by nose cone. Shave the rat's neck. Make an incision about 2 cm long down the midline of the neck, ending just before the sternum. Do a blunt dissection through the interstitial tissue. Continue the blunt dissection through the strap muscles down the trachea. Separate the muscles on either side of the trachea with blunt curved forceps. Insert forceps beneath the trachea, bringing tips through and facing upward, thereby separating the trachea from the underlying muscles. The forceps now hold the trachea slightly above the strap muscles. Using an electrocautery, make an opening in the trachea large enough to insert the tracheo-catheter. (The tracheo-catheter should be a 2-cm section of PE 240 tubing covered 3 mm from either end with a shorter piece of silastic spaghetti.) Carefully insert the end of the catheter into the opening, keeping forceps under trachea but held slightly toward the chin, in order not to obstruct passage of the catheter. Push the catheter toward the lungs until the collar is completely inside the trachea, suture under the trachea, remove the forceps. Tie a double knot around the trachea and catheter at the level of the trachea opening, to prevent catheter slippage. Clip the wound closed with two or three autoclips. Stitch once through the wound above catheter. Knot once below catheter, then bring thread round catheter and knot below external collar of catheter to prevent slippage of catheter.

3. While the infant's learning of voluntary control over his skeletal muscles merits much more study than it has received, this process is obscured by rapid maturational changes. Furthermore, the infant cannot communicate by speech. At a later age, the learning of additional control over the skeletal musculature involves an enormous amount of transfer of training. Studying the learning of voluntary control over the viscera by adult subjects may minimize the foregoing difficulties.

4. An alternate possibility is that there is something about certain meditational states that either has an anti-homeostatic effect or, as work by Wallace, Benson, and Wilson (1971) suggests, directly produces certain visceral changes. Personal conversation with Professor Bal K. Anand has also suggested the latter possibility.

17

LARRY E. ROBERTS, J. MICHAEL LACROIX
and MARION WRIGHT

Comparative Studies of Operant Electrodermal and Heart Rate Conditioning in Curarized Rats

INTRODUCTION

This chapter describes some research currently underway in our laboratory on the operant conditioning of two autonomic systems, the electrodermal and the cardiac. However, before discussing the research, we would like to comment briefly on why these experiments were carried out.

Most psychophysiologists would agree that autonomic systems are regulated to a significant degree by neural processes that perform specific functions in behavior. For the most part, however, these functions are not well understood, although frequently suggested possibilities include the regulation of motivational or attentional arousal (Lacey and Lacey 1970; Overmier 1966), or the initiation and execution of movement (Black 1971a). In this chapter, we shall refer to the study of neural processes that regulate autonomic responding as the study of the "functional organization" of the autonomic nervous system.

In our laboratory we have approached the study of functional organization through an analysis of the mechanisms of classical and operant autonomic conditioning. We have been particularly committed to experiments that compare the relationship of different autonomic responses to one another and to overt behavior during conditioning.

This research was supported by grants from the Ontario Mental Health Foundation (345) and the National Research Council of Canada (A132), to L. E. Roberts. We thank Martha Tuckett for technical assistance, and A. H. Black for his comments on an earlier draft of this chapter.

since these appear to provide more information about the organization of responding than do experiments that consider various autonomic responses separately. Some of our completed work on classical conditioning is reported in Chapter 9, where evidence is presented to indicate that the electrodermal and cardiac systems of the rat are organized very differently with respect to motivational processes and movement control mechanisms. Briefly, the nature of this difference is that sudomotor pathways appear to be more closely coupled with motivational systems than with movement control processes, whereas the reverse appears to be true of autonomic pathways that determine heart rate. Our research on operant conditioning is described in the present chapter.

Initially, our research on operant autonomic conditioning had two purposes. The first of these was to determine whether the mechanisms of operant electrodermal and heart rate conditioning are different, as is apparently true in classical conditioning. Differences in the mechanism of classical conditioning do not necessarily imply differences in the mechanism of operant conditioning, since these two procedures may achieve control of autonomic responding in very different ways. The second purpose of our experiments was to shed some light on the nature of the processes that control electrodermal activity and heart rate in the rat. We planned to approach this second goal by comparing the relationship of electrodermal and heart rate responses to movement during and following operant autonomic conditioning, and by extending these analyses to other autonomic systems and to measures of central nervous system (CNS) activity. Our utilization of operant techniques to study the organization of electrodermal and heart rate responding does not differ in principle from recent applications of operant conditioning methods to the study of brain waves and other measures of CNS electrical activity (Black 1972a).

Any study of functional organization approached through an analysis of operant conditioning assumes that operantly conditioned autonomic responses can be shown to have electrophysiological and behavioral correlates, and that study of these correlates will provide important information about the neural systems that control autonomic activity during conditioning. However, an influential series of experiments by Miller and his colleagues on the specificity of visceral learning during and following conditioning under curare, particularly the transfer studies (see DiCara and Miller 1969b; DiCara and Weiss 1969), has suggested that the effect of conditioning may be specific to the autonomic response that is reinforced. Miller has interpreted specificity of learning to mean that visceral responses may be conditioned independently of central neural processes that regulate autonomic responding under more normal circumstances (Miller 1969).

The implications of specificity of learning for the study of functional organization are profound. One implication of practical significance is that if specificity is the rule rather than the exception, we may learn relatively little about the processes that control autonomic responding through an analysis of operant autonomic conditioning. Another implication is that operant conditioning may provide a mechanism whereby the functional organization of the autonomic nervous system may be modified in a quantitative or perhaps even a qualitative way. This is precisely what is meant by suggestions that operant conditioning might shape the way in which autonomic arousal attending emotional or other psychological states is expressed, or that operant conditioning might uncouple an autonomic response from its normal correlates and control mechanisms (Goesling and Brener 1972; Miller 1969).

These speculations are, of course, justified only to the extent that specificity of visceral learning is a well established empirical phenomenon. However, the principal evidence for specificity has come from research on curarized rats, the repeatability of which now appears to be in doubt (Chapter 16 Miller). In the present chapter, we describe our attempts to operantly condition electrodermal and heart rate responses in curarized rats. It will quickly become apparent that we, too, have had difficulty demonstrating operant control in the curarized preparation.

We begin with a description of experiments in which operant conditioning was attempted. Then, some experiments on the effects of curarization on electrodermal activity and heart rate will be discussed.

EXPERIMENTS ON OPERANT CONDITIONING

We used a curarized preparation in our experiments because there was, until recently, reason to believe that muscular paralysis facilitated conditioning and contributed substantially to the dissociation of autonomic operants from their usual behavioral correlates (Miller 1969). Our curarization procedure may be described briefly, as follows.

In our experiments on electrodermal conditioning, male hooded rats weighing 270 to 520 gm were injected intraperitoneally with 1.2 mg/kg d-tubocurarine chloride and infused intramuscularly at 1 mg/kg/hr throughout the experimental session. Subjects were fitted to a face mask cut from a rubber balloon as soon as they began to experience difficulty in breathing, and were respirated at 70 breaths per minute with an inspiration:expiration ratio of 1:1 and a peak pressure of 18 to 20 cm of water (DiCara 1970). The same general procedure was followed when heart rate was operantly conditioned. However, the subjects in these experiments were male albino rats (370 to 480 gm) given 3.6 mg/kg curare and infused at 2 mg/kg/hr. This preparation was cho-

sen to approximate that used by Fields (1970a,b) after some preliminary experimentation with hooded rats given 1.2 mg/kg curare failed
to provide clear evidence of learning. In all experiments, rats were
accommodated on a plastic platform tilted 7° head-down and enclosed
in an acoustically insulated chamber with an interior heated to 78° F.

The reinforcing stimulus in all experiments was a brief electric shock
to the tail, applied by operant procedures similar to those developed
by Fields (1970a,b) for conditioning of the PP, PR, and RR intervals
in the rat's electrocardiogram. Ideally, it would have been desirable to
apply precisely the same conditioning procedure to each response system, varying only the response (electrodermal or cardiac) that was reinforced. However, technical limitations and certain properties of electrodermal and heart rate responding necessitated the use of different
methods with each autonomic system. The methods employed, however, may be considered variations of a more general shaping procedure.

Skin Potential Experiments

Our research on operant conditioning of the skin potential (SP)
response employed a yoked-control procedure. In this procedure,
experimental rats received a brief tail shock for every spontaneous SP
response above a chosen amplitude ("criterion responses"). Yoked-
controls received the same pattern of shock as their experimental part-
ners, but for these subjects punishment was independent of behavior.
Operant conditioning was expected to produce greater suppression of
criterion responding in experimental subjects than in yoked-controls.[1]
To be interpretable, this effect must persist well into extinction, since
group differences during punishment training could be due to differential unconditioned effects of shock or to a variety of artifacts for
which there is no convincing control.

Each experiment was carried out in the following way. After curarization and application of the appropriate electrodes, subjects were
given 30 minutes of adaptation during which heart rate and electrodermal activity were allowed to stabilize. Near the end of adaptation, a
distribution of 200 consecutive, spontaneous SP responses was collected
and used to determine criterion response amplitude. A typical distribution is illustrated in Figure 17.1, where the results obtained from a
single rat are portrayed. Criterion amplitude was chosen to ensure that
a predetermined proportion of the rat's responses would be followed
by shock when conditioning began. In Figure 17.1, for example, the
value chosen as criterion amplitude (3.0 mv) identified all responses
falling in the upper 75% of the amplitude distribution as criterion responses. This proportion, which we shall refer to as "punishment density," was varied systematically across four experiments, since earlier

work (Roberts 1972) suggested that it might be an important determinant of whether conditioning takes place. Once selected, criterion amplitude remained unchanged for the duration of the experiment; punishment density, however, was allowed to deviate from its nominal value as training progressed. In Fields' (1970a) terminology, this may be described as a constant criterion shaping procedure in which the reinforcement criterion is computed on the basis of response amplitude rather than interresponse time.

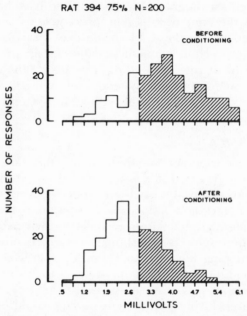

FIGURE 17.1. *Distribution of 200 SP response amplitudes before and after punishment training in the curarized rat. Distributions were taken from adaptation and extinction, respectively. All responses above the broken line (criterion amplitude) were criterion responses.*

At this point a decision was made regarding whether the subject would be an experimental or a control. If the rat's temporal rate of criterion responding during the last 10 minutes of adaptation matched that of a previous experimental run at the same nominal density of punishment (for example, 75%), he became that animal's yoked-control. If not, he became an experimental.

The remainder of training was divided into six consecutive periods, each 12 minutes long. During the first of these, which we shall refer to as the Operant Level Period or Period 0, the subjects were left undisturbed while electrodermal activity was recorded. For the next 48 minutes (Periods 1 to 4), shocks were delivered following criterion responses for experimental subjects, or whenever the experimental had been shocked, in the case of yoked controls. Shock was administered to experimental rats on the ascending limb of the SP response, as soon as criterion amplitude was surpassed. Experimentals were punished for all responses exceeding criterion amplitude, although a time constant of 1 second in the RC circuit used to detect criterion responses exempted almost all responses elicited by shock from further punishment. Conditioning was followed by 12 minutes of extinction, during which the shock circuitry was turned off (Period E).

The results from four experiments that differed with respect to punishment density are summarized in Figure 17.2. In these studies, criterion amplitude was chosen to identify either 10, 35, 60, or 75% of the subject's largest responses as criterion responses before training began. The punishing stimulus was a 2.3 ma, 27 msec tail-shock, monitored oscilloscopically through a 1 K-ohm resistor in series with the shock electrodes.[2] Inspection of the upper panel of Figure 17.2 shows that, contrary to expectation, experimental rats did not differ from yoked-controls in the frequency of criterion responding during conditioning or extinction, at any punishment density. Statistical tests applied to measures of the degree of suppression produced by conditioning (criterion responding in Period 0 minus criterion responding during Period E) also failed to reveal a statistically reliable difference between experimental and control rats in any study, or when the results from all studies were combined. Clearly, these findings do not support the idea that operant conditioning had taken place.[3]

Although experimental and control rats did not differ with respect to the frequency of criterion responding during conditioning, a reliable difference did occur in the 35, 60, and 75% studies when responses falling below as well as above criterion amplitude were counted (total response frequency). We found that punishment increased total response frequency in experimentals but not in controls, and that this effect was due entirely to an elevated rate of subcriterion responding in the experimental group. Consequently, experimental rats punished for at least 35% of their responses displayed *proportionately* fewer punished responses during training than did yoked-controls. This effect is apparent in the lower panel of Figure 17.2, where criterion responding is represented as a proportion of the total number of responses emitted by the subject (relative response frequency) during each conditioning stage. This result might be interpreted as evidence for operant conditioning, since the effect of punishment training in experimental rats was to reduce the relative frequency of responses that were followed by shock. However, suppression of relative frequency appeared during the first minute of punishment training and disappeared before 1 minute of extinction had been carried out. This

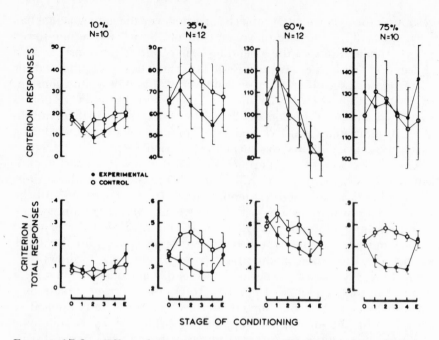

FIGURE 17.2.   *Effect of punishment training on electrodermal responding in curarized rats. Upper panel shows the average number of criterion responses emitted by each rat during 12-minute stages of conditioning. Lower panel represents criterion responding as a proportion of total responding. Since it was impossible to distinguish responses elicited by shock from responses that would have occurred spontaneously had shock been omitted, all responses in the electrodermal record were counted when computing response frequencies. The bars are ± 1 SE of the mean. The percentages above each panel denote nominal densities of punishment; N denotes the number of experimental yoked-control pairs.*

is shown in Figure 17.3, where the transitions from Periods 0 to 1 and Periods 4 to E are portrayed for the 35, 60, and 75% studies combined. It is exceedingly unlikely that acquisition and extinction effects of this rapidity can be attributed to operant conditioning, particularly when one considers that the rats typically displayed fewer than eight criterion responses during the minutes in which acquisition and extinction took place. Studies currently in progress are investigating the possibility that suppression of relative frequency may have been an unconditioned effect of punishment on electrodermal responding.

The experiments considered up to this point have examined the effect of punishment density on operant electrodermal conditioning. However, we have explored the effect of shock intensity as well. In one study, experimental rats were punished with a 1 ma shock for all responses falling in the upper 35% of their amplitude distributions. The results for 12 experimental yoked-control pairs were the same as those reported for the 35% group of Figure 17.2, where 2.3 ma was used. In a second study, experimental rats received a .4 ma shock for all responses falling in the upper 75% of their amplitude distributions. This intensity of shock appears to be just above the sensory threshold in our preparation. The results for 12 experimental yoked-control pairs were identical to those obtained when experimental rats were punished with a 2.3 ma shock for criterion responding (75% group, Figure 17.2). Clearly, these findings do not support the idea that learning failed to occur in our earlier work because an optimal intensity of shock may not have been used.

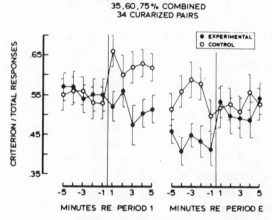

FIGURE 17.3. *Transitions from the Operant Level Period to Conditioning (left panel) and from Conditioning to Extinction (right panel). Criterion responding is represented as a proportion of total responding. The bars are ± 1 SE of the mean.*

Experimental and control rats did not differ with respect to heart rate in any of the above experiments. In both groups, heart rate increased from 445 to 463 bpm following the introduction of shock (p < .01) and decreased significantly thereafter, falling to 453 bpm during extinction. Thus, although we do not believe that the effect of punishment on the relative frequency of criterion SP responding can be attributed to operant conditioning, the effect was specific to the electrodermal system.

Heart Rate Experiments

The procedure used to operantly condition heart rate may be described by referring to Figure 17.4, where the results from a single subject are portrayed. After curarization and application of the appropriate electrodes, the subjects were left undisturbed for 60 minutes while heart rate and electrodermal activity stabilized. At this point, the circuitry used to measure RR intervals was switched on and a distribution of 200 intervals was compiled. If the rat was to be trained to decrease its heart rate, the 10th percentile RR interval was chosen as criterion (broken line in Figure 17.4), and all intervals shorter than this were followed by shock when punishment training began. If, on the other hand, the rat was to be trained to increase its heart rate, the 90th percentile RR interval was chosen as criterion and all responses longer than this value were subsequently followed by shock. In either case, distributions of 200 intervals were recompiled and the criterion interval recomputed approximately once every minute, in order to hold the probability of a criterion response (and, therefore, of shock) as constant as possible throughout the experiment. Thus, in contrast to the procedure used during electrodermal conditioning, where the response criterion denoted a particular amplitude that remained unchanged throughout training while punishment density varied, the response criterion during heart rate conditioning denoted a particular RR interval and was readjusted throughout training to hold punishment density within a fairly narrow range. In Fields' (1970a) terminology, this may be described as a variable criterion procedure, applied to interresponse time.

Following adaptation, the subjects were left undisturbed for an additional 30 minutes while the operant level of heart rate and electrodermal responding was ascertained. The subjects were then given 105 minutes of conditioning, during which a .5 ma, 27 msec shock was delivered 1.2 msec after the completion of each criterion RR interval. Conditioning was followed by 60 minutes of extinction, during which the shock circuitry was turned off.

A total of 24 rats completed heart rate training. However, five of these rats failed to respond electrodermally during the experiment, even when shock was introduced. We decided at the beginning of the study to complete the training session for each of these animals, but to treat their results separately, since there was reason to believe that the presence or absence of electrodermal responding might be an important predictor of conditioning success.

The changes in heart rate which occurred during conditioning are reported in Table 17.1, where heart rate during the Operant Level Period has been subtracted from heart rate during the first 30 minutes of extinction for each rat. When the results were considered without respect to the status of electrodermal responding, the difference between the bidirectional groups was statistically unreliable (t = 1.22, p > .10). However, the performance of electrodermally active and inac-

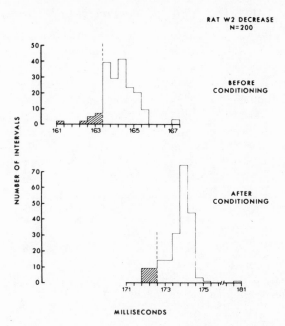

FIGURE 17.4. *Distribution of 200 RR intervals before and after punishment for fast heart rates. All intervals falling below the broken line (criterion interval) were punished.*

tive rats appeared to be different. When electrodermal responding was absent (right hand panel, Table 17.1), the bidirectional difference was again unreliable and was in a direction opposite that expected, had operant conditioning taken place. On the other hand, the bidirectional difference was significant and in the expected direction when electrodermal responding was present (p < .025, left hand panel, Table 17.1). Of course, the differential performance of electrodermally active and inactive rats must be interpreted with caution, owing to the small number of rats in our inactive group. One possible interpretation is that the bidirectional difference observed in electrodermally responsive rats was sympathetically mediated and did not occur when peripheral sympathetic ganglia were blocked by an overdose of curare, as may occasionally happen when a large dose of curare is used (Guyton and Reeder 1950). An alternative and more likely possibility is that electrodermal inactivity may be indicative of a physiological or CNS state (shock or unconsciousness) that impedes the progress of conditioning or prevents it altogether. These and other possibilities can be pursued experimentally should the quality of the electrodermal record prove to be a useful predictor of performance in future studies of operant heart rate conditioning.

TABLE 17.1   *Effect of punishing the RR interval**

SP active		SP inactive	
Increase	*Decrease*	*Increase*	*Decrease*
39	−30	−51	12
11	−31	− 4	−24
−19	−11	−76	
− 8	−10		
−16	−49		
35	−50		
−10	−75		
−10	−35		
−36	− 2		
−29			
M − 4.3	−32.6	−43.7	−6.0
t − 0.54	− 4.21	− 2.1	−0.3
p ns	< .01	ns	ns

$t = 2.5$ $t = -1.24$
$p < .025$ ns

*Heart rate during the Operant Level Period is subtracted from heart rate during the first 30 minutes of Extinction for each rat.

The heart rates of rats that were electrodermally responsive are portrayed for all segments of training in the upper panel of Figure 17.5. Although there were no differences between the bidirectional groups during the Operant Level Period, rats punished for long RR intervals displayed significantly faster heart rates by the end of conditioning than did rats punished for very short interbeat intervals. The groups did not differ significantly with respect to the number or pattern of shocks they received, indicating that these variables cannot account for the obtained result. However, while these findings are favorable to an interpretation of operant conditioning, there were some discrepancies between our results and those of previous studies of operant heart rate conditioning in which punishment procedures were used (DiCara and Miller 1968a; Fields 1970b). Unlike the earlier studies where most if not all rats changed in the rewarded direction, only a small minority of subjects trained to increase their heart rates in our study (3 of 10) actually did so. The remainder of the rats in the increase group were not remarkably different from rats that were trained to decrease their heart rates. Another anomaly is that although Fields (1970b) observed extinction of bidirectional effects within 30 minutes following punishment training, our bidirectional differences remained undiminished 60 minutes after training ended. This leads one to wonder whether random allocation of subjects may have failed to prevent fortuitous assignment of rats with an upward or downward trend in heart rate to the respective bidirectional groups. These discrepancies suggest that

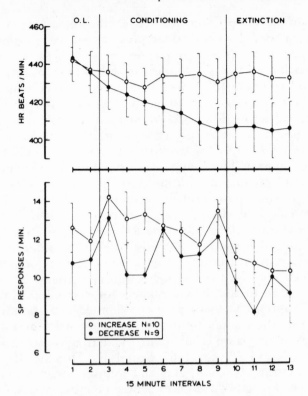

FIGURE 17.5. *Effect of punishing long and short RR intervals on heart rate (upper panel) and electrodermal activity (lower panel) in curarized rats. All rats were electrodermally active. The bars are ± 1 SE of the mean.*

further research is necessary before our results can be attributed confidently to operant conditioning.

The SP data for animals that were electrodermally active are shown in the lower panel of Figure 17.5. Although rats trained to increase their heart rates tended to display higher rates of electrodermal responding than rats that were trained to decrease their heart rates, this difference was not statistically reliable, nor did it change systematically over the course of conditioning. Response frequency increased significantly following the introduction of shock, and decreased significantly when the shock circuits were turned off during extinction, in both groups. Thus, the effect of punishment for fast or slow heart rates was specific to cardiac activity.

Discussion

Operant conditioning is a process that produces changes in behavior which are due to the relationship between a response and a reinforcer, rather than to some other feature of the experimental situation. Moreover, operantly conditioned responses are assumed to be strengthened by positive reinforcement or weakened by punishment, and to persist for a period of time after reinforcement or punishment training is discontinued. Unfortunately, our experiments on electrodermal conditioning failed to satisfy all of these requirements. Punishment for SP responding reduced the relative frequency of punished responses in experimental subjects compared to yoked-controls; however, this effect disappeared less than 1 minute after punishment training was terminated. The change was not enduring. Our experiments on heart rate conditioning, on the other hand, were more successful, but only when electrodermally responsive rats were considered. Moreover, failure of electrodermally responsive rats to increase their heart rates when punished for long RR intervals, and the persistence of bidirectional differences undiminished by 60 minutes of extinction, made us reluctant to accept an operant conditioning interpretation for these subjects until further research had been carried out.

It is reasonable to ask why punishment for electrodermal responding failed to suppress the temporal rate of criterion responding in our experiments, when suppression has been reported by other investigators on three previous occasions (Crider, Schwartz, and Shapiro 1970; Johnson and Schwarz 1967; Senter and Hummel 1965; also see Grings and Carlin 1966, and May and Johnson 1969). Unfortunately, the presence of several differences between our experiments and these studies with respect to the nature of the punishing stimuli (shock versus loud noise), the preparations studied (normal human subjects versus curarized rats), and various details of the shaping procedures (definition of criterion responses and the inclusion of shock-free periods) makes it difficult to determine why the outcomes were discrepant. However, perhaps the most obvious possibility is that learning may have been prevented in our studies by the use of a curarized preparation. This is suggested by earlier reports of sympatholytic effects of curare on some autonomic systems, at least when large doses of the paralyzing drug are used (Black 1971a; Guyton and Reeder 1950), and also by the fact that the list of investigators reporting failures to operantly condition heart rate in curarized animals has grown quite long in recent months (Chapter 13, Brener et al.; Chapter 16, Miller and Dworkin) even though the evidence for operant control of heart rate in noncurarized subjects is extensive and apparently beyond dispute (Engel 1972; Schwartz 1972; Chapter 12, Black; Chapter 19, Brener; Chapter 8, Obrist et al.). In the next section, we examine some effects of curarization on electrodermal activity and heart rate, and consider whether these might have been responsible for our failure to demonstrate operant conditioning of electrodermal activity in our earlier work.

EXPERIMENTS ON THE CURARIZED PREPARATION

Inspection of the oscillographic records from our experiments on operant conditioning suggested to us that curarization affected electrodermal activity and heart rate quite differently. Like many other researchers who have studied the curarized preparation, we found the heart rates of our rats unusually high and relatively invariant, even when a low dose of curare was used (1.2 mg/kg). On the other hand, the electrodermal records of rats given 1.2 mg/kg were not noticeably deviant from the recordings obtained from noncurarized, partially restrained rats during previous research on classical conditioning (Roberts and Young 1971). However, some impairment of electrodermal function did appear at higher doses of curare, where 11 of 36 rats (31%) given 3.6 mg/kg during research on operant heart rate conditioning failed to respond electrodermally, even when shock was introduced. By comparison, only 5 of 155 rats (3%) were found to be electrodermally inactive in our experiments on operant SP conditioning where the lower dose of curare was used.[4] These observations led us to compare the effects of curarization on electrodermal responding and heart rate more directly, in the following way. This experiment also compared the effects of curare with those of another paralyzing drug, succinylcholine chloride (Anectine), as a first step toward developing an improved preparation for the study of learning.

We began by implanting EKG electrodes subdermally on each side of the rib cage of male hooded rats. Wire leads ran from these electrodes beneath the skin to a headcap cemented to the rat's skull, so that connection with a cardiotachometer could be made and heart rate recorded in the normal state. Approximately 10 days following surgery, the subjects were partially restrained in a rat holding device (Roberts and Young 1971) for 105 minutes while electrodermal activity and heart rate were recorded. Partial restraint tended to arouse the rats, since apart from a single 30-minute period of adaptation given 48 hours earlier, they had never been restrained before.

Twenty minutes after recording began, each rat received .2 cc. isotonic saline IP. Twenty minutes after this they received either d-tubocurarine (1.2 or 3.6 mg/kg), succinylcholine (4 or 12 mg/kg), or another injection of saline. Rats receiving curare were infused at the same rates used in our experiments on operant conditioning (1 and 2 mg/kg/hr for the low and high doses, respectively); rats given 4 or 12 mg/kg succinylcholine were infused at 4 and 8 mg/kg/hr, respec-

tively. All subjects receiving a paralyzing drug were artificially respirated by the same methods used in our experiments on learning.
Thirty-five minutes after paralysis or a second injection of saline, all
rats received a dose of atropine (2 mg/kg) which appeared sufficient
to produce complete vagal blockade. This dose was selected after a
series of preliminary experiments on another sample of rats, in which
the effects of .5 mg/kg to 4 mg/kg atropine on heart rate were
explored.

The results regarding heart rate are shown in the upper panel of
Figure 17.6. Administration of either d-tubocurarine or succinylcholine
increased heart rate from 370 to 480 bpm, after which a gradual
decline occurred. Atropine subsequently raised heart rate to a level
(again 480 bpm) that was not reliably different from the heart rates
displayed by rats given atropine without a paralyzing drug. With one
exception, there were no differences in heart rate among the four dosages of paralyzing drug at any point in the experiment. The exception
was that, following atropinization, rats previously given 1.2 mg/kg
curare were found to have significantly higher heart rates than rats
given 3.6 mg/kg curare or nonparalyzed controls. Within-subject standard deviations in heart rate are also reported in Figure 17.6. Paralysis
by curare was followed by a moderate reduction in heart rate variability
($p < .01$), whereas succinylcholine had a smaller and statistically unreliable effect on this measure. Atropine, however, sharply reduced heart
rate variability in rats given either paralyzing drug ($p < .01$). The combined action of atropine and curare or succinylcholine on heart rate
variability was more potent than atropine alone.

The lower panel of Figure 17.6 shows that the effect of paralysis
on electrodermal activity was quite different. Although we had
expected some rats would be rendered electrodermally unresponsive
by 3.6 mg/kg curare, spontaneous activity was present in all subjects
given this dose of paralyzing drug. Moreover, these subjects did not
differ significantly at any point in the experiment from rats given 1.2
mg/kg curare or either dose of succinylcholine, or from non-paralyzed
controls. However, paralysis by 3.6 mg/kg curare was followed by a
statistically reliable decrease in electrodermal responding below the
pre-curare rate, whereas paralysis by other drugs was not. This suggests that some rats receiving 3.6 mg/kg curare might have become
electrodermally unresponsive had they been studied for a longer
period of time, as was done during our research on operant heart rate
conditioning. The same pattern of results was obtained when the
amplitude of SP responding was analyzed, although these data are not
reported in Figure 17.6. Atropine abolished electrodermal responding
in all groups, as was expected, since the postganglionic sudomotor fiber
is cholinergic in the rat. Thus, succinylcholine and d-tubocurarine had

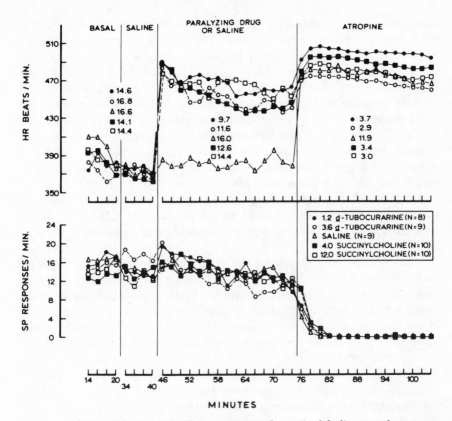

FIGURE 17.6. *Effect of d-tubocurarine and succinylcholine on heart rate (upper panel) and electrodermal activity (lower panel) in curarized rats. All rats were given atropine in the 75th minute of the session. The numbers in the upper panel are mean within-subject standard deviations in heart rate.*

relatively little effect on SP responding, although there was some evidence for a suppression of electrodermal responding at 3.6 mg/kg curare. However, all doses of paralyzing drug affected heart rate markedly.

The mechanism of the effect of d-tubocurarine on heart rate is not clear. One frequently mentioned possibility is that elevated heart rates may be due to the vagolytic action of the drug, an effect that has been well documented in cats (see Chapter 18, Howard et al.) and dogs (Black 1971a). However, the pronounced effect of atropine on heart rate and heart rate variability clearly indicates that some vagal function is left or has recovered after 30 minutes of curarization, even when 3.6 mg/kg curare is given. This result is consistent with the report by Hahn (Chapter 15), who found that the heart rate response to direct stimulation of the vagus nerve was, on the average, decreased only 20% by 3 mg/kg d-tubocurarine in rats. The failure of rats given curare to differ from rats given succinylcholine, a drug with apparently little or no vagolytic action at least in cats (Chapter 18, Howard et al.), further suggests that blockade of parasympathetic pathways is not entirely responsible for the effect of curare on heart rate. Admittedly, our knowledge of the ganglionic blocking effects of d-tubocurarine and succinylcholine in rats is very incomplete, particularly at the dosages typically used in studies of visceral learning. However, the results of Figure 17.6 suggest that paralysis of the respiratory and skeletal musculature and the consequences of positive pressure ventilation, or the histaminic or other pharmacological properties of d-tubocurarine, are more important determinants of the cardiovascular state of curarized rats, than are the possible ganglionic blocking effects of the paralyzing drug.

Whatever the mechanism of the effect, the markedly deviant heart rates displayed by rats given 1.2 or 3.6 mg/kg d-tubocurarine suggests some obvious limitations of the curarized preparation for the study of operant heart rate conditioning. It is quite possible that the acquisition of operant control may be retarded or prevented by unusually strong baroreceptor or chemoreceptor modulation of heart rate under curare, or by partial blockade of sympathetic and parasympathetic cardiac control fibers. However, even if these factors failed to prevent learning from taking place, they might limit the extent of control, or insure that control is established by a mechanism which is different from the mechanism involved when conditioning is carried out in the normal state. In view of these possibilities, failure to operantly condition heart rate in curarized rats may have little bearing upon the question of whether operant control can be established in noncurarized preparations. We believe that the evidence for operant conditioning of cardiovascular responses in noncurarized human subjects is extensive and convincing, although the mechanism of conditioning remains a matter of considerable dispute.

However, our failure to demonstrate operant electrodermal conditioning after several attempts cannot be explained by an appeal to sympatholytic or other effects of curare on the sudomotor control system. Although our evidence for impairment of electrodermal function by large doses of curare is conflicting, the fact remains that we have been unable to distinguish the electrodermal records of subjects given 1.2 mg/kg curare from those recorded from partially restrained, noncurarized rats. Moreover, the cardiovascular effects of curare, or possible central nervous system effects of the drug, are not sufficient to prevent at least some forms of learning from taking place. This is demonstrated by the results of Figure 17.7, where the outcome of an experiment on classical conditioning in the curarized rat is described.

The subjects in this study were curarized, infused, and artificially respirated by the same methods used during our experiments on operant SP conditioning, and they received precisely the same reinforcing stimulus (2.3 ma, 27 msec tail-shock) used in those studies. Differentiation between positive and negative trials was apparent and statistically reliable after eight conditioning trials or approximately 1 hour of training, which is how long our experiments on operant conditioning lasted (CS+ vs CS− x Trials Interaction, p < .05). By the end of training, 17 of the 21 rats studied displayed larger responses to CS+ than to CS− (p < .01, sign test), and for 10 of these 17 animals, differentiation was statistically reliable when within-subject analyses were carried out. Thus, rats paralyzed by 1.2 mg/kg curare are capable of learning at least a simple Pavlovian discrimination. However, it is interesting to note that although differentiation occurred with respect to SP, it did not occur with respect to heart rate. Once again, the effect of curarization on electrodermal activity and heart rate was different.

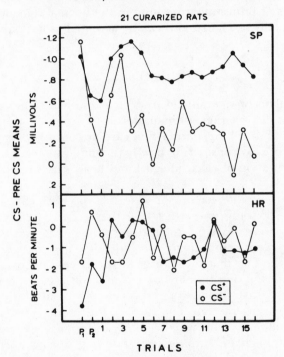

FIGURE 17.7. *Classical conditioning in the curarized rat. The CSs were a clicker or a tone, counterbalanced across subjects with respect to positive and negative trials. The CS-US interval was 20 seconds; intertrial interval averaged 3 minutes. The letter P on the abscissa denotes a pretest trial in which unconditioned responses to the CS were evaluated before conditioning began. The first shock was given on the last pretest trial.*

A final reason for questioning the idea that curarization may have prevented learning during our experiments on operant SP conditioning is that we have been unable to demonstrate operant control when punishment training is carried out in the normal state. The results from one experiment on the noncurarized rat are reported in Figure 17.8. The procedure followed during this study was identical to that employed when curarized rats were punished for 75% of their largest responses, except that a lower shock intensity (1 ma) was used. There is no evidence for a suppression of either the temporal or relative rate of criterion responding by punishment training in Figure 17.8, even though suppression of relative frequency during training was found when conditioning was carried out at this punishment density in the curarized rat (cf. Figure 17.2). The discrepancy may have been due to the use of a lower shock intensity, although this seems unlikely since .4 ma shock suppressed relative frequency when rats were punished for 75% of their largest responses while curarized. However, more data on the effects of punishment training in the normal state are required before the results of Figure 17.8 can be accepted as definitive.

CONCLUSION

The experiments on operant electrodermal and heart rate conditioning described in this chapter were undertaken to study the functional organization of the electrodermal and cardiac control systems. We conclude, therefore, by considering briefly the implications of our findings for the organization of electrodermal and heart rate responding in the rat.

One finding of interest in our research was that changes in electrodermal responding and heart rate that occurred during operant conditioning were specific to the response that was reinforced. Although we were reluctant to conclude that the changes were due to learning, the fact that they were uncorrelated with one another is consistent with the outcome of our research on classical conditioning, which suggests that the neural processes that control electrodermal activity and heart rate in the rat are different (see Chapter 9). However, we do not know whether these differences extend to central processes that regulate autonomic responding during operant conditioning, or whether they reflect specificity only in peripheral control systems themselves. Nor can we be sure that specificity will be retained when response relationships are studied in the normal state or in preparations paralyzed by drugs that do not disturb cardiovascular function. These questions, as well as the question of whether the bidirectional differences we observed during heart rate conditioning are due

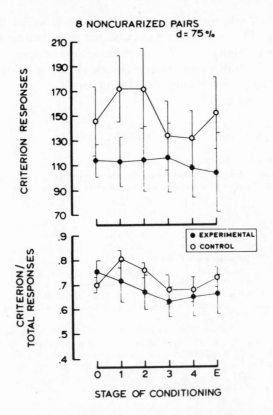

FIGURE 17.8. *Effect of punishing SP responding in the noncurarized rat. Punishment density was 75%. The bars are ± 1 SE of the mean.*

to learning and can be predicted from the integrity of the electrodermal record, remain to be answered by further research.

One implication of our findings, however, seems quite clear. Whatever their function in behavior, the neural processes that control electrodermal responding in the rat do not appear to be obedient to a principle of operant conditioning, when punishment training is carried out in the curarized state. Moreover, our failure to achieve control of these processes does not seem to have been due to sympatholytic effects of curare on sudomotor arousal, or to cardiovascular or possible central nervous system effects of the paralyzing drug. These conclusions are supported by our inability to differentiate the electrodermal records of rats given a low dose of curare from recordings obtained in noncurarized animals, and by the fact that the curarized animal is clearly able to learn a Pavlovian discrimination. Whether the electrodermal system of the rat will remain differentially sensitive to operant and classical conditioning when different preparations and training procedures are employed is an unresolved problem that deserves further study. The question seems well worth pursuing, since, unlike heart rate and many central nervous system responses that have recently been operantly conditioned (Black 1972a), electrodermal functioning appears to be highly dependent upon a non-motor process (Roberts and Young 1971).

NOTES

1. This assumes that the classically-conditioned and unconditioned effect of shock is an increase in electrodermal arousal, not a decrease. However, as will be apparent later, we have reason to believe that the unconditioned effect of shock may be more complex than this.

2. Shock was a capacitor discharge (100 μf charged to 150 v) through a series of resistance totalling 48 K-ohms. Contact area was .5 cm^2. The lowest value of shock that will consistently elicit an SP response in the curarized rat appears to be about .2 ma. A 3.2 ma, 1-second shock produces good differentiation between positive and negative trials during CER training in partially restrained rats, with no responding to CS- and little or no disruption of the operant baseline. A 5.8 ma, 1-second shock also produces good differentiation during CER training, but there is generalization between CS+ and CS- and the operant baseline may be suppressed from 2 to 5 days (Roberts and Young 1971).

3. The 60% group of Figure 17.2 was an attempt to replicate an earlier study (Roberts 1972, Experiment 1) in which operant conditioning appeared to have occurred. However, in that study, experimental rats were found to display significantly smaller SP response amplitudes during the Operant Level Period than their yoked-controls ($p < .01$). When this difference was eliminated, as happened in all experiments reported in Figure 17.2, criterion responding was not suppressed by punishment training at any punishment density.

4. A total of 12 rats given 3.6 mg/kg curare for heart rate training was discarded prior to conditioning because of heart rate instability, death, or equipment problems. Of these 12 rejected rats, 6 were electrodermally inactive. If we add these 6 rats to the 5 others that were electrodermally unresponsive but completed punishment training, 11 of 36 or 31% of the total sample was electrodermally inactive when given 3.6 mg/kg curare. Although this is substantially higher than the percentage observed during research on electrodermal conditioning where a lower dose of curare was used, the difference cannot be interpreted unequivocally as a dosage effect, since the subjects in the two experiments were drawn from different strains.

18

JAMES L. HOWARD, RICHARD A. GALOSY,
CLAUDE J. GAEBELEIN, and PAUL A. OBRIST

Some Problems in the Use of Neuromuscular Blockade

INTRODUCTION

The most common method of separating autonomic nervous system and striate muscular response components of behavioral acts has been the use of pharmacological blockade of the skeletal response system, usually through the use of d-tubocurarine. The implication in studies using curare is that the major, if not only, change produced in the organisms by curare or curare-like drugs is muscular blockade. However, the mixed results obtained in both operant and classical conditioning of curarized organisms have led to this basic assumption being questioned. To the extent that curarization alters the physiology of the organism, other than by simply preventing nerve impulses from reaching the muscle, then to that extent the usefulness of curare as a tool may be compromised. The problems in using curare may be segregated into two classifications: (a) those problems directly associated with producing and maintaining a paralyzed organism including the criteria of muscular blockade and artificial respiration; and (b) those problems associated with the side effects produced by the drugs including ganglionic blockade, promotion of histamine release, and alteration of sensory processes.

The preparation of this chapter was supported by research grant MH-07995 NIMH, and institutional grant HD-03110 NICHD, USPHS.

CRITERIA OF MUSCULAR BLOCKADE

Several criteria have been used to show that paralysis has been produced by curare. One has been absence of observable movement (Harlow and Stagner 1933), including absence of respiratory movements (Hahn 1970). A second major way of showing paralysis is electromyogram (EMG) monitoring (Black and Lang 1964). EMG activity would seem to be the more stringent criterion since it can be found in the absence of observable movement (Black 1967b; Howard et al. unpublished data). However, studies employing EMG monitoring (e.g., Black and Lang 1964; DiCara and Miller 1968a; Gaebelein et al. 1972; Yehle, Dauth, and Schneiderman, 1967) have differed widely in their choice of recording sites and sensitivity of measurement, suggesting that some of the inconsistency among experimental results might be due to investigators inadvertently using different levels of curarization.

Choice of recording site is important because the drugs affect the neuromuscular junctions in different parts of the body at different thresholds (Grob 1967; Koelle 1970). For instance, when a competitive blocking agent such as d-tubocurarine is used, peripheral muscles will be paralyzed at lower dosage levels than will more cranial muscles. The sensitivity with which EMG is recorded is an important consideration because if too low a gain is employed, EMG activity will be missed. Howard (pilot data) employed two EMG recording sites, the gastrocnemius muscle of the hindlimb and a cervical neck muscle, and two gain settings, 150 uv/cm and 10 uv/cm. EMG activity always disappeared in the gastrocnemius at lower dosage levels than in the cervical neck muscle, and when all trace of EMG activity disappeared at the lower gain setting, EMG activity could still be observed at the higher gain setting. This EMG activity could be suppressed by increasing the amount of curare infused, demonstrating that it was not artifactual.

A further complication is posed by the intrafusal, or gamma, fiber system. The gamma efferent system alone has been shown to support skeletal muscular conditioning (Buchwald and Eldred 1962; Buchwald et al. 1964), and it was suggested that the gamma fiber system has a higher threshold than the extrafusal muscle fiber system to the blocking effect of curare (Buchwald et al. 1964). These observations support the view that if *all* muscular activity and feedback from it is to be blocked, then very high gains and optimal recording sites must be used to monitor EMG. However, it is necessary to point out that when absence of EMG activity is used as a criterion for muscular blockade, it is difficult to assess whether an amount of the drug in excess of that needed is being delivered to the animal. Since overcurarization can potentiate all of the side effects of the drugs, it is essential to carefully titrate the infusion to just produce neuromuscular blockade.

RESPIRATION

A requisite for maintaining a "normal" curarized organism is proper ventilation. Respiratory parameters of major concern include rate and volume, inspiration-expiration (I:E) ratio, and lung compliance. The basic concern is to maintain normal blood gas levels of O_2 and CO_2. The importance of monitoring respiratory function has been emphasized by reports that baseline heart rate (HR) can be set at almost any level which the experimenter desires by adjusting respiratory rate and volume (Howard, unpublished data; Brener, personal communication; Miller and DiCara 1967; Hahn 1970). For example, Hahn (1970) routinely adjusts respiratory rate and depth until HR falls within a certain preset range. Conditioning changes are then assessed from the baseline. It would seem that this is putting "the cart before the horse", since the primary concern should be with maintaining normal pO_2 and pCO_2 with HR and other response measures allowed to assume whatever values are normal for that animal. For a more complete discussion of the respiration of curarized animals, see Chapter 19 by Brener.

GANGLIONIC BLOCKADE

All of the agents used for neuromuscular blocking also have some effect on ganglionic transmission (Grob 1967; Guyton and Reeder 1950; Koelle 1970). Black (1967) directly tested the possibility that cardiac innervations were modified by curare. Under sodium pentobarbital anesthesia, three dogs were implanted with vagal stimulating electrodes and the HR deceleration to direct nerve stimulation was tested after the animals had been administered progressive doses of d-tubocurarine. All three dogs showed an attenuation of the deceleration to vagal stimulation as the level of curarization increased. Black (1967b) also prepared two chronic animals: one with vagal stimulation electrodes and one with sympathetic stimulation electrodes. After recovery, instrumental conditioning of HR was begun under curare. The HR response to direct nerve stimulation was also periodically assessed. It was found that as depth of curarization increased, both the conditioned response and the response to direct nerve stimulation diminished at approximately the same rate. Grob (1967) states that "d-tubocurarine blocks conduction in autonomic ganglia rendering them unresponsive to preganglionic nerve stimulation." He also states that "the parasympathetic ganglia, particularly in the vagus nerve, are more sensitive than are the ganglia supplying sympathetic fibers." Furthermore, d-tubocurarine, which is the most often used agent, has the greatest effect on sympathetic ganglia of any of the commonly used curarization agents and the second greatest on the parasympathetic system—only Flaxedil has a greater effect—(Koelle 1970).

To explore this issue, we have recently completed an assessment of the ganglionic blocking effects produced by d-tubocurarine chloride, dimethyl d-tubocurarine iodide, and succinylcholine chloride. Stimulating electrodes were implanted under sodium pentobarbital anesthesia on the cervical vagus, the preganglionic fibers entering the right stellate ganglion, and the motor nerve innervating the sartorius muscle in 16 cats. When the thoracic cavity was entered to allow access to the stellate ganglion, the animal was placed on positive pressure ventilation through an endotracheal tube. Throughout the experiment, peak expired CO_2 was maintained at 5% by adjusting rate and volume of respiration. Recordings were made of integrated EMG, HR, blood pressure from the femoral artery, expired CO_2, and rate and volume of respiration. Body temperature was maintained at 101.5° F by warming the animal with a heating pad. Following surgery, the HR response to both a 5-second vagal (40 Hz, 3 to 5 volts, 4 msec pulse duration) and a 10-second sympathetic (6Hz, 10 to 20 volts, 4 msec pulse duration) stimulation was determined, and stimulation levels were selected which produced large decelerations and accelerations respectively. These stimulation levels were then used throughout the remainder of the experiment. The EMG response in the sartorius muscle following a 5-second femoral nerve stimulation (100 Hz, 0.1 to 0.8 v, 4 msec pulse duration) was also assessed, and stimulation parameters were fixed for the remainder of the experiment. At this point the animal was assigned to one of four infusion groups each consisting of four cats: saline, d-tubocurarine chloride, dimethyl d-tubocurarine iodide, or succinylcholine chloride. The drug selected for the session was infused through a catheter in the femoral vein. Infusion, at a rate below that necessary to cause complete paralysis, was begun, and the HR and EMG responses to direct nerve stimulation were determined every 15 minutes as the infusion rate was gradually increased. After complete muscular blockade was obtained, as evidenced by the complete block of evoked EMG, the infusion was terminated and the neuromuscular junction was allowed to recover.

Figure 18.1 shows the evoked EMG response for each of the drug conditions before the infusion of any drug (Pre-Drug), at the point of maximum block of evoked EMG (MAX Block), and during recovery. There was no significant difference among groups during the Pre-Drug period, although the group that was to get succinylcholine showed a significant decrement in response magnitude over seconds. At the point of maximum blockade, all neuromuscular blocking drugs produced a complete and equivalent suppression of evoked EMG activity, whereas, after the passage of the same length of time and volume

EVOKED MUSCLE RESPONSE

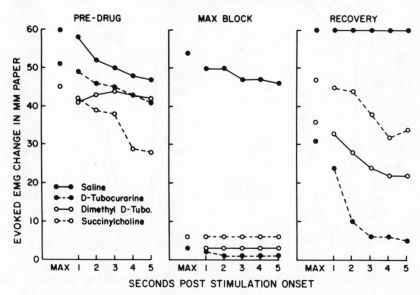

FIGURE 18.1. *Average evoked muscle response to suprathreshold electrical stimulation prior to the infusion of the drugs, during neuromuscular blockade, and 90 minutes after the termination of the infusion. MAX on the abcissa indicates the largest change in EMG observed during the 5-second stimulation period. See text for details.*

of infusion, the saline control group's response was unaffected. Ninety minutes after cessation of infusion the evoked EMG response had recovered differentially in the three experimental groups.

Figure 18.2 shows the heart rate change evoked by direct sympathetic and parasympathetic nerve stimulation in each drug condition. There were no significant differences among the heart rate responses evoked by direct stimulation of the sympathetic preganglionic fibers at any point for any group. However, base level HR was affected (-30 bpm) at the point of maximum EMG block in the d-tubocurarine group, and the maximum acceleration of HR following stimulation showed a similar decrement in comparison to Pre-Drug and Recovery conditions.

Results from vagal stimulation indicated that during the Pre-Drug condition all of the drug groups responded with a rapid, significant decrease in HR of approximately 100 bpm which returned to base level within 5 seconds following the offset of stimulation. At maximum EMG blockade under d-tubocurarine the HR response to vagal stimulation was completely blocked, while that of other groups was not significantly

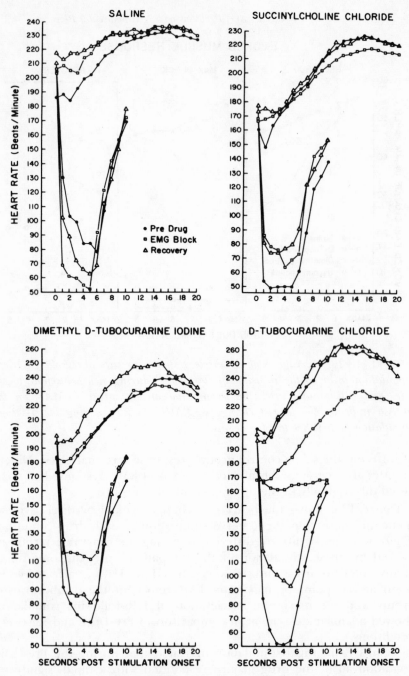

FIGURE 18.2. *Average heart rate responses to suprathreshold electrical stimulation of the sympathetic and parasympathetic innervations of the heart prior to, during, and following neuromuscular blockade for each of the drug conditions. See text for details.*

affected. Recovery data showed that the HR response of cats in all drug conditions had recovered to the same degree.

The results of this experiment and those of others suggest that experimenters need to be aware of the ganglionic effects of curarization agents at least in interpreting the results that they obtain. The results also confirm the notion that d-tubocurarine is the least desirable compound for neuromuscular blockade if autonomic nervous system responses are to be measured, because it has the most potent effects on ganglionic transmission—however, see also Hahn Chapter 15.

HISTAMINE RELEASE

Another property that curarization compounds have is that of releasing histamine (Douglas 1970; Everett 1948; Koelle 1970). Histamine causes widespread changes in the body including stimulation of the smooth muscle of arteries and veins, capillary dilation and increased permeability, brisk dilation of cerebral blood vessels, perhaps a direct stimulatory effect on sensory nerve endings responsible for pain, and bronchiolar constriction (Douglas 1970). The overall effect on the cardiovascular system of the changes produced in the arteries, veins, and capillaries is species dependent. Blood pressure increases in the rodent due to strong arteriolar constriction which is not compensated for by dilation elsewhere. Blood pressure decreases in the cat and dog, because the slight constriction of arteries and veins produced by histamine is overwhelmed by the dilation of the minute blood vessels. Although the curarization agents do not act entirely like a massive dose of injected histamine, the histamine releasing properties of d-tubocurarine are substantial and should probably be considered in speaking of the curarized preparation (Everett 1948). Observation in this laboratory suggests that dimethyl d-tubocurarine and succinylcholine also possess histamine releasing properties, at least in terms of stimulating bronchial secretions.

SENSORY PROCESSES

One of the assumptions that experimenters using curare have made is that their subjects are conscious and that their sensory apparatus is functioning normally. This assumption is apparently based on a few studies in humans and a very confusing animal electroencephalogram (EEG) literature. Two studies using one human each (Leuba, Birch, and Appleton 1968; Smith et al. 1947) and one study using six humans (Unna and Pelikan 1951) have reported that complete (first two studies) or incomplete (third study) muscular paralysis does not impair consciousness or impede sensation.

Studies which have monitored EEG in animals under curare in an attempt to specify arousal level provide inconsistent results. Such investigations have reported everything from arousal to slow wave sleep patterns in curarized animals (Bovet and Longo 1953; Gellhorn 1958; Girden 1948; Hodes 1962; McIntyre, Bennett, and Hamilton 1951; Morlock and Ward 1961; Okuma, Fujimori, and Hayashi 1965). Black, Carlson and Solomn (1962), in their survey of the literature, found that the EEG pattern displayed by the animal under curare could be affected by species, method and speed of injection, dose level, and adequacy of the artificial respiration. Okuma and his co-workers (1965) demonstrated that variations in ambient temperature, with body temperature constant and normal, could alter EEG pattern. Within a range from 25° C to 33° C, EEG patterns resembled those of animals in light or deep sleep. When ambient temperature was outside this range, the animals displayed a low voltage, high frequency pattern characteristic of arousal (or paradoxical sleep).

Hodes (1962) did one of the most careful and complete studies of the effect of curare compounds—Flaxedil, d-tubocurarine, and succinylcholine—on EEG. He concluded that all of the agents produced a sleep pattern in the animal within a short time, and that cortical synchronization became progressively greater over the course of the session. Furthermore, although desynchronization of the cortical EEG could be readily produced by minor stimuli at first, as the duration of neuromuscular block extended into several hours even extremely strong noxious stimuli were unable to provoke the arousal reaction. At all times, CO_2 levels in expired air, blood pressure, rectal temperature, and other vital signs were maintained within the normal range. Hodes concluded by cautioning against the use of terms such as "unanesthetized," "waking," "vigilant," "alert," and "normal" in describing the curarized organism. Therefore, the question of the arousal state of the animal under curare in a conditioning state still remains unanswered.

Finally, it has been shown that a strong possibility exists that curarization affects the action(s) of acetylcholine in various sensory nerve endings and receptors (Koelle 1970). Overall, it seems that no clear statement regarding the state of the sensory system under curare can yet be made.

SUMMARY

In view of the physiology and pharmacology of curare reviewed above, it is apparent that none of the experimenters utilizing curare as a tool have controlled all the variables which might influence their results. Few studies have monitored the effectiveness of neuromuscular block by measuring EMG. Very few studies have measured the amount of ganglionic block produced by curare or even indicated awareness of the possibility that such a ganglionic block effect might be modifying the results. No studies have tried to ascertain systematically what effect the histamine releasing properties of curare might have on the results. The importance of *normal* respiratory parameters has been largely ignored as has the influence of ambient temperature, rate of infusion, and the gamma-efferent muscle spindle system. At present, it is not even known what the EEG arousal state of animals is during conditioning under curare. With this many "loose ends" it is not surprising that there are contradictions in the results obtained using curare as a tool.

IV

Human Operant Conditioning

In this section, research on the operant conditioning of autonomic responses in human subjects is discussed. The focus of attention in these chapters is quite different from that of the chapters in the previous section. A quick examination of the chapters reveals two main themes. The first is an analysis of operant autonomic training procedures, especially those that are required to establish "voluntary control." This interest is reflected in the papers by Brener, Schwartz, and Lang. The second theme is the use of operant conditioning techniques therapeutically. This is reflected in the chapters of Engel and Bleecker and of Shapiro.

It is interesting to note that the contributors to this section display a fair degree of consensus regarding their theoretical approaches to learned cardiovascular phenomena. For example, the concepts and models of the motor skills literature are generally deemed to provide a useful conceptual framework within which to examine the learning of cardiovascular responses. The relative emphasis on the role of feedback in the development of cardiovascular control seems to mark a renewed interest in mechanisms of learning and a shift away from the simple use of conditioning procedures as a tool.

The points of major focus are somewhat different among the chapters comprising this section. Brener attends primarily to the application of an explanatory model to the analysis of learned cardiovascular phenomena and emphasizes the role of exteroceptive feedback in the development of response discrimination and subsequent control. Lang, also working within a motor skills framework and employing a computer-controlled environment, reports on the effects of manipulating certain feedback parameters on the control of heart rate. A theoretical appreciation of learned cardiovascular control in terms of the operation of the processes of reinforcement contingency and biological constraint is described in the chapter by Schwartz. Shapiro broaches a number of questions relating to the application of reinforcement and feedback procedures in the treatment of chronic elevation in blood pressure. Finally, Engel and Bleecker describe a compelling series of observations relating to the clinical application of feedback procedures in the training of control over cardiac arrhythmias in a clinical population.

19

JASPER BRENER

A General Model of Voluntary Control Applied to the Phenomena of Learned Cardiovascular Change

INTRODUCTION

The past 10 years have witnessed a prolific growth in the literature relating to learned control of cardiovascular processes. For the most part, investigators have attended to demonstrating that the activities of this and other visceral response systems may be modified by operant reinforcement and feedback procedures. Although such demonstrations fly directly in the face of hitherto prevalent theories regarding the principles of visceral learning, this burgeoning literature has been noticeably devoid of any significant theoretical reorientation.

A provocative aspect of this new literature is that it purports to demonstrate behavioral properties in the cardiovascular system that were hitherto believed to be exclusive attributes of the somatic response system. The question has necessarily arisen as to whether the mechanisms involved in voluntary and operant cardiovascular modification are the same as those involved in equivalent modification of somatomotor activity. This issue represents the focal point of the present chapter.

In attempting to describe the learning mechanisms that underly the development of voluntary control, the most profound obstacle to be overcome resides in the entrenched meaning of traditional concepts employed in the description and analysis of these processes. These obstacles are exaggerated, where the attempt is to describe the develop-

The research reported here was supported by NIMH Grant 17061.

365

ment of voluntary control over activities that have previously been considered to be members of an involuntary class. Despite the acceptance of voluntary cardiovascular events that is implicit in the experimental literature of the past 10 years, the redefinition of such basic concepts as "voluntary" and "involuntary" that these phenomena demand has not yet been made explicit.

One indisputable implication of this literature is that the traditional view of a structurally-based operant-respondent dichotomy is no longer tenable. The cardiovascular system displays easily demonstrable voluntary *and* involuntary characteristics. In deference to this observation, the terms "voluntary" and "involuntary" as employed in this chapter refer only to the conditions under which a given instance of a response is observed, and have little to do with the structural attributes of the response apparatus in question. In other words, these terms describe observational procedures and not functional attributes of specific effector systems or their associated neural control circuits. In the present context a voluntary response is defined as one that is systematically influenced by instructions. The development of instructional control is assumed to be dependent upon the execution of certain training procedures to be specified below. An involuntary response, on the other hand, is defined as the reliable consequence of a narrowly-delineated class of eliciting stimuli. This form of control is assumed to be independent of any other prior conditions. Thus given instances of the same topographically restricted response may be classified as voluntary or involuntary, depending on the procedures employed for the demonstration of those particular instances.

It is proposed then that "voluntary" and "involuntary" represent two independent dimensions in the classification of behavior, rather than opposite poles of a linear continuum. It is further assumed that in principle all responses, regardless of their structural attributes, are amenable to both voluntary and involuntary control. In this context, the task of investigators in the area of learned cardiovascular control is seen as the specification of the conditions under which the voluntary characteristics of cardiovascular behavior may be reliably demonstrated. The mode of attack adopted with respect to this problem is necessarily determined by the model of functioning assumed to underly voluntary control processes. Two similar but distinctive empirically-based approaches are discernible.

Perusal of the literature on learned cardiovascular control in humans indicates that the terms "operant conditioning," on the one hand, and "voluntary control" or "feedback", on the other, are employed interchangeably. While these procedures, both involving the presentation of response-contingent stimuli, are virtually indistinguishable, the analytical models associated with them differ in a significant fashion.

Whereas the strict operant conditioning approach posits the response-contingent event (reinforcing stimulus) as the final cause of behavior change, the feedback approach attempts to account for the processes by which response-contingent events lead to behavior change. In other words, the principle of reinforcement which is axiomatic in the conditioning approach is derived from more basic axioms in the feedback approach. Thus, the feedback approach permits a finer-grain analysis of the voluntary control process. It suggests feasible lines of enquiry into the structural basis of such control processes, and, more than any other approach, it violates the traditional notion of volition by offering a mechanistic analog of this antiscientific and pervasive psychological concept.

A MODEL OF VOLUNTARY CONTROL

A voluntary response has been defined as one that is systematically influenced by instructions. The model proposed here attempts to account for the processes underlying the development of instructional control of motor activities. In agreement with the general theme of the literature relating to learned motor control and to cardiovascular control in particular, it is assumed that feedback processes are fundamental to the development of voluntary control.

At an introspective level we may satisfy ourselves that compliance with an instruction (emanating from one's self or someone else) to execute an act does not depend upon being able to specify the efferent motor programs for that act. However, there are discriminable sensory consequences associated with the occurrence of all responses that we classify as voluntary. Our ability to discriminate the occurrence of voluntary acts is assumed to rest upon activation of interoceptive afferent pathways by the effectors involved in the act. When individuals are deprived of such intrinsic feedback from an effector, they are also robbed of the illusion that they can voluntarily control responses of that effector (Laszlo 1966). In this context, it is of significance to note that, although we can readily discriminate the stimulus antecedents of many involuntary responses, the responses themselves are frequently indiscriminable.

The topographical dimensions and intensive characteristics of a response are very precisely defined in terms of the interoceptive[1] feedback array contingent upon that response. James (1890) proposed that with repeated elicitation, the afferent information consequent upon a response is stored centrally as the response image (RI). Both the RI and the immediate sensations contingent upon its occurrence are functions of the afferent system serving the effectors involved in that response. The RI is, therefore, simply a stored representation of the pattern of afferent stimulation produced by past occurrences of the response. The ability of an individual to identify a given response in his repertoire is assumed to depend on a comparison of the immediate feedback consequent upon the response with the established image for that response.

James further proposed that elicitation of an RI leads inevitably to the activity represented in the image. This proposition is adopted in the present model. Specifically, it is proposed here that, as a function of certain procedures to be specified below, instructional stimuli acquire the ability to elicit an RI and that activation of the RI leads to a state of nervous system imbalance resulting in the production of the response specified by the image. Von Holst (1954) has provided evidence that the termination of a motor act is dependent upon the matching of afferent stimuli consequent upon the response with a central copy of the neural motor program underlying the response. Where there is a disparity between the afferent feedback consequent upon the response and the central copy of the motor program, additional motor signals are generated until the comparator achieves a null state. In the present model, the RI is assumed to represent the standard against which neural feedback from the periphery is compared.

In summary, then, a voluntary act is initiated through the activation of an RI by some external (instructional) stimulus. Activation of the RI produces a specific pattern of activity in some central motor controller. This pattern of activity leads to the occurrence of effector action and consequent interoceptive feedback. The interoceptive afferent signals are compared to the pattern of excitation specified by the RI. If they are in accord, the act is completed; if not, additional motor signals are generated until the comparator achieves a null state.

The model in terms of which these processes are achieved is described in Figure 19.1. Two primary central structures are identified, the central sensory integrator (CSI) and the central motor controller (CMC). Interaction of these two structures controls the activity of an effector (Eff) via the motor nerves (M). Regulatory feedback from the motor apparatus occurs via three major pathways: the central feedback (CF) pathway, which feeds information from the CMC to the CSI; the interoceptive afferent (IA) pathway, which transmits information from the interoceptors (I) serving the Eff to the CSI; and, the exteroceptive afferent (EA) pathways leading to the CSI. Two EA pathways are described. In EA_1 the environmental energy produced by the Eff acts directly upon an exteroceptor (E) feeding the CSI. An example of this form of exteroceptive feedback would be seeing one's arm move. EA_2 is an exteroceptive feedback pathway which transmits response-produced energy to an exteroceptor following transformation of such energy into a form which is detectable by that exteroceptor. The trans-

ducer employed to transform response-produced energy into exteroceptive stimulus energy may receive its input from the environmental
consequences of the act (a) such as the presentation of a tone when
movement of a subject's limb interrupts a light beam, or it may receive
its input from some biological probe (b) such as the electrocardiogram
(EKG) being employed to operate a light stimulus on each R-wave. The
latter exteroceptive feedback pathway, EA_2(b), is inevitably employed
in the training of voluntary visceral control since the effectors of this
response system do not produce environmental stimuli that are directly
amenable to exteroception. The interaction of the various components
of this model are described below with reference to the processes
deemed here to be necessary to the development of instructional control over cardiovascular and other motor activities.

Calibration

The procedure of calibration involves the systematic pairing of exteroceptive stimuli with the interoceptive feedback stimuli consequent
upon an act. During the normal development of motor control, this
pairing operation occurs naturally in the consistent and near-
simultaneous occurrence of activity in the IA and EA_1 pathways following the occurrence of a response. The sensorimotor integration that
occurs as a function of such stimulus pairing is also known to be
dependent upon the response in question deriving from activity in the
CMC rather than the action of some external force operating directly
upon the effector or its peripheral motor nerves. Thus Held (1965)
has observed that adaptation to prism-induced sensorimotor rearrange-
ment does not occur in cases of passive movement. This contingency
is handled in the present model by the central feedback pathway. During the development of voluntary control, this pathway is assumed to
serve an enabling function. Following activity in the CMC, signals are
transmitted to the CSI via the CF pathway. This serves to activate the
CSI so that the immediately following IA and EA signals impinging
upon it acquire an association. This property of the CF pathway
ensures that associations are formed only between signals that arise as
a function of the motor activities generated by the organism and not
between extraneous exteroceptive signals and interoceptive signals that
may arise as a function of passive movements of the organism. Later
in training, such CF signals may well provide the major source of feedback during the behavioral regulation[2] (Festinger et al. 1967).

The primary function of the calibration processes is to establish in
the EA stimulus the property of eliciting the pattern of excitation in
the CSI previously dependent upon the IA signals acting upon this
structure (the RI). Secondary to the formation of this learned association is the demonstrative ability of the organism to discriminate in-

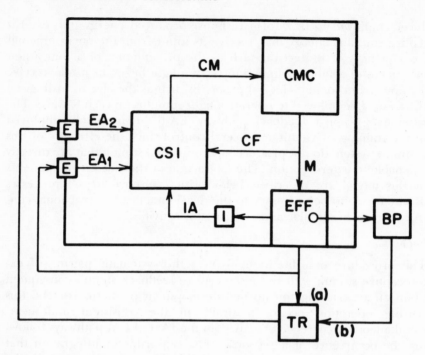

FIGURE 19.1. *Voluntary control model. (See text for explanation.)*

ABBREVIATIONS

CMC	= Central Motor Controller	BP	= Biological Probe
CF	= Central Feedback Pathway	E	= Exteroceptor
M	= Peripheral Motor Pathway	EA₁	= Directly activated exteroceptive afferent pathway
Eff	= Effector		
I	= Interoceptor		
IA	= Interoceptive Afferent Pathway	EA₂	= Indirectly activated exteroceptive afferent pathway
TR	= Transducer activated by (a) environmental effector-produced energy, and (b) internal effector-produced energy.	CSI	= Central Sensory Integrator
		CM	= Central Motor Pathway

stances of IA stimulation that have been paired with the EA referent from instances of IA stimulation that have not been paired with the EA stimulus (Kamiya 1969). There is also evidence to suggest that following calibration, instances of the previously paired IA activity will give rise to central activity similar to that produced by the EA stimulus with which that IA event has been previously paired. Thus Hefferline and Perera (1963) noted that when subjects had been trained to discriminate the occurrence of a virtually imperceptible muscle twitch with which an auditory stimulus had been paired and the auditory stimulus was faded out, subjects continued to discriminate the muscle twitch but also reported hearing the tone.

It will be recognized that exteroceptive feedback may occur simultaneously in a number of modalities and may be direct (EA_1) and/or indirect (EA_2). A form of indirect exteroceptive feedback that is essential to the development of instructional control over a motor activity is the verbal labeling of an act. In this case the experimenter simply tells the subject whenever he emits a particular response. Alternatively the experimenter may prelabel an EA stimulus, e.g., "When you hear the high-pitched tone your heart rate is high and when you hear the low-pitched tone your heart rate is low." This latter procedure is a form of sensory preconditioning. In both cases, however, the verbal label is considered to be a form of exteroceptive feedback, and its consistent pairing with the IA consequences of an act establish in such verbal stimuli the property of eliciting the RI.

Initiation of a Voluntary Act

Following calibration, an EA stimulus (including verbal feedback stimuli) will elicit the RI. This pattern of excitation in the CSI is assumed to operate on the CMC via the central motor (CM) pathway so as to elicit a specific pattern of activity transmitted to the Eff via the peripheral motor (M) pathway. The pattern of stimulation delivered via the CM pathway to the CMC is based upon the characteristics of the RI. It is assumed here that this pattern of CM stimulation results in the activation of those CMC circuits that were previously implicated in the production of the IA signals forming the RI in question.

Termination of the Voluntary Act.   Consequent upon Eff action that has been evoked by the presentation of a calibrated EA stimulus, feedback occurs in the IA pathway to the CSI. Here the resulting pattern of stimulation is compared to the pattern of activity represented in the RI. If the two patterns match, the RI is deactivated and the act completed; if they do not, additional motor signals are generated until a null state is achieved by the comparator mechanism.

It must be reemphasized that these processes are assumed to operate only during the development of voluntary motor control. Thus, it will be recognized that the functions of the different components of the motor control mechanism change as training proceeds. Initially the IA pathways provide a basis for the formation of the RI. Once the RI is established and has come under the control of an external stimulus, the function of the IA pathways is to transmit information on the basis of which Eff action may be evaluated and regulated. Central *feedback* (CF) initially serves to enable the formation of associations between EA and IA stimuli consequent upon Eff action. Once voluntary control over the Eff has been established and well practiced, such CF activity provides the primary feedback pathway in the regulation of the activity. Exteroceptive feedback, which is initially contingent upon Eff action and serves to calibrate the correlated IA feedback later in training, provides the initiating stimulus for the act in question.

In simple terms, this model proposes that compliance with an instruction to execute an act depends upon the ability of the instruction to evoke a memory (image) of the sensory consequences of the act. This ability in turn is assumed to rest upon the prior pairing of the words denoting the act with the internal sensations consequent upon the act. Finally, completion of the act is assumed to rely upon the comparison of sensations arising from present instances of the act with the image (memory) of previous instances of such sensations. The application of this model as an understanding of learned cardiovascular control is facilitated by a consideration of two common cases of deafferentation. These are referred to here as interoceptive and exteroceptive deafferentation and are illustrated respectively in Figures 19.2a and 19.2b.

Mott and Sherrington (1895) were the first to empirically document the observation that intrinsic deafferentation of an effector apparatus leads to loss of voluntary control over that effector. This preparation is illustrated schematically in Figure 19.2a. Although subsequent work (Taub, Bacon, and Berman 1965) has indicated that Sherrington overstated the effects of deafferentation, it is generally conceded that interruption of the afferent neural pathways will lead to a substantial impairment of performance involving the effectors served by those nerves.

Another common form of deafferentation that leads to a severe impairment of voluntary activity is observed in deaf humans and is illustrated schematically in Figure 19.2b. Such individuals have intact neural afferentation from the vocal apparatus, but, because of structural deficits, are not provided with the normal channels of exteroceptive feedback. In such cases individuals do not learn to produce articulate speech unless they are submitted to certain remedial procedures.

Although both these forms of deafferentation lead to some impairment of voluntary activities in the effector systems involved, the nature of the deficits and their treatments are substantially different. In both cases the provision of additional exteroceptive feedback serves to correct the impairment of voluntary control. Illustrations of the arrangements of afferent prosthesis for the cases of interoceptive and exteroceptive deafferentation are presented respectively in Figures 19.2c and 19.2d.

An example of the type illustrated in Figure 19.2c is the maintenance of postural and ambulatory responses in patients with tabes dorsalis. Such individuals, deprived of neural feedback from the lower limbs, are almost totally reliant on exteroceptive feedback (visual and/or auditory) for the control of these effectors. In the absence of visual feed-

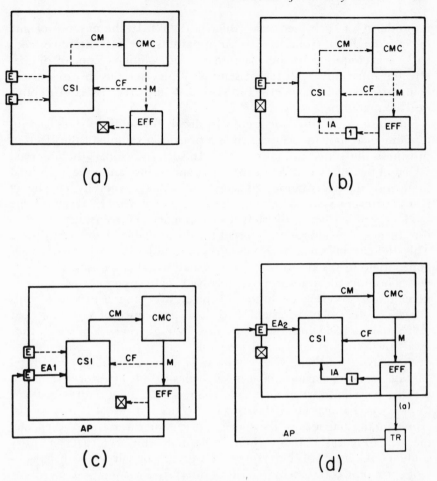

FIGURE 19.2. *Illustrations of disturbances in the voluntary control mechanism produced by (a) interoceptive and (b) exteroceptive deafferentation. The provision of exteroceptive feedback illustrated for interoceptive deafferentation in (c) and for exteroceptive deafferentation in (d) leads to restoration of voluntary motor control via the pathways indicated by solid lines (——————).* ABBREVIATIONS: *Same as in Figure 19.1, plus: AP = Afferent Prosthesis*

back a patient with tabes dorsalis is unable to maintain an erect posture. In such cases then, where interoceptive feedback is absent, exteroceptive feedback provides a functional substitute. The response image in this case is defined in terms of certain response-contingent exteroceptive stimulus changes, and the motor adjustments produced are relatively gross. In other words, afferent prosthesis in such cases is employed as a "crutch" to maintain performance, and its availability does not lead to learning (calibration) which eventually results in the redundancy of such feedback. (Bilodeau 1969) In the absence of any intrinsic feedback from an effector apparatus, the exteroceptive feedback is prerequisite to the maintenance of voluntary control of that effector apparatus. A different state of affairs pertains in cases where voluntary control of an effector system is impaired by exteroceptive deafferentation.

Substitution of visual or tactile feedback for auditory feedback in teaching deaf individuals to speak is a practical example of the afferent prosthesis illustrated in Figure 19.2d. In such individuals the observed deficit in voluntary control of the vocal apparatus cannot be attributed to intrinsic deafferentation, since deaf individuals generally have intact neural afferent systems serving the vocal apparatus. In terms of the model proposed here, this deficit in voluntary control is attributed to the absence of a calibrating referent for the available intrinsic feedback. This deficit, in turn, prevents the formation of response images appropriate to the production of articulate vocal responses. However, by calibrating the interoceptive feedback patterns in terms of some nonauditory referent, voluntary control over the activities of this effector system may be established. The procedure of enabling deaf individuals to feel vibrations in the fingers (Guberina 1955) which vary as a function of intensity and frequency of the audible consequences of the activities of their vocal apparatus is such a calibrating procedure. Certain sensations associated with activities in this effector system are reliably paired with certain tactile changes in the vibratory feedback display. As a function of this procedure the individual learns to discriminate the activities of the speech musculature in terms of their tactile consequences. Then, when presented with a target vibratory stimulus, the appropriate response image will be elicited with its consequent motor component. A critical difference between the effects of afferent prosthesis in such cases, compared to cases in which interoceptive deafferentation is present, is that in cases of exteroceptive deafferentation, when the exteroceptive prosthesis is withdrawn, voluntary control of the effector apparatus is maintained. In such cases, then, afferent prosthesis serves functions other than that of a performance crutch. The exteroceptive feedback does not substitute functionally for interoceptive feedback, but rather it calibrates the intrinsic feedback in terms of an external referent. Following calibration, variations in the referent system may be employed to elicit specific motor activities of the response system in question; in this case, the vocal apparatus.

It is assumed here that learned control of cardiovascular activity occurs according to the mechanisms described in this last example (Figure 19.2d). Given the apparent paucity of interoceptive feedback from the cardiovascular effectors when compared to that of the striate muscles, it could be argued that the mechanisms described for interoceptive deafferentation (Figures 19.2a and 19.2c) are more appropriate. At an empirical level, however, this alternative does not glean much support. The next section of this chapter describes a series of experiments on learned cardiovascular control that are relevant to these considerations.

THE VOLUNTARY CHARACTERISTICS OF HEART RATE

Although it is readily conceded by numerous investigators that heart rate changes may be systematically produced by verbal instructions (Brener and Hothersall 1966; Engel and Chism 1967a; Hnatiow and Lang 1965) in the presence of exteroceptive feedback of heart rate performance, few experiments report the influence of verbal instructions on heart rate in the absence of such feedback. So deeply entrenched are the prejudices against the possibility that heart rate may be controlled in the absence of exteroceptive feedback that this simple control procedure has been omitted almost without exception.

Brener, Kleinman, and Goesling (1969) did, however, observe that when naive undergraduates were instructed to successively increase and decrease their heart rates in the absence of any special feedback conditions, they did comply with these instructions. Although the differences between the mean increase and decrease heart rates were small (about 3 bpm), they were statistically reliable and were displayed by 9 of the 10 subjects submitted to the procedure. In a further experiment by these investigators, this effect was replicated and a practice effect was observed. Subjects who received no exteroceptive feedback displayed greater heart rate control on the second of two training sessions than they did on the first. In terms of the model proposed above, these observations may only be accommodated by drawing the inference that the subjects had developed appropriate heart rate response images. This in turn assumes the availability of interoceptive feedback associated with cardiovascular activity to the central sensory integrator and also the past calibration of such feedback in terms of the labels "heart rate increase and decrease." The nature of this calibration experience is subject only to speculative description. However, it would appear that heart rate increases are more subject to instructional and operant control than are decreases (Brener 1966; Engel and Hansen 1966).

Since most individuals report discriminable thoracic and auditory as well as other localized sensations during tachycardia, it could be argued that these collateral sensations serve to identify the heart rate increase response for the subject. Such sensations may, in turn, become associated with sensations arising from correlated striate muscle responses and also with environmental stimuli which provide the context of discriminable tachycardic episodes. The basis for a chain of associations leading to the verbal labeling of heart rate increases may, therefore, be considered to be available. Because bradycardic responses are relatively infrequent during normal functioning and because such responses are not associated with readily discriminable sensations, the verbal labeling of this response and hence its amenability to instructional control is relatively retarded. In view of these considerations, it seems unlikely that in the present cases instructions to increase and decrease heart rate elicited response images based on cardiovascular feedback. Rather it may be assumed that these instructions activated motor programs that were directed towards producing those sensations (striate muscle, respiratory, etc.) previously identified as "heart rate increases" during increase trials, and motor programs directed at eliminating such sensations during decrease trials. Regardless of the basis of the observed control, however, it will be recognized that these evidences support the classification of heart rate as a voluntary response in terms of the definition proposed earlier—it was systematically influenced by instructions. Although statistically significant, the magnitude of the observed heart rate effects was small relative to the normal limits of heart rate variation. In view of the procedures employed in these demonstrations this is not surprising.

Heart rate increments are generally imbedded in a complex of other activities including vigorous somatomotor adjustments. Since the subjects in these experiments were specifically instructed not to move or breathe irregularly while controlling their heart rates, it could be argued that they were receiving antagonistic instructions, in addition to being deprived of the most discriminable elements of the peripheral feedback associated with the tachycardic response complex, viz., a high level of proprioceptive stimulation.

In order to test this possibility a further experiment was run in which naive subjects were instructed to increase and decrease their heart rates in the absence of exteroceptive feedback, but also in the absence of any verbal constraints on movement. These subjects displayed mean increase-decrease heart rate differences of 7.05 bpm—over twice the magnitude of subjects who had received antagonistic instructions. Obrist et al. (Chapter 8) have reported a similar result—the greater the verbal constraints placed on somatomotor activity during learned heart rate control, the poorer the control. However, in accordance with the observations made by these investigators, where somatomotor activity was not verbally constrained, it was manifestly exhibited and bore a close correlation to the observed heart rate changes. In view of this, it seems reasonable to assume that the instruction to increase heart rate leads to a general motor activation with all of its attendant symptoms and the instruction to decrease heart rate leads to a general motor quiescence. In terms of the proposed model, this general motoric adjustment is specified in terms of, and regulated via, the easily discriminable peripheral feedback available from the striate muscles. This mode of parallel somato-cardiovascular regulation has previously been suggested by Smith (1967).

Because the instruction to control heart rate leads to a general behavioral adjustment of which heart rate is only one component, it might be expected that instructions to control other components of the general response would lead to similar adjustments with a similar heart rate effect. Since systematic respiratory changes had been observed to accompany the heart rate control evidenced in the experiments described above, it was decided to investigate the influence on heart rate of instructing subjects to control their respiratory activity. Under this procedure it was observed that subjects displayed a mean heart rate 8 bpm higher when they were hyperventilating than when they were hypoventilating[3]. In view of the similarity in the magnitude of the heart rate difference produced by these instructions, it might be concluded that similar response images and consequent motoric adjustments are produced by respiration and heart rate control instructions. Thus, although heart rate does display the characteristics of a voluntary response in the absence of any special conditions, it would appear that its voluntary characteristics are supported not by feedback of cardiovascular activity per se, but rather by a feedback constellation derived from the behavioral complexes in which heart rate responses are imbedded.

If we assume that both sets of instructions gave rise to similar states of general motoric activation or quiescence (viz., that they are functionally equivalent), then it should also follow that the provision of exteroceptive feedback identifying a desired performance goal should result in similar performance changes, regardless of whether respiration or heart rate instructions are given. In order to test this possibility an experiment was performed in which one group of subjects was instructed to increase and decrease their respiratory activity, and another group to increase and decrease their heart rate activity so as to produce 1 of 2 auditory stimuli. Regardless of whether subjects received respiration or heart rate instructions, on increase trials a high-pitched tone occurred whenever the subject's heart rate exceeded the upper quartile of his heart rate distribution, and on decrease trials a low-pitched tone occurred whenever the subject's heart rate fell below the lower quartile of his heart rate distribution. Subjects were informed that the occurrence of the appropriate tone signified that they were complying well with the instructions. The influence of this feedback procedure upon heart rate change for subjects given respiration and heart rate instructions is illustrated in Figure 19.3, together with the data from the previous two experiments in which no exteroceptive feedback was given. It will be seen that the provision of exteroceptive feedback of heart rate performance greatly enhanced the heart rate control exhibited by subjects given heart rate instructions, and had practically no effect on the heart rate difference induced by respiration instructions. The interpretation of this disparity in the effects of exteroceptive heart rate feedback is critical to the analysis of voluntary control proposed here.

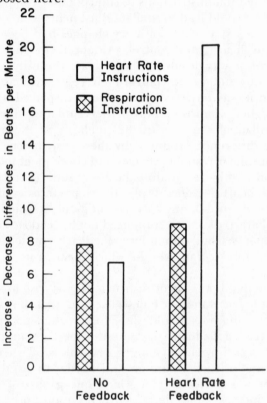

FIGURE 19.3. *Increase-decrease heart rate differences as a function of different combinations of instructions and feedback.*

It will be remembered that in terms of the proposed model, the primary function of an instruction is to specify the internal sensations that are consequent upon the act referenced in the instruction. In so doing, the instruction leads to the specification of a behavioral goal. Exteroceptive feedback, as it is employed in these experiments, also functions to identify instances of the desired act by virtue of its contiguity with the internal sensations deriving simultaneously from the act. In view of this, it will be appreciated that the efficacy of instructions in determining behavioral change resides in the past calibration of the internal sensations associated with the act in terms of the labels employed in the instructions. This, in turn, rests upon the relative discriminability of the sensations deriving from the act. On the other hand, the extent to which exteroceptive feedback is effective in promoting behavioral change to instructions depends upon the degree to which the internal sensations identified by the feedback stimuli are similar to those identified by the instructions. Where there is a lack of correspondence, facilitation of performance by exteroceptive feedback would not be expected. However, where the sensory consequences of the act are relatively indiscriminable and, by virtue of this, poorly calibrated, in terms of the instructional labels, exteroceptive feedback serves an augmenting function defining the behavioral goal more adequately and thereby facilitating performance.

Relative to heart rate responses, respiratory responses are easily discriminable. It is suggested, therefore, that in the case of the group that received respiration instructions and heart rate feedback, the behavioral goals specified by the instructions on the one hand and by the exteroceptive feedback on the other were in conflict. Since the response images associated with heart rate instructions are not as well formulated due to a lack of specific calibration of the intrinsic feedback associated with this response, exteroceptive feedback was the primary descriptor of the desired activity and led to a substantial enhancement of heart rate control. In summary, then, it may be concluded that instructions to alter heart rate in the absence of any special conditions leads to the production of a general motor adjustment of which heart rate changes represent one component. Similar heart rate changes may be produced by instructing subjects to control their respiration which is another component of the general motor adjustment complex. Heart rate control is, however, substantially improved by the provision of exteroceptive heart feedback, whereas the provision of such feedback does not enhance the heart rate changes associated with respiration instructions. The latter observation is explicable in terms of a conflict between the behavioral goals specified in the instructions on the one hand and by the exteroceptive feedback on the other.

Exteroceptive feedback may facilitate heart rate control in either or both of two ways. Such feedback may substitute for a lack of available intrinsic feedback; i.e., it may act as a performance crutch or, alternatively, it may serve to calibrate the available intrinsic feedback by defining the internal sensations associated respectively with high and low heart rates. Evidence in support of the latter possibility derives from an experiment by Brener, Kleinman, and Goesling (1969) who provided individuals with different amounts of exteroceptive feedback during training, and then tested their abilities to control their heart rates in the absence of such feedback.

Three groups of subjects were given increase and decrease heart rate trials on each of two sessions. On three trial pairs (a trial pair consisted of an increase followed by a decrease trial) interspersed among the training trials in each session, tests of heart rate control in the absence of exteroceptive feedback were made. On the other six trial pairs in each session, subjects received exteroceptive feedback of heart rate on 1 of 3 schedules. Subjects in the 100% group received feedback on all non-test trials, in the 50% group, on half of the non-test trials. Subjects in the 0% group did not receive any exteroceptive feedback during the experiment. The amount of heart rate control as measured by the mean intermedian inter-beat-interval (IBI) differences recorded during the increase and decrease test trials of the second session (no exteroceptive feedback available) were a direct function of the amount of exteroceptive feedback provided during training. This relationship is illustrated in Figure 19.4. In other words, the greatest heart rate control was exhibited by subjects who had received exteroceptive feedback on 100% of training trials, and the poorest control was exhibited by subjects who did not receive any exteroceptive feedback during training. It should be clear that this result is in accordance with predictions based upon the calibration model. Subjects who had most exteroceptive feedback available learned to distinguish the feelings associated with high and low heart rates best and were, hence, best able to control their heart rates in the absence of such feedback.

If it were true that learning to discriminate the activities of the cardiovascular system were an important prerequisite to the control of these activities, we might expect individuals trained to discriminate cardiovascular states to be better at controlling such states than individuals who were not provided with such training. This topic forms the substance of another experiment.

Evolving a procedure to test the discrimination of cardiovascular feedback poses innumerable technical problems. If the interest is to specifically investigate the discrimination of cardiovascular feedback, rather than feedback associated with correlated activities (such as respiration or muscle action), then requiring individuals to indicate when, for example, their heart rates are high or low is unsatisfactory. Under such a procedure, individuals have available to them a variety of feedback sources, any of which could be employed as the discriminandum. In view of this, we opted to test the ability of individuals to discriminate their pulses. The instructions were, very simply, to press a button whenever and as soon as a heart beat had been sensed. The assessment of discrimination employing this procedure also poses a number of problems. At first, we believed that we could obtain the requisite information by counting the different sequences of heart beat (HB) and buttonpress (BP) events. If a heart beat was followed by another heart beat without the interposition of a button-press, this would indicate that the subject had not discriminated the heart beat; if a button-press was followed by another button-press without the interposition of a heart beat, the subject had "seen" a heart beat that had not occurred. However, if a heart beat was followed by a button-press, this would represent evidence of discrimination.

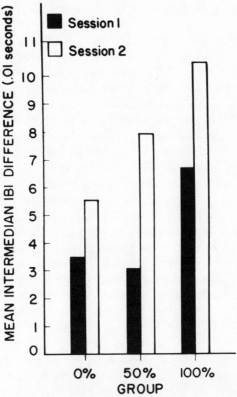

FIGURE 19.4.   *Mean differences in median IBI's recorded during heart rate increase and decrease trials in the absence of exteroceptive feedback following training under different schedules (0%, 50%, and 100%) of exteroceptive feedback.*

Although we obtained good learning curves employing this measure with a number of HB-BP sequences increasing systematically as a function of the subject's exposure to exteroceptive feedback, this was largely a function of the subject learning to press the button at approximately the same rate as his heart. We, therefore, decided to employ a measure of the latencies between heart beats and button-presses. This measure was based on the assumption that if the occurrence of heart beats and button-presses were not synchronized, the distribution of heart beat:button-press latencies would be rectangular in form, provided that appropriate corrections for truncation of the latency distribution by the IBI distribution were made. In other words, each button-press would have an equal chance of falling anywhere in the interval between two successive heart beats. If, however, the subject displayed a clear mode in the latency distribution, this would constitute evidence that he was using some sensory consequence of the heart beat as a cue for his button-presses.

Two groups of seven subjects each were run over each of three sessions. On the first two sessions, experimental subjects were submitted to the heart beat discrimination procedure; and control subjects, to a similar task that did not involve discrimination of the pulse. On the final session, all subjects were required to produce high and low heart rates with and without augmented sensory feedback of heart rate.

The discrimination sessions were broken down into seven blocks of four trials each. On the first three trials in each block, subjects were required to listen to a brief tone that occurred on each R-wave and to associate it with the internal sensations produced by the heart beat. On the fourth trial, no tones were presented and the subject was required to press the button whenever and as soon as he sensed each heart beat. Control subjects heard an irregular sequence of tones during the three trials of each block in the discrimination series and were required, on the fourth trial, to press the button so as to reproduce the temporal distribution of tones heard on the previous three trials. Evidence of discrimination was contained in the observation that the experimental subjects displayed a significant increase in the proportional frequency of the modal category of the latency distribution from the first to the second discrimination session. Heart rate control was assessed employing the same procedure for all subjects. The session consisted of four blocks of four trials each. Each block was comprised of alternate increase and decrease heart rate trials. On two blocks, subjects were provided with exteroceptive feedback of heart rate, and, on the other two blocks, subjects received no exteroceptive feedback. It was found that subjects who had been submitted to the pulse-discrimination procedure displayed better heart rate control under both feedback conditions, with the group differences reaching statistical significance on the second block of feedback and no-feedback trials. The results are illustrated in Figure 19.5. These data then provide support for the hypothesis that exteroceptive feedback may function to calibrate intrinsic feedback associated with cardiac activity, and that such calibration leads to a subsequent enhancement of heart rate control.

THE INTERACTION BETWEEN INSTRUCTIONS AND FEEDBACK

It will be appreciated that, in terms of the model of voluntary control presented here, instructions and exteroceptive feedback represent two sides of the same coin. In order for instructions to be effective, they must be cast in terms of the exteroceptive referent that has been employed to calibrate the intrinsic feedback from the response in question. Calibration, therefore, serves to provide an interface between the motor control mechanism and the environment. In computer language, the calibration system represents a compiler that translates the specific demands of the environment into the machine language of the motor control mechanism, assumed here to be framed in terms of interoceptive feedback signals. By examining the constellation of activities produced by various instructions it is possible to draw inferences regarding the prior calibration of interoceptive feedback in terms of the referent system employed in the instructions. Then, by manipulating exteroceptive feedback arrangements, it is also possible to recalibrate the system so that a given instruction will lead to alternative behavioral outcomes. Thus, it would be perfectly feasible to construct a training procedure whereby, on the issuance of a single foreign language command, one group of subjects would stand up and another group would sit down. In a sense, instructions to control visceral responses represent a foreign language to the human organism. In order to establish specific response-controlling properties in such instructions, appropriate calibration procedures must be performed. In particular, the subject needs to learn which states of the response apparatus are denoted by the symbols employed in the instructions.

Several reported observations are germane to these considerations. For example, it has been shown by a variety of investigators that blood pressure may be brought under voluntary control under conditions of exteroceptive feedback (Brener and Kleinman 1970; Shapiro et al. 1969). In these studies, significant blood pressure control in the absence of correlated heart rate changes was observed. The exteroceptive feedback employed to guide performance in these studies was specific to blood pressure variations. However, in subsequent studies, Schwartz (1972) has shown that when exteroceptive feedback is provided to subjects contingent upon associative and dissociative heart rate and blood pressure changes, parallel and antagonistic changes in these two aspects of cardiovascular activity may be produced upon command. Similarly, it is generally recognized that heart rate and respiration co-vary to a significant extent and that learned heart rate control is usually accompanied by systematic changes in respiration (Brener and Hothersall 1966; Shearn 1962). When, however, subjects are trained to control their respiration while also controlling their heart rates, it is observed that this relationship is not immutable (Brener and Hothersall 1967). Recently, Levenson and Strupp (1972) demonstrated that, although it is extremely difficult to establish heart rate control in the absence of its normal respiratory correlates, when subjects were provided with feedback of both heart rate and respiration, they exhibited significantly more respiration-independent heart rate control than when dual feedback was not provided.

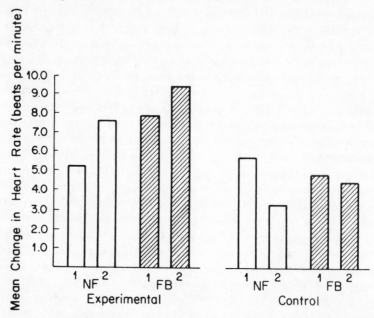

FIGURE 19.5.   *Mean differences in heart rate between Increase and Decrease trials in successive blocks (1 and 2) of Feedback (FB) and No-feedback (NF) heart-rate control trial blocks in one group previously trained to discriminate their pulses (Experimental) and another group (Control) not provided with such training.*

It can be argued, therefore, that the precise nature of the behavioral adjustment produced by an instruction may be controlled by appropriate manipulations of the exteroceptive feedback in terms of which the target behavior is defined. Two obvious constraints impose limits on the generality of this principle. These are, first, the biological constraints implicit in the functional and structural interrelationship of certain behavioral processes. Thus, it would seem extremely unlikely that a procedure could be devised to simultaneously increase striate muscle activity and decrease cardiovascular activity. On the other hand, increases in cardiovascular activity may well be established in conjunction with somatomotor quiescence. Presumably this type of dissociative learning forms the basis of diseases, such as essential hypertension, where the abnormality is not specified as much by instantaneous levels of cardiovascular activity but rather in terms of the somatomotor context in which these levels are evidenced.

The other constraint is imposed by the past calibration of intrinsic feedback from a given effector apparatus. Thus, in the experiment previously reported, where subjects were told to control their respiration and were provided with a heart rate goal, it was observed that the degree of heart rate control was not increased over the level displayed in the absence of such feedback. In this case it is assumed that the exteroceptive heart rate feedback described a behavioral goal that was not readily assimilable with the goal specified by the respiration instructions. These instructions had, over a long history of respiratory control, come to refer to internal sensations different from those identified by the exteroceptive heart rate feedback.

In order to further investigate the relationship between feedback and instructions, a series of experiments (Brener and Shanks 1972)[4] was performed in which subjects were instructed to increase and decrease either their heart rates (HRI) or blood pressures (BPI) under three feedback conditions: no feedback (NFB), heart rate feedback (HRFB), and diastolic blood pressure feedback (BPFB). In the two by three design, 10 naive undergraduates served as subjects in each of the six experimental groups. These groups are identified by the symbols BPI/NFB, HRI/NFB, BPI/BPFB, HRI/BPFB, BPI/HRFB, HRI/HRFB. Thus, for example, the BPI/HRFB group received instructions to control their blood pressures and feedback contingent upon heart rate variations. Each subject was run for one session during which he was required to increase the specified activity for seven consecutive trials, and then to decrease it for another seven trials. Rest periods were interspersed before, between, and following the blocks of experimental trials. In each group, the order of increase and decrease trials was counterbalanced, with five subjects receiving increase trials first and five receiving decrease trials first. In 4 of the 6 groups, feedback was provided to subjects during each training trial. On "increase" trials, a tone came on whenever and as soon as the feedback activity (either heart rate or blood pressure) exceeded a criterion value approximating the upper quartile of the subject's pretraining distribution on that measure. On "decrease" trials, the feedback tone occurred when the feedback activity fell below a criterion based upon the lower quartile of the subject's preconditioning distribution.

It is important to note that two groups of subjects received instructions to control one activity, either heart rate or blood pressure, and received feedback contingent upon variations in another activity, either blood pressure or heart rate. All subjects were led to believe that the feedback they received indicated success in complying with the instructions. Therefore, subjects in the BPI/HRFB and HRI/BPFB groups were told that the feedback reflected changes in the activity referred to in the instructions. Throughout the training procedure continuous recordings were made of heart rate, diastolic blood pressure, chin electromyogram (EMG), and respiratory activity[5]. The data were analyzed by subtracting the mean heart rate, blood pressure, EMG, and respiration scores obtained on decrease trials from the corresponding measures obtained on increase trials to yield a set of four difference scores for each subject.

A positive difference score indicated that the subject had displayed greater activity during increase than decrease trials on the measure in question. Figure 19.6 presents the median difference scores for each measure of activity for each group of subjects. It will be seen from these data that all median difference scores are positive, indicating that, in general, subjects displayed higher levels of activity during "increase" than during "decrease" trials in all responses monitored. Of the 60 subjects in this experiment, 51 displayed higher heart rates, 47 displayed a higher respiratory index, 42 displayed a higher EMG score, and 40 displayed higher diastolic blood pressures on increase than on decrease trials. This tendency indicates the power of the increase and decrease components of the verbal instructions. It also accords with a previous observation of ours (Brener and Goesling 1967) that instructions to decrease a feedback stimulus associated with subnormal heart rates did not lead to heart rate increases as substantial as those produced by instructions to increase a feedback stimulus associated with supernormal heart rates.

It will also be observed that the constellation of activities produced by each instruction/feedback combination is different. Close examination of these data reveals certain consistencies:

1. In general, greater difference scores are evidenced in the performances of groups which received feedback than in groups which did not.

2. Heart rate instructions led to a significantly larger EMG difference than did blood pressure instructions ($z = 2.66$, $p<.01$).

3. Significantly greater blood pressure differences were observed under conditions of blood pressure feedback than under conditions of either heart rate feedback ($Z = 2.08$, $p<.05$) or no feedback ($Z = 3.15$, $p< .01$).

4. Significantly greater respiratory differences were observed under conditions of heart rate feedback than under conditions of either blood pressure feedback ($Z = 2.71$, $p<.01$) or no feedback ($Z = 2.62$, $p<.01$). These general findings are made clearer by reference to Figure 7 and 8 which illustrate respectively the influence of instructions averaged across feedback conditions, and the influence of feedback conditions averaged across instructional conditions.

In terms of the model of voluntary control proposed here, these data warrant the following interpretations. The substantial EMG component elicited by heart rate instructions reaffirms the previous suggestion that

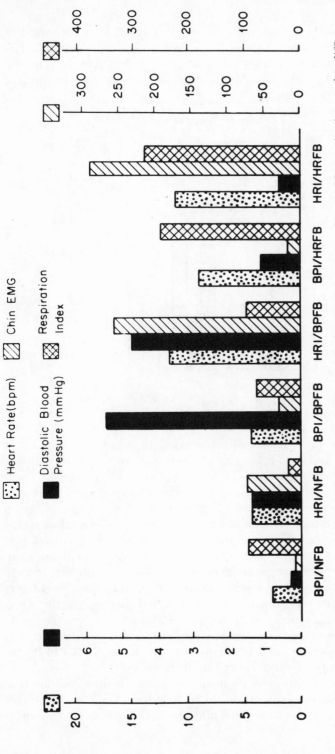

FIGURE 19.6. *Increase-Decrease differences in heart rate, diastolic blood pressure, chin EMG, respiration under different combinations of instructional feedback conditions.*
ABBREVIATIONS

BPI = Blood Pressure Instructions   BPFB = Blood Pressure Feedback
HRI = Heart Rate Instructions   HRFB = Heart Rate Feedback
NFB = No Feedback

in the absence of exteroceptive feedback this response is identified in terms of, and regulated via, feedback from the striate muscles. The production of substantial heart rate changes may, however, be achieved in the absence of correlated EMG changes as, for example, in the case of the BPI/HRFB group.

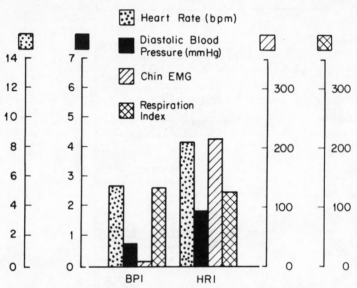

FIGURE 19.7. *Response profiles produced by Blood Pressure (BPI) and Heart Rate (HRI) Instructions.*

The provision of heart rate feedback led to a facilitation of heart rate differences and a more specific enhancement of respiratory differences. The fact that this response was specifically influenced by feedback contingent upon heart rate variations would tend to indicate that such respiratory changes are an integral aspect of the motor program identified by such feedback. In other words, the behavioral adjustments necessary for the production of exteroceptive heart rate feedback had a large respiratory component. This activity was not a significant component of the motor program identified by blood pressure feedback.

Blood pressure feedback tended to have a specific effect in enhancing blood pressure differences. It will be noted that significant blood pressure differences occur only under conditions of such feedback. The combination of heart rate instructions (associated with a substantial respiratory component) and blood pressure feedback HRI/BPFB also led to the induction of large heart rate differences.

Although this analysis is by no means complete, it does indicate that the behavioral adjustments produced by voluntary control procedures are a joint function of instructional and feedback influences. The influence of instructions would appear to depend on the discriminability of activities associated with the response referenced in the instruction. Thus, heart rate instructions gave rise to large EMG changes. It is assumed here that, in the absence of exteroceptive stimuli identifying the behavioral goal, subjects identify increases and decreases in heart rate in terms of such proprioceptive feedback. The behavioral adjustments produced by an instruction in the absence of exteroceptive feedback may, therefore, provide an indication of the interoceptive discriminanda employed by individuals to identify the activity specifically referenced in the instruction. Since blood pressure instructions did not of themselves produce significant blood pressure differences, we must assume that interoceptive feedback from the activity complex in which this response is imbedded have not been previously calibrated in terms of an external referent.

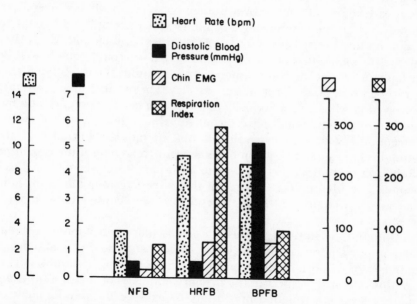

FIGURE 19.8. *Response profiles associated with No Feedback (NFB), Heart Rate Feedback (HRFB), and Blood Pressure Feedback (BPFB) conditions.*

The constellation of activity changes induced by the provision of exteroceptive feedback is considered here to provide an indication of the behavioral correlates (components of the motor program) associated with the production of the response upon which the feedback is contingent. Thus, it was observed that heart rate feedback gave rise to substantial respiratory differences. Although these differences were associated with corresponding large heart rate differences, the relationship between these two aspects of behavior does not appear to be immutable. In the HRI/BPFB group, for example, substantial heart rate changes were evidenced in the absence of corresponding respiratory changes.

CONCLUSIONS

An attempt has been made here to describe the processes of learned cardiovascular control in terms of a general model of voluntary behavior. Within the framework of this model, the development of instructional control over an activity is seen to depend on the subject learning the association between the words employed in the instruction, and on the sensory consequences of the acts to which those words refer. Particular emphasis has been given to the development of verbal control over cardiovascular behavior, because words represent the most pervasive source of control over human behavior. It will be recognized, however, that the exteroceptive stimulus which is employed initially to calibrate the internal sensations associated with an act and which later serves to initiate that act need not be verbal—it could equally well be a light or a tone or some other simple stimulus. It is assumed that precisely the same mechanisms as have been described here are involved in what we traditionally call "operant conditioning." Undoubtedly, reinforcing stimuli have incentive value although, with very few exceptions, such incentive value is not an intrinsic property of the stimulus but rather a function of some prior treatment of the organism. Reinforcing stimuli are also, for the most part, exteroceptive feedback stimuli that identify occurrences of the correct response and, presumably, serve to calibrate the interoceptive sensory consequences of such responses.

Although the study of learned cardiovascular control has an obvious and important practical goal in its clinical application, it also has a number of important nonapplied implications which should not be overlooked. With respect to the primary emphasis of the present chapter it provides a unique opportunity to explore the development of motor control. Unlike the striate musculature, the cardiovascular effectors and other visceral response systems do not have a history of instructional control. They represent an almost virgin territory with respect to the influence of instructions and response-contingent feedback and, as such, their study provides a powerful source of knowledge concerning the development of voluntary control in general.

In addition to providing a tool for the investigation of general principles of behavior, operant and voluntary cardiovascular techniques promise to shed light on the functional organization and dynamic characteristics of cardiovascular control. Thus the arrangement of exteroceptive feedback following the occurrence of constellations of activity rather than changes in a single modality (Schwartz, 1972) may be employed to investigate biological constraints on the plasticity of learned cardiovascular change. Alternatively, by making feedback contingent upon more restricted changes in cardiovascular activity and by examining the nature of behavioral changes in related response systems, the nature of normal behavioral integration may be examined.

NOTES

1. Sherrington (1906) distinguished between proprioception which was specific to the striate musculature and interoception which referred to feedback from the autonomic effectors. This distinction is not observed here so as to maintain the apparent functional equivalence of the different internal feedback pathways in the execution of voluntary activities.

2. Such central feedback mechanisms have also been proposed to account for the acquisition of motor control over deafferented effectors (Taub and Berman 1968).

3. Engel and Chism (1967b) have reported that requiring subjects to breathe at rates 25% higher and lower than their mean respiratory rates did not produce significant heart rate differences. It should be noted that Engel and Chism paced the respiration rates of their subjects, whereas no pacing was employed in the present case. Experiments in our laboratory have validated this observation of Engel and Chism, and it would appear that when the rate of respiration is artificially controlled, subjects compensate for the changes in rate by moderating volume with a consequent stabilization of pulmonary air turnover. In the absence of the rate constraint, however, subjects comply with instructions to increase and decrease respiratory activity by hyper- and hypoventilation respectively.

4. This research was collected by Emily M. Shanks as part of her doctoral dissertation, University of Tennessee.

5. The amplified EMG signal was rectified and fed to a voltage-to-frequency converter which provided a numerical reading reflecting the integrated EMG level exhibited by the subject on each trial. Respiration was recorded by a rather unorthodox method. Respiratory activity was sensed using a nasal thermistor. This probe was employed to produce a voltage which increased during expiration and decreased during inspiration. The output voltage of the transducer circuit was fed to a voltage-to-frequency converter which provided a numerical respiratory index at the end of each trial. This index varied as a direct function of the total expiratory activity. In other words, the longer the time the subject spent expiring and the greater the volume of his expiration, the higher was the numerical index. Thus the index varied inversely as a function of respiration rate, but directly as a function of magnitude. Although this is an anomalous measure, as is indicated in the text, it was systematically and significantly influenced by the independent variables employed in this study. It was, for example, observed that of the 60 subjects employed in this experiment, 47 displayed a higher respiratory index during decrease trials than during increase trials. To simplify the presentation of these data, the respiratory difference scores (increase − decrease) were multiplied by −1.

20

PETER J. LANG

Learned Control of Human Heart Rate in a Computer Directed Environment

INTRODUCTION

Over the last decade a number of investigations have shown learned changes in heart rate associated with the administration of contingent heart rate feedback. In studies of animal subjects these experiments have followed the strict form of the instrumental conditioning paradigm (Miller 1969). Thus, animals are placed in a restricted environment over which the experimenter has almost total stimulus control. In general the response repertoire of the animal is also drastically reduced through the administration of curare. Primary reinforcers (most notably, direct stimulation of the medial forebrain bundle) are then administered contingent on the desired heart rate changes. Shaping schedules can be used to augment initially small responses, and dramatic increases or decreases in heart rate have been reported. Furthermore, the method allows for considerable response specificity, and organs which normally covary can be adjusted independently, with what appears to be remarkable precision.

Studies of heart rate feedback with human subjects defy such concise description. While successful demonstrations antedate the animal studies (Lisina 1958; Shearn 1962; Hnatiow and Lang 1965), the magnitude of reported effects has been more modest (particularly if we consider heart rate deceleration) and the psychophysiological interpre-

This research was supported in part by grants from the National Institute of Mental Health (MH-10993, MH-35,324) and the Wisconsin Alumni Research Foundation.

tation of the obtained changes has not been obvious. Most investigators are inclined to consider the results of feedback studies as evidence of instrumental conditioning. However, the operant paradigm is applied to the human subject only with great difficulty. Ethical considerations prevent the subject isolation and stimulus control needed for efficient instrumental learning. Human volunteers go only where they want to go, and powerful reinforcers cannot generally be used to control their behavior. Instead, we enter into a kind of social contract with the subject. The "reinforcers" (mild shocks, unpleasant tones, nudes, and nickels) are often simply counters which provide information on success rate, within the context of an overall instructional set. Thus, shaping cannot be used in quite the same way as with an animal subject. Our control is limited, and the human subject's response to a detected change in the schedule of reward may be to angrily "give up," or to reinstruct himself to strive for different (perhaps lower) goals than those proposed by the experimenter.

Furthermore, we cannot simply eliminate most of a subject's response repertoire with curare or physical restraints. He learns heart rate control with an intact somatic system, including the partially covarying respiratory apparatus. It is unlikely that we can just ignore these somatic events. They may have to be independently trained, or special instructions given, if success is to be achieved.

Finally, there are vast individual differences in motor skill, and there may be similar variation in the ability to control a viscus. It is possible that many subjects are poor visceral learners. I mean this in the sense that there are "natural" athletes, and others who, despite prodigious practice, continue to be "duffers." I have suggested elsewhere (Lang 1970) that the target population for practical visceral training might well be made up of such poor learners. It is not unreasonable to assume that, if heart rhythm and blood pressure can be modified through learning, deviation in directions dangerous to health would be unlearned in response to normal environmental contingencies. In other words, individuals with psychosomatic illnesses could be a population with a specific visceral learning deficit.

All these considerations suggest that the training of human subjects to control their own heart rate resembles only metaphorically the operant conditioning of animals. The greater intellectual capacities of the human subject and the freer conditions under which he performs radically changes the learning situation. Thus, the literature on human skills learning (Bilodeau 1966; Fitts and Posner 1968) is, I believe, more relevant to developing self-control of the viscera, than is research on animal conditioning. In any event, we need to pay more attention to such things as the subject's instructional set and the optimal characteristics of the feedback display (relative to the information processing capacity of human subjects). We need to know more about the effect of social motivation on performance, and the role of individual differences. Furthermore, we need to consider the role of language mediators and somatic muscle activity, not as something to be ignored or eliminated, but as response systems which often covary with cardiovascular change and which could facilitate the visceral learning of intact subjects.

CURRENT RESEARCH

Our research effort is broadly oriented toward the above goals. Specifically, we are interested in training human subjects to bring their heart rhythm under instructional control. In the present paper, I will describe our computer based procedure. I will also report some new findings relevant to the optimal characteristics of feedback displays, as they relate to different heart rate learning tasks, and will consider the role of incentives in visceral learning. I would like to emphasize at this point that these data were collected recently and are, in some cases, only partially analysed. Thus, any conclusions must be considered tentative, and requiring the benediction of subsequent, cross-validating research.

Computer Programmed Procedure

Our present research program is built around a machine controlled experimental procedure. A Digital Equipment Company LINC-8 or PDP-12 administers and times the entire sequence of experimental stimuli. It is used to present instructions, generate a feedback display, record data from two physiological systems, and provide summaries of the subjects' performance at the end of the experiment.[1] This controlled environment permits an unusual degree of precision in the execution of an experiment. It is expected to greatly facilitate the replicability, between subgroup samples and across different experiments, necessary to the extended study of biofeedback effects.

The feedback display that we presently employ has the following characteristics. The subject is seated in a reclining chair before a large oscilloscope screen. Each heart cycle initiates a moving line, starting at the left, which extends itself across the screen at a constant rate. In the standard program, this line is turned off by the next electrocardiogram (EKG) cycle, a horizontal marker is briefly illuminated at the terminus, and within microseconds a new line starts across the screen. Thus, the length of successive horizontal lines is exactly proportional to the length of each successive R-R interval.

The screen also contains a fixed, vertical line running from top to the bottom of the screen. This is the subject's target. If the subject is asked to speed his heart rate, his job is to terminate the horizontal line before it crosses the target. If his task is slowing, the horizontal line must extend past the target for a success to be recorded. Each success is underscored for the subject by the appearance of the work "good" on the screen, at the completion of the cycle. The display is illustrated in Figure 20.1.

The target line is initially set at the subject's median R-R interval. This is done during a 1-minute period, at which time the subject is asked to perform the desired task (speed or slow) without feedback. The target may be altered subsequently, depending on subject performance. The schedule is as follows: If during feedback trial, a slowing subject's median heart interval should exceed that of the previous trial, a new target is set for the next feedback period, which is midway between his previous median and his current median. A similar adjustment to a less difficult target is made for subjects who show "poorer" performance on a trial. We call this schedule the "rule of halves." It is designed to prompt improved performance without making discouraging demands.

The format of the experimental session is the same for all subjects. Following the attachment of a respiration sensor and the heart rate electrodes, the adjustments of heart cycle and respiration input levels, and a brief rest period, control of the experiment is assumed by the computer. Three minutes of baseline data are acquired. The subject is then instructed to attempt heart rate control (speed or slow depending on the task, for a 1-minute period). He is subsequently instructed to use the feedback display for the same purpose, and the display is then presented for 3 minutes. After termination of the display, subjects are asked to continue control (speeding or slowing for 1 minute). Subjects are then given a 1-minute rest. This sequence of feedback trial, transfer trial, and rest is repeated five times during an experimental session.

Experimental Studies

Several experiments employing this basic procedure are currently underway. Both normal college students and patients with heart disease serve as subjects. A primary concern of this research is the establishment of basic parameters which modulate performance. While there are many demonstrations of human learning through biofeedback, we do not yet know much about the dimensions of this task. A great variety of procedures have been employed. Information has been fed back through various modalities. Investigators have simulated the operant paradigm, signaling subjects only when they make a successful or unsuccessful response. Others present continuous analogue representations of the viscera being trained. Various combinations have also been used, e.g., analogue feedback with an operant administration of palp-

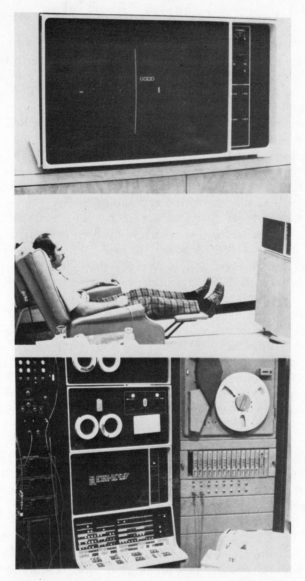

FIGURE 20.1. *The feedback display as it appears on the subject's monitor is shown in top photograph. The long, verticle line represents the target. The short verticle line indicates the point at which the last "R" wave terminated a sweep line. As this mark exceeds the target line (heart slowing task), the word* Good *is presented. The short horizontal line at the right shows the point of initiation for the next sweep.*

A subject is shown in the center photograph, observing the feedback display. The computer is shown at the bottom. The experimenter's monitor displays the instruction: "The feedback display will now be presented to help you decrease your heart rate."

able reinforcers. Most of these procedures have resulted in some success. However, the critical elements of the task have not been
delineated. We do not know what parameters to emphasize in order
to augment the current, modest learning effects, and produce a training program of clinical value.

In line with the above goal an initial focus of our research has been
an analysis of the feedback itself, the effects of altering its frequency
and specificity on the degree of heart rate change achieved. We are
guided in part by earlier studies of motor learning. Thus, Trowbridge
and Cason (1932) studied the effects of feedback in a line drawing task.
Subjects made over 100 drawings, in an effort to reproduce a standard
target line. A group receiving precise, directional information (in deviations of ⅛ inch) showed superior performance to a group that received
only a digital, correct/incorrect feedback. In her early paper on vasomotor control, Lisina (1958) reported a similar effect. Initial efforts
to shape vascular change through shock avoidance were unsuccessful;
however, control of both vasoconstriction and vasodilation was obtained
when subjects were permitted to watch their continuous vasomotor
changes on the polygraph during conditioning.

Bilodeau and Bilodeau (1958) systematically evaluated frequency of
information feedback (knowledge of results) in a motor task. Subjects
were required to adjust a lever within one hundredth of a degree of
an arc. Different groups were told their direction and magnitude of
error, either every trial, every third trial, or after every fourth trial.
The group receiving knowledge of results every trial showed clear
superiority in performance over the less frequently informed groups.
In this study, the absolute number of feedback trials determined the
level of performance; the number of interspersed trials in which no
information was provided had no effect on learning.

The above results suggest that frequent and precise feedback enhances learning. However, it is also possible that analogue presentations of a rapidly changing viscus, such as the heart, may represent
input at a rate too rapid for a subject to process. Furthermore, other
research in motor learning suggests that the degree of transfer
achieved may be negatively related to amount of feedback. Thus Lincoln (1954) compared the effects on a tracking task of continuous
analogue feedback versus a summary error score at the end of a trial.
Subjects were instructed to turn a crank handle at a constant rate. Subjects receiving analogue feedback observed a dial while performing.
Both groups learned the task, although the subjects receiving only summary scores did so at a somewhat slower rate. However, on those criterion trials which were administered with no feedback, the summary
score group was superior in performance to subjects who had watched
the dial. Lincoln suggested that close attention to the external dial pre-

vented the analogue feedback subjects from attending to their own internal, kinesthetic cues. They were not tuned to their own intrinsic feedback, but to an external crutch. When denied this support, their performance deteriorated. On the other hand, subjects receiving only summary scores were forced to increase their sensitivity to internal cues, which facilitiated their performance when all external information was withdrawn. It is not unreasonable to assume that similar effects may apply in visceral learning.

In a recent experiment from our laboratory, Robert Gatchel studied the effects of varying frequency of feedback information on learning to accelerate and decelerate heart rate. It will be recalled that the computer heart rate display involves a moving horizontal line, initiated by an EKG cycle and terminated by the subsequent cycle. This constitutes a true analogue representation of heart rate (with the moving line acting as a real time clock) and, thus, the highest frequency of feedback input. However, the program can be modified such that not the next, but any specified succeeding cycle terminates the clock line. Thus, information about heart rate may be fed back to subjects at any frequency, as accumulations of several successive R-R intervals. The target line is of course adjusted to the new learning unit, and the spatial characteristics of the display remain constant.

In the present experiment three feedback frequencies were assessed, 1-beat, 5-beat, and 10-beat units. The 1-beat unit is continuous feedback. A 5-beat accumulation approximates the length of a respiratory cycle, and might be expected to have special characteristics for that reason. The 10-beat unit represents a gross summary of performance, and is uncorrelated with other natural rhythms of the body. From a cybernetic point of view, the 1-beat group is favored. However, the considerations of processing rate limits and special requirements for transfer mentioned earlier, suggest that larger learning units could be more efficient.

All experimental groups were compared with a control group that worked with a similar moving line display, which was generated by the computer rather than the subject's heart. Under this condition, the subject's task was to monitor the lines and press a microswitch whenever a line terminated on the designated side of the display target line (to the left for speeding controls, and to the right for slowing controls). If the subject pressed his button within 300 microseconds of line termination, the word "good" was illuminated as it was for the successes of feedback subjects. Previous research (Lang, Sroufe, and Hastings 1967) has shown that this type of tracking task has unconditioned effects on heart rate very similar to those generated by a feedback trial.

Ten college student subjects were assigned to each group, and each subject was seen for a total of six sessions. The previously described standard format was used in all sessions. All subjects performed the tracking task during sessions 1 and 2. Controls also continued tracking during the subsequent four sessions. The other groups were administered two speeding and two slowing sessions, randomly assigned within blocks of two.

Results and Analysis

Subjects mean heart rates for the first speeding session are presented in Figure 20.2. The data include the initial resting rate and all subsequent feedback trials. The superiority of the 1-beat group is clear. The effect is somewhat enhanced in session 2 (Figure 20.3). It will be noted that the 10-beat group now also shows some learning, relative to tracking controls. Analysis of variance and planned contrasts of means confirmed these findings. All feedback groups generated faster rates than tracking subjects (F = 5.99, 1/36, p < .025). In addition, subjects receiving continuous analogue feedback (1-beat group) show faster heart rates than the two feedback groups (F = 4.26, 1/36, p < .05).

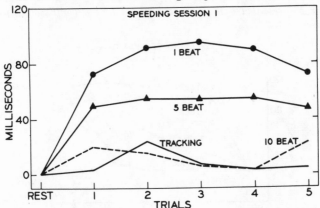

FIGURE 20.2.   *Speeding session 1. Changes in average R-R interval length over feedback trials for the tracking and three feedback groups.*

These differences were also observed when subjects were instructed to continue heart rate speeding in the absence of further feedback. Transfer period performance during session 2 is shown in Figure 20.4, expressed as deviations from the median R-R interval at initial rest. Feedback subjects were again superior to tracking (F = 5.17, 1/36, p < .05). The 1-beat group was marginally superior to the other heart control task subjects (F = 4.11, 1/36, p < .10).

These data demonstrate that success at the speeding task varies systematically with frequency of information feedback. Continuous analogue feedback produced the greatest heart rate change. The 5- and 10-beat samples produced less change. These differences persisted dur-

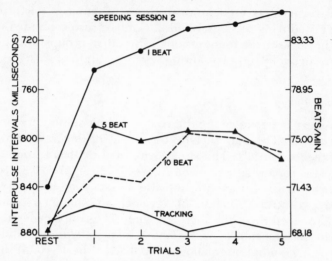

FIGURE 20.3.   *Average heart rhythm for all experimental groups during speeding Session 2, presented both in R-R interval length (milliseconds) and beats per minute.*

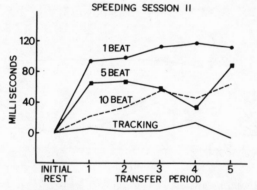

MEDIAN INTERPULSE INTERVALS DURING TRANSFER PERIODS
EXPRESSED AS DEVIATIONS FROM INITIAL REST

FIGURE 20.4.   *Speeding Session 2 transfer trials, presented as change in R-R interval length. Transfer trials immediately followed feedback. Subjects were provided with no exteroceptive information about their heart rate during these periods.*

ing transfer trials, and there was a tendency for all feedback groups to improve over sessions ($F = 3.88$, 1/36, $p < .10$).

The results for the heart rate slowing task present a different picture. Feedback trial performance for this task is shown in Figures 20.5 and 20.6. As for the speeding task, feedback resulted in performance superior to that of tracking controls ($F = 8.67$, 1/36, $p < .01$). However, there is no significant differences between feedback groups. Furthermore, the feedback trained subjects are not different from tracking controls during transfer. There is a significant trial's effect for the slowing task (F = 17.51, 4/144, p < .001), suggesting some tendency to improve within a session; however, no significant improvement was found over sessions.

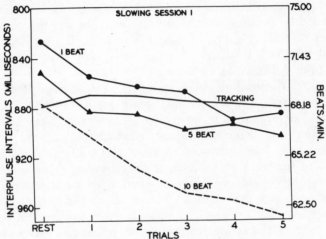

FIGURE 20.5.   *Average heart rhythm for all experimental groups during slowing Session 1, presented both as R-R interval length (milliseconds) and beats per minute.*

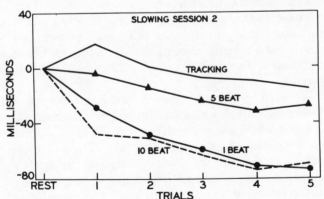

FIGURE 20.6.   *Slowing Session 2 changes in R-R interval length for all experimental groups.*

These results imply that heart rate slowing and heart rate speeding depend on very different mechanisms. The speeding data follow a pattern that might be predicted for a motor performance task, i.e., more frequent information prompts greater success (Bilodeau and Bilodeau

1958). The slowing results support a general feedback effect, but, in contrast to speeding, they do not suggest that slowing performance is finely tuned to information input.

The effects of information frequency on speeding transfer were the same as for feedback trials. The 1-beat group showed a faster heart rate than the 5- or 10-beat groups. Thus, low information rates did not yield greater transfer, as suggested by some motor skills research (Lincoln 1954). Furthermore, significant transfer was not obtained for any heart rate slowing group. Relative to their resting rate, subjects who had received feedback showed no slower heart rates during transfer than did tracking controls.

Changes in respiration were examined to determine if this system paralleled the speeding and slowing heart rate differences. An analysis of median respiration rate during feedback trials revealed no differences among the three individual feedback frequencies. However, respiration rate was significantly faster for the combined feedback groups than for tracking subjects. During slowing there was a similar lack of respiration rate differences between feedback groups, and the combined feedback groups did have slower respiration during actual feedback trials than did tracking subjects when working on their task. Furthermore, variance in respiration cycle length was significantly greater for all feedback groups, during both speeding and slowing, relative to tracking subjects. Again, there were no differences in respiration cycle length variances between groups receiving the different frequencies of feedback information.

Thus, change in respiration rate or variability in cycle length does show some covariance with the successful use of heart rate feedback. However, it is not uniquely associated with speeding, nor does it vary systematically with feedback frequency (as heart rate does during speeding trials).

We have recently observed some other interesting differences between speeding and slowing. In Figure 20.7, average performance during feedback trials are presented graphically for a small group of subjects (N = 6) studied over several weeks. These subjects received repeated speeding and slowing sessions following the already described standard format, using a 5-beat sweep display.[2]

These subjects were drawn from introductory psychology classes and originally participated to receive extra course credit. Subsequently, they were paid a flat salary of $2.00 per session for continuing in the experiment. After three speeding and four slowing sessions had been completed, they were permitted to work for additional monetary incentives. In these "piece work" sessions, two successful 5-beat sweeps resulted in 5 cents being paid to the subject. Furthermore, any feedback or transfer trial in which the subjects median performance exceeded his previous maximum, resulted in an additional 50 cents.

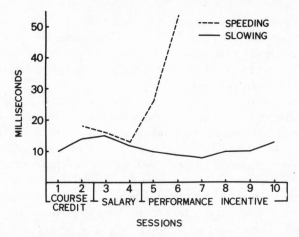

FIGURE 20.7. *Performance over speeding and slowing sessions of six college student subjects, seen over a period of several months. Heart rate is shown as change in average R-R interval length from the initial rate for that session. On this figure improved performance (either speeding or slowing) is indicated by an upward movement in the curve. Note that little difference between speeding and slowing sessions is apparent until the performance incentive (extra money for correct responses) was instituted.*

As can be noted in Figure 20.7, with the onset of incentive sessions subjects immediately improved speeding performance, often increasing their heart rates 60 to 70 beats over resting levels. However, no positive change in slowing performance was observed, despite the fact that rewarded practice in slowing continued over six individual sessions.

Discussion and Conclusions

The observed differences in speeding and slowing performance could be an effect of initial values. Subjects in these experiments were well habituated to the laboratory and average rest period heart rates were quite low (less than 70 bpm). It could be argued that further reductions would press built-in physiological limits, and, thus, for slowing trials, they could not be large. Analogously, the failure to find a difference in feedback frequency for slowing subjects could be attributed to the smaller overall change, which would make it difficult to observe the subtler effect of differential information.

The correlation between resting rate and change during slowing trials does not provide great support for this hypothesis ($r = .36$). A very small percent of the variance is accounted for by this relationship—no more than by the relationship between resting rate and speeding performance ($r = .47$), in which direction this limitation presumably does not exist. Nevertheless, the resting rate of the subject relative to his own range of rates may be more important than his rate relative to the group of subjects. That is to say, each subject has a certain normal range of heart rates over a 24-hour day. During the rest period of the experiment, subjects may have been near the bottom of their own range. This limitation on performance would not necessarily be reflected in a between subjects correlation.

Except for anecdotal reports of exceptional men (yogi, and the like), there have been no studies of learned changes in heart rhythm in which subjects have exceeded rates that occur normally in response to other stimuli or states. An individual's range of rates over a 24-hour period may represent a limited area within which feedback training can change heart rhythm. Super-normal control may be the consequence of a genetic, athletic ability and may not be something that the average person can expect to acquire. To determine with certainty whether such limits exist, and if there are true directional differences within it, we will have to examine subjects with habitually fast or slow rates and broad and constricted ranges, and to systematically evaluate the speeding and slowing performance of individual subjects at different base levels within their known 24-hour range.

It is possible that the differences between speeding and slowing represent a differential involvement of striate muscle mediators. That is to say, the data for speeding are similar to what we would anticipate for a motor task. The differential effects of information frequency may reflect the fine tuning of respiratory changes, particularly respiration depth, (see Sroufe 1971b) and muscle tension. This implies that the mechanism of slowing is more clearly autonomic learning (perhaps a function of direct vagal innervation), and that the relationship of autonomic control to information frequency is different than for the striped musculature. There is no conclusive evidence for or against this possibility in these experiments. Both groups showed some evidence of respiratory change correlated with success in the heart rate task. However, the relationships were different for speeding and slowing, and it is not clear from these preliminary data what role respiration played in heart rate change for either task.

We are currently beginning to explore some of these possibilities. We are also interested in the effects of arousal reducing instructions on heart rate slowing (e.g., autogenic training, Jacobsen's relaxation procedures), both separately and in tandem with heart rate feedback. It seems likely that arousal level exerts some limiting influence on heart rate slowing. One might hypothesize that the failure of subjects to improve when large monetary incentives were offered was due to the excitement and stress occasioned by the procedure, which acted to inhibit the subject's efforts to slow heart rate.

With Dr. William Troyer, we have also begun work on the evaluation of heart rate speeding and slowing among patients with ischemic heart disease. While it is too early to report definitive results, we have been surprised to note that—in contrast to college students—these older, patient subjects seem to have more difficulty increasing rate than decreasing heart rhythm. We should know soon whether this phenomenon is determined by the presence of disease, or is simply an effect on learning of increasing age.

Our present experimental program is now about one year old, and we are beginning to reap the benefits of the procedural uniformity provided by the computer. A replication has been completed of the experiment described earlier, on information frequency and heart rate speeding. It resulted in a clear cross validation of the initially observed effects and encourages our view that a computer directed laboratory provides unusual procedural stability. We believe that this system will be a powerful tool in the analysis of the instructional control of heart rate. We also hope to define methods applicable to the therapeutic control of cardiac rhythm, that it may become a useful aid in the treatment of cardiovascular disease.

NOTES

1. The programs used in this precedure were written by Michael Falconer. The design of specialized, ancillary hardware and machine maintenance was accomplished by Kent Hayes.

2. Tom Cheng, Linda Gannon, Robert Gatchel, Jean Holland, and Craig Twentyman assisted in running these subjects.

21

GARY E. SCHWARTZ

Toward a Theory of Voluntary Control of Response Patterns in the Cardiovascular System

INTRODUCTION AND REVIEW

Common sense tells us that it is indeed adaptive for animals, including man, to have evolved a highly specialized and automatic system for keeping its tissues alive and healthy. For all practical purposes, the total plumbing comprising the cardiovascular system is "involuntary" in that it performs its complex functions without requiring conscious effort or "will"—hence, under normal circumstances we need not divert attention from our daily activities to maintain and control our heart rate, blood pressure, and so forth. Furthermore, when all systems are working properly, there is little conscious experience of these functions to compete with those sensory and cognitive processes necessary for registering and processing information from the environment. Only under conditions of extreme emotional or physical exertion (e.g., the throbbing heart beat in fear) or with certain diseases (e.g., the pain of angina pectoris) does feedback from the cardiovascular system enter consciousness and modify ongoing behavior.[1] On the whole, it seems self-evident that were it necessary for man to consciously perceive and control all the complexities of maintaining blood flow throughout the body, he would have neither the time, nor the ability, to do much of anything else. On the other hand, not so obvious is the realization that by keep-

Preparation of this chapter was supported in part by a grant from the Milton Fund of Harvard University and by the Advanced Research Project Agency of the Department of Defense and monitored by the Office of Naval Research under Contract N 00014-70-C-0350 to the San Diego State University Foundation.

ing the systems away from conscious or voluntary control, man could not easily make serious bodily mistakes that would disrupt the intricate balance necessary for maintaining the internal structures. In other words, the biological constraints of the homeostatic mechanisms serve not only to protect man against environmental changes and demands, but also against himself.

Contrary to this evolutionary, biological approach to cardiovascular activity, most of the recent research on the voluntary control of physiological responses through feedback and reward has assumed, and emphasized, the similarity of all bodily processes (both somatic and visceral). Whether the theoretical model be learning to press a bar for food (the traditional operant conditioning model—Miller 1969; DiCara 1970b) or learning to shoot a golf ball into a hole (a motor skills model—Brener Chapter 19; Lang Chapter 20), the idea is essentially the same: to posit that all responses have some potential to act independently, both centrally and peripherally, and, therefore, can be selectively brought under voluntary control when provided with the appropriate contingencies of feedback and reward.[2]

Support for this position grew as research began to uncover specificity of learning in the autonomic nervous system of curarized rats on a par with that normally observed in the skeletal system (e.g. Miller and Banuazizi 1968). In early work with humans on operant conditioning of electrodermal activity (Kimmel 1967; Shapiro, Crider, and Tursky 1964) and heart rate (Hnatiow and Lang 1965; Engel and Hansen 1966), the major theoretical issue was also whether these responses could be "directly" conditioned (assumed to be the case for somatic responses), or if the autonomic changes were "mediated," that is, caused by other responses such as overt motor movements or cognitive events (Katkin and Murray 1968; Crider, Schwartz, and Shnidman 1969). However, since at the level of brain it becomes meaningless to talk about any overt response, either visceral or somatic, as being "not mediated" neurophysiologically, the concept of "direct" conditioning or control comes to have little theoretical or practical use. With the luxury of hindsight it can be seen that the mediation issue was a negative research endeavor in this context, for it attempted to "blame" autonomic learning on something else, rather than to raise the more positive and important questions concerning the specific psychophysiological mechanisms underlying autonomic control.

On the other hand, the concept of mediation does prove to be of value when specifically applied to self-regulation of blood pressure, because in order for blood pressure to change, something in the plumbing of the cardiovascular system must "cause" it to change. The term "plumbing" is not used here facetiously, because the pressure of a liquid in a closed circulatory system is, in fact, directly determined by the operating characteristics of the pump, the tubing, and the state of the liquid itself. Consequently, if a person is given feedback and reward for lowering his blood pressure and his pressure does decrease, he has in some way reduced his cardiac output or peripheral resistance, or both. That is—since pressure is at all times a complex, changing sum or integral of these factors—when a subject is given feedback and reward for specific changes in pressure, he is really receiving the feedback and reward for some *pattern* of cardiovascular effectors, those responses over which he has neural and/or hormonal control. Unfortunately, in order to actually investigate such ongoing patterns of activity, it becomes necessary to be able to: (a) continuously monitor all the relevant factors, which in the case of blood pressure is technically exceedingly difficult; and, (b) calculate the relationships between the functions in a systematic and meaningful manner. Given these difficulties, coupled with the state of knowledge and the theoretical climate at the time, it is not surprising why operant-feedback researchers did not intially address themselves to these questions.

The first published report demonstrating operant control of blood pressure was performed in rats paralyzed by curare (DiCara and Miller 1968c). Using a signalled shock escape-avoidance paradigm for criterion changes in systolic blood pressure, it was found that subjects in the increase group learned to raise their systolic pressure about 30 mmHg above their initial resting level of 139 mmHg, while the subjects reinforced for systolic decreases dropped their pressure about 27 mmHg. In addition to the large magnitude of these effects, of particular interest was the finding that the changes in systolic blood pressure occurred independent of both heart rate and body temperature. Although this finding of specificity was viewed with some surprise, the authors did not enumerate why they did—or did not—expect that only the systolic pressure would change, nor did they speculate as to what was the cause of the pressure changes.

Dissociation of systolic blood pressure from heart rate was subsequently replicated in a series of studies in humans (Shapiro et al. 1969; Shapiro, Tursky, and Schwartz 1970a; Brener and Kleinman 1970), although the magnitude of these effects were smaller than those obtained in the curarized rat. Unlike the DiCara and Miller (1968c) blood pressure paradigm and subsequent animal experiments (e.g., Plumlee 1969; Benson et al. 1969), relatively long trial periods were used in the human blood pressure work (e.g., 1 minute) so as to require more tonic as opposed to phasic changes in autonomic activity. Again, the human researchers did not go on to explain why specificity effects were obtained, nor what the mechanisms of the learning could be.

To further evaluate the systolic blood pressure-heart rate dissociation question, Shapiro, Tursky, and Schwartz (1970b) reversed the procedure; subjects were given binary (yes-no) feedback for increases and decreases in heart rate (modeled after their binary blood pressure system) while at the same time monitoring systolic pressure. They found that under these conditions subjects learned to increase and decrease their heart rate without simultaneously changing their systolic pressure. In addition, when Shapiro, Tursky, and Schwartz (1970b) selected out their best learners in both the heart rate study and in the earlier blood pressure study, they still found no evidence for simultaneous learning in the corresponding function. As a result, the authors concluded that the operant changes in blood pressure were not caused by changes in heart rate, and that other variables, such as stroke volume and/or peripheral resistance, were probably involved.

However, more questions were raised than answered. For example, why did systolic pressure change without also changing heart rate? Does this imply that these functions are unrelated such that reinforcement for one leads to simultaneous random reinforcement for the other as well, and vice versa? Is it possible to teach subjects to simultaneously control their systolic blood pressure and heart rate in the same direction or make them both go in opposite directions, and how would this be done? Why does it appear that decreases in systolic pressure—and heart rate—are more easily learned than increases? Are there any constraints in systolic pressure control such that heart rate would also be affected? Altogether, is it possible to determine under what conditions combinations of functions will be learned, and how is this related to the specific nature of the physiological systems involved?

DEVELOPMENT OF THE INTEGRATION— DIFFERENTIATION MODEL

In lieu of these and related questions, an initial model was formulated to help provide a combined behavioral-biological framework for understanding and predicting learned patterns of physiological activity (Schwartz 1971b, 1972). Like many theoretical conceptions, the core of the model is inherently simple and makes reasonable common sense, whereas the actual application of the approach quickly reveals the complexity of the interactions and the emergence of new, yet to be solved problems. However, this need not necessarily hamper the heuristic value of the formulation; for, as it turns out, the phenomena under investigation are inherently complex.

Central to the model are the concepts of (a) contingency and (b) constraint. The term contingency is borrowed from operant conditioning (Skinner 1953), but is used more broadly here to refer to the systematic following of any behavioral event (a response, such as a bar-press, a golf swing, or a heart rate change) by either an environmental event (an external stimulus, such as food or a tone), or a biological event (an internal stimulus, such as afferent signals from stretch receptors in the muscles). Used in this manner contingency simply means "information" about a behavioral response. However, close examination reveals that as information "contingency" can serve two different purposes, and, therefore, should be subclassified into two general forms. One form of information can be called "state contingency," stimulation that tells the organism the state of his own behavior. This aspect of contingency is similar to the concept of "feedback," particularly continuous or "analogue" feedback (be it internal or external) as employed in the biofeedback area. However, the second form of information is more selective and can be called "task contingency," stimulation that tells the organism that it has "done the right thing." Task contingency would be similar to the traditional binary or "digital" concept of contingency used in operant conditioning: "You have made the correct response."[3]

It follows that a "reinforcer," when it is presented "contingently" (as opposed to randomly or "noncontingently"), is a special case of a task contingency where the digital information contains incentive value as well (Estes 1972). Thus, food for a hungry animal can be used as a reinforcer, as can be a tone for a human—if it signifies monetary reward, or in some cases simply success in doing the task. In most learning situations, an organism usually has both state and task forms of contingency or information available to him; he knows the state of his limbs, and he knows when he has done the right thing with them to obtain—or in the case of punishment to avoid—the incentive. Similarly, if a person is given analogue meter feedback for beat-by-beat changes in heart rate and then is told to make the needle of the meter go to the right (and therefore earn a bonus, or just succeed), he now also has both state and task contingencies operating—with incentive value as well. However, it should be clear that in the case of most autonomic, as opposed to somatic, processes, if the subject is given only task information (e.g., binary reinforcement) his *conscious* awareness of his own behavior is limited to that supplied by the digital shaping procedure itself.

Although traditional learning theory maintains that the precise nature of the contingency is crucial for the learning of "simple" behaviors, such as pressing a bar (Skinner 1953), the implications and applications of these principles to the learning of multiple responses are yet poorly understood and documented. If for the moment the analysis is restricted to the simplest use of contingency, that being the digital (yes-no, or up-down) case of task contingency, then one approach to the problem of pattern learning is to carefully analyze what else is being simultaneously "reinforced" when feedback and reward (contingency and incentive) are given for a particular function (Schwartz 1972). Systolic blood pressure and heart rate are good responses for illustrating this general approach, because both functions show discrete bursts of activity that can readily be reduced to digital response units.

With every normal heart contraction, blood pressure rises and reaches a systolic peak, its magnitude determined by a complex interaction of heart rate, stroke volume, and peripheral resistance (Rushmer 1961). If average (mean) levels are specified for heart rate (HR) in bpm and for blood pressure (BP) in mmHg, it is possible to classify at each heart beat whether HR and BP values are above (^{up}) or below ($_{down}$) their tonic levels. Therefore, at each heart beat only four coincidence patterns are possible: BP ^{up} HR ^{up}, BP $_{down}$ HR $_{down}$, BP ^{up} HR $_{down}$, and BP $_{down}$ HR ^{up}.

If systolic blood pressure and heart rate were naturally related over time, such that increases in one were always associated with increases in the other (BP ^{up} HR ^{up}) and vice versa (BP $_{down}$ HR $_{down}$), then when an experimenter chose to give feedback and reward for one (e.g., BP ^{up}) he would unwittingly provide the identical contingency for the other as well (HR ^{up}). Therefore, from learning theory it would be expected that both functions should, in fact, learn simultaneously, and in the same direction. Although not totally satisfactory, the term integration has been used to refer to such a case where two autonomic functions increase and decrease together in "sympathetic-like" directions (Schwartz 1972).

If these two functions were so related that whenever one increased the other simultaneously decreased (BP ^{up} HR $_{down}$) and vice versa (BP $_{down}$ HR ^{up}), then if feedback and reward were given for one (e.g., BP ^{up}) the other would simultaneously receive the opposite contingency (HR $_{down}$). Here, it would also be expected that both functions would learn, only now they should change in opposite directions. This case has been previously referred to as differentiation, where two functions move in "opposite directions" (Schwartz 1972).

However, neither of these results were empirically obtained. Therefore, according to learning theory, it would follow that systolic blood pressure and heart rate must be unrelated such that digital feedback for one results in some form of simultaneous, but random, reinforcement of the other. Although it is physiologically the case that blood pressure rises and reaches peak systolic at each normal heart contraction, the operant-feedback data suggest that at any given point in time, the magnitude of the pressure rise cannot simply be related to the duration of the preceding heart cycle. Were the relationship between BP and HR truly random, the frequency of the four possible BP-HR patterns would each occur only 25% of the time. When learning of one function occurs without simultaneous learning in another, this has been referred to as specificity of learning.[4]

Close scrutiny reveals that two somewhat separable factors are involved: (a) the exact nature of the relationship between two or more responses; and, (b) the precise manner in which the contingency is given. Learning theory would dictate that the behavioral relationship between responses should, in part, be defined by the nature of the reinforcing procedure itself. Simply stated, in order to predict simultaneous learning of patterns of functions, it makes sense that their relationship must in part "be seen through the eyes of feedback and reward" (Schwartz 1972). This theoretical point of view proves to be especially valuable, for it suggests a practical way to define and measure patterns of responses in real time: by arranging separate independent contingencies (or shaping procedures) for each function in question and then determining the degree to which reinforcement for one is simultaneously accompanied by reinforcement for the others (simple "and" logic circuit). In addition, by not actually presenting the feedback and reward, it is possible to assess these behavioral relationships over time without directly influencing the subject.

A second advantage to this approach is that it provides a workable procedure for providing feedback and reward for specific patterns of functions. To the extent that patterns of responses are naturally learned when simultaneously reinforced, one approach to teaching a subject to control specific patterns of functions is to deliberately provide the subject with feedback and reward for the desired pattern. Returning to the systolic blood pressure and heart rate example, if when using a digital response definition procedure, it is found that these functions rise and fall together 50% of the time (BP ^{up} HR ^{up} and BP $_{down}$ HR $_{down}$ responses each occurring only 25% of the time), then it should be theoretically possible to teach subjects to integrate their systolic blood pressure and heart rate—voluntarily raise or lower both functions simultaneously—or differentiate them—voluntarily make them go in opposite directions—by providing the digital feedback for the desired pattern of responses. Furthermore, to the extent that each pattern occurs equally likely, learning theory would predict that each of the four patterns can be learned equally well.

To summarize, it is hypothesized that (a) the relationships between physiological responses over time, coupled with (b) the exact nature of the contingency administered, each determine the degree to which learned specificity or patterning occurs. Although this formulation may provide a useful first step in the prediction and control of multi-autonomic functions using operant-feedback techniques, it must be incomplete, for it treats physiology as if it operates in a vacuum, without constraints (Schwartz 1972). By constraint is meant any causal restriction that inhibits, or augments, the direction and time course of physiological activity over time. One class of constraints has been broadly described as "changing operant baselines" (Crider, Schwartz, and Shnidman 1969.) In most operant autonomic studies to date, researchers have plotted their data relative to some preexperimental baseline obtained at the beginning of the experiment, implicitly assuming that this baseline reflects a stable, non-changing operant level. However, this assumption is not usually viable when applied to autonomic functions, for over the course of a session many factors not related to the contingency variable per se, such as initial excitation, sensitization, and habituation, may influence autonomic activity over time.

For example, in a replication of a single session systolic blood pressure experiment, lights and tones were used as feedback and slides of nude females, landscapes, and monetary bonuses were used as rewards (Shapiro, Tursky, and Schwartz 1970a). Three experimental groups were used. Included were not only the traditional increase and decrease reinforcement groups, but also a third group of "random reinforcement" subjects who were given comparable instructions, feedback and reward, but for whom the blood pressure contingency was removed by randomly presenting half the stimuli for BP^{up}s and half for BP_{down}s. The results for this group show that systolic blood pressure naturally rises above the initial baseline, and then eventually returns to baseline under the particular conditions of this experiment. Since the learning effect occurs above and beyond the constraints of these noncontingency factors, the interpretation of the shape and time-course of the increase and decrease groups cannot be accurately evaluated without taking into account this changing baseline. Clearly, knowledge of baseline constraints can help improve the ability to predict the shape and time course of learned autonomic control.

When more than one function is considered concurrently, the question of constraints becomes even more important, and more complicated. For example, if the functions differ in the way they respond to the experimental situation, thus producing different changing baselines, these differences must be evaluated in order to compare learning across functions. Another possible type of constraint concerns the relative ease with which subjects can learn to control specific patterns of functions. In the systolic blood pressure-heart rate example, it was predicted from learning theory per se that subjects should be able to integrate, as well as differentiate, these functions to a similar degree. However, this prediction would fail if physiological constraints were preventing heart rate and blood pressure from changing independently, either by keeping them together or by pulling them apart. In this manner, the discrepancy between the predicted and measured extents of learning would uncover the ways in which the constraints were operating. Conversely, by independently assessing the nature of the constraints beforehand, it should be possible to improve the ability to predict the ease with which subjects can learn to control different patterns of physiological activity.

Speculations as to how various physiological, environmental, and cognitive constraints can influence the learned control of patterns of cardiovascular activity will be presented later in the chapter. However, before outlining these complications, some experimental data specifically addressed to the prediction and control of patterns of cardiovascular activity through feedback and reward will be discussed.

CONTROL OF PATTERNS OF SYSTOLIC BLOOD PRESSURE
AND HEART RATE THROUGH FEEDBACK AND REWARD

To assess the behavioral relationship between systolic blood pressure and heart rate, as well as provide feedback and reward for specific BP-HR coincidence responses, a system for detecting each of the four BP-HR patterns per beat was developed (Schwartz 1972; Schwartz, Shapiro, and Tursky 1971) using a digital detection procedure described in Figure 21.1. A digital (task contingency) procedure was developed because: (1) The earlier research had used digital feedback procedures, and it was important to make comparisons across studies as meaningful as possible. (2) Digital analyses are easy to understand and evaluate using solid state programming equipment (Grason Stadler 1200) (on-line computer facilities are necessary for more complex wave form analyses). (3) The equipment developed for measuring systolic and diastolic blood pressure (Tursky, Shapiro, and Schwartz 1972) was restricted in that phasic, beat-by-beat changes in pressure can only be reliably detected as digital events (above or below the constant pressure in the cuff), although tonic (median) pressure can be accurately ($\pm$ 2 mmHg) obtained as interval data. Parenthetically, the technical constraint of the blood pressure recording system was a fortuitous accident, for it dictated the use of a simple model for reducing complex functions to easily understood and theoretically relevant digital units.

However, this procedure has some inherent complications which should be briefly outlined before considering the data, especially since the definition of a "response" is an important determinant of contingency effects. First, whether or not BP or HR is classified as above or below a given value depends on where this criterion value is set with regard to the total distribution of pressures and rates. It is only when the tonic levels for each function are set at their correct median values—half the values being above the tonic level and half below it—that it is possible to accurately assess the true phasic distribution of the four BP-HR coincidence responses. For example, if at the start of a given trial the blood pressure and heart rate levels are set at their

EKG

Cardiotachometer

Korotkoff sounds

ID marker

Feedback-reward marker

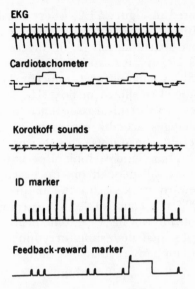

FIGURE 21.1. *Representative portion of a polygraph record of the integration-differentiation (ID) system in operation. Shown are the electrocardiogram (EKG), heart rate (HR) displayed through a cardiotachomoter, Korotkoff sounds measured at a constant cuff pressure, and two marker channels. Dashed lines represent the approximate levels of the three electronic switches. The presence or absence of a Korotkoff sound relative to the constant pressure in the cuff indicates whether blood pressure (BP) is up or down, while HR is rated up or down relative to the median HR. After each heart cycle (except during a reward) one of four possible marks appears on the ID marker channel. The longest and shortest marks indicate integration, with $BP^{up}\ HR^{up}$ producing the longest mark and $BP_{down}\ HR_{down}$ producing the shortest mark. The other two marks indicate differentiation, with $BP^{up}\ HR_{down}$ producing the third longest mark, and $BP_{down}\ HR^{up}$ producing the second shortest mark. The bottom channel indicates which one of the four possible combinations is eliciting feedback (short mark) and reward (long mark). In this example, feedback is occurring for $BP_{down}\ HR^{up}$ differentiation. (from Schwartz 1972)*

respective medians, but the subject immediately raises his tonic blood pressure level by 4 mmHg so that he is now almost always above the constant cuff pressure level, then he will be producing almost 100% BP^{up} responses, and the system will only detect $BP^{up}\ HR^{up}$ and $BP^{up}\ HR_{down}$ coincidence responses. This will occur even though phasically his blood pressure is likely waxing and waning around its new tonic value. Therefore, subjects can learn to increase or decrease their blood pressure and heart rate in this system by either changing the phasic relationships between the functions, or by changing the tonic values, or by changing some combination of both. The extremes of this are schematically illustrated in Figure 21.2, where it can be seen that two functions (A and B) can wax and wane together phasically (phasic integration), but move apart tonically (tonic differentiation—the combination shown in box II), or they can be phasically moving in opposite directions (phasic differentiation) yet tonically be moving together (tonic integration—together shown in box III). It should be stressed that this is not purely a procedural issue since, to the extent that the phasic and tonic changes actually represent different physiological processes with different constraints, the degree to which a subject learns to change the phasic and/or tonic aspects of a single function or pattern of functions will depend on: (a) exactly what the criteria of feedback and reward is; and, (b) the nature of the constraints involved. For example, it is conceivable that learning to increase levels of circulating epinephrine will increase tonic heart rate without necessarily affecting vagally-mediated sinus arrythmia, phasic heart rate changes that often accompany regular breathing.

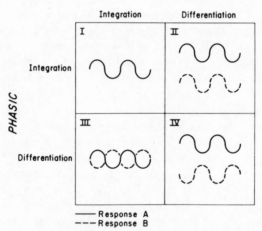

FIGURE 21.2. *Sine waves illustrating differences between tonic and phasic integration and differentiation for two hypothetical responses (A and B). (From Schwartz 1971b)*

An experiment was designed to empirically assess both phasic and tonic constraints in the feedback and reward situation (Schwartz 1972). Forty male subjects were given: (a) a standard series of five resting trials with cuff inflation (each trial 50 beats long, trials separated by 20 to 30 seconds of no stimulation-cuff deflation); and, (b) five trials of random reincorcement where feedback and reward occurred equally likely for each of the four BP-HR patterns. Then, all subjects received 35 conditioning trials where feedback and reward were given for 1 of the 4 coincidence patterns. In this way, it was possible to measure the frequency and sequence of the phasic coincidence patterns during rest and in response to random stimulation, and at the same time assess tonic reactions to random stimulation, including the degree to which changes in tonic values in one function were related to tonic changes in the other. Finally, to make the experiment as comparable to the earlier studies as possible, similar instructions and incentives were employed.

Examination of the data, in conjunction with the earlier findings, proved to have solid predictive value in terms of the degree and time course with which subjects were able to learn to control patterns of systolic blood pressure and heart rate (see Figure 21.3). First, in light of the earlier data it was predicted that the curves would "look" as if it was easier to lower blood pressure and heart rate than to raise them (particularly when the level reached after random reinforcement —the procedure used in the present experiment—is used as the baseline). This was based on the observation that both systolic blood pressure and heart rate tend to adapt during the session, especially using as a baseline those values obtained after the first five trials of feedback and reward (which typically produces an initial increase in tonic levels in both BP and HR). It was further expected from the previous data that the curves would show heart rate dropping more than blood pressure, because when mmHg and beats per minute (bpm) are compared on the same axis (a reasonable scale to use in light of the magnitude of effects obtained and the equivalent nature—± 2 mmHg or ± 2 bpm—of the tracking procedure) systolic blood pressure appears more stable and shows somewhat less of a decrease than does heart rate. These results can be seen on the left panel of Figure 21.3, showing large decreases in blood pressure and heart rate, with BP_{down} HR_{down}, integration training (p < .0001), plus a slightly greater drop in heart rate relative to blood pressure for each of the two integration conditions (p >.05).

Close examination of the integration curves reveal some interesting additional findings. One is that, unlike the earlier systolic blood pressure-heart rate data (where learning did not appear until about 10 to 15 trials), the learning of integration patterns occurs almost immediately. Second, comparing increase to decrease conditions, the magnitude of the effects for both blood pressure and heart rate are now somewhat larger than those obtained when each was singularly reinforced and specificity of learning occurred! Although the integration subjects received on the average 50% less feedback and reward per trial (since BP^{up} HR^{up} and BP_{down} HR_{down} were found to each represent but half of the total ups and downs for the functions alone), they nonetheless learned more quickly, and produced somewhat larger changes. This does not appear simply to be a "partial reinforcement" effect, because, as shown on the right of Figure 21.3, differentiation training, which also resulted in about 50% less feedback and reward, yielded smaller effects and required more trials to evidence learning. According to the model, these data imply that systolic blood pressure and heart rate are somewhat constrained in this situation, tending to be more tonically integrated than differentiated.

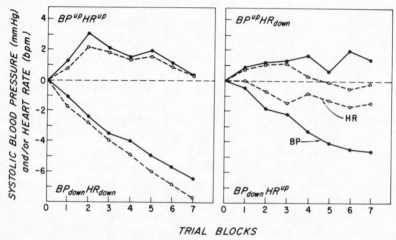

FIGURE 21.3.   *Average systolic blood pressure and heart rate for subjects receiving feedback and reward in the four coincidence patterns. On the left are the data for the two integration conditions; on the right are the data for the two differentiation conditions. Solid lines are BP, dashed lines are HR. Each point is the mean of 10 subjects, 5 trials each, set to zero by the last random reinforcement trial. Beats per minute and millimeters are therefore on the same axis. (from Schwartz 1972)*

Analysis of tonic reactivity to random reinforcement provides further support for this conclusion, and since it "preceded" the training period, it has important predictive value. The data indicate that median levels of blood pressure and heart rate tend to naturally change together ($r = 0.36$, p. $< .05$). For example, if a subject reacted to the beginning reinforcement trials with a large tonic increase in blood pressure, his heart rate tended to show a comparable rise in level. However, since this relationship accounts for less than 15% of the variance, it shows that there is inherent room for change. Consequently, learning can occur in the opposite direction, as indicated by the significant ($p < .0001$), although smaller, magnitude effects obtained with differentiation feedback and reward. It should be noted that were this relationship not actually constrained and, therefore, causally linked in the nervous system, then, despite the observed concurrence of the two functions, learning of integration and differentiation would have been equally likely. The pattern reinforcement procedure serves to uncover the degree to which a correlation actually represents a causally linked relationship.

Analysis of the phasic (beat-by-beat) changes during both rest and random stimulation revealed that the frequency of the four coincidence responses were equally likely, about 25% each. This supported the prediction that in order for specificity of blood pressure and heart rate to have been obtained in the earlier studies, systolic blood pressure and heart rate must be randomly related, at least from a digital reinforcement point of view. However, close analysis of the sequence of response patterns over time reveals that the relationship is not truly random. Rather, the data showed that heart rate was about 90° out of phase and in front of systolic blood pressure, which simply stated says "first comes the heart, then comes the pressure." This sequence is roughly as follows, repeating itself about every 10 beats: BP_{down} HR_{down}, BP_{down} HR^{up}, BP^{up} HR^{up}, BP^{up} HR_{down}, and finally BP_{down} HR_{down}, etc. For example, the data showed that when a BP_{down} HR_{down} pattern changes, 70% of the changes go to a BP_{down} HR^{up} pattern. Therefore, to the extent that BP_{down} HR_{down} patterns consistently precede the BP_{down} HR^{up} pattern, reinforcement for the latter produces consistent, although delayed, reinforcement for the former as well. This is an example of a response chaining factor. A similar analysis can be applied to the BP^{up} HR_{down} condition. As the results in Figure 21.3 confirm, subjects reinforced for BP_{down} HR^{up} patterns tend to lower both responses as well, while subjects reinforced for BP^{up} HR_{down} patterns tend to raise both functions as well. On the other hand, with natural tonic integration acting as a further constraint, it would be predicted that the response chaining factor would have less influence when integration BP-HR patterns were directly reinforced.

These findings illustrate the complexity involved in simultaneously evaluating the tonic and phasic properties of multisystems, particularly in relationship to contingency and constraint factors. Space does not allow a detailed analysis of the possible predictions involved, for example, in determining which of the two differentiation conditions should be more readily learned (Schwartz 1971b). However, if it is assumed that the findings are reliable and reflect on interaction of contingency and constraint variables, then the data provide new information concerning pattern learning and control in the cardiovascular system. Further experiments parametrically manipulating both contingency (e.g., response definition, shaping procedures, etc.) and constraint (e.g., drug studies, exercise conditions, etc.) factors are needed to tease out the various effects.

Altogether, the data demonstrate that it is possible for human subjects to develop some control over the relationship between their systolic blood pressure and heart rate when they are provided with feedback and reward for the desired pattern of blood pressure and heart rate. When the behavioral relationship of these functions is analyzed, and when natural constraints are taken into account, it is possible to understand and predict the resulting pattern of learned control. However, these initial findings need to be carefully applied to other systems and other problems before being justified in considering the generality of the conclusions. The following studies on diastolic blood pressure and heart rate provide some additional support for these ideas.

CONTROL OF PATTERNS OF DIASTOLIC BLOOD PRESSURE AND HEART RATE THROUGH FEEDBACK AND REWARD

Whereas phasic changes in systolic pressure are not usually directly mediated by heart rate (more so by contractility changes—Obrist et al. 1970b), phasic changes in diastolic pressure can readily be a direct cause of heart rate change, since the longer the pause in a given beat, the longer time there is for the pressure to continue falling after the systole (all other things being equal). These brief phasic changes occur despite the fact that the tonic level of diastolic pressure is in large measure determined by peripheral resistance factors (e.g., arteriolar tone). Hence, if a subject were given digital feedback and reward for brief as well as more sustained changes in diastolic pressure (a characteristic of the current blood pressure system), it would be predicted that he would learn to control both his heart rate *and* peripheral resistance, since both systems would be partially integrated with the feedback and reward.

Unlike the earlier systolic blood pressure-heart rate specificity findings, when a similar digital feedback and reward procedure was applied to the control of diastolic pressure per se—using similar instruction, trial periods, and so forth—it was found that simultaneous learning in heart rate also occurred (Shapiro, Schwartz, and Tursky 1972). The results are particularly interesting because: (a) whereas the diastolic blood pressure begins to diverge by the first trial block, reaching almost half its maximum learning by the third block of trials, heart rate does not begin to evidence learning until after the third block of trials; and, (b) the magnitude of the heart rate learning is much reduced when compared to direct (100% correct) digital feedback for heart rate itself (Shapiro, Tursky, and Schwartz 1970b). Thus, the data suggest that the initial stages of learned diastolic blood pressure control probably reflect changes in peripheral resistance, whereas in the later stages of training cardiac changes may add to the total magnitude of the pressure differences observed.

According to the model, were diastolic pressure and heart rate completely integrated from a reinforcement point of view, then heart rate would have shown learning comparable to the early heart rate reinforcement study. This was not the case. However, since partial heart rate learning was in fact observed, it would be predicted that heart rate and diastolic pressure must be partly, but not completely, integrated. Analysis of the frequency of the four possible BP-HR coincidence responses revealed that $BP^{up} HR^{up}$ and $BP_{down} HR_{down}$ tend to occur on the average about two-thirds of the time, thus confirming the prediction.

What implications do these findings have for determining the extent and ease with which subjects can voluntarily integrate or differentiate their diastolic pressure and heart rate? If the observed relationship between diastolic pressure and heart rate reflects causally linked processes, it would be predicted that: (a) subjects should be readily able to learn to further integrate their diastolic blood pressure and heart rate when given feedback and reward specifically for integration responses; and, (b) subjects should find it difficult (especially when compared to the earlier systolic blood pressure-heart rate findings) to differentiate their diastolic blood pressure and heart rate when given feedback and reward for differentiation responses. One further prediction is also in order. Although a random reinforcement group was not employed in the Shapiro, Schwartz, and Tursky (1972) study, it can be inferred what random reinforcement might look like by simply averaging across the increase and decrease curves separately for each response. This would inflate the estimate slightly, to the extent that it is easier for subjects to increase rather than decrease their responses against the changing baseline. Nonetheless, the results suggest that while average heart rate tends to drop over the experiment (as did average systolic pressure), the average over 35 trials for diastolic pressure is an increase. Hence, if this constraint difference between the two systems is strong, it should maintain itself despite the contingencies of reinforcement imposed.

With these considerations in mind, an experiment was performed using the same experimental design; tracking procedures for tonic blood pressure and heart rate; digital pattern recognition system; number of resting, random, and conditioning trials; and instructions as those in the previous systolic blood pressure-heart rate study (Schwartz 1972). However, an additional 10 subjects were run in a complete random reinforcement condition (the 35 conditioning trials were actually a continuation of random reinforcement). The results of this experiment are depicted in Figure 21.4 (Schwartz, Shapiro, and Tursky 1972), and support the predictions of the model. First, it can be seen that integration reinforcement again leads to more rapid learning of both blood pressure and heart rate, while the heart rate results in particular are now almost twice the size of those observed when diastolic pressure per se controlled the feedback and reward. Second, it can be seen that, although diastolic pressure and heart rate in the random reinforcement condition show a similar pattern over trials, the curves diverge as expected, with the pressure on the average being about three units above heart rate (see Figure 21.4). Finally, it can be seen that there was little evidence for learned differentiation of diastolic blood pressure and heart rate, especially when the curves are appropriately compared with the results of the random reinforcement group.

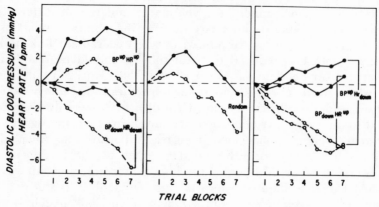

FIGURE 21.4. *Average diastolic blood pressure and heart rate for subjects receiving feedback and reward in the four coincidence patterns and complete random reinforcement. On the left are the data for the two integration conditions; in the center are the data for the one complete random reinforcement group, and on the right are the data for the two differentiation conditions. Solid lines are BP, dashed lines are HR. Each point is the mean of 10 subjects, 5 trials each, set to zero by the fifth random reinforcement trial. Beats per minute and millimeters of mercury are therefore on the same axis. (Redrawn from Schwartz, Shapiro, and Trusky, 1972)*

Altogether, these findings point to the differences in mechanisms and constraints involved in the voluntary control of systolic versus diastolic pressure, and the data provide further support for the heuristic and predictive value of the model. Of course, it is conceivable that longer training, different instruction, and/or different feedback procedures could produce stronger evidence for learned differentiation of diastolic pressure and heart rate. As will be discussed below, the current formulation does help provide a framework for predicting what some of these changes in procedure might be, as well as the likelihood of actually obtaining larger effects. However, before turning to these issues, some recent experiments on the interaction of constraints, cognition, and contingency factors will be considered, for they point out additional complications that must be taken into account in order to more fully understand and predict the nature of learned patterns of cardiovascular activity.

INTERACTION OF CONSTRAINT, COGNITION, AND CONTINGENCY FACTORS IN THE VOLUNTARY CONTROL OF HEART RATE

When a subject sits quietly in a soft lounge chair and no aversive consequences are likely to occur in the situation (the typical biofeedback condition), it would be expected that his heart rate would be at its low end relative to the total range of heart rates possible under different states—varying from deep sleep to active exercise. To the extent that floor and ceiling effects do occur in a given individual for a given function, then, if a subject is already at his low end, this should be reflected in both his reactivity as well as in his ability to voluntarily raise and lower this function; increases should be more readily produced than decreases.

The concept of range and range correction has received systematic attention by Lykken and associates (Lykken et al. 1966), who basically argue that in order to compare one individual with another or one function with another, one must know where the function is relative to its own possible range. Parenthetically, it occurred to the writer that this analysis provides a handy explanation for the law of initial values (Wilder 1957), a "law" that, at least for the cardiovascular system, apparently holds only when intense stimuli or situations are used within subjects. If the Lykken range concept is applied to Wilder's observations, it can be seen that if stimulation is so intense that it pushes a given subject to his maximal response amplitude (his ceiling), then the higher his initial base level, by necessity, the smaller will be the increment to reach his peak response (therefore producing a negative correlation between baseline and change). However, if stimulation does not consistently produce peak responses—as is the case for most mild to moderate stimuli used in psychophysiology—then this would produce a significant additional source of variance which would dilute or eliminate Wilder's observations.

To the extent that a subject's range is further limited by the physical and psychological situation imposed on him, the "effective" range for a given subject must be assessed in order to more accurately evaluate his capacity for change. In other words, when applied to the question of magnitude of effects and biofeedback, it is suggested that the effective range must be determined for the particular state required of the subject. For instance, if a subject in instructed to sit quietly, breathe regularly, and not tense his muscles, and then is told "raise your heart rate," his maximum response should be somewhat constrained, since the peak is now lowered by the imposition of the immobile psychophysiological state. Of course, were he allowed to move around, or exercise, this would expand his range dramatically. For example, as recently demonstrated by Obrist and colleagues (Obrist et al. 1973b), if via instructions subjects are allowed freer use of somatic strategies (both excitatory and inhibitory), this leads to larger self-produced heart rate increases and decreases through feedback and reward.

To explore the question of effective range, both in and out of the laboratory setting, Bell and Schwartz (1972a) conducted an experiment designed to assess reactivity and voluntary control under conditions expected to yield relatively large changes in autonomic activity. Heart rate was chosen for this initial study, primarily because it was the only cardiovascular function that could be easily and accurately measured outside of the laboratory setting without resorting to telemetry, tape recording, or other more expensive biomedical systems. Rather, a structured protocol was developed for obtaining heart rate under standard conditions in the field, and Harvard undergraduates were trained to take their own pulses. Although the pulse-taking procedure has problems of possible inaccuracy and falsification of data, it does have one advantage in that the pulse rates are all taken when the subjects are in a similar psychophysiological state (attending to pulsations in the artery, standing still, counting the heart beats). In other words, the measurement procedure reduces the number of other activities the subject might be engaged in while taking the measures, hence reducing variance across situations.

To assess cardiac reactivity in the laboratory, subjects were given two mental effort tasks, each 1-minute long (e.g., subjects were instructed to continually subtract the number 33 from the larger number 985 as quickly as possible, without resorting to clever short cuts), and two attention tasks (e.g., subjects were told to watch a series of randomly flashing lights). Relative to quiet sitting resting base rates, the former environmental rejection (Lacey 1967) plus later verbalization (Johnson and Campos 1967) tasks produced large 12 bpm increases in mean heart rate, while the latter environmental intake (Lacey 1967) without verbalization (Johnson and Campos 1967) tasks produced smaller −1.5 bpm decreases in rate.

Using analogue beat-by-beat meter feedback from the cardiotachometer and full instructions about the nature of the task, Bell and Schwartz (1972a) found that subjects were able to voluntarily raise their heart rate by 9 bpm and lower it by -4 bpm. These results, including the out of laboratory pulse rates, can be seen in Figure 21.5. The data clearly show that, by and large, the range of heart rate increases and decreases observed in the laboratory closely parallel the reactivity ranges, as well as the normal range of heart rates observed during the day outside the laboratory (when a subject is taking his own pulse). For example, feedback rest and out of the laboratory pre-lunch heart rates were at comparable levels (respectively 72.5 and 72.8 pbm) and they were correlated (r = 0.486, p < .05). In fact, the mean time of day during which the subjects were run in the laboratory (12:40 p.m.) compares favorably with the mean time of day at which they report eating lunch (12:30 p.m.). Similarly, feedback up (80.9 bpm) was close to and correlated with the afternoon walk heart rate (79.3 bpm), (r = 0.450, p < .05); feedback down (69.0 bpm) was bracketed by and correlated with heart rate on retiring (67.8 pbm), (r = 0.474, p < .05). With the exception of two extreme conditions (in which psychophysiological state is markedly altered), "on awakening" (while supine in bed) and "postrunning" (after 1 minute running in place) the feedback rest, up and down heart rates fall very near the normal range of heart rates that subjects produce over the course of a "typical" day. Also, these data illustrate that resting heart rates in the laboratory are close to the low end of normal heart rates occurring during the day. Hence, as predicted above, it is no wonder why decelerations (both elicited by external stimuli and self-generated) are smaller under these conditions than heart rate changes observed for acceleration tasks.

Given that effective range constraints can operate and thereby influ-

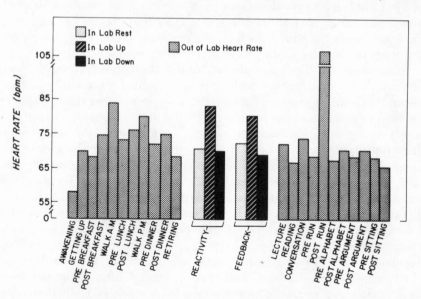

FIGURE 21.5. *Mean heart rates for 20 subjects out of the laboratory compared with those for in-laboratory reactivity and feedback tasks. (from Bell and Schwartz 1972a)*

ence magnitude of learned control, the next question that arises is "what combination of instructions and contingency will enable the subject to reach, or even exceed, his effective range?" Returning to the previous blood pressure-heart rate studies, it will be recalled that these subjects were given minimal instructions concerning the nature of the experiment. They were simply told that their task was to control their physiological activity by making the lights and tones (feedback) occur as often as possible, and to do so without moving around or breathing irregularly. However, they were not told what the response was, nor were they told in what direction the response was to change. Under these conditions, subjects produced "learning curves" in that relative increases or decreases in autonomic activity grew over time.

Although it is often assumed that such learning curves represent the development of new voluntary control, it is theoretically possible that part, if not much, of the changes observed for a given function (or pattern of responses) reflect the subjects ability to assess what set of cognitive or somatic changes—behaviors already in the subjects repertoire—occur with the presentation of the task information and cause the feedback and reward to occur more frequently. According to the model, it would be predicted that the degree to which the external feedback is integrated with the underlying psychophysiological strategies of the subject will, in part, determine the degree to which the subject will learn to use these strategies to control the response in question. Of course, subjects might also use such strategies because they had previously used them in the past, or because they were instructed by the experimenter to do so, either explicitly or implicitly.

Since these strategies are already under the control of the subject, it would be expected that with appropriate instructions the subjects should be able to produce immediate, and possibly maximal, changes in the desired autonomic response. In the Bell and Schwartz (1972a) study, with the hope of maximizing effects in a short time period, subjects were specifically told that the cardiotachometer feedback was their heart rate, and that their task was to raise their heart rate to one cue and lower it to another. (A third cue meant simply rest.) To make the results comparable to earlier studies, subjects were told to sit still and breathe regularly. Subjects were also tested in their ability to raise and lower their heart rate without feedback, both before (pre) and after (post) exposure to the feedback trials. The results showed that without feedback, but with full instructions, subjects could voluntarily raise their heart rate by 7.5 bpm, and lower it by−0.5 bpm in the prefeedback period. Although the addition of feedback tended to further raise the increase condition and produce larger reliable heart rate decreases, this effect was also immediate, occurring on the first 1-minute feedback trial. Hence, no "learning curve" was found, despite the fact that some "learning" had occurred (during the post-feedback period, subjects were able to maintain their enhanced heart rate control without the external meter display).

Based on these findings Bell and Schwartz (1972b) repeated the earlier full instruction group except that included this time was a second group of subjects told to "control the meter, make it go to the right." However, they were not told that it was their heart rate, and that they were to increase their rate. Whereas the former group showed an immediate 8 bpm increase in heart rate feedback which replicated the Bell and Schwartz (1972a) results, the latter group showed a gradual learning curve over the 8 minutes of feedback, which approximated but did not completely equal the performance of the fully informed group. Altogether, these data suggest that instructions and associated cognitive strategies can play a significant role, at least in single session heart rate operant-feedback studies.

As to the possible nature and mechanism of these more central cognitive and somatic strategies, it should be pointed out that in the earlier blood pressure-heart rate research using uninstructed subjects, it was generally found that subjects reported that they had no idea what condition they were in, nor did they indicate any consistent classes of thoughts or feelings related to their raising or lowering various patterns of activity. However, it was not until the subjects were specifically taught to lower both their blood pressure and their heart rate simultaneously (Schwartz 1972) that they began to consistently report feelings of relaxation calmness, and floating sensations associated with the task. In other words, as subjects began to lower combinations of functions (decrease arousal in multi-autonomic responses) consistent global reports of relaxation emerged in previously uninstructed subjects. Looking back at these data the results make intuitive sense, since relaxation generally means decreased activity in many systems simultaneously, including somatic and cognitive processes, as well as reduced activity in cardiovascular, electrodermal, metabolic, and other bodily processes. It would be predicted by the model that to the extent that selective patterns of activity reflect more specific central mechanisms, then in the process of trying to self-produce these autonomic patterns the subjects will learn to generate the accompanying underlying central state.

Instructions can enhance or short circuit this process. In the initial Bell and Schwartz (1972a) experiment, although no explicit statement was made to this regard, it was found that subjects consistently reported using thoughts of excitement, sex, fear, tension, and anger during the up trials—and never during down trials—while they consistently reported using thoughts of happiness, daydreaming, well being, contentment, relaxation, and tranquility during the down trials—and never during up trials. The problem, however, is interpreting these data! For example, do these data mean that: (1) the thoughts were mediating or causing the heart rate changes (Katkin and Murray 1968); or, (2) they contribute to, but reflect only a part of, other mechanisms that raise and lower heart rate; or, (3) they are simply epiphenomena having no cause at all?

The approach taken here is that feedback does play an important role in directing the subject to generate specific brain processes that control the effectors measured as behavior. However, to the extent that many different central mechanisms can produce similar overt effects at the periphery, it becomes imperative to explore different relationships from the point of view of the mechanisms involved. In Bell and Schwartz (1972a), although the reactivity tasks did bracket the eventual feedback effects, heart rate increases in reactivity did not correlate with feedback! In other words, how much a person accelerated during mental arithmetic did not actually predict how much his heart rate would raise with feedback, even though the effective range for the group was predicted by the mental effort tasks. The same applied to the deceleration conditions, and, furthermore, accelerations did not correlate with decelerations. These data suggest that the variables determining cardiac acceleration to mental effort tasks are different than those involved in the feedback condition, and that the mechanisms of acceleration are different than those of deceleration, supporting the conclusion of Engel (1972).

However, more important was the fact that acceleration during the pre-feedback voluntary control period (full instructions but no feedback) did predict success during both feedback and post-feedback. In other words, the strategies set up by the instructions "raise your heart rate" were reliable and were related to what subjects actually did with feedback. It might be mentioned at this juncture that situational stereotypy of this type was dramatically shown in the out of laboratory pulse data, where correlations from day one to day two for most tasks were highly reliable and significant, whereas correlations from one task to another, even in the same day, were mostly nonsignificant.

To explore this question further, the Bell and Schwartz (1972b) study also included a third group of subjects who were specifically instructed to make themselves "aroused" by "thinking arousing thoughts," and told that the feedback would help them find those thoughts that would make them most aroused. The complete experimental design consisted of a pre-feedback phase; one group told to "control-and-raise" heart rate, the second group to "think-arousing-thoughts," and the third to just sit quietly (all without feedback). Then during feedback, the control-and-raise group was told to use the meter to help raise their heart rate; the think-arousing-thoughts group was told to use the meter to help think arousing thoughts; and, the third "control-alone" group was told to control the meter, make it go to the right (but were not told that it was their heart rate, or that the direction was up). Finally, all subjects were given a post-feedback period, and were all told that their task was to raise their heart rate.

The results for pre-feedback were most interesting, because although the group specifically instructed to think-arousing-thoughts did produce immediate heart rate accelerations as expected, the magnitude of these changes were only half the size of those obtained by subjects specifically told to raise their heart rate! Of course, the group stold to sit quietly showed no heart rate changes. However, by the end of the feedback training, both the control-and-raise group and the control-alone group (which, as previously mentioned, showed a learning curve during feedback) produced higher heart rates than the think-arousing-thoughts group. Finally, during post-feedback, when all subjects were specifically told to raise their heart rate, significant differences between groups disappeared. These data support other data (e.g., Schwartz 1971a) finding that arousing thoughts per se do not necessarily produce large magnitude heart rate changes. Altogether, the data suggest that arousing imagery itself is not the primary mechanism for self produced heart rate increases. Rather, it can be hypothesized that (a) "control" instructions may initiate the self generation of somatic control processes that affect heart rate through central and peripheral mechanisms, and (b) focusing attention on the self generation of imagery per se may inhibit the active generation of motor activity, thereby minimizing the magnitude of self regulated heart rate increases.

However, the strongest evidence concerning the question of similarity of mechanisms is to be found when the individual groups are compared across the three conditions. As expected, in the control-and-raise group, heart rate increases during pre-feedback predicts success during feedback, and both conditions are highly correlated with post-feedback performance (rs around .90). However, turning to the think-arousing thoughts group, while pre-feedback accelerations during thinking do correlate with heart rate changes during feedback, neither condition correlates with post-feedback changes when the new "heart rate control" instructions are given. Finally, pre-feedback (resting) values do not correlate with feedback accelerations for the control-alone group, but performance during feedback does predict later control during post-feedback. To summarize, specific use of thinking arousing thoughts cannot simply be the mechanism for raising heart rate in typical single session heart rate biofeedback studies. Furthermore, uninformed subjects developing heart rate control appear to learn mechanisms that are similar to those used by subjects who are directly instructed to control their heart rate. As discussed below, the nature of the physiological relationships plus the characteristics of the feedback suggest that one primary mechanism in learned heart rate control involves central somatic control, thus supporting the cardio-somatic position advanced by Obrist and colleagues as one major determinant of heart rate change (Obrist et al. 1970b).

It appears that range constraints and instructions each influence control of responses in the cardiovascular system, and it is readily apparent how these factors further complicate the picture when control of patterns of responses are to be understood. However, the nature of the feedback adds an additional complexity, since—to the extent that patterns of responses are naturally integrated, and feedback is provided for one of them—the others will be receiving a similar contingency. Furthermore, the precise nature of the feedback can either augment, or diminish, the similarity with regard to other changing functions. For example, in the present series of heart rate studies, analogue meter feedback of heart rate was used. But to the extent that subjects showed sinus arrythmia, then when subjects receive meter feedback for heart rate, they were also receiving feedback and reward for respiration! Consequently, this pattern of feedback should enhance the degree to which subjects consciously or unconsciously manipulate their breathing. In an earlier heart rate study (Shapiro, Tursky, and Schwartz 1970b), when digital feedback was compared with analogue feedback, it was noted that the latter seemed to produce much more respiratory involvement. However, the explanation for this observation was not then realized.

The current formulation indicates that relationships between responses over time coupled with the exact nature of the feedback and reward each determine, in part, what patterns of functions will be learned. It is suggested that analogue feedback for heart rate serves to accentuate the respiratory relationship and, to the extent that cardiac increases and decreases reflect more central somatic control processes as well (e.g., Black 1971a), subjects will learn to also control their somatic system. It might be worth mentioning at this point that one of the best overall predictors of heart rate control during feedback in the Bell and Schwartz (1972b) situation was the number of hours a person exercised regularly each week! Furthermore, separate group analyses showed that this especially applied to the control-alone group where subjects' attention was not diverted from their somatic activity as was the case in the think-arousing-thoughts group, which showed no such relationship.

Like the strategy developed for the analysis and modification of patterns of blood pressure and heart rate, similar integration and differentiation procedures are needed to assess, and possibly modify, such cardio-somatic relationships. Similar strategies have been advanced by Black (1971a) for the control of patterns of electroencepholographic (EEG) activity, and Fetz and Finocchio (1971) for the integration and differentiation of motor activity with single motor neurons in the brain.

DISCUSSION AND THEORETICAL SPECULATIONS

By expanding the general concepts of contingency and constraint, and systematically applying them to two or more functions simultaneously, it is possible to provide an initial framework for predicting and controlling patterns of cardiovascular activity through feedback and reward. Specifically, it is suggested that both the qualitative and quantitative nature of learned pattern control are in large measure determined by the interaction of three factors: (1) the characteristics of the interrelationships between bodily functions over time; coupled with (2) the exact nature of the contingency involved; in the context of (3) biological, cognitive, and environmental constraints. For ease of discussion, the first two factors will be considered in combination, followed by an analysis as to how they interact with different constraint conditions.

Analyzing the Nature of Physiological Relationships from an Operant-Feedback Point of View

Different characteristics of the feedback (contingency) may affect the degree to which different patterns of responses are learned. For example, analogue meter feedback for beat-by-beat changes in heart rate can also act as feedback for respiratory inhalation and exhalations in sinus arrythmia. On the other hand, digital feedback for changes in rate above a certain criterion may reduce the relationship between respiration and heart rate, especially if the feedback is so deliberately programmed that half the time criterion heart rate changes are reinforced when the subject is breathing in, and half the time for breathing out (assuming that the relationship between phasic changes in heart rate and breathing is not perfect). In other words, the goal would be to provide partial, although contingent, reinforcement for heart rate, and at the same time provide some form of random reinforcement for respiration. However, if under these experimental circumstances it was found that respiration still changed, this would suggest that underlying central connections linking heart rate and respiration were operating. To more directly explore these mechanisms, one strategy would be to test subjects for their ability to directly integrate or differentiate their heart rate and respiration through the use of pattern feedback and reward. Were it found that integration was easy to obtain, whereas differentiation was quite difficult, this would provide strong support for a causal link between phasic heart rate and respiratory changes.

However, since phasic changes and tonic changes may reflect different processes, both neural and hormonal, then, when a subject is given analogue feedback for heart rate per se he is, in fact, receiving complex integrated information about vagal, sympathetic, and hormonal influences, those "mediating" processes over which he has actual control. Clearly, through the use of specific drugs and surgical procedures, it is possible to uncover the exact mechanism that the subject is using to control his rate (Weiss and Engel 1971). However, what happens if it is desirable for a subject to learn to directly control only one of these processes, or some specific pattern? The theory would suggest that it is necessary to make the feedback more directly integrated with the underlying neural and/or hormonal processes. One way to do this is to directly record neural impulses from the vagus, or to monitor levels of circulating catecholamines on line and provide feedback and reward specifically for these changes (the latter being particularly technically difficult). Another technique is to use specific pharmacological blocking agents, and then give feedback for the remaining heart rate changes. For example, if it were desirable to teach a subject to control cardiac sympathetic levels, atropine, a cholinergic blocking agent, could be administered to effectively cut out parasympathetic vagal influences on heart rate itself. This would greatly eliminate the more phasic changes in heart rate due to such factors as sinus arrythmia, and allow more direct control of other mechanisms to be learned.

Ideally, through proper response definition, it should be theoretically possible to compute what aspect of the total signal reflects a given process, and to provide the subject with such feedback directly, without resorting to physiological or pharmacological intervention. One example is the use of running averages to remove phasic components. By selecting a sampling rate to encompass sinus arrythmia, the phasic arrythmia changes would be averaged out of the feedback, and only the more tonic changes would show up as significant changes in the contingency. In this manner it may be possible to train subjects more directly to modulate the slower, but longer lasting, components determining heart rate.

However, there are many problems in looking across systems that need to be solved. Whereas it is relatively easy to compare across responses such as heart rate and systolic pressure, since they share some common elements in terms of periodicity, it is more difficult to compare, for example, changes in heart rate with slower tonic changes in peripheral resistance due to alterations in arteriolar tone. In the light of these problems, it is not clear whether it will be possible to fully understand and predict the nature of pattern learning that will occur by simply looking at the empirical relationship between systems. Possible solutions that come to mind include: (a) arbitrarily placing systems on a similar time base (e.g., using running averages across multifunctions and comparing degrees of tonic integration); or, (b) using normalization or other statistical techniques, such as range correction. However, at least at a theoretical level, these solutions are not wholly satisfactory.

One other aspect of contingency that deserves mention is the question of inherent power functions in sensory transmission. Stevens (1970, 1972) has pointed out that the discrimination of sensory input, both external and internal, obey different power functions. Furthermore, these differences occur even at the level of the peripheral sensory effectors involved (e.g., the power function for the eye differs from that of the ear). The present theory suggests that the more directly integrated the external feedback is with the underlying neural processes, the more direct and immediate will be the learning. Considering the example of beat-by-beat feedback for heart rate, if the analogue feedback were intensity modulated and presented visually versus auditorily, the subject would be processing the information through two different power functions which, by definition, would be more or less similar to the underlying processes involved. Hence, one difference between modalities of sensory input may be the degree to which they naturally enhance or distort the senory information related to the particular autonomic function.

Applying this idea to a "single" system, the question becomes "what power function for heart rate is best for learning heart rate control?" Should it be greater than 1, less than 1, or what? Clearly, it is possible to build a power function generator that would allow one to experimentally manipulate this information. According to theory, it may be possible to empirically uncover the power function of the underlying afferent information system for a particular autonomic function by determining the best overt power function for external feedback (taking into account the way in which specific external sensory systems influence the feedback).

It should be noted that a power function generator in common use in psychophysiology is the standard cardiotachometer which converts period (time between beats) into an inverse rate function (beats per minute). Although there is debate as to which system—period or rate—more closely approximates the way in which the nervous system senses its own heart contractions, it makes intuitive sense at least that the brain could easily track the time between each beat, whereas it would be less likely to have built a complex computer for converting each heart beat into beats per minute to match the form used by the average physician taking pulses by hand! Regardless of intuitive theoretical explanation, the question is clearly an empirical problem, one amenable to experimental test (eg., which power function of feed-back produces greater heart rate control?). Khachaturian and his co-workers (Khachaturian et. al. 1972) have recently found that period analysis provides a more accurate, and less distorted analysis of heart cycle data.

With regard to comparison across sensory systems, the simple inte-gration analysis assumes that there are no underlying neurophysiologi-cal reasons for one external sensory system to be better equipped for voluntary control of a given autonomic function than another. However, this assumption may be questioned on biological grounds (e.g., Seligman 1970). For example, it could be argued that the best way to give blood pressure feedback is by producing inverse pressure changes in a pressure cuff. By using this procedure, the experimenter would be maximizing the similarity of power functions between the external feedback device and an internal afferent system probably involved in normal pressure reception, and the external feedback mo-dality would direct the subject's attention to this natural source of blood pressure feedback.

Although speculative in nature, these concepts are useful to the ex-tent that they illustrate the potential for systematically evaluating the integration of contingency variables with ongoing physiological changes, and are open to direct empirical test. The theoretical specula-tions outlined below are meant to be viewed in a similar light.

Evaluating Change with Regard to Biological Constraints as they Interact with Contingency and Cognition

As hinted at in the opening paragraph of the chapter, and documented by experimental research, it makes good sense to view learning in the cardiovascular system in terms of its biological structure and function. In the same way that a person can handle different physical loads depending upon the muscle groups he uses, different components of the cardiovascular system probably have different capabilities for change, and these factors need to be taken into account. By classifying constraints into four basic categories (state, neural circuitry, organ, and reward) it is possible to speculate as to how such constraints will in-fluence learning in the cardiovascular system.

By state constraints are meant the effects of such factors as time of day, drugs, situation, instructions, and so forth on the physical and psychological "state" of the organism. For example, requiring a subject through instructions to sit in a quiet, relaxed position without resorting to respiratory or muscular movement, and then asking him to raise his heart rate puts him in a state that is clearly not optimal for raising heart rate. Interestingly, the addition of feedback, especially analogue feedback, may put the subject to some extent in a "conflict" situation, since on one hand the subject is receiving feedback for increased somatic involvement and metabolic demands, yet on the other hand he is specifically instructed to consciously "ignore" this aspect of the contingency.

Similarly, variables, such as sex of the experimenter and the social situation, may alter the state of the subject and, thereby, alter the degree to which his cardiovascular system may change. Also, physical factors can act as state variables. For example, it might be hypothesized that room temperature would have specific state effects on subjects given the task of self-producing increases or decreases in peripheral blood flow related to skin temperature. Finally, drugs like curare clearly influence state (e.g., by eliminating peripheral somatic feedback), and this may have specific state effects on cardiovascular control.

To the extent that state variables can change the levels and variability of cardiovascular responses, and possibly alter their interrelationships, this will alter the kinds of patterns of responses that will be acquired. It is for this reason that state variables are considered crucial to the prediction and control of patterns of responses. Also, transfer from state to state may be questionable, since different processes may be acquired under different states. In this regard, the whole notion of state dependent science takes on added significance (Tart 1972).

Of course, state effects operate because of specific brain structures and interconnections. However, the purpose of isolating neural circuitry constraints per se is to highlight such specific processes as homeostasis that will influence the development of cardiovascular control. Similarly, the extent to which heart rate, for example, is centrally integrated with the somatic system is an important neural circuitry constraint, since it helps explain why heart rate increases under resting conditions are so readily obtained.

Not so obvious is the fact that state and task demands may change these relationships in very specific ways. For example, the relationship between heart rate and mean blood pressure depends in part on the kind of exercise performed. In active (isotonic) exercise (e.g., running, swimming, or "flight"), heart rate increases markedly to supply increased blood to the muscles and brain, while pressure may drop —or, relatively speaking, rise less—since blood flows into the muscles. However, in passive (isometric) exercise (e.g., the posture for "fight"), blood pressure markedly rises due to increased venous constriction yielding increased contractility, while heart rate drops—or, relatively speaking, rises less—due to the baroreceptors attempt to reduce pressure by turning on the vagal inhibition of heart rate (Lind et al. 1964). This observation is very important, not only because it illustrates how task demands may effect relative changes in two systems, but also because it provides a possible mechanism for learned differentiation of blood pressure and heart rate under different states. For example, it would be predicted that if subjects were tested for degree of voluntary control of patterns of blood pressure and heart rate under these two different exercise conditions, they would be better able to produce the specific exercise-related differentiations than a generalized integration of these functions, a conclusion opposite to the findings previously generated for "resting" conditions (Schwartz 1972).

By organ constraints is simply meant the relative maximum and minimum changes possible across all different situations. Whereas state effects restrict the total range possible for a given organ (here called the effective range), the concept of organ constraint refers to Lykken's use of range correction for determining true peak and trough values per individual per function (Lykken et al. 1966). However, "true" peak and trough values still involve some neurocirculatory constraints, since maximum heart rate increases, for example, are limited by a normally functioning vagal control system and sino-atrial pacemaker. If this were changed through injury, disease, or drugs, the peak (and trough) values would change accordingly.

Finally, some discussion of possible "reward" constraints are in order. Miller (1969) early noted that if the reward was too strong, learning appeared to be impeded. This observation would here be explained as the effect of changing state through intensity of reward. However, little discussion has been offered concerning the biological implications of different forms of reward for learning specific bodily processes. Seligman (1970) has pointed out that the learning of many overt behaviors are "reward specific," that is, the animal is "prepared" to make certain associations between behavior, external stimuli, and rewards, and "contraprepared" to make others. It seems likely that similar effects will apply to more basic visceral and neural learning as well. Peper (1970), for example, has documented that the unconditioned effect of light stimuli as feedback serves to inhibit the voluntary production of alpha (since if alpha is followed by light feedback, the light will block the alpha); however, turning the light off with the occurrence of alpha has the opposite effect, resulting in the production of long trains of alpha enhancement. Similarly, one can speculate what effects warm versus cold feedback stimuli might have on the voluntary control of peripheral vasodilation and constriction, the hypothesis being that the former would enhance control of vasodilation, while the latter would inhibit voluntary vasodilation but enhance vasoconstriction.

This list is speculative in nature and by no means exhaustive (e.g., individual differences in all of these variables have not been presented). However, it does point out the need for considering such factors in the control of both "single" and multicardiovascular functions. To the extent that the heart is considered to actually be a complex "multiresponse" system itself (Obrist et al. 1970b), the issues of integration and constraints take on added significance.

CLINICAL IMPLICATIONS OF PATTERN LEARNING

The combined behavioral-biological approach to biofeedback outlined here has a number of implications for treatment (see also Schwartz 1973a). One is that the clinician should carefully evaluate how he administers feedback to an individual patient, in order that he be more able to precisely determine, and control, what the patient will and will not learn. The simple assumption that by using an operant procedure, the learning will be "specific" is not always justifiable. This does not mean that the clinician must be concerned with obtaining "pure" learning effects from a scientific point of view. In fact, the clinician is mainly concerned with any combination of functions or factors that will produce large, long lasting, generalizable, and safe effects. Thus, if for a given hypertensive patient, biofeedback training in general muscle relaxation alone produced the most rapid and massive decreases in pressure, this would have obvious clinical value.

On the other hand, the therapist may be concerned with what else is changing when a person is provided with feedback for a given function. In fact, there are instances where the therapist may well be interested in patterns of responses. For example, the desired goal for those hypertensive patients having normal heart rates may be to lower stroke volume and/or peripheral resistance rather than to change heart rate per se. However, in reducing pain in patients suffering from angina pectoris, the desired goal may not be to lower just blood pressure, or heart rate, but rather both functions simultaneously; since, by decreasing rate and pressure, the heart requires less oxygen and this leads to reduced pain, e.g., lowering the product of heart rate and blood pressure through direct stimulation of the baroreceptors (Braunwald et al. 1967). In this case, directly training the patient to lower both pressure and rate through BP_{down} HR_{down} feedback may be a useful strategy. Similarly, the importance of understanding mechanisms when feedback and reward is applied to cardiologic problems has been illustrated by Weiss and Engel (1971) and Engel (1972). Pattern analysis in the context of biological constraints can add further insights into these issues.

Further comment on feedback control of high blood pressure is in order. As mentioned earlier, there is reason to distinguish between phasic and tonic activity, not just for statistical purposes, but for reasons involving underlying processes as well. If a subject has high diastolic pressure due to chronic peripheral constriction (tonic level, even under resting conditions, is above the normal range), but is given

feedback for small phasic changes in diastolic pressure around this high
level, he may well learn to control his heart rate rather than to modify
the peripheral resistance factors, since this feedback is more directly
integrated with the phasic heart rate changes (Schwartz, Shapiro, and
Tursky 1972). In other words, just because there is an observable blood
pressure change does not necessarily mean that this is what the subject
needs to change and therefore what should be reinforced. Blood pressure is an integrated measure, at all times the sum total of the state
of the plumbing of the cardiovascular system. It is suggested that more
emphasis should be placed on attempting to diagnose the underlying
mechanisms contributing to the given problem. In behavioral terms,
this amounts to not simply treating the "symptom," but rather trying
to treat the "cause."

Different problems may require different solutions. One may be to
use running averages to eliminate distracting phasic changes from the
feedback so that the underlying tonic changes may be more directly
reinforced. Another approach might involve the use of two blood pressure cuffs, and only reinforce the pattern of systolic BP_{down} diastolic
BP_{down}. This pattern reinforcement procedure would insure that the
subjects were always reinforced for drops in mean pressure, which is
not solely dependent on either heart rate or contractility.

Of course, it is conceivable that concerns over the precise nature of
the feedback are not really critical, because the subject will, through
trial and error, learn to lower all the systems coupled in any way with
the feedback and to lower all of them to their own biological minimum.
Although this writer has emphasized the contingency of patterns as
an important factor, in the final analysis the question is an empirical
one.

Concerning the question of biological constraints, it follows that if
it is possible to clinically evaluate the flexibility or variability of the
function(s) in question, it may be possible to assess whether biofeedback
will have any significance on purely physiological grounds. For
instance, if a patient has fixed hypertension due to arterial sclerosis
such that his pressure is always high, then it would seem unlikely that
self generated neural or hormonal control will have any consistent
marked effect on lowering pressure to normal levels. Evaluating the
potential for organ change (e.g., by taking sleep measurements) may
be one useful screening technique. From this point of view, early diagnosis of the individual for preventive feedback training before the
organ system is seriously damaged is a reasonable direction for application to psychosomatic disease.

Finally, brief mention should be made concerning the possibility
of learned behavioral-physiological integration or "coordination"
(Schwartz 1973b). Although the study of learning processes involving

behavioral systems has traditionally occurred separately from research on autonomic learning, the present formulation, when followed to its logical conclusion, leads to a somewhat unusual conception. That is, to the extent that overt behavior and underlying autonomic changes are naturally integrated in specific situations, such as the expression of anger and patterns of blood pressure and heart rate, (Ax 1953), then if the former is consistently reinforced, the latter may also be receiving a similar contingency, and therefore may "learn" as well. Hence, if a hypertensive person has learned certain maladaptive ways of dealing with his environment behaviorally, such as inhibiting anger expression and thereby maintaining blood pressure, (Hokanson, Burgess, and Cohen 1963), but is simply taught to lower his blood pressure in the laboratory, this may have little "generalization" outside the laboratory, because the individual has, in fact, not learned to control the appropriate behavioral-physiological complex. Creating more comprehensive treatment programs that directly train new, more adaptive behavioral-physiological coordinations may be an alternative strategy to consider (e.g., using biofeedback in anger situations modeled in the laboratory).

SUMMARY AND CONCLUSIONS

Beginning with findings of specificity of learning in the cardiovascular system, and attempting to understand them in the context of learning theory and biology has led to the evolution of the research presented here, as well as the development of a general theoretical approach for understanding and predicting learned patterns of cardiovascular activity. Although it seems fair to conclude that some progress has been made on both empirical and theoretical grounds, it is clear that many complexities have been unearthed which require further experimental and theoretical consideration. Furthermore, the extent to which two or more responses need to be behaviorally integrated in order for pattern learning to naturally occur is not yet known. Nor does current data or theory fully explain how it is possible for specificity of learning to emerge from partially integrated systems if long term training procedures are employed.

However, one strong conclusion that seems justified at this time is that the systematic application of operant-feedback patterning procedures can help make it possible to determine the nature of autonomic and central nervous system constraints and their modification *in the intact organism*. This point has been independently drawn by Black (1971a) and Fetz and Finocchio (1971), the goal being to use these procedures as analytic tools. It is suggested that the present theoretical approach may offer a framework in which to determine the relative

440   HUMAN OPERANT CONDITIONING

importance of feedback and reward in producing the kinds of patterns that emerge, both in basic and applied research settings. Finally, the importance of viewing voluntary control of patterns of cardiovascular activity in biological perspective is stressed, although the question as to whether or not it is really possible, or adaptive, for man to learn to counteract these natural constraints is up to future research to decide.

NOTES

1. This is not meant to imply that other unconscious feedback loops (such as baroreceptor mechanisms emphasized by Lacey 1967) cannot influence behavior, but, rather, that under normal circumstances they do not directly enter consciousness as competing stimuli.

2. Since this general distinction is carefully considered in a number of chapters in this volume, no further discussion of it will be presented here. Rather, this chapter takes an eclectic point of view, tending to favor a conceptualization of voluntary control of patterns of cardiovascular activity as representing the learning of a specialized skill, yet retaining some of the terminology of operant conditioning to the extent that it emphasizes the precise nature of contingency effects.

3. Although as here defined contingency is equivalent to information and feedback, the reader preferring the latter terms may wish to distinguish between "state" and "task" components (or uses) of information and feedback.

4. These definitions depart somewhat from those generally used in biology, where the term integration refers to any consistent pattern of unified activity, regardless of direction, while differentiation refers to a separation of one response from others (here called specificity). However, except when referring to specific experiments where it is essential to verbally distinguish between directions of change, the term integration will be used more broadly to refer to any consistent association of functions over time.

22

DAVID SHAPIRO

Operant-Feedback Control of Human Blood Pressure: Some Clinical Issues

INTRODUCTION

In the past 10 years, rapid advances have been made in basic research on the environmental regulation of visceral processes in man by means of biofeedback and instrumental learning techniques (Barber et al. 1971a). While this research has not moved much beyond the stage of simple demonstrations of the phenomena, it is clear that many properties of behavioral plasticity observed in responses of the skeletal muscles can also be shown in responses of the viscera. The wide variety of responses that can be altered, and the apparent power of the techniques to bring about consistent increases and decreases in autonomic response frequency and magnitude has encouraged further basic research on some of the factors affecting the efficiency of learning in normal human subjects. Among the topics currently under investigation in my laboratory are self-control and the maintenance of learning after feedback training, effects of different kinds and amounts of feedback, response definition, and type of incentive.

The research to date taken together with the recent evidence indicating that *different* patterns of cardiovascular responses can be selectively modified by feedback and reinforcement in human subjects (Schwartz 1972) has encouraged new applications of these methods to the control of symptoms in psychosomatic and autonomically-mediated disorders.

Supported by: NIMH Grants K3-MH-20,476 and MH-08853; Office of Naval Research, Psychophysiology Program, under Contract N00014-67-A-0298-0024, NR 309-012

PSYCHOSOMATIC DISORDERS: GENERAL ISSUES

A major focus of interest has been on the potentiality of instrumental learning concepts and biofeedback techniques in research on the etiology, maintenance, and modification of psychosomatic symptoms, in particular in cardiovascular disorders. Miller (1969) has argued that evidence of the instrumental learning of visceral responses removes the major basis for assuming that psychosomatic symptoms that are autonomically mediated are fundamentally different from so-called hysterical (sometimes considered purely psychogenic) symptoms that represent somatomotor and central nervous system processes. Regarding the etiology of psychosomatic disorders, theorists have emphasized one or some combination of such causative factors as constitutional vulnerability, organ response learning, stimulus situation, emotional reaction pattern, and personality profile (Lachman 1972). However, no really systematic extension of instrumental learning concepts to specific psychosomatic disorders has been attempted to explain the selective differentiation of symptoms through reinforcement. Miller (1969) gives an example of a child who is reinforced by being kept at home from school on the basis of a particular physiological symptom, and who, thereby, avoids an important examination for which he is not prepared. Depending on the particular concerns of the parent, the child may be reinforced for such symptoms as gastric distress, headache, skin rash, respiratory symptoms, cardiovascular changes, or muscle tension. With repetitive reinforcement, and the possible generalization of the learned reactions to other situations, a workable model of psychosomatic etiology might be constructed.

As to evidence of the experimental induction of psychosomatic symptoms in animals by instrumental conditioning methods, this critical research has as yet achieved only limited attention. In squirrel monkeys, sustained reactions in mean blood pressure were observed by making the avoidance of shock contingent on elevations in blood pressure (Benson et al. 1969). The degree to which such learning could also progress to the point of organic pathology is a problem meriting further study.

Whether or not selective instrumental reinforcement will turn out to serve as a realistic mechanism for psychosomatic symptom formation, it may not be unreasonable to attempt to modify symptoms, whatever their etiology, by this means. In research on squirrel monkeys having behaviorally-induced high blood pressure, sustained reductions in mean pressure could be achieved by training under a schedule in which these changes prevented the delivery of noxious stimuli (Benson et al. 1969). In a sense, the rationale for such an approach to symptom alleviation is not fundamentally different from that for the use of drugs to alleviate symptoms in many disorders. To the degree that the symptom is in itself harmful, as in elevated blood pressure which may contribute to vascular lesions, symptom relief is quite beneficial. The major difficulty of drugs, of course, is that of toxic or other detrimental side effects, which should not figure significantly in the use of conditioning techniques. In any discussion of the usefulness of instrumental techniques in the control of abnormal physiological responses, a number of critical questions have to be posed, and these will be discussed in the remainder of this chapter.

CLINICAL GOALS

Given the particular individual patient and his illness, and having defined the physiological measure to be controlled (see next section), a goal must be set in terms of desired or appropriate change. Blanchard and Young (1973) have argued that the results for changes in cardiovascular functioning in operant-feedback studies have been of a *statistically* rather than a *clinically* significant magnitude. For their purposes, they defined a change in response as clinically significant "if it is equal to either 20% of the base rate or, in the case of an abnormally high response, the change is such so as to return the response to the normal range." However, the setting of arbitrary percentage of absolute limits is probably not realistic in a clinical situation. In some instances, such as in high blood pressure, even a relatively small percentage reduction in pressure may turn out to have important health implications for the patient. In the use of heart rate control, as another example, relatively small changes in rate may be finely critical in diminishing the frequency of irregular heart beats (Weiss and Engel 1971). It is probably not magnitude of change, per se, but rather the relative effectiveness and cost of the behavioral procedure, as compared with others, and its ability to maintain a desired effect over a reasonable course of time, with or without other auxiliary means of treatment.

APPROPRIATE PHYSIOLOGICAL MEASURE

A second issue concerns the choice of physiological function appropriate to control using instrumental methods. Thorough knowledge of the physiological mechanisms underlying the particular symptom and disorder, and the consequences of changes in the symptom in the total physiological economy of the individual is obviously critical. Both indirect and direct approaches are possible. For example, Weiss and Engel (1971) investigated a variety of heart rate training procedures—speeding, slowing, and maintenance of rate in a certain range—and their effects on premature ventricular contractions (PVCs).

In some patients, they attempted to elucidate mechanisms controlling heart rate and arrhythmia by means of autonomic nervous system drugs. The arrhythmia was shown to be mediated by sympathetic nervous system activity in a few patients, and in others by parasympathetic activity. Weiss and Engel concluded: "The flexibility of operant conditioning is demonstrated by the fact that PVCs were reduced whether they were mediated primarily by the sympathetic or by the parasympathetic nervous system. This underscores the fact that operant conditioning can be used to alter pathologic conditions mediated by different mechanisms." (Weiss and Engel 1971, p. 319)

Direct feedback for the symptom itself was also involved in some of the Weiss and Engel procedures, although the value of this method of control—for example, by reinforcing PVCs on schedules which should generate low rates of the responses—has not been thoroughly studied.

To illustrate this problem in another illness, Raynaud's disease is an example in which the choice of an appropriate and relevant physiological function is complex and rests in large measure on basic information about the physiology of blood flow and temperature control in the hands and feet. Raynaud's disease is an idiopathic bilateral paroxysmal contraction of the arteries and arterioles of the digits, not occurring in the course of other diseases such as scleroderma, precipitated by cold or emotion, and relieved by warming (Harrison et al. 1966). In my laboratory, we have provided two patients feedback for increases in blood volume using a reflectance photoplethysmograph. The first patient showed large increases in blood volume and pulse volume, and he reported less pain and increased feelings of warmth in his toes (where the device was attached). (Incidentally, this patient reported that images of the sun and heat helped him warm his toes.) The second patient had a severe problem, including tissue damage that was not alleviated by feedback training.

In another laboratory, Richard Surwit (personal communication) used feedback of skin temperature rather than blood volume as the primary technique in a single patient who achieved considerable success by this method. Further inquiry into the physiology of blood flow in the digits and local mechanisms of control will serve to clarify the basis for proceeding with one function or another. Moreover, detailed study of the vasomotor (and other physiological) reactions of specific patients with Raynaud's disease to different stimuli—thermal and emotional—is needed to determine means of enhancing the possibility of clinical improvement in these patients. Similar psychophysiological diagnostic procedures are probably desirable in other psychosomatic illnesses as well.

In the case of blood pressure control, the obvious target behavior would seem to be blood pressure itself, and a decision has to be made whether the measure should be systolic, diastolic, or mean pressure. This decision rests on the availability of instruments for detecting the different indices of pressure and for providing feedback. Medical and physiological considerations as to the stage and variety of hypertensive illness and its duration and severity have a bearing on this decision as well. After choosing the specific measure, as with any other application, further questions arise concerning the time course and amplitude of the response that is fed back or reinforced. Consider the fact that successive changes in pressure are often directly linked with changes in respiration and heart rate. Should these phasic changes be reinforced, or is it desirable to block them out and insist on fluctuations going beyond respiratory-induced values?

Alternative bodily functions related to blood pressure control are also to be considered. Inasmuch as muscular tension may be a factor in the maintenance of high blood pressure, the appropriate strategy in some patients may call for muscular relaxation training, autogenic training, meditation exercises, or muscle tension feedback (Jacobson 1938; Luthe 1963; Wallace, Benson, and Wilson 1971; Budzynski, Stoyva, and Adler 1970). At a Bombay hospital, a group of Indian investigators using a yogic exercise called "shavasan" have reported significant reductions in pressure in about half a sample of 47 patients with hypertension of various etiologies. The yogic exercise is described as follows:

> The patient lies in the supine position, lower limbs 30 degrees apart and the upper making an angle of 15 degrees with the trunk, with the forearms in the midprone position and fingers semiflexed. The eyes are closed with eyelids drooping. The patient is taught slow, rhythmic diaphragmatic breathing with a short pause after each inspiration and a longer one at the end of each expiration. After establishing this rhythm, he is asked to attend to the sensation at the nostrils, the coolness of the inspired air and the warmth of the expired air. This procedure helps to keep the patient inwardly alert and to forget his usual thoughts, thus becoming less conscious of the external environment, thereby attaining relaxation. The patient is asked to relax the muscles so that he is able to feel the heaviness of different parts of the body. This is achieved automatically once the patient learns the exercise. The exercise is performed for 30 minutes. An experimental supervisor checks that there is no movement of any part of the body, except rhythmic abdominal movements. Physical relaxation is checked from time to time by lifting the extremities and letting them go, to observe their flaccidity. Most of the patients learn the exercise correctly in about three weeks. The pulse, blood pressure, and respiration were recorded before and after the exercise. After patients learn the exercise correctly, the respiratory rate is usually between 4 and 10 per minute. (Datey et al. 1969, pp. 325-326)

Procedures such as these may possibly be facilitated by various techniques of monitoring muscle tension and providing feedback for reductions. Furthermore, a relaxation procedure may be combined with biofeedback and reward for reductions in blood pressure itself.

In other instances, particularly in the early "labile" phase of hypertensive illness, increased overall activity of the sympathetic nervous system may be a primary factor (see Gutmann and Benson 1971). Instrumental techniques could be applied to the reduction of several indices of sympathetic nervous response. It may be hypothesized that such *general* physiological functions as sympathetic activity are more readily subject to control, because they involve a number of common elements that are likely to be integrated at higher levels of the nervous system. In support of this conjecture, Schwartz (1972) found larger decreases—or increases—in heart rate *and* systolic blood pressure when feedback and rewards were given for the simultaneous occurrence of decreases—or increases—in *both*, as compared to earlier results when only one or the other function was reinforced (Shapiro, Tursky, and Schwartz 1970b). A total pattern of complete muscular relaxation plus reduced sympathetic activity would seem to be an ideal physiological condition for achieving reductions in blood pressure. The role of feedback in this case may be to cue the subject about any increases in sympathetic *or* somatomotor responses. This may be considered a "negative biofeedback" approach as compared with the "positive biofeedback" usually given for increases in the desired response.

On the other hand, modifying a global pattern of activity means that some unwanted accompanying change may also be augmented. While unpublished data in our laboratory (Schwartz, Shapiro, and Tursky 1972) suggests that it is difficult to dissociate such closely integrated responses as diastolic pressure and heart rate (either simultaneous increase or decrease) with a small amount of training, such response discrimination is theoretically possible, unless there are rigid constraints of anatomy or physiology. The strategy of training would be to go from the general to the specific, at first utilizing as many common response tendencies and then selectively controlling the specific response independently of the others.

In this connection, Kimble and Perlmuter (1970) describe the process of acquiring voluntary control over involuntary responses as one that is:

> . . . always accompanied with the aid of supporting responses already under voluntary control. The desired response is elicited initially as a part of a larger pattern of reactions. With practice the supporting responses gradually drop out, an accomplishment that required a careful paying of attention to the desired behavior and a simultaneous ignoring of the others. With still further practice the now voluntary reaction becomes capable of being performed without deliberate intent. What was once involuntary and later

became voluntary is now involuntary again, in the sense of being out of awareness and free of previous motivational control. (p. 382)

These authors cite an old study by Bain in 1901 to exemplify the process of developing voluntary control of ear movement. Bain elicited the movement by electrical stimulation of the retrahens muscle in order to provide subjects with the sensations accompanying this movement. The electrical stimulation was not effective in and of itself, and subjects needed to practice by making large facial contortions, lifting their brows, and grimacing at first, then detecting the desired movement, and subsequently differentiating it from the massive reaction. Kimble and Perlmuter (1970) point out that it was important for the subjects to focus attention on the responses to be performed and to ignore the unwanted elements of the behavior. They add, ". . . the subjects specifically stated that this did *not* mean trying to inhibit these other responses and that when they did try to do so it only made the responses occur more vigorously." (p. 375)

The methods described by Schwartz, Shapiro, and Tursky (1971) and Schwartz (1972) for measuring ongoing complex patterns of autonomic, or other, responses can be applied in examining such processes of differentiation as they may operate in blood pressure control. Biofeedback and instrumental training could maximize learned blood pressure control by maximizing the differentiation process. Whether the Kimble-Perlmuter model of voluntary control pertains equally to visceral response patterns and to somatomotor responses is a problem for further research.

CLINICAL MANAGEMENT

Patient motivation and cooperation are issues that bear on the selection of suitable candidates for treatment, choice of proper and effective incentives, and design of comprehensible instructions and explanations about the techniques. Inasmuch as biofeedback training as a means of treatment will probably involve many hours of supervised and unsupervised practice, means have to be devised to see that it is carried out. We usually assume that people will do what is good for them to improve their health; yet, we also know they often neglect to prevent or treat their illnesses unless there is a great deal of discomfort and pain, or severe disability. The problem of consistent acceptance and delivery of health care applies across the board in medicine. It is important, therefore, to recognize that shortcomings of biofeedback training may be due to the failure to apply it consistently, rather than to any inherent deficiencies of the method. The idea of physiological self-control without pills is one that has not as yet achieved wide acceptance in the medical establishment or in the public.

The importance of expectancy has been suggested by results of an unpublished biofeedback study (Sirota, Schwartz, and Shapiro). We were interested in the effects of voluntary control of heart rate in an anticipatory fear situation. While all subjects changed their heart rate in the desired direction as a function of instructions, feedback, and rewards, the training had an effect on perception of the anticipated noxious stimulus (painful shocks) only for those subjects who reported an awareness of their heart rate in everyday fear situations. It could be hypothesized that instrumental training was effective for subjects who saw a connection between heart rate and the stimulus situation. Similarly, if a patient believes there is a relationship between his success in autonomic self-control and his illness, will the effectiveness of the feedback method be enhanced?

This leads to a related issue—the role of placebo or suggestion effects. From a research standpoint, adequate no-treatment and placebo controls have to be carried out to evaluate the efficacy of biofeedback and instrumental conditioning over and beyond the operation of suggestion. Random feedback or feedback for irrelevant responses can also be employed as control procedures. From a clinical standpoint, however, if the total machinery of biofeedback can help people overcome symptoms and illness on the basis of suggestion per se, it is of great value, so long as it can operate consistently and results in real therapeutic value. Any behavioral manipulation that provides an alternative or auxiliary means of therapy may be beneficial. Research on the physiological effects of hypnosis and suggestion (Barber 1970) may allow more systematic exploration of these procedures in conjunction with operant-feedback methods.

FEEDBACK TECHNIQUES

The transformation of physiological information into sensory analogues is a basic psychophysical and psychophysiological problem. Some investigators prefer to maximize information by continuously changing displays which closely match the physiological dimensions, while others prefer to categorize the information into a small number of groupings. The pros and cons of using one sensory modality or another depend on such factors as ease of discrimination of stimulus changes, and the type of matching of such changes with the physiological phenomenon. The mathematical transformation of physiological dimension into feedback is an issue that has received little formal investigation. For example, heart period which is the inverse of heart rate may be the more significant function from a physiological standpoint, and could be more effective in autonomic learning (see Khachaturian et al. 1972). Similar questions can be raised about the most suitable transformation of blood pressure, although the limitations of measuring techniques have restricted most of our research to the use of binary feedback. In heart rate control, a few studies have addressed themselves to the differential effectiveness of varying amounts of feedback (Brener, Kleinman, and Goesling 1969; Shapiro, Tursky, and Schwartz 1970b; Lang, Chapter 20).

PROBLEM OF TRANSFER

Of particular importance from a clinical standpoint is the transfer of learning from the laboratory situation to everyday life situations. Some investigators have explored the use of intermittent or partial reinforcement schedules (Greene 1966; Shapiro and Crider 1967; Shapiro and Watanabe 1971), but the evidence is too scanty to conclude that partial reinforcement increases resistance to extinction in the case of visceral responses.

From a clinical position, the ability of the patient to develop self-control in the absence of feedback is critical, at least for some extended period of time. "Booster" feedback training sessions can also be employed to reinstate the learning, if there has been an indication of extinction. Weiss and Engel (1971) in their study of PVC control phased out the feedback gradually in the range contingency procedure, making it available all the time at first, then 1 minute on and 1 minute off; then 1 on, 3 off; and, finally, 1 on, and 7 off. "By this procedure, the patient was weaned from the light feedback and made to become aware of his PVCs through his own sensations." (p. 302) Hefferline and Bruno (1971) describe a technique of slowly fading out the feedback as a means of transferring external to internal control. Some evidence for the short-term maintenance after training of learned control of diastolic pressure in normal subjects has been presented (Shapiro, Schwartz, and Tursky 1972).

A stickier issue concerns the need of patients to control their reactivity to their usual stressful environment. In most cases, the biofeedback procedure is applied in a resting, nonstimulating laboratory setting. Will the patient be able to transfer this training to the relevant situations in everyday life? A study previously discussed (Sirota, Schwartz, and Shapiro) attempted to explore a new methodology which used feedback training in attempting to facilitate adaptation to noxious events. An earlier unpublished study (Shapiro, Schwartz, Shnidman, Nelson, and Silverman 1972) combined feedback and reinforcement with a variant of a desensitization procedure in attempting to facilitate the adaptation of phobic subjects to the feared stimuli—snakes. Procedures such as these may be needed in patients with psychosomatic disorders to increase the potential of transfer.

AUTONOMIC AWARENESS

The role of awareness of one's own physiological responses in visceral learning has also been treated as a significant theoretical and physiological issue, and various methods of increasing this awareness have been considered as further means of facilitating self-control (see Chapter 19, Brener). The definition of awareness and the creation of experimental procedures to study its relationship to other variables poses very complex methodological problems. While some writers make a simple translation between autonomic control and awareness, the two seem to represent processes that are not always parallel and that can be independent. Homeostatic control of blood pressure and many visceral processes is essentially reflexive, and not associated with conscious sensations or awareness—or learning, for that matter. As Ádám (1967) points out, interoceptive impulses provide normal afferent feedback control of the normal functioning of organs and symptoms from which they arise. On the other hand, there is also relatively well-developed environmental regulation of certain biological functions, such as hunger, thirst, micturition, and defecation, which involves some conscious recognition of bodily sensations. Early in life significant learning takes place in developing this essential control.

In certain pathological conditions, there may be some recognition of internal processes, such as the awareness of minor degrees of hypoxia in patients with heart disease (see Ádám 1967). In essential hypertension, patients commonly complain of a dull pounding headache, dizziness, weakness, palpitations, and other nonspecific symptoms (Harrison et al. 1966). These may provide useful cues to patients, and it may be worthwhile to explore, in the laboratory, relationships between these sensations and accompanying changes in pressure and other physiological measures.

In the early stages of abnormal visceral functioning, it may be speculated, interoceptive signals result in conscious sensations, alerting the individual to the need for readaptation. With prolongation of abnormal function, internal afferent processes become reorganized—including those that relay to higher nervous centers—new homeostatic levels are derived, and consciousness is less disturbed. The resetting of the baroreceptors in maintaining higher levels of blood pressure is a related example of this internal physiological reorganization.

It seems obvious that natural tendencies are built into the organism to keep awareness of internal visceral functions to a minimum, and of the external environment to a maximum. However, disturbed bodily sensations may arise readily where physiological dysfunction occurs. Differences between normals and patients in autonomic awareness of symptom and non-symptom related physiological functions should be evaluated in further research. In patients with arrhythmias, Weiss and Engel (1971) emphasize the importance of "CNS (central nervous system) processing" as an essential element for successful learning of PVC control. This processing enables the patient "to recognize the PVC and to provide the motivation and flexibility necessary to enable learning to occur."

The complex interrelationship of awareness and control is reflected in the apparently inconsistent findings on the role of personality or individual differences in autonomic perception and in the effects of specific instruction regarding the response to be controlled in regard to learned visceral control (see Blanchard and Young 1973; Engel and Hansen 1966; Blanchard, Young, and McLeod 1972; Bergman and Johnson 1972). Clearly, the usefulness of training patients to become aware of their symptoms, perhaps at different stages of biofeedback training, needs careful study.

The role of attentional processes has been discussed previously regarding the development of voluntary control. The degree to which attention and concentration bear directly on awareness of actual bodily sensations arising from visceral processes is not well understood. Kimble and Perlmuter (1970), in their analysis of the problem of volition, note that the elimination, reduction, or distortion of kinesthetic feedback interferes with but does not prevent voluntary behavior. They emphasize centrally located feedback loops, which they translate as "images," in the production of voluntary action. The role of central imagery in developing feedback control of the viscera is currently under investigation (Bell and Schwartz 1972b). How such central imagery corresponds with actual sensations arising from the viscera also needs to be studied more extensively.

HYPERTENSION RESEARCH

In the remainder of this chapter, I will briefly review our specific efforts to date in applying operant-feedback methods to the lowering of blood pressure in patients with essential hypertension. As will be obvious, the actual research with such patients has barely scratched the surface of many of the issues raised above.

An early interest in this illness was stimulated by its widespread prevalence, which is estimated to be about 15% of the general population, and its relationship to other disorders. Elevated arterial blood pressure increases the risk of coronary artery disease, cerebrovascular accidents, atherosclerosis, and nephrosclerosis (Herting and Hunter 1967). Ninety to 95% of all cases of hypertension are "essential," having no known physical etiology, and these cases are considered to be related to and aggravated by behavioral, social, and environmental conditions (see Gutmann and Benson 1971). It has been hypothesized that hyper-reactivity of the sympathetic nervous system may be a major factor in the elevation of blood pressures, as it is often associated with increased heart rate, high cardiac performance, and other related functions.

In view of the assumed environmental and autonomic nervous sys-tem components of essential hypertension, a behavioral method such as operant-feedback autonomic training could offer a nonsurgical, non-drug method of lowering pressure, especially where there are undesired or intolerable side effects. Any lowering of blood pressure reduces the risk of disease, and the potential of biofeedback or other behavioral methods in the early stages of hypertensive illness was par-ticularly intriguing.

The work to date with patients is modeled after the measurement and biofeedback procedures described by Shapiro and his colleagues (Shapiro et al. 1969). Subsequent developments in the procedures and studies in normal subjects on factors affecting learned control of sys-tolic and diastolic blood pressure are described in Chapters 5 and 21.

Benson and his associates (Benson et al. 1971) summarize the appli-cation of operant-feedback techniques to the lowering of systolic blood pressure in seven hypertensive patients, five of whom had essential hypertension. Of the other two, one did not have elevated systolic pres-sure and the other had renal artery stenosis. The latter patients showed little or no decrease in systolic pressure as a result of the conditioning procedure. The five patients responding positively to the procedure showed decreases of 34, 29, 16, 16, and 17 mmHg with 33, 22, 34, 31, and 12 sessions of training, respectively. These changes were measured only under laboratory conditions, and no reliable pressure readings were taken outside the laboratory, although there was an indi-cation of carry-over of training in several patients.

This was a study to demonstrate the bare possibilities of applying the techniques, and the therapeutic usefulness of such methods remains to be evaluated in more systematic clinical research. As men-tioned earlier, nonspecific placebo effects have to be considered, in addition to simple adaptation to the laboratory situation, as alternative explanations of any obtained reductions. The latter possibility seems remote, inasmuch as little or no reduction in pressure was observed in the patients after as many as 15 control sessions under resting condi-tions with no feedback or rewards.

Certain features of these preliminary data can be highlighted. The average amount of within-session decrease in systolic pressure for the patients was about 5 mmHg, about the same as in normals. (In resting control conditions, no such reductions were observed.) Given the over-all effect, this means that the training tended to carry over from session to session. Close inspection of the individual curves suggests a pattern of successive cycles of decreasing pressure, followed by increase, and then a new lowering trend. Apparently, at times, certain events in the life of the patient, or other factors presently not understood, disturb the decremental process, and the pressure bounces back, although not necessarily to the original level. Then, the pressure starts to reduce again over sessions. In some respects, the data resemble a process of successive habituation cycles, interspersed with points of sensitization. The feedback-reward technique may facilitate the process of habituation to the laboratory situation. Whether noncontingent or random feedback, attempts at voluntary control without feedback, or simple muscular relaxation alone could achieve the same results are problems currently under investigation. (This work is being done at the Boston City Hospital with Drs. Herbert Benson and Gary Schwartz).

The problem of transfer of training outside the laboratory is best exemplified by a patient studied in my laboratory at the Massachusetts Mental Health Center. The patient, a 35-year-old mental health worker, appeared to be highly motivated after being diagnosed as essential hypertension, with a pressure of 160/110 mmHg taken during a regular physical examination by his physician. The patient knew about our work and decided to try the procedure before being put on anti-hypertensive medications. He was given feedback for reductions in diastolic pressure after six resting control sessions in which he fluctuated from 80 to 105 mmHg, diastolic. Over nine training sessions, he steadily reduced his pressure from over 100 to about 85 mmHg. Following these sessions, we tried a variety of other procedures, such as autogenic phrases and progressive relaxation in addition to feedback, but the patient began oscillating in pressure between 85 to 95 mmHg. His systolic pressure was recorded in a final session, and it ranged from 135 to 130 mmHg over a 35-minute period. Following these sessions, he returned to his physician for a second physical examination, and he was recorded again at 160/110 mmHg and was put on drugs.

Although it is hazardous to draw any conclusions from this case, a number of speculations can be offered. The patient seemed to be able to adapt to the laboratory situation with the aid of feedback training, although placebo effects cannot be ruled out. Was he unable to transfer this learning to other relevant situations or was his hyperreactivity confined to the medical examination? The latter could be a classically conditioned response unique to the physician taking his pressure. However, it seems likely that other stresses in this patient's environment would have also yielded abnormal responses.

Several approaches are suggested. (1) More extensive, long-term training and greater reductions in basal pressures under resting conditions may be needed. Then, partial reinforcement and training without feedback could be instituted to transform external into internal or self-control so as to effect permanent reductions. (2) In cases exhibiting hyperreactivity that appears to be stimulus-bound, some combination of a desensitization procedure and biofeedback could be combined to facilitate adaptation to real-life situations, perhaps through the use of stresses that are imagined in the laboratory. (3) Feedback training could be instituted in a stimulating or a mildly stressful environment, such as that produced by noise or distracting tasks, as a means of building up resistance to and reducing abnormal physiological responses to general stresses, and possibly to specific stresses. (4) Other clinical procedures discussed previously (meditation, relaxation, autogenic training, yogic exercises) could also be combined with feedback procedure to facilitate learning.

The above possibilities are mentioned to indicate some other directions in clinical application that may be useful to investigators working in different settings, with diverse individual cases, and from a variety of points of view. Needless to say, it is too early to draw any firm conclusion about the future role of biofeedback and operant techniques in treating hypertension. Too little data have been collected, and our present efforts are, by and large, still focused on demonstrating the potential usefulness of the techniques.

Finally, inasmuch as diastolic pressure is commonly viewed as being more critical in certain later stages of hypertension because of its closer relationship to peripheral resistance (Harrison et al. 1966), further research is needed to determine the usefulness of biofeedback procedures for lowering diastolic pressure in such patients. Initial studies in our laboratory at the Boston City Hospital indicate that it is difficult to reduce abnormally high diastolic levels. Part of the difficulty may be related to some unreliability in obtaining accurate and consistent measures of diastolic pressure in repeated sessions. Learned control of diastolic pressure has been observed in a single-session study of normal subjects, with consistent changes occurring in most subjects (Shapiro et al. 1972). Furthermore, systolic pressure may, in fact, be the meaningful index. Comprehensive data were obtained in the Framingham Study to examine the contribution of various indices of blood pressure to the risk of coronary heart disease in a prospective study of more than 5,000 men and women (Kannel, Gordon, and Schwartz 1971). The investigators concluded that "the association between antecedent blood pressure and the incidence of coronary heart disease is actually stronger for systolic than for diastolic pressure." For these reasons, our present strategy is to work with patients showing some lability in their pressure, concentrating on reductions in systolic pressure.

CONCLUSION

Operant-feedback approaches to the control of cardiovascular functions are currently under intensive exploration as a means of alleviating symptoms of various psychosomatic and other disorders that are autonomically mediated. For illnesses such as hypertension, which is believed to affect more than 20 million Americans, the importance to public health of behavioral and environmental methods of controlling high blood pressure, or of preventing the disorder from reaching a serious stage, is obvious. The state of the art, however, is still undeveloped, and much remains to be done in systematic research on the basic techniques themselves. We need to know more about the role of different types and amounts of biofeedback; the matching of feedback with appropriate physiological indices; the proper selection, use, and scheduling of reinforcers; the transfer of training to real-life situations; and the possibilities of enhancing self-control. The techniques of feedback and operant conditioning open up many new possibilities of investigating the integration of physiological processes and central nervous system factors affecting their regulation. Perhaps the most significant development will be in further basic research in "mind-body" interrelationships.

From a clinical point of view, evaluation of the effectiveness and therapeutic value of operant-feedback techniques needs to be established in careful research employing no-treatment and other suitable controls. While basic research on the techniques will help point the way toward more effective application, it is clear that only the most critical questions can be put to careful test. The appetite for application and clinical relevance is great, and the purpose of this chapter was to offer a discussion of issues that might be of value in work with individual patients and in carrying out useful clinical research. To the extent that biofeedback and instrumental learning techniques will be seen not as a solution unto itself of psychophysiological disorders but rather as a means of further elucidating some of the behavioral and environmental factors controlling such disorders, this chapter will have attained its goal.

23

BERNARD T. ENGEL and EUGENE R. BLEECKER

Application of Operant Conditioning Techniques to the Control of the Cardiac Arrhythmias

INTRODUCTION

It is the intent of this chapter to review a number of studies which we and our colleagues have carried out in an attempt to evaluate the clinical application of operant conditioning techniques in the control of cardiac arrhythmias. The research we will be describing here also was designed to enable us to learn more about the control mechanisms of the heart; however, that aspect of our work has been reviewed elsewhere (Engel 1972). Any considerations of mechanisms in this chapter will be limited to speculations about how operant conditioning procedures might be useful diagnostically ·or how these procedures might be therapeutically useful, both as adjuncts to other forms of therapy and by themselves.

CLASSIFICATION OF THE CARDIAC ARRHYTHMIAS[1]

Physiology of Impulse Formation and Conduction in the Normal Heart

Electrical impulse formation is possible throughout the cardiac conduction system, since most cardiac cells have the unique property that they can depolarize spontaneously. The cells in each area of the cardiac conduction system have characteristic rates of depolarization. Normally, the sino-atrial (SA) node has the greatest rate of depolarization. The rate and pattern of cardiac contraction is determined by this pacemaker. Impulses which originate in the SA node subsequently

456

spread through specialized conduction pathways to all parts of the atria and also to the atrioventricular (AV) node.

The cells of the AV node have relatively long refractory periods. Impulses from the AV node are conducted by way of the common bundle (His bundle) through the bundle branches. The bundle branches divide into many fine Purkinje fibers which conduct the electrical impulses to the ventricles, thereby leading to the contraction of these main pumping chambers of the heart. The fibers in the His-Purkinje system exhibit the slowest rate of spontaneous depolarization.

Because of the major differences in conduction among different regions of the heart, one can observe that some cells are depolarizing at times when other cells are repolarizing. This condition creates the possibility that an intracardiac, reverberatory circuit could emerge if a region was depolarized by a normally conducted impulse, subsequently repolarized and then was prematurely depolarized by abnormally prolonged impulses which were being transmitted through adjacent cells. This phenomenon, which is called a reentry mechanism, is important in understanding the cardiac arrhythmias.

The autonomic nervous system innervates the heart at the SA node, the atria, the AV node, and the ventricles (James 1967). Vagal stimulation slows heart rate by decreasing the rate of depolarization of the fibers in the SA node, the atrium, and the AV node. Vagal stimulation also causes modest increases in the conduction velocity of impulses in the atria, and it causes significant decreases in conduction velocity through the AV node. Beta-sympathetic stimulation increases the rate of depolarization, and it increases conduction velocity at all levels of the conduction system.

Cardiac arrhythmias

A cardiac arrhythmia is defined as any abnormality in the site of impulse formation, in the spread of impulses through the conduction system, in the rate at which the heart beats, or in the rhythm with which the heart beats. In the following discussion we will consider the cardiac arrhythmias in terms of two broad classes, ectopic rhythms and conduction defects.

Ectopic Rhythms. When a region of the heart is depolarized by an impulse which has already mediated a normal beat, this region is said to have been depolarized through a reentry mechanism. When this reentrant depolarization leads to the generation of another impulse, the second impulse will be premature, since it will occur too soon after the normal beat to have permitted the ventricles to fill with blood. Premature beats occur rarely in the normal heart. They are common in the injured heart since injury often results either in an increased refractory period of the affected tissue or abnormal conduction patterns in the region of the injured tissue. In either case, the affected tissue depolarizes abnormally late in the cardiac cycle. The interval between the normal and premature beat is called the coupling interval, and it tends to be constant for a given ectopic focus. Since there are a number of factors that can influence the vulnerability of an ectopic focus to a reentering impulse, it is uncommon to see every normal beat followed by an ectopic beat.

Ectopic beats take their name from the locus of their source; e.g., premature atrial contractions (PACs); junctional beats, i.e., the AV nodal-ventricular junction; and premature ventricular contractions (PVCs). Most PVCs are coupled to the preceding normal beat, and, therefore, are probably mediated by a reentrant mechanism. When each normal beat is followed by a PVC, a very regular rhythm, which is called bigeminy, results.

On rare occasions, a ventricular ectopic focus emerges which discharges spontaneously, and which is isolated from normal depolarization by a form of electrical block. This ectopic focus is called a parasystolic focus, and it gives rise to parasystolic beats. These beats have no temporal relationship to the normally conducted beats; however, they do have a fixed temporal relationship to one another. Ventricular rhythm in this case is mediated by two independent pacemakers, the normal one and the parasystolic one. Occasionally, the normal and parasystolic beats coincide to produce a fusion beat.

Tachyarrhythmias.   A tachycardia may be mediated by rapid firing of the SA node or by rapid, repetitive discharge of an ectopic focus. Such an ectopic focus will become the dominant pacemaker and will "capture" the heart rhythm. Tachycardias are usually classified as supraventricular, if the dominant focus is proximal to the ventricles; junctional, if the focus is in the AV nodal-ventricular junction; or, ventricular, if the pacemaker is in the ventricle. Supraventricular tachycardias include: (1) sinus tachycardia in which the pacemaker is the SA node, in which atrial rate ranges from about 100 to 140 bpm, and in which each atrial depolarization leads to a ventricular depolarization; (2) atrial tachycardia which is mediated from an atrial ectopic focus, which is associated with atrial rates which range from about 140 to 220 bpm, and which is associated with one-to-one atrial-ventricular depolarization; (3) atrial flutter in which atrial rate ranges from about 220 to 300 bpm, at which rate the atrium is no longer capable of beating effectively, and at which rate ventricular rate no longer follows atrial rate on a beat-to-beat basis; and, (4) atrial fibrillation in which atrial rate is in excess of 300 bpm, at which rate atrial contraction and conduction patterns are totally disorganized. Atrial fibrillation is the most common cardiac arrhythmia. Ventricular tachycardia is a serious arrhythmia, because it may lead to ventricular fibrillation which is the most serious arrhythmia since it is incompatible with survival.

Bradyarrhythmias. The slow rate observed in patients with bradycardia may be caused by defective impulse formation in the SA node (Rubenstein et al. 1972), or by a defect in impulse conduction—in which case, ventricular rate is partly or wholly determined by a lower, slower pacemaker. This second case is discussed more fully below.

Conduction Defects. The other major class of arrhythmias includes those cardiac abnormalities which are characterized by impaired impulse conduction. The impairment may manifest itself in the electrocardiogram (EKG) by a temporal prolongation of the conduction time between atrial and ventricular depolarization—i.e. by a prolonged P-R interval—or by evidence of bundle branch block. A detailed discussion of all possible conduction defects is beyond the scope of this chapter (see Hecht 1971 for such an analysis). However, we will briefly consider heart block, which is a major subclass of conduction defects.

Heart Block. This category includes three distinct subcategories. First degree heart block is defined in the EKG by the presence of P-R intervals of greater than 0.20 seconds and by one-to-one atrial-ventricular depolarization patterns. Second degree heart block includes two subclasses: Mobitz type I or Wenckebach block in which successive beat-to-beat P-R intervals become progressively longer until, finally, an atrial contraction is not followed by ventricular depolarization and this cycle is repeated; and, Mobitz type II block which is characterized by fixed P-R intervals and by occasions when atrial contractions are not followed by ventricular beats. In Mobitz type I block the defect is in the conduction path between the atrium and the AV node, whereas in Mobitz type II block the defect is in the His-Purkinje system. Third degree heart block is characterized by complete atrioventricular dissociation. The atria beat normally—i.e., about 75 bpm—whereas the ventricles beat abnormally slowly—40 bpm or slower, depending on the site of the ventricular pacemaker.

RESEARCH FINDINGS

Patients with Ectopic Rhythms

Patients with premature ventricular contractions have been studied extensively in our laboratory. This arrhythmia has been of particular clinical interest because of the association of PVCs with sudden death and coronary artery disease (Chiang et al. 1969; Lown and Wolf 1971), and because drug therapy often does not surpress these ectopic beats satisfactorily. Premature atrial contractions have not been associated with serious cardiac prognoses, and until now we never have trained patients with premature atrial or nodal contractions to control these ectopic beats.

Since the results of one study in which patients were trained to control PVC frequency have been published (Weiss and Engel 1971), we will only summarize its major clinical findings. That study reported the results with eight patients, five of whom showed evidence of being able to learn to decrease the prevalence of their PVCs in the laboratory, and four of whom showed evidence of being able to maintain this behavior outside the laboratory. Among these four patients we have followed only one in our clinic beyond the period cited in the published report. The patient we have followed was reported then to have 1 to 6 PVC/min, two months after study. After about five years her PVCs continue to be rare, and she does not require any antiarrhythmic medication. During 5-minute rhythm strips taken in the clinic, she rarely has any PVCs.

Among the patients who failed to show any evidence of control in the laboratory, two probably had hearts which were diseased irreversibly, and which could not respond to therapy. One patient had a cardiomyopathy with a severely enlarged heart, and the other had an extremely, electrically unstable heart which produced multifocal PVCs of at least four different electrical configurations, and which posed difficulties for heart rate (HR) and PVC detection and made accurate feedback to the patient difficult.

We subsequently have studied another patient with PVCs. This patient was a 27-year-old woman with Marfan's syndrome, an inherited connective tissue disorder clinically characterized by abnormalities of the skeletal system, the eye, and the cardiovascular system. Since she was 20, this patient experienced progressive congestive heart failure which was unresponsive to medical management. At 25 she had a mitral valve replacement for severe mitral regurgitation which controlled her congestive heart failure. However, she has continued to have as many as 20 PVCs/min despite therapy with quinidine and procainamide. Because of these persistent, frequent PVCs which were not controlled medically, she was referred to our laboratory.

This patient was first trained to control her heart rate. This training comprised three stages: First, she was trained to slow HR, then to speed HR, and, finally, to slow and speed HR cyclically. After this training was completed, she was trained to maintain her HR within a narrow range. Because a PVC is followed by a compensatory pause, the feedback during this stage of training gives the patient information about each ectopic beat (see Weiss and Engel 1971, for a detailed discussion of this procedure).

Figure 23.1 summarizes her PVC and HR levels during this study.

During pretraining, control sessions over each of two days, this patient emitted averages of 12 PVC/min and 18 PVC/min, respectively. She was able to speed HR more consistently than to slow HR, and she was able to differentially slow and speed HR. PVC frequency was not related to absolute HR. She stated that during initial training, besides gaining the ability to control HR, she had learned to recognize PVCs; and, she said that she was able to decrease PVC frequency. In the course of training, PVC frequency decreased to less than 0.5 PVC/min. During range training when she was primarily trained to control PVCs directly, she emitted almost no PVCs. Follow-up testing during the following nine months has shown no PVCs, except for one occasion just after completion of training when she had about 1 PVC/min. These laboratory results are corroborated by several, continuous, 10-hour tape recordings of her EKG outside of the laboratory. Presently she is active, works as a secretary, and does not require antiarrhythmic medications.

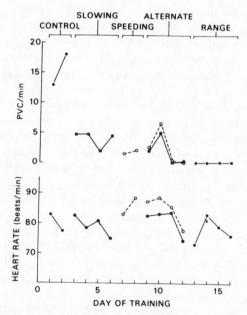

FIGURE 23.1. *Daily averages during training to control HR and PVCs. Each day comprises three to five, 1024-second training sessions. During control (o–o) days the patient received no feedback nor did she attempt to exercise any cardiac control. During slowing (o–o) and speeding (o---o) days the patient was trained to slow and to speed her HR respectively. During alternate days the patient was required to speed and to slow her HR cyclically for 256 seconds each during each 1024-second training session. During range (o–o) training the patient was required to maintain her HR within a 5 or 10 beat range.*

Patients with Tachyarrhythmias

Ventricular tachycardia is much less common than supraventricular tachycardia, and it is a very serious arrhythmia since it may lead to ventricular fibrillation which is usually fatal. This arrhythmia, therefore, requires emergency treatment and does not lend itself to laboratory conditioning.

We have seen three patients with various supraventricular tachycardias. Their data will be presented in detail.

Patient with Sinus Tachycardia[2]

This patient was a 53-year-old woman who had persistent sinus tachycardia which was not secondary to thyroid, adrenal, or hematological disease. Barbiturates, digitalis, and small doses of quinidine and phenothiazine, which were administered during the preceding four years, had not been effective in the control of her arrhythmia. Her pulse rate, whether recorded by the patient, her family, her physician, or laboratory personnel, never fell below 80 bpm and averaged 106 bpm on 50 observations over four years. The patient participated in 21 experimental sessions, during which she was always trained to slow her heart. The results (Figure 23.2) indicate clearly that the subject learned to slow her rate from rest. Her baseline HR fell from 86.3 bpm during the early training sessions to 68.5 bpm during the later sessions.

During the last nine sessions we alternated periods of feedback with periods of no feedback. In sessions 12 to 15 the feedback was present for 1 minute and not present for the next minute (1:1); during sessions 16 to 18 the feedback light was functional for 1 minute and not functional for the next 3 minutes (3:1); during sessions 19 to 21 the light was functional for 1 minute and not functional for the next 7 minutes (7:1). All of these cyclic-alternation sessions lasted 48 minutes. The purpose of the cyclic-alternation sessions was to determine whether the patient had developed internal cues to keep her rate slow regardless of whether the extrinsic feedback was available. We found that she did equally well whether the light was functional or not (Figure 23.2). She said that she kept the light on by relaxing and that she concentrated on her heart beat, which she had learned to sense.

In order to learn whether the effect we were observing in the laboratory was unique to the situation, the patient saw her private physician each week (he was not informed about her progress in the laboratory). His records show that she maintained her rate at about 75 bpm during these visits (Figure 23.3). Furthermore, her blood pressure fell from about 140/80 mmHg before training to 115/75 mmHg by the end of training.

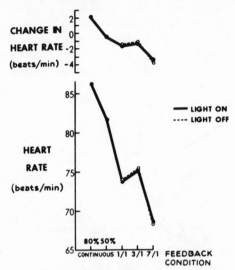

FIGURE 23.2.   *Mean heart rates and mean changes in heart rate from baseline levels in a patient with sinus tachycardia being trained to slow her heart rate. Numbers on the abscissa refer to various stages of training: 80%, continuous feedback with the trigger set so that maintenance of baseline heart rate would result in successful performance 80% of the time; 50%, continuous feedback with the trigger set so that maintenance of baseline heart rate would result in successful performance 50% of the time; 1:1, alternate 1-minute periods of feedback and no feedback during which the patient was instructed to slow her heart rate; 3:1, alternate 3-minute periods of no feedback and 1-minute period of feedback; 7:1, alternate 7-minute periods of no feedback and 1-minute periods of feedback. Performance is equally good with (o-o) and without (o---o) feedback. (From Engel 1972–Copyright © 1972, The Society for Psychophysiological Research)*

Patient with Supraventricular Tachycardia[2]

This patient was a 41-year-old man who reported that he always had had symptoms of rapid pulse and palpitations. A diagnosis of paroxysmal atrial tachycardia was made 10 years before our study. During the last eight years before the study his tachycardia became constant. He was admitted to the hospital this time because the tachycardia had led to exercise intolerance, paroxysmal nocturnal dyspnea, orthopnea, and evidence of mild congestive heart failure unresponsive to digitalis and diuretics.

His heart rate ranged between 130 and 140 bpm. During 15 hospitalizations at the University of California and 10 at Stanford University, no underlying cardiac disease could be found nor did treatment with metaraminol, edrophonium, diphenylhydantoin, Xylocaine®,

digoxin, vagal stimulation, guanethidine, or direct-current cardiover-
sion produce reliable or prolonged amelioration of his arrhythmia.
Physical and laboratory findings reflected left ventricular enlargement
and failure without evidence of congential heart anomalies or acquired
valvular heart disease.

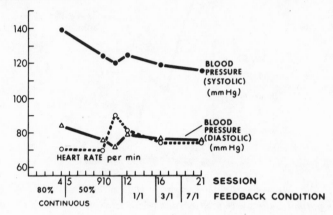

FIGURE 23.3.   *Systolic (o-o) and diastolic (Δ-Δ) blood pressure and heart
rates (o---o) recorded by the patient's physician. See Figure 23.2 for
definition of abscissa.*

   This patient participated in one control session and 25 experimental
sessions. The training periods lasted about 30 minutes, and the subject
was always taught to slow his rate. He usually had two sessions each
day. Because his heart rate was relatively stable in the early stages of
our study, we provided him with an oscilloscopic display of a cardiotachometer signal rather than a light feedback. The face of the oscilloscope was calibrated in beats per minute (80 to 140 in early sessions
and 60 to 120 in later ones), so that he always knew not only his cardiac
rhythm but also his absolute rate. During the final eight sessions we
replaced the oscilloscope with the light-feedback system. We also
recorded his cardiac activity on the ward by means of a telemetry/tape
system. Our results are based on one continuous 10-minute sample
taken from each hour in a 17-hour period, three days a week.[3]
   Figure 23.4 shows the changes in HR during training. This patient
was usually able to slow his rate from rest, and was even more effective
when using the light feedback than when using the oscilloscope feedback.
   This patient's HR recorded in the laboratory paralleled that recorded
by telemetry (Figure 23.5). The low rate during Session 10, for example, was primarily the result of frequent periods of sinus arrest. By
the tenth experimental day the patient had established a regular HR
which was about 15 bpm below that of the control period.

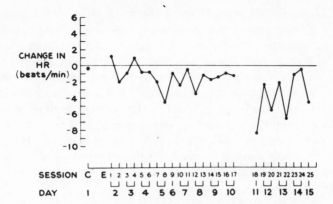

FIGURE 23.4. *Changes in HR from baseline during one control (no feedback training) and 25 slow training sessions given over 15 days. During sessions 1 to 17 (days 2 to 10), feedback was a calibrated oscilloscope face; during sessions 18 to 25 (days 11 to 15) feedback was a light.*

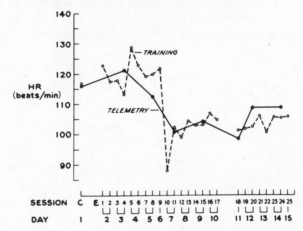

FIGURE 23.5. *Heart rate levels during laboratory training sessions and during ward telemetry recordings. See Figure 23.4 for definition of abscissa.*

There were other signs of significant change in cardiac function. By day 15, digitalis was discontinued when his HR slowed and diuresis also occurred. His heart size decreased as recorded by roentgenograms, his venous pressures were within normal limits, and his liver became smaller. Simultaneously, his exercise tolerance increased, his clinical status shifted from functional Class III to Class I, and his cardiogram was interpreted as a normal sinus rhythm.

About three weeks after the completion of the training sessions and discharge from the hospital, an additional five sessions were scheduled. On two of those occasions his HR was about 60 bpm, and on the other three occasions his HR was 120 to 160 bpm. During the training period of one of these sessions he converted his heart rhythm, when he abruptly terminated an episode of supraventricular tachycardia at a rate of 156 bpm to a normal sinus rhythm at a rate of 66 bpm (Figure 23.6). He recognized when his rate was elevated, and said he believed that the increase was transient. Further evidence of significant changes in the patient occurred during visits to the outpatient department and cardiac clinic over the succeeding five months. His rate ranged from 60 to 75 bpm, and an EKG taken about three months after his last laboratory training session showed a sinus rhythm with a rate of 65 bpm. At the time of this clinic visit there had been no return of his symptoms of congestive heart failure.

Patient with a History of Paroxysmal Atrial Tachycardia (PAT) and Episodes of Sinus Tachycardia

This 36-year-old practical nurse had been evaluated in the outpatient cardiac clinic because of episodes of rapid HR which were associated with syncope and diaphoresis. On at least two occasions prior to study these episodes were documented electrocardiographically to be consist-

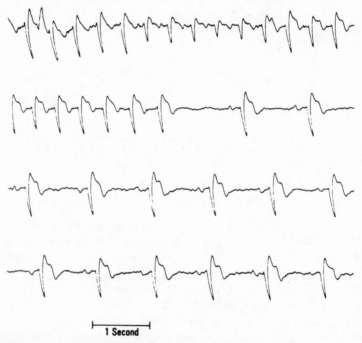

1 Second

FIGURE 23.6. *EKG rhythm strip during spontaneous conversion from PAT to normal sinus rhythm within a training session.*

ent with paroxysmal atrial tachycardia (PAT). Atrial rate was 180 bpm, and the rhythm was converted to normal sinus with carotid massage. She reported that she experienced approximately one episode of PAT every month over a period of two years. She also reported episodes of what we presume to be sinus tachycardia with HR between 120 to 130 bpm. These episodes were not related to physical activity. A complete endocrine evaluation had been normal. There were no signs of congestive heart failure. Her heart was not enlarged clinically, and her electrocardiogram was essentially normal. The only medical therapy administered was diazepam, 5 mg three times per day, when needed.

The patient was trained to control HR and the results of this training are graphed in Figure 23.7. Although she slowed HR in 10 of 20 slow training sessions, the magnitude of her HR changes was small and her performance was not consistent. The patient was then trained to speed HR. She learned this response easily, and often was able to speed HR between 15 to 20 bpm above her baseline rate. By learning to increase her HR she stated that she experienced less anxiety with a faster HR. During differential training she correctly modified HR during sequential 256-second speeding and slowing phases of each 1048-second alternate training sessions.

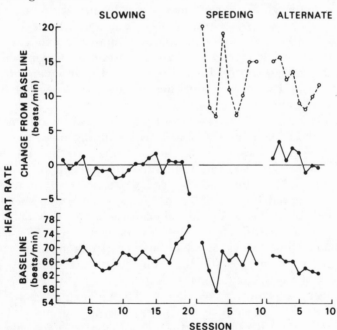

FIGURE 23.7. *Changes in HR and baseline HR levels during slowing training (o-o), speeding training (o- -o) and alternate slowing and speeding training. Abscissa is session number within each training condition.*

During these training sessions, she said that she gained confidence in her ability to control her HR and that she "knew" she could significantly decrease a rapid HR. This control was evident in follow-up testing in the laboratory.

In the six months since the completion of training she has experienced only one episode of rapid heart rate which she states she was able to slow voluntarily, and for which she did not require medical treatment.

Patients with Atrial Fibrillation

We have recently studied a group of six patients with atrial fibrillation (Bleecker and Engel 1973). The primary purpose of that study was not clinical. It was designed to clarify some of the physiological mechanisms underlying learned control of cardiac function (Engel 1972). The results of this study indicated that digitalized patients with atrial fibrillation can learn to modify ventricular rate (VR) voluntarily. This control of VR seems to be mediated at the atrioventricular node by modification of vagal tone to the heart. In this study there also were some findings of clinical interest, and we will review our results with one patient in detail.

This patient was a 57-year-old man with a history of rheumatic heart disease characterized by mitral stenosis and aortic insufficiency. In 1951 and in 1958 he underwent mitral commissurotomies to relieve his mitral stenosis. Since 1950, he has had atrial fibrillation which has required digoxin to control his normally rapid ventricular rate. Prior to this study he had been maintained on a stable dosage of digoxin and hydrochlorothiazide.

This patient received a total of 40 training sessions during which he was trained to slow his VR, speed his VR, and, finally, to cyclically slow and speed his VR. During this last phase of training he was required to slow his VR for 4 minutes, then speed his VR for 4 minutes, and then to slow and to speed VR again for 4 minutes each. The patient slowed his VR in 12 of 12 sessions, and he speeded his VR in 13 of 16 sessions. He was able consistently to slow or to speed VR approximately 10% above or below baseline levels. Figure 23.8 shows interval histograms of all of his ventricular beats during the baseline and training phases of four representative sessions. As can be seen, the training histograms are shifted to the left relative to the baseline histograms during speeding training indicating faster VR, and they are shifted to the right relative to baseline during slowing training indicating slower VR. These shifts indicate shorter and longer R-R intervals, respectively. Although the histograms are skewed, they are unimodal.

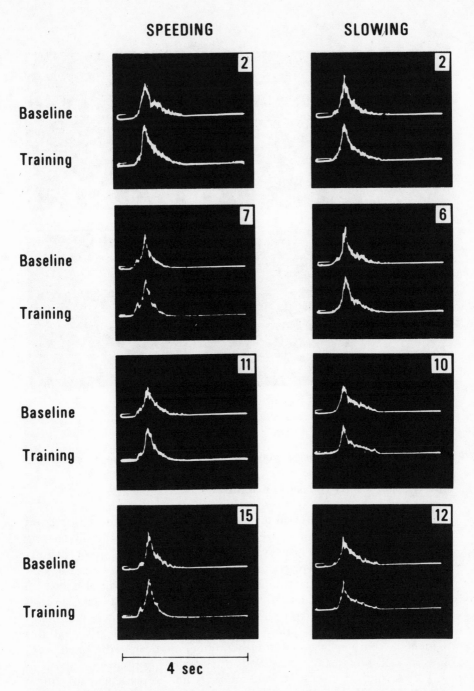

FIGURE 23.8. *R-R interval histograms during progressive stages of slowing and speeding training (Number on histogram refers to training session number). (From Bleecker and Engel 1973)*

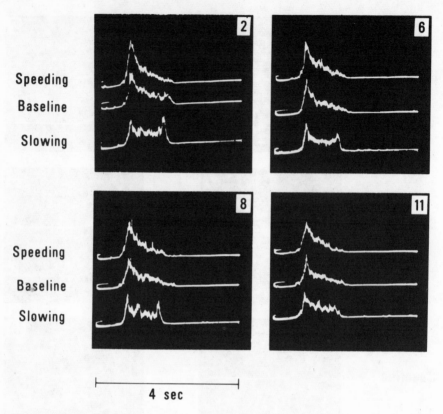

Speeding

Baseline

Slowing

Speeding

Baseline

Slowing

4 sec

FIGURE 23.9.   *R-R interval histograms during progressive stages of alternate training sessions the second modal peak during slowing occurs at a ventricular rate of approximately 40 bpm. (From Bleecker and Engel 1973)*

Figure 23.9 shows interval histograms from the baseline slowing and speeding phases of four representative sessions from the alternating sessions. A consistent tendency for bimodal distributions to occur during the slowing phases of training only is clearly discernible. The second mode in these distributions occurs at an R-R interval of about 1.5 seconds, which is equivalent to a VR of 40 bpm. Figure 23.10 is a series of rhythm strips taken from the baseline, slowing, and speeding phases of alternate session 2. These rhythms strips show clearly that this patient is voluntarily generating a number of beats with fixed, prolonged R-R intervals of 1.5 seconds during slowing phases only.

This second grouping of R-R intervals may represent a junctional escape pacemaker which is considered to be caused by pathologic AV block in atrial fibrillation (Urbach, Grauman, and Straus 1969). This patient was chronically maintained on a stable dosage of digoxin. There is no evidence of digitalis toxicity during immediately preceding baseline recording periods, nor during temporally contiguous periods of VR speeding. One may conclude that this junctional escape pacemaker was either caused by direct modification of the AV node during voluntary slowing of VR, or that learned modification of VR was additive to that of digitalis thereby unmasking latent digitalis toxicity.

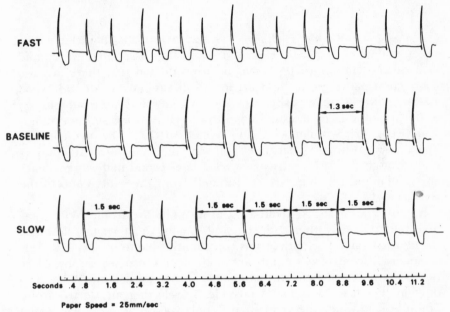

FIGURE 23.10. *EKG rhythm strip showing junctional escape rhythm only during slowing phases of an alternate training session.*

Patients with Conduction Defects

As we have discussed previously, conduction abnormalities include a number of complex arrhythmias. We have studied only two kinds of conduction defects, third degree heart block and the Wolff-Parkinson-White Syndrome (WPW). Complete reports describing these findings are now in preparation; therefore, these studies will be summarized here only.

Third Degree Heart Block. Three patients with this diagnosis were trained to speed VR. None of the patients increased VR consistently. In one case, pharmacological studies indicated that the cardiac lesion was in the atrioventricular node, and that the VR probably was mediated by a junctional pacemaker. A second patient produced premature ventricular contractions, and, since this arrhythmia is not associated with compensatory pauses in patients with complete heart block, the emergence of these ectopic beats was associated with increased ventricular rate. The data from this last patient, incidentally, offer further evidence that extrinsic, autonomic nerves to the ventricles do not mediate chronotropic responses (Engel 1972). A third patient was unable to alter his ventricular rate. The results of this study indicate that the connections from the atrioventricular node to the ventricle are necessary for the mediation of learned control of ventricular rate.

Wolff-Parkinson-White Syndrome.   This arrhythmia is characterized by preexcitation of the ventricles, and it is often associated with rapid tachycardias (James 1970). It has been postulated that there are two conduction pathways to the heart in this disease (Wolferth and Wood 1933). However, many aspects of the anatomy and electrophysiology of this hypothesized, accessory conduction pathway are still not understood (Durrer, Schuilenberg, and Willens 1970). The two-pathway hypothesis postulates that one pathway mediates normal conduction through the atrioventricular node. The second pathway mediates aberrant impulses which are transmitted from the sinus node to the ventricles.

A patient with type A, Wolff-Parkinson-White Syndrome (WPW) was first trained to slow, then to speed, and, finally, to alternately slow and speed heart rate. The patient was consistently able to modify HR. Differential HR control was significant in 20 of 21 alternate sessions. After rate training, the patient was taught to control normal and WPW conduction. Feedback was made possible by selecting an electrocardiograph lead in which the ventricular depolarization of WPW conducted beats and normally conducted beats were opposite. The patient learned to increase and to decrease WPW and normal conduction reliably. During the last phase of training, the patient learned to increase normal conduction without feedback. Pharmacologic studies suggested that the mechanism of this control of conduction was by modification of vagal tone to the heart. It should also be noted that analyses of the changes in HR and the changes in conduction patterns indicated that these two responses were uncorrelated. Thus, the degree to which this patient could control cardiac conduction was not mediated by his ability to control HR (Bleecker and Engel 1973).

DETERMINANTS OF LEARNING

Our laboratory results to date have been largely positive. Most of the patients we have studied have been able to learn some degree of control over their arrhythmias. Some of our findings have been especially encouraging because follow-up data have indicated that the effects learned in the laboratory have carried over to outside environments, and because the patients seem to be able to retain the skills they learned in the laboratory even after many years. In this section we will summarize those factors which we believe are especially important in our training procedures or in the patients themselves, and which mediate successful learning.

Training Procedure

We believe that there are three factors in the training procedure which contribute to the successful performances we have seen. One factor is the presence of a percentage time meter in the patient's room. This meter is calibrated from zero to 100, and it runs whenever the subject's feedback light is on. At the end of a training session this clock tells the subject how well he has done. Many subjects have reported that the clock provides them with an additional incentive to "try harder to keep the light on." Since the clock is functional only during the earlier stages of training when the subject is being taught to slow or to speed his heart, its major role is probably to facilitate the maintenance of the motivational level of the patient during these initial learning stages.

A second factor which seems to contribute importantly to successful performance is the differential training procedure. A number of patients have indicated to us that their successful performance during these cyclic alternation periods was the factor which most convinced them that they truly were able to control their hearts. These patients stated that they regarded their performances during the unidirectional conditioning sessions as encouraging; however, they believed that their performances during the alternating sessions comprised irrefutable evidence of their abilities to control their hearts. The laboratory data also seem to support the notion that the differential training sessions were important, since some of the greatest changes in cardiac function occur during these training sessions, and these changes seem to be maintained subsequently.

The third factor which appears to be important in patient training is the differential feedback procedure. During these sessions, the subjects are alternately given feedback information and then not given feedback information. Our purpose in including this procedure was to wean the patient from the gadgetry, because the clinical value of the conditioning depended on the subject being able to perform successfully in nonlaboratory environments. Apparently this technique was successful, since the patients report that their ability to perform without feedback is strong evidence *to them* that they have developed their own intrinsic cues, and that they "know" when their hearts are beating normally *and* abnormally, and that they "know" how to change the rhythm in either direction.

Patient Characteristics

Elsewhere we have proposed six factors which seem to us to be important in learning to control PVCs (Weiss and Engel 1971). These factors seem to be important in the learning of any arrhythmia. The factors are: (1) Peripheral receptors which are stimulated by the cardiac response of interest. In the initial stages of training this function is subserved by the feedback light. Eventually the patient learns to recognize information provided by other receptors. (2) Afferent nerves which transmit information from the receptors to the central nervous system (CNS). (3) CNS factors which enable the patient to recognize the information transmitted about the heart, and which provide the patient with behavioral characteristics—e.g., motivation—necessary to mediate learning and to maintain performance. (4) Efferent nerves to the heart which are capable of producing the desired changes in cardiac function. (5) A heart which is capable of beating more regularly. There are many patients in whom the disease is too severe to permit any significant changes in cardiac function to occur. We already have reported two instances in which we believe this was true (Weiss and Engel 1971). (6) A homeostatic system which will tolerate a more normal function of the heart. In the case of the cardiac arrhythmias this factor should not be a significant limitation. However, there are other diseases of the heart which may be theoretically modifiable by conditioning, but which practically are difficult or impossible because hemodynamic requirements preclude such changes. For example, a patient with coarctation of his aorta will not be able to maintain a reduction in his cardiac output, because his peripheral circulation will be too severely compromised.

PROJECTIONS

In this section we will assess the status of the clinical application of operant conditioning of cardiac function, and we will indicate some additional experiments which have been suggested by our results.

We believe our results show clearly that patients can be taught to regulate their cardiac arrhythmias, and that some patients can initiate and maintain this learned behavior outside of the laboratory. These results are sufficiently encouraging to warrant two kinds of studies: One set of studies should be directed at procedural issues; and the second set should be concerned with clinical applications to other cardiovascular diseases.

Procedural Questions

We believe that efforts should be made by other investigators to try to replicate our results. Once this has been done—we presume successfully—a number of studies should be designed to optimize the training procedures from a clinical point of view. Some questions which these studies should answer are: (1) What responses must a patient be taught—e.g., we taught all our patients to control their heart rates; however, it is possible that one might be able to teach patients rhythm control directly. (2) What criteria can be used to decide that a patient is ready to move to another stage of training—our criteria usually have been intuitive rather than rational. (3) What is an optimal training procedure—we have tended to mass practice with several daily sessions over a few weeks; however, fewer sessions or longer training periods might be better. (4) Should one include "refresher" courses—our limited experience indicates that patients retain their skills without intervening training sessions; however, we have not followed all of the patients we have studied, nor have we studied great numbers of patients. (5) Can technicians be trained to implement the training procedures—we have trained all the patients we have seen. However, it is impractical to expect that there will be sufficient professional workers available to carry out these procedures, and skilled technicians working under appropriate supervision are necessary to make the training procedures practical.

The five questions we raised above do not exhaust the procedural problems which are yet unsolved. However, these questions do illustrate the magnitude of work yet to be done before one can begin to regard our techniques as therapeutic in any practical sense. Hopefully, others who have speculated about clinical applications of operant conditioning procedures to cardiovascular or other diseases will also consider the relevance of questions, such as we have raised, to their own work.

Additional Applications to Cardiac Diseases

There are a number of cardiac diseases which are medically controlled by autonomic drugs. It would be interesting to study the possible application of operant conditioning procedures to any or all of these. For example, beta-adrenergic blockade with medications such as propranolol is employed in several cardiac disease states including supraventricular arrhythmias (atrial flutter, atrial fibrillation, paroxysmal atrial tachycardia, and tachyarrhythmias and ventricular irritability due to digitalis intoxication), angina pectoris, hyperdynamic beta-adrenergic circulatory states, as an adjunct in the therapy of hypertension, and in other disorders of adrenergic control of the heart. Operant cardiac training might prove to be either a useful therapeutic technique or an adjunct to present forms of therapy in these conditions. It would be interesting to try to teach patients with angina pectoris to reduce their heart rates and possibly simultaneously to reduce blood pressure. Such control would be expected to enable these patients to voluntarily reduce the frequency and severity of the chest pain associated with this disorder. This training could be used to resolve individual episodes of pain and might circumvent the side effects of chronic administration of propranolol in these patients such as bradycardia, congestive heart failure, and even hypoglycemia.

Other arrhythmias may be studied in the hope of further clarifying the physiology of these disorders and thereby establishing a better rationale for their treatment. For example, Mobitz type I—the so-called Wenckebach block—should be modifiable through conditioning, whereas Mobitz type II heart block should not be so controllable. These and other arrhythmias frequently complicate the recovery from an acute myocardial infarction and may cause therapeutic problems (e.g., DeSanctis, Block, and Hutter 1972; Rotman, Wagner, and Wallace 1972).

In addition to the experiments which we have proposed to test the clinical merit of operant conditioning techniques, and to add to the general knowledge about additional potential applications of these techniques, there is another class of experiments that is suggested. It would be interesting to evaluate the role of learned control of cardiac function as a tool in diagnostic procedures or as means of refining a drug regimen. An example of an experiment to evaluate the use of the conditioning techniques as a diagnostic adjunct would be among patients scheduled for diagnostic, His bundle recordings (Scherlag, Samet, and Helfant 1972). It is possible that if these patients also were trained to differentially control their heart rates, the assessment of their nodal conduction patterns might be improved. An example of a test of the application of conditioning as an adjunct to pharmacological therapy would be in the case of patients who are treated to slow HR with propranolol or digoxin. Would the hearts of such patients be able to function effectively on reduced amounts of these drugs if the patients also were trained to slow their heart rates? Might the management of patients with refractive PVCs be improved by combining drug therapy and operant conditioning?

NOTES

1. We wish to acknowledge our deep appreciation to Miss Jeanette Williams who helped us greatly by typing the final draft of this manuscript when our secretary was taken ill.

2. This patient was seen by Dr. Bernard T. Engel in collaboration with Dr. Kenneth L. Melmon.

3. Ordinarily, a 17-hour average would be of dubious value since diurnal variations in heart rate are considerable. However, in the early stages of the study this patient had little or no change in cardiac rate. Only by the third telemetry day (the fifth experimental day) did any diurnal variations appear. These variations were frequent periods of sinus arrest and occasional sustained episodes of rates of about 60 bpm. Such periods occurred most frequently about 6:00 to 8:00 a.m.

V

Heart Rate — Attentional and Motivational Processes

The three chapters in this section focus on heart rate and its relation to several behavioral processes, particularly sensorimotor processes. The chapter by Clifton details several experiments evaluating orienting and conditioning in newborns the purpose of which is to determine whether heart rate can be used to index developmental status. The results are somewhat inconclusive and indicate the methodological difficulties faced in working with the newborn. Elliott's chapter is a more general critical review of the use of heart rate to index motivational and emotional states as well as in sensorimotor processes. Where relevant, experimental data is presented. Such a review is overdue particularly in the light of the mounting evidence indicating that heart rate is not a simple index of arousal and affective states. The chapter by the Laceys presents some new experiments concerning sensorimotor processes where they evaluate not only phasic heart rate changes but intracardiac cycle effects within the framework of their neurophysiological afferent feedback model. In several places in the chapter, as well as in an addendum to the chapter, some recent criticisms that have been directed at the afferent model are discussed.

24

RACHEL KEEN CLIFTON

Cardiac Conditioning and Orienting in the Infant

INTRODUCTION

Three Paradigms for Investigating Cognitive Processes in the Infant: Orienting, Habituation, and Conditioning

When a newborn baby is examined by the pediatrician, the assessment of central nervous system (CNS) development is crude at best. The elicitation of various reflexes and the observation of the baby's responses during the examination constitute a gross means of determining the intactness of the nervous system. The detection of prenatal and perinatal brain damage is extremely difficult in the newborn, unless there is a disease present that is known to produce such impairment, or the damage is so great that the brain stem has been affected. Histological work (Conel 1952) has indicated that important anatomical changes in the cerebral cortex take place during the early postnatal months. The problem of tying readily observable behavioral responses to these anatomical changes remains.

The human newborn has few responses that can readily be used to indicate cortical functioning. He is nonverbal and motorically immature; he has rapidly shifting states of arousal, and no feeling of

Portions of the research reported in this paper were supported by grants MH-18107 and HD06753 to the author, and fellowships from the Government of Quebec to Andreé Pomerleau-Malcuit and the Canadian National Research Council to Gerard Malcuit. The author deeply appreciates these colleagues' collaboration, as well as that of Christina Appleton, who aided in data collection and analyses. The author would like to thank the pediatric and nursing staff of the Cooley Dickinson Hospital in Northampton, Massachusetts for their cooperation.

obligation to cooperate with the experimenter. For the past decade, researchers have heavily employed physiological responses as a means of tapping the infant's responses to sensory stimulation. Heart rate, respiration, basal skin conductance, and evoked potentials are among the responses that have been used to reflect the infant's reception and processing of sensory input. Reviews of psychophysiological responding in infants are available by Graham and Jackson (1970), Lewis (1972), and Steinschneider (1967). This chapter will deal primarily with the use of the cardiac response in studies of habituation, orienting, and conditioning. These three paradigms may reveal the infant's mental organization of repetitive, novel, and contingent events, respectively.

The cardiac response has been extensively used to study habituation to auditory, visual, and tactile stimuli during the first year of life. Heart rate (HR) changes in newborns can reflect differences in auditory stimuli varying in duration (Clifton, Graham, and Hatton 1968); intensity (Steinschneider, Lipton, and Richmond 1966); and rise time (Jackson, Kantowitz, and Graham 1971). Concomitant HR changes have been found in older infants for visual stimuli varying in complexity (McCall and Kagan 1967); facial arrangements (Kagan et al. 1966); and apparent depth in a visual cliff situation (Campos, Langer, and Krowitz 1970). Maturational changes in the direction of the cardiac response to auditory stimuli have been observed (Clifton and Meyers 1969; Hatton 1969). Arousal state also influences direction and amplitude of HR change to sensory stimuli (Lewis, Bartels, and Goldberg 1967; Jackson, Kantowitz, and Graham 1971). In general, HR has provided a means of reflecting the infant's reception and discrimination of a wide variety of stimulus change. Furthermore, repeated stimulation generally produces a decrement in both amplitude and duration of HR change (Bartoshuk 1962b; Clifton, Graham, and Hatton 1968), while dishabituation elicits levels of responding similar to the initial response (Berg 1972; Bartoshuk 1962a).

Investigators interested in the infant's habituation to stimuli used HR change as a response measure primarily because it worked; i.e., orderly changes in HR reflected changes in the presented stimuli. With the exception of Lipton and his co-workers (Lipton, Steinschneider, and Richmond 1961, 1964, 1966), who sought to characterize individual infants on the basis of their autonomic responding, most investigators did not consider HR an intrinsically interesting response. Indeed, 50 data points per trial are not desirable, if a simple head turn or knee jerk would yield the same information about central processing of stimuli. Although this attitude is, for the most part, still prevalent, there are two aspects of cardiac responding itself that bear further investigation. One is that the directionality of HR change may differentiate reactions arising from different arousal systems (orienting versus defense);

and, secondly, that autonomic responses may yield unique information not available from somatic responses.

Directionality of HR Change

The meaning of the directionality of the HR response in infants has been explored by Graham and Jackson (1970). They discussed Sokolov's (1963) two arousal systems, the orienting reflex (OR) and the defense reflex (DR), that are mobilized in specific situations for different purposes. The OR, primarily elicited by novel stimuli, serves to enhance environmental intake by the organism's sensory systems. The DR, primarily elicited by intense stimuli, serves to inhibit the reception of such stimuli, thereby lessening their effect. Although many physiological changes are involved in the elicitation of both reflexes, HR is one of the few components that differentiates between them. HR acceleration is a component of the DR, while HR deceleration is a component of the OR (Graham and Clifton 1966; Graham and Jackson 1970). This is relevant for understanding infant behavior, since a developmental shift from acceleratory to deceleratory responses has been observed from the newborn period up to three or four months of age. Clifton and Meyers (1969) found HR deceleration in four-month-olds to the same square wave stimulus that had elicited acceleration in the newborn. The older infant's deceleratory response has been further documented with a variety of auditory stimuli (Berg 1972; Berg, Berg, and Graham 1971; Hatton 1969). Likewise, the newborn's acceleratory response to both tactile and auditory stimuli has been reported by many investigators (Lipton, Steinschneider, and Richmond 1961; Bridger 1961; Bridger and Birns 1963). At the time of Graham and Jackson's review (1970), no clear HR deceleration to any stimulus had been reported in the newborn, but these authors noted that stimuli presented to newborns usually had sudden onsets, were fairly intense, and stimulated the less mature sensory modalities. Additionally, newborn subjects generally had been sleeping or in unspecified states of arousal.

At least three studies have recently reported HR deceleration in newborns. A checkerboard pattern (Sameroff, Cashmore, and Dykes 1973), pure tones and white noise with slow rise times (Kearsley 1973), and a low frequency square wave and vestibular stimulation (Pomerleau-Malcuit and Clifton 1973), to be described later in this paper, have all been found to produce slowing of cardiac rate in neonates. It is noteworthy that the Ss were awake in all three studies. Although Lipsitt and Jacklin (1971) reported deceleration to olfactory stimuli in sleeping newborns, Jacklin (1972) was unable to replicate this finding in a later study. Lewis, Bartels, and Goldberg (1967) had suggested that state might be the major determinant of the direction of HR change to stimulation, and the source of the developmental shift from birth to the older infant, since newborns are more apt to be tested when asleep. Graham and Jackson (1970) reviewed studies using 6- and 12-week-old infants, awake and sleeping. Both age and state affect phase and direction of the HR response, with acceleration appearing to some tones in sleeping Ss. Jackson, Kantowitz, and Graham (1971) reported deceleration in awake newborns to pure tones with a slow rise time on the first second of the first trial block, but failed to replicate the finding in a second study. This same stimulus elicited sustained deceleration in awake, older infants. To further complicate the acceleration-deceleration picture, Gregg, Clifton, and Haith (1973) reported HR acceleration when newborns actively scanned a simple wedge-shaped stimulus or tracked a moving stimulus. In light of the most recent data, an interaction hypothesis appears most appropriate. That is, the newborn's deceleratory response is less common than the acceleratory response, is specific to certain types of stimuli, and appears primarily when such stimuli are presented to awake subjects. Thus, neither arousal state nor type of stimulus is the whole story. Finally, as Jackson and his co-workers (1971) noted, the problem of a change in direction of response to the *same* auditory stimulus remains unanswered, even though HR deceleration to some stimuli is possible for the newborn.

Autonomic Conditioning in Infants

The importance of finding HR deceleration in the newborn is twofold. The newborn's ability to orient must be reconsidered. In addition, the role of the OR in other developmental processes, such as learning, should be explored. When Sameroff (1971) reevaluated the difficulty in demonstrating classical conditioning in newborns, he suggested that the newborn's apparent inability to orient might be responsible for his unstable conditioning performance. In this respect, Sameroff adhered to the Soviet view that the formation of a conditioned response (CR) is preceded by an OR to the conditioned stimulus (CS) (Polikanina and Probatova 1958; Sokolov 1963). Sameroff (1971) reviewed a number of OR components including motor orientation (head turning, visual fixation), cessation of motor activity, respiratory slowing, and desynchronization of electroencephalogram (EEG). He noted that all of these OR components had been observed in newborns, leaving the HR component as the only response not found. As indicated previously, deceleration is difficult but not impossible to obtain. In a more recent review, Sameroff (1972) suggested that using a CS that elicited an OR, rather than defensive acceleration, would facilitate classical conditioning in the newborn.

The literature on classical conditioning of human infants indicates that most studies attempted to condition defensive motor responses to noxious stimuli. Favored response systems include eye blink to a puff of air (Morgan and Morgan 1944; Lintz, Fitzgerald and Brackbill 1967); eyelid closure to a bright light (Wenger 1936); and foot withdrawal to shock (Lipsitt 1963; Wenger 1936; Wickens and Wickens 1940). As Lipsitt (1967) noted, successful conditioning had often involved an appetitive unconditioned stimulus (UCS) rewarding sucking or head-turning (Lipsitt, Kaye, and Bosack 1966; Marquis 1931; Siqueland and Lipsitt 1966). There is a striking gap in the use of autonomic responses as the conditioned response. Despite a large literature reporting classical conditioning of autonomic responses in adult humans and animals of various species, there are few such studies with human infants. Brackbill and colleagues (Brackbill, Fitzgerald, and Lintz 1967; Fitzgerald et al. 1967), in a series of studies with older infants, used pupillary dilation and constriction as the CR. Brackbill (1972) and Forbes and Porges (1972) found evidence of trace conditioning of HR in the newborn, using a sequence of two tones. Brackbill found that HR variability increased on test trials compared to no-stimulus control periods, while Forbes and Porges reported HR deceleration during extinction at the point where the UCS was omitted. Apparently the only published newborn study using autonomic responses is from Lipsitt and Ambrose (see Lipsitt 1969), who found temporal conditioning with the CR defined as a change in behavior in either respiration, HR, or motility. Since HR can be rapidly conditioned in a variety of subjects (Fehr and Stern 1965; Black, Carlson, and Solomon 1962; Wood and Obrist 1964), and it is very responsive to external stimulation in habituation studies with infants (Bartoshuk 1962a,b; Keen, Chase, and Graham 1965), it is possible that HR change may prove to be an easily obtainable CR in the infant.

What would be the value of one more demonstration of classical conditioning in the newborn? In other words, what is special about conditioning an autonomic response as compared to other responses? Concomitant recording of autonomic responses when motor responses are being either classically or instrumentally conditioned may indicate that the infant is responding to manipulated contingencies earlier than motor responses alone show. More important, discontinuities between autonomic and motor responses may reflect immaturity of the CNS. Polikanina (1961) conditioned both autonomic and somatic responses to ammonia vapor in prematures. Discontinuity in responding was displayed by the youngest premature infants, such that autonomic responses were elicited prior to the establishment of defensive motor responses. Once the latter were well-established, autonomic responses tended to disappear. As prematures were tested at older ages, this discontinuity disappeared. Papousek (1967) observed that slower conditioning in the newborn allowed a finer analysis of all phases of the learning process; this may be particularly true as conditioning is explored with premature infants. Concomitant recording of both autonomic and motor responses, as well as conditioning of autonomic responses alone, offers a fruitful attack on the development of learning processes.

STUDIES OF THE ORIENTING RESPONSE

In this section, two studies of the OR will be presented. The first study sought to optimize the elicitation of the OR in newborns through careful selection of stimuli. The second study utilized two tactile stimuli, both of which elicited head-turns. However, in one case, a contralateral head-turn escaped a noxious stimulus; while, in the other case, an ipsilateral turn oriented *S* toward a stroke on the cheek. These head-turns were expected to parallel HR responses of opposite directionality in response to escape and approach stimuli.

As previously noted, the typical neonatal HR response to sensory stimuli has been reported as acceleration. Because these stimuli have often been arousing—airstream to the abdomen—(Lipton, Steinschneider, and Richmond 1961), or intense—115 db tone— (Bridger 1961), or had sudden onsets, they were likely to elicit a DR. Jackson, Kantowitz, and Graham (1971) presented awake newborns with low to moderately intense pure tones with controlled rise times, a stimulus calculated to remove many startling qualities present in previous stimuli. Their failure to find HR deceleration to this auditory stimulus indicated a need to extend testing to other sensory modalities and to stimuli that might have adaptive value to the organism.

In the first study (Pomerleau-Malcuit and Clifton 1973), three sensory modalities were stimulated in both waking and sleeping newborns, before and after feeding. Tactile stimulation to the face and vestibular stimulation were considered to be similar to sensory experiences of the fetus in utero, and would elicit responses from relatively more mature sensory systems (Conel 1952; Humphrey 1965). The third stimulus, a low frequency, low intensity square wave, was selected on the basis of previous work (Eisenberg et al. 1964; Hutt et al. 1968) that suggested broad bandwidth stimuli whose fundamental frequencies are within the range of human speech frequencies can provide the most effective stimulation for the newborn's ear. Two state factors, level of arousal and prandial condition, were varied. The same stimulus may have a different impact on the organism, depending on the particular behavioral or physiological state at the time of stimulation. Lenard, von Bernuth, and Prechtl (1968) established that ease of eliciting responses to tactile, pressure, and auditory stimuli varied with state of wakefulness, whereas noiciceptive reflexes were elicited readily in all three states studied (regular sleep, irregular sleep, and quiet awake). Stimulus modality may interact with arousal state to determine amplitude and direction of the cardiac response.

All infants were obtained from the newborn nursery at the Cooley Dickinson Hospital in Northampton, Massachusetts. Forty-six full-term newborns (mean age = 58 hours) were tested: Thirty-six Ss were in a state of quiet or active sleep, and 10 were in a spontaneously alert, awake state. Half the Ss in each state group were tested before feeding, and half after feeding. Tactile stimulation consisted of stroking S's forehead with a camel hair artist's brush. For the vestibular stimulation, S lay on a platform that tilted through a 12° arc. The arc of S's head movement was 2 inches up from a level position, then 2 inches back down to level, with each directional movement lasting 5 seconds. There was no pause at the apogee, so the effect was one of continuous movement for 10 seconds. The auditory stimulus was produced by an Eico audiooscillator driving an inexpensive amplifier and loudspeaker with a 40 Hz square wave, 65 db over a background noise level of 55 db (re 0.0002 dynes/cm²). This signal was subjected to spectral analysis by means of a Kay Sonagraph to determine its auditory characteristics more specifically. The signal's energy was found to be concentrated around 1,300 Hz, with a frequency range between 600 and 2,500 Hz. Despite the lack of energy at 40 Hz, the stimulus was clearly identifiable as such due to the pitch of the residue effect (Schouten, Ritsma, and Cardozo 1962).[1] Each S received three consecutive trials of each type of stimulus, for a total of nine trials. Each stimulus trial lasted 10 seconds, with intertrial intervals randomly varying between 40 and 60 seconds.

The electrocardiogram (EKG) was detected by three electrodes placed in a triangular array on S's chest, with one active lead high on the sternum, the other active lead and the ground on the lower ribs, 2 or 3 in from the midline. The EKG signal was amplified and shaped by a Datascope Carditron (Model 650), then fed into a Revox 77A audio tape recorder, operating at 3¾ ips. A brief (7 msec) pip for each r spike was recorded on Channel 1 of the tape recorder. On Channel 2 the onset of each stimulation period was recorded, so that HR information could be time-locked to stimulus presentations. The data were fed through a small computer, a PDP 8/I, that timed the interval between each heart beat. In addition, the weighted average HR per second was computed for 1 second before each stimulus onset, and 18 seconds after onset. Data were punched on IBM cards by the computer (see Clifton 1974 for detailed description and available programs). Poststimulus second-by-second scores were adjusted for prestimulus level with the following formula: $AD = D - b_{dx}(X - \bar{X})$, where AD = adjusted difference, D = postonset HR minus prestimulus HR, $b_{dx} = -.26$, and $\bar{X} = 121.68$. Statistical analyses were performed on these adjusted scores for the 10 seconds during stimulation periods.

The results were analyzed separately for sleeping and awake babies. For sleeping Ss, the shape of the response is primarily accelerative to all three types of stimulation (see Figure 24.1). Cardiac acceleration to tactile stimulation peaked at poststimulus second 5, and returned to base level by second 9. An analysis of the variance yielded a main effect of seconds [$F(9,270) = 3.46$, p<.01], with a significant quadratic trend accounting for 67% of the variance. The response to vestibular stimulation, although primarily accelerative, was preceded by a brief deceleration lasting 3 seconds. The biphasic response was reflected in significant quadratic [$F(1,17) = 9.77$, p<.01] and cubic trends [$F(1,17) = 5.55$, p<.05] on the seconds variable. Response to the auditory stimulus appeared to be acceleratory, but was statistically unreliable and smaller than responses obtained previously to a 300 Hz square wave (Clifton, Graham, and Hatton, 1968).

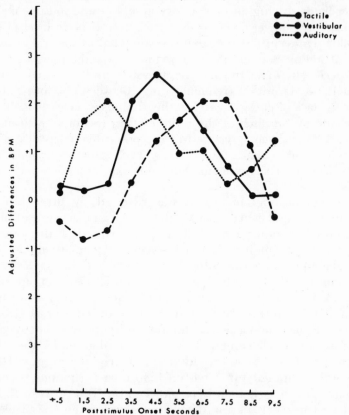

FIGURE 24.1. *HR response of sleeping infants to three different types of stimuli. Each curve is averaged over three trials (From Pomerleau-Malcuit and Clifton 1973, with permission from the publisher). Data are plotted at the midpoint of each time interval.*

For the awake Ss, the feeding variable affected the stability of the cardiac response. After feeding, there was no reliable response to any stimulus. Before feeding, HR deceleration appeared in response to auditory and vestibular stimulation, while acceleration appeared to tactile stimuli (see Figure 24.2). Since HR deceleration was of major interest, the responses to auditory and vestibular stimuli were tested separately. Reliable deceleration was indicated by the seconds effect $[F(9,36) = 5.23, p<.01]$ and the linear trend on seconds $[F(1,4) = 17.99, p<.025]$. A decelerative response to vestibular stimulation was also found in sleeping babies tested before feeding, but it was found only when the vestibular stimulus was presented first. In other words, when the order of stimulus presentation was vestibular, auditory, and tactile, a reliable Feeding X Seconds interaction $[F(9,90) = 2.29, p<.05]$ was obtained, with curves in the same direction as awake Ss. A decelerative response was found to auditory stimulation in sleeping babies tested *after* feeding, but, again, only when the auditory stimulus came first.

In agreement with previous work, cardiac acceleration was found to be more easily elicited than deceleration. However, when state of wakefulness and feeding condition are controlled, HR deceleration to certain types of stimuli may be elicited. But, without additional measures of the OR, it is not clear that the HR deceleration shown in this study was a component of the OR. That is, HR deceleration is multidetermined, and the presence of such deceleration does not necessarily imply an OR. In a subject suspected of an inability to orient, HR deceleration should not be assumed to be an OR component. If a stimulus was known to elicit behavioral orienting, and behavioral measures as well as cardiac responses were obtained, this would offer more evidence that such deceleration was an OR component.

Pomerleau-Malcuit, Malcuit, and Clifton (1972) recorded cardiac and behavioral reactivity to facial stimulation that elicited approach and avoidance responses. One stimulus, stroking the cheek near the mouth, produced ipsilateral turning, an approach response usually referred to as the rooting reflex (Prechtl 1958). A second stimulus, a light pinch on the ear, produced contralateral head-turning, a defensive response. These approach and defensive responses are congenitally organized patterns of behavior and have been described in neurological studies (Peiper 1963; Sainte-Anne Dargassies 1962). Defensive reflexes appear earlier in fetal development and are elicited more rapidly and easily than positive responses in the newborn (Humphrey 1970). Although these two response patterns involve a similar motor activity, headturning, they serve different functions for the organism. The approach response may be considered to be a behavioral component of the OR, just as head-turning to sound and to visual orienting are OR components. The escape response is defensive behavior to a noxious stimulus, and may be considered an index of a DR. By recording cardiac as well as behavioral responses to these two types of stimulation, Pomerleau-Malcuit, Malcuit, and Clifton (1972) attempted to differentiate the OR and DR arousal systems, thus establishing the presence of both systems in the neonatal period.

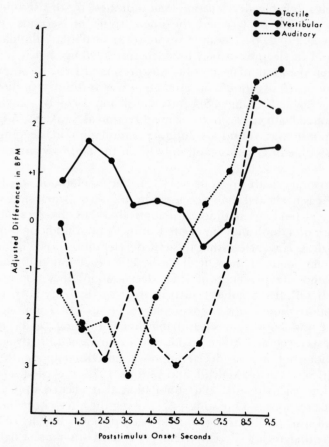

FIGURE 24.2. *HR response to tactile, vestibular, and auditory stimulation by awake infants before feeding (N = 5) (From Pomerleau-Malcuit and Clifton 1973, with permission of the publisher).*

Full-term newborns (mean age = 51 hours) with no history of labor or delivery complications—Apgar scores 8 to 10—participated in the study. All Ss were tested in light or deep sleep: 12 within 1 hour before the 2:00 p.m. feeding, and 12 within 1 hour after this feeding, Infants who became alert or began crying during the procedure were dropped from the sample (N = 9). Before administering any tactile stimulation, the side preference for head position, left or right, was determined by two procedures: (a) The spontaneous head position was noted; and, (b) S's head was centered by experimenter (E) to the midline position, and allowed to return to the preferred side. For all Ss in this experiment, the preferred head position was to the right. Thus, cheek and ear stimulation were always applied on the left side of S's face, as this was the more available side. If Ss had been stimulated on the right side, it would have been necessary to center their heads before starting ear or cheek stimulation. Head-centering itself can result in tactile and movement stimulation that may interfere with the response to ear and cheek stimulation (Turkewitz et al. 1969).

Each S received eight cheek and eight ear stimulations, randomly delivered with the restriction that no more than three consecutive stimulations could occur at the same location. To administer cheek stimulation, E stroked S's cheek just beyond the corner of the mouth and perpendicular to it, once per second for 6 seconds *or* until S responded with a behavioral movement. The following movements were scored during each trial: ipsilateral and contralateral head turning, sucking motions, mouth opening, grimacing, arm and leg abduction movements, and crying. If S made none of the responses described, he was scored as making no response on that trial. Ear stimulation was a pinch on S's left ear lobe, delivered by E once per second for 6 seconds, or until S responded with one or more of the behavioral movements indicated above. One E always administered the tactile stimulation, while a second E pressed a hand switch that recorded onset and offset of stimulation. Both Es scored the infants' motor responses to the stimulation. The minimum interstimulus interval (ISI) was 25 seconds from onset to onset of a stimulus trial; the maximum ISI was 2 minutes, with the usual ISI between 30 and 40 seconds. After a light signalled E that the minimum ISI had elapsed, E administered the stimulation as soon as S was not moving, sucking, or vocalizing, and heart rate was steady.

Cardiac responses were recorded, reduced, and analyzed with the same equipment and procedures just reported for Pomerleau-Malcuit et al. (1972), with one exception. When prestimulus levels were tested, Ss tested before feeding were found to have significantly lower levels of HR ($\overline{X}$ = 110.1 bpm) than Ss tested after feeding ($\overline{X}$ = 120.4 bpm). Evans and Anastasio (1968) have questioned the practice of adjusting scores for initial level effects when the variable under consideration (e.g., feeding) may have produced group differences in initial level. For this reason, before and after feeding groups were tested separately for homogeneity of regression coefficients among the 16 trials at each postonset second. No F ratios were significant, indicating homogeneity of linear regression within both groups. Postonset scores were corrected for prestimulus level within each feeding group with the formula previously given, except $b_{dx} = -0.56$ for before feeding Ss and -0.36 for after feeding Ss.

To identify relationships between cardiac and motor responses, the overt behaviors were classified as follows:

Cheek stimulation:

    a. approach type behavioral responses, such as ipsilateral head-turning, mouth opening, sucking

    b. no behavioral response, i.e., a nonresponse trial

Ear stimulation:

    a. escape type response, such as contralateral head-turning, grimacing, arm and leg abduction movements

    b. no behavioral response, or nonresponse.

Trials on which S gave an overt response opposite to the expected movement (e.g., escape response to cheek stimulation), and trials (N = 4) on which Es disagreed in scoring the response were not considered. According to these criteria, 25 cheek stimulations and 4 ear stimulation trials were dropped, out of a maximum of 192 trials for each type of stimulus. There was no difference in the percentage of behavioral responses before and after feeding.

In order to compare HR responses with behavioral responses, the trial data on the 16 stimulus trials for each S were categorized into one of the four categories indicated above. Four of the 24 Ss did not make any approach responses to cheek stimulation, leaving 20 Ss to be analyzed for "Cheek" trials. Although all Ss made avoidance responses to ear stimulations, only 13 of the total 24 also made no response to this stimulus on some trials. By excluding Ss having no trials in some categories, a within subjects design was created to test cardiac activity to the same tactile stimulus when overt responses were present and absent. An average HR curve was computed over the trials in each category for each S, so that each S contributed only once to each category.

The cardiac response curves for nonresponse and response trials are presented in Figure 24.3. Ear stimulation produced HR acceleration regardless of whether S made an overt movement or not. A main effect of seconds [$F(9,108) = 8.92$, $p<.001$] with reliable linear, quadratic, and cubic trends [$F(1,12) = 6.57$, $p<.05$; $F = 10.00$, $p<.01$; $F = 27.73$, $p<.001$, respectively] were present. Although greater amplitude of acceleration appeared when an overt response was made, this difference was not reliable. However, when peak amplitude, rather than the whole curve was tested ($t = 2.24$, $p<.05$), this difference was reliable. On the other hand, making an overt response reversed the direction of cardiac change to cheek stimulation [$F(1,19) = 31.33$, $p<.001$, for response type and $F(9,171) = 4.58$, $p<.01$ for Response Type X

Seconds interaction]. Cardiac acceleration accompanied approach responses, while cardiac deceleration appeared when no overt response was made. Separate analyses of variance on these response categories were necessary in order to determine if the deceleration on nonresponse trials was simply the absence of acceleration. Both curves were reliable.. For the approach response trials, a seconds main effect [F(9,171) = 2.65, p<.01] with significant quadratic and cubic trends on seconds was found, and for the nonresponse trials, seconds [F(9,171) = 2.53, p<.01] with a highly reliable cubic trend [F(1,19) = 11.33, p<.005 on seconds].

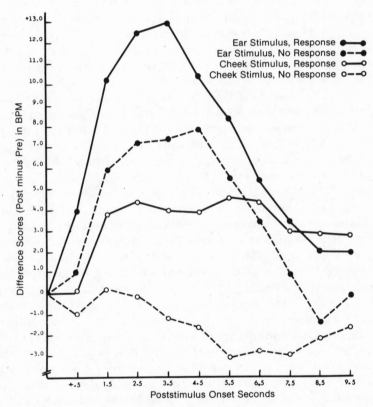

FIGURE 24.3. *HR response to onset of ear (N = 13) and cheek (N = 20) stimulation according to type of overt behavior to stimulus (From Pomerleau-Malcuit, Malcuit, and Clifton 1972).*

The HR response of the four Ss excluded from the cheek stimulation analysis because they had not made approach responses was an accelerative, inverted-U shaped response, similar to that of Ss making an approach response. They did not show the decelerative HR response. Perhaps these infants who never made overt approach responses to cheek stimulation were in a deeper sleep state and responded with an accelerative defense reaction.

These data indicate the interrelatedness of motor and cardiac responses in the newborn. As predicted, the ear stimulation produced defense responses and cardiac acceleration, with overt movement amplifying the latter. With tactile approach stimulation, the picture is unclear. The presence or absence of an overt response predicted the direction of HR change, but this differentiation may have been due to a number of different processes. Overt movements may, in general, produce or be correlated with cardiac acceleration, so that the "true" HR response to cheek stimulation is HR deceleration that appears when no movement effects overlay it. In other words, the HR acceleration to the approach stimulus on "response" trials may have been secondarily produced by body movement.[2] Indirect support for this position comes from studies measuring HR during movement. Chase, Graham, and Graham (1968) found that HR increased in anticipation of exercise and during exercise in adults. In infants, HR increased during sucking and immediately preceding sucking (Clifton 1974; Gottlieb and Simner 1966). Bridger and Birns (1963) found that gentle head-rocking by E and sucking on a sweetened pacifier, both considered to be soothing stimuli, increased HR over resting levels.

While it is likely that head-turning may have produced acceleration to the approach stimulus in the present study, other possibilities must be considered. Turkewitz and his colleagues (Turkewitz et al. 1970) recorded HR, eye movements, and finger movements to white noise at seven intensity levels. They concluded that there was nonequivalence among these responses and questioned whether a unitary OR exists in the infant. Their finding of nonconcordance between HR acceleration and eye and finger movements might be accounted for by the HR measure—a comparison of the time between the first and seventh beats preceding and following stimulus onset (about 2 or 3 seconds pre- and postonset). This measure cut short the full time-course of the cardiac response. Furthermore, the concordance measure (percent of trials on which two responses occurred together) probably did not detect relationships that would be evident in a second-by-second analysis of cardiac curves on trials when movement did and did not occur. Finally, since nonaccelerations received a score of zero, possible deceleratory responses may have been overlooked.

The data presented here on response to ear stimulation corroborates previous research, in finding that cardiac responses to stimulation occur in the absence of overt movement. Lipton, Steinschneider, and Richmond (1960, 1965) reported that restricting motor activity by swaddling decreased some infants' cardiac and respiratory responses as expected, but actually increased other infants' physiological responding. Swaddled newborns accelerated to a tactile stimulus—a cool air-stream to the abdomen—even when no movement was observed. The problem of somatic-cardiac relationships continues to be of theoretical significance for all investigators of cardiovascular activity, but full understanding of the mechanisms involved must await further data.

Studies of HR Conditioning

A series of three studies investigating HR conditioning in infants will be described. The first study deals with newborns, the remaining two with infants two to three months of age. The primary purpose of the initial study was to demonstrate classical conditioning of HR in newborns; the remaining studies extended the paradigm to older infants and attempted to overcome methodological difficulties encountered earlier.

Newborn HR conditioning

The first study (Clifton 1974) was an appetitive conditioning procedure involving contingent tone and glucose presentations. The Ss were 14 healthy, full-term neonates, mean age of 59.4 hours. An additional 20 infants had incomplete sessions. Nine sessions were interrupted because Ss refused to accept the nipple (the UCS) for three consecutive trials; this was usually due to a change in arousal state, either to crying or deep sleep. Experimental errors accounted for four more aborted sessions, and poor EKG records accounted for the remaining seven sessions. All Ss were tested between 12:00 noon and 2:00 p.m., i.e., within the 2-hour interval before the 2:00 p.m. feeding. Written permission was obtained from each mother. Refusal rate was 22%. The major reason given for refusal was that of the breast-feeding mother who did not wish to reduce her infant's appetite by a glucose offering between feedings.

The auditory stimulus (CS) was a 72 db (re 0.0002 dynes/cm^2), 300 Hz square wave produced by an Eico audiogenerator. This signal was fed through a speaker placed about 18 in from S's head. The UCS was a manual presentation of a 5% glucose solution obtained from the newborn nursery. The CS and a light indicator to E for UCS presentations were timed and programmed by a BRS film programmer and associated logic modules. The EKG was recorded and reduced in the manner previously described under the OR studies, except that scores were not adjusted for prestimulus levels. Analyses of variance with appropriate trends on unadjusted scores were used. Trend analyses are not sensitive to prestimulus level differences and will indicate reliable responses to the stimulus (Seconds effect), group differences in response (Groups X Seconds interaction) and trial effects (Groups X Trials X Seconds), independent of prestimulus level differences.

Two groups of Ss were compared: a Conditioning Group and a Random Control Group. All Ss received nine identical base or preconditioning trials. The first three trials consisted of UCS alone; Ss were allowed to suck on a bottle of 5% glucose for 10 seconds. These trials attempted to establish the unconditioned response (UCR) to this stimulation in this age infant. The next six trials consisted of tone alone, with three more glucose presentations randomly interspersed. After this base period, the Conditioning Group received 30 trials of an 8-second tone, a 6-second ISI, and a 10-second glucose presentation overlapping with tone for 2 seconds. Thus, total length of a conditioning trial was 16 seconds. Random Control Ss received tones at the same intervals as the Conditioning Ss, but glucose was randomly presented—the exact time being determined by consulting a table of random numbers. Following these 30 trials, all groups were given six extinction trials of tone alone. Intertrial intervals (tone onset to onset) randomly varied between 30 and 60 seconds.

The first test for conditioning was the determination of HR change during the ISI. The 6-second ISI allowed the examination of response to the tone on each trial. Thus, the possibility of a CR to the tone developing over trials was tested by comparing group responses to the tone on the first and last three-trial blocks of conditioning trials. An analysis of variance for 1 prestimulus second through 6 postonset seconds was conducted. No main effects or interactions were significant. Although there was HR acceleration to the tone during the six base trials, this habituated by the first conditioning trials. Response curves for both groups on first and last blocks of conditioning appear in Figure 24.4. Although some slight acceleration (3 bpm) reappeared for the Conditioning Group on the last block of trials, this was not significant. Figure 24.4 also shows the HR acceleration to the nipple mentioned earlier. This effect seems to have become accentuated by the end of conditioning (Compare Trial Blocks 1 and 10 on seconds 6 to 16 for the Conditioning Group).

The second test of conditioning compared the last trial of conditioning with the first trial of extinction during the period when Conditioning Ss were normally sucking on the bottle. On the first extinction trial beginning at the sixth second following tone onset, the Conditioning Group progressively slowed in HR, reaching a peak deceleration of 20 beats at the 16th postonset second (see Figure 24.5). Statistically, this effect appeared as a Groups X Trials X Seconds interaction [$F(12,144) = 6.63$, $p<.01$], and a linear trend on seconds for this interaction [$F(1,12) = 9.41$, $p<.01$]. The Control Group did not show HR deceleration during this period.

To further establish that the Conditioning Group decelerated on the first extinction trial, a separate analysis of variance and trend analysis

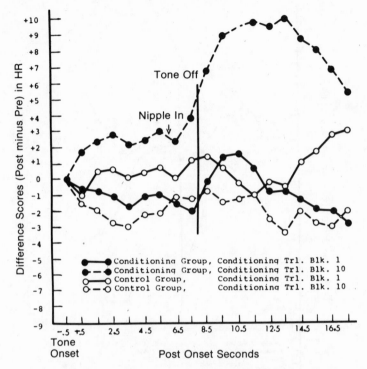

FIGURE 24.4. *Cardiac response of Conditioning and Control Groups on the first and last trial blocks of conditioning (From Clifton 1974).*

on seconds 6 to 18 was done for each group. Conditioning Ss showed a main effect of seconds, with the linear trend accounting for 88% of the variance. The Control Ss had no reliable effects or trends. When data were trial-blocked into three-trial blocks, the same interaction was significant (Groups X Trial Blocks X Seconds F = 2.41, p<.05), but trends were not reliable. The effect is diluted when the first three trials of extinction are considered, rather than the first trial. When trial-blocked data were followed by separate *anovas* on the two groups, the same results were found as for the first trial on extinction.

The results of this study were discouraging in that there was no evidence for a CR to the tone. If classical conditioning is defined in the strict sense of a CR developing to a previously neutral CS, then conditioning was unsuccessful. However, the large deceleration during extinction can be interpreted as an OR to the absence of an expected event, the UCS. This interpretation agrees with Sokolov's model (Sokolov 1963, p. 41) in which the disturbance of a temporal sequence of events will elicit an OR. The appearance of an OR during extinction may offer indirect evidence of learning in the newborn. In his discus-

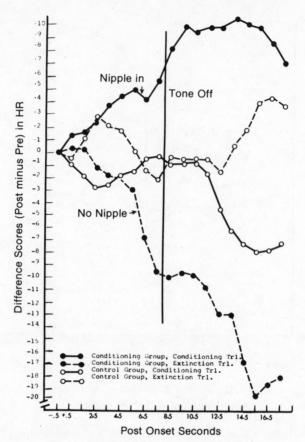

FIGURE 24.5. *Cardiac response of Conditioning and Control Groups on the last conditioning trial and first extinction trial (From Clifton 1974).*

sion of the difficulty in classically conditioning the newborn, Sameroff (1971) suggested that more experience with stimuli is required before the infant can differentiate and then integrate his responding to stimuli in different modalities. I would propose that the newborn can integrate stimuli from two modalities, that he is sensitive if the stimuli occur in a time-locked sequence, but that he does not transfer a response originally elicited by the UCS to a neutral stimulus, the CS. His processing of the stimulus sequence may be determined by disrupting the temporal relationship, as during extinction, and by looking at his response to the disruption.

Sokolov (1963, p. 247-249) outlined the following sequence of events in the OR's role in classical conditioning. The CS must first elicit the OR, or conditioning will be slow and difficult. During conditioning, the OR becomes a stable, nonhabituating response to the CS, as *S* learns the CS is a signal stimulus. If conditioning continues for a long period, the OR may eventually habituate, as S performs some well-learned CR. The conditioning of the OR to the CS can be interpreted as S's learning a "get ready" response for the anticipated UCS. In many classical conditioning studies the ISI is too short to see whether HR deceleration occurs to the CS, particularly if the UCR is an acceleration to some noxious stimulus. In HR conditioning studies using ISIs of five seconds or longer, the development of the response can be followed on both reinforced and nonreinforced (or probe) trials. If Sokolov's analysis of the OR's role in conditioning is correct, the adult literature should reveal HR deceleration as the usual cardiac response to the CS. This should be true, regardless of whether the UCS is noxious and produces an acceleratory UCR, or is pleasant and produces a deceleratory UCR.

Many studies using adult Ss have, in fact, reported a HR deceleration to the CS, even with a shock UCS (Hastings and Obrist 1967; Wood and Obrist 1964), or a biphasic or triphasic response with a predominant deceleratory component (Headrick and Graham 1969; Wilson 1969). A number of studies have reported HR acceleration, but their findings have been questioned by Headrick and Graham (1969) regarding high shock level (Westcott and Huttenlocher 1961), and type of respiration control employed (Fuhrer 1964; Smith 1966; Zeaman and Smith 1965). At this stage, there seems to be fair agreement that HR deceleration is the most typical cardiac response found to the CS in a classical conditioning experiment. However, many varied explanations have been tendered as to why deceleration appears. Geer (1964) suggested that HR deceleration to the CS is the reappearance of the *unconditioned* OR to the CS. Headrick and Graham (1969) obtained a triphasic response consisting of a small deceleration and small acceleration, followed by a larger deceleration immediately before UCS (shock) onset. Interpretations were given for all components, with strong evidence that the third component was a *conditioned* OR. By contrasting the form of the response to CS during adaptation trials preceding conditioning with the response to the CS during later conditioning, Headrick and Graham showed that the deceleration was not an unconditioned OR. They also pointed out that even studies reporting HR acceleration as the response to the CS have a deceleration immediately prior to UCS onset. Although Wilson's data (1969) were not in conflict with Headrick and Graham's, his interpretation was quite different. He suggested that the final form of the conditioned HR response is a composite resulting from the original response to the CS, the direction of the response to the UCS, and the length of the ISI. Wilson described how various components of the conditioned HR response could be shaped through manipulation of external variables, but he did not offer an explanation of the internal mechanisms responsible for the conditioned deceleration. Obrist and colleagues have offered an explanation in terms of the parasympathetic nervous system. They claimed that anticipation of an event, be it pleasant or unpleasant, produces a parasympathetic alerting reaction, one of the consequences being HR deceleration (Obrist, Wood, and Perez-Reyes 1965; Hastings and Obrist 1967).

Whether one chooses words like "preparatory set" (Grings 1960), conditioned OR, sensitization to the CS (Dykman 1967), or vagal enervation (Obrist, Wood, and Perez-Reyes 1965), the concept of a readiness or anticipation of the UCS is the key idea. The newborn infant apparently fails to develop the typical anticipatory deceleration during the ISI shown by adults. He shows no sign of "getting ready" or preparing for the UCS. His response might rather be characterized as a "What happened?" response when the UCS doesn't come at the expected moment. If this analysis is correct, then elicitating a deceleratory OR during extinction may be a more sensitive means of determining what has been learned in the conditioning situation than looking for the development of a CR to the CS.

HR Conditioning in Older Infants

Appleton (1972) extended the conditioning procedures of the newborn study to 2½- to 3-month-old infants (mean age = 82 days, N = 14). Older babies might show responses more typical of adults, i.e., development of a CR to the CS, as well as an OR during extinction. The newborn study was essentially replicated with minor changes. Tone and glucose again served as CS and UCS respectively; however, the tone was a 1300 Hz sine wave and was continued throughout nipple presentation rather than the 2-second overlap in the earlier study. A conditioning trial consisted of tone onset, a 6-second ISI, a glucose presentation lasting 8 seconds, and tone offset with nipple withdrawal at 14 seconds following tone onset. The Conditioning Group had 24 conditioning trials, preceded by three trials of glucose alone, and followed by three extinction trials of tone alone. The Random Control Group had the same initial three glucose trials and extinction trials, and heard tones at the same intervals during conditioning as the Conditioning Group. Presentation of glucose randomly varied between 31 and 41 seconds.

As with the newborns, the HR response to the UCS was an acceleration that was maintained until the nipple was withdrawn. The groups did not differ in their response on initial UCS trials. Unlike the newborns, the older babies responded with HR deceleration to the tone initially. This developmental shift agreed with previous data on HR response to tones in this age group (Berg 1972; Clifton and Meyers

1969). But, again, like the newborns, the response to tone habituated over trials for both groups, with no evidence for a CR to the CS. Analyses of variance comparing HR during the 6-second ISI on first and last trial blocks of conditioning found no group differences over trials. Group curves on the last trial block of conditioning were quite flat, with great error variance.

During conditioning trials it was not appropriate to analyze beyond 6 seconds due to HR acceleration during the UCS in the Conditioning Group. When groups were compared for the entire 14-second tone period on extinction trials 1 and 2, a Group X Trials X Seconds interaction was significant [$F(13,156) = 2.21$, $p<.01$]. The Conditioning Group showed a fairly flat curve on extinction 1, but deceleration appeared on trial 2 that peaked around seconds 6 to 7, approximately when Ss had been receiving the bottle (see Figure 24.6). Follow-up analyses on this interaction showed the Conditioning Group when tested alone maintained the Trials X Seconds interaction [$F(13,78) = 2.44$, $p<.01$], while Control Ss showed no reliable response on these trials. The decelerative response was further substantiated by the quad-

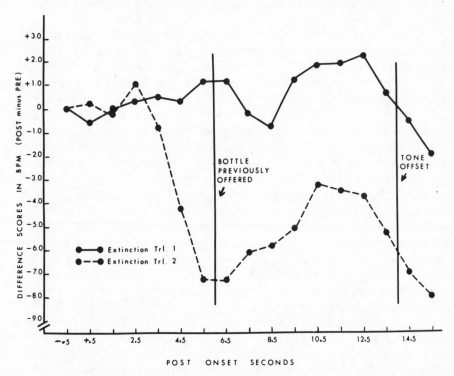

FIGURE 24.6. *Response of 3-month-old infants to the CS on the first two extinction trials (From Appleton 1972).*

ratic component of seconds [F(1,6) = 8.65, p<.05]. The greater down-ward trend on extinction trial 2 was reflected by a Trials X Seconds interaction on the linear component of seconds [F1,6) = 5.64, p<.10]. The deceleratory response during extinction was ephemeral; the third extinction trial was quite flat, showing only slight, unreliable accelera-tion.

These results are similar to the newborn study in that Conditioning Ss responded differently from Controls only during extinction trials, and the response was HR deceleration. The timing of the deceleration for the age groups differs. The newborns showed a large sustained drop in HR to the nonappearance of the UCS, while the older infants began decelerating during the tone, and had a much shallower, briefer HR decrease. Perhaps the offset of the CS, coming at 8 seconds, pro-vided a signal of the trial's end for the newborns better than the con-tinuing tone in the second study. However, the newborns started decelerating before tone offset, indicating time-locked behavior to nip-ple presentation (see Figure 24.5). In conclusion, Appleton's study offered somewhat tenuous evidence for older infants' learning of the CS-UCS contingencies, in that the effect appeared on only one trial and was quite brief on that trial.

Although these studies showed that the HR response was sensitive to stimulus sequences, a major methodological problem concerning the UCS should be discussed. The glucose presentations were difficult to make with many Ss. Nine newborns and seven older babies had incom-plete sessions due to nipple refusal for three consecutive trials. Even cooperative Ss included in the final sample all had occasional trials with no sucking, although the nipple was accepted. This difficulty was prob-ably due to glucose's dependence on hunger for its effectiveness. Many infants were not hungry even when 2 to 3 hours had elapsed since the previous feeding. Most newborns have not established a regular feeding schedule, or even strong sucking behavior. When obtaining mothers' permission prior to testing, we found that incidental observa-tions by the mother on her infant's feeding behavior were quite predic-tive of the baby's performance. For example, if a mother said that her baby was typically hungry and easy to feed, then the baby usually main-tained sucking during the experiment. But, if a mother said her baby was difficult to feed and wasn't eating well, this observation was usually borne out by nipple refusal in the experiment. With older babies, mothers were instructed to bring their infants to the laboratory midway between feedings. Pilot work indicated this time to be better than immediately before feeding. Although hungry infants eagerly accepted glucose, they became frustrated with the nipple withdrawal on each trial and soon rejected it altogether. At midway between feedings, they were not so satiated that a sweet solution was unattractive, nor so hungry that interrupted sucking was upsetting.

A second problem with glucose was that manual presentation inevitably introduced inaccuracy in time of UCS onset. The ISI, nominally 6 seconds, actually varied with E's reaction to the indicator signal. An ideal UCS would be independent of hunger state, automatically controlled and presented to S, and would elicit a reliable HR response on each trial. Since vestibular stimulation had produced large HR responses independent of feeding and arousal state (see Pomerleau-Malcuit and Clifton 1973) a rocking UCS was adopted. Pomerleau-Malcuit, Malcuit, and Clifton (1972) essentially replicated the Appleton (1972) study, substituting rocking for glucose. A commercial cradle was motorized, with onset and duration of rocking controlled by a Digibit Film programmer and logic modules. An infant seat was anchored in the cradle, so that S was rocked in a semi-reclining rather than supine position. The cradle moved from side to side through a 22° angle of displacement, with S's head moving through a 5-in arc. The CS was a 75 db, 1,700 Hz sine wave produced by a BRS audiogenerator, presented in free field through a speaker about 8 ft from S.

Mothers were asked to bring their infants at a time when their babies were usually alert and not hungry. A total of 46 infants were tested, but 23 infants did not complete the session due to crying on three consecutive trials. An additional three infants had interrupted sessions because of equipment problems, leaving 20 Ss in the final sample (10 per group). Infants ranged in age from 15 to 17 weeks, with a mean of 15.6 weeks. All Ss were awake throughout the procedures.

Experimental Ss had three base trials of tone alone, 24 conditioning trials consisting of an 8-second tone, 6-second ISI, and 10-second rocking. Three extinction trials of tone alone ended the session. Control Ss had the same base and extinction trials. During conditioning they received tones at the same intervals, but the UCS was randomly presented during each trial. One restriction on this randomness was made in order to determine the Control Group's HR response to rocking over trials. Although the Experimental Group's response to rocking was available on every trial since the UCS came at a specified time, the Control Group's response was normally lost, as only tone onsets were recorded. To compare the groups' responses to UCS, rocking was presented and recorded approximately 20 to 25 seconds after CS presentation on conditioning trials 1 to 3, 12 to 14, and 22 to 24 for the Control Group. Intertrial intervals varied between 30 and 50 seconds, and were the same for both groups.

The UCR to rocking was a 5 to 6 bpm deceleration for both groups that did not habituate over trials [seconds $F(12,216) = 9.25$, $p<.01$, with significant linear and quadratic trends on seconds]. As in the experiments reported previously, no systematic response to the tone appeared in the Experimental Group. Both groups initially decelerated to tone and habituated over trials. Figure 24.7 presents the data for all conditioning trials, blocked into three, eight-trial blocks for each group. Although Experimental *S*s appeared to habituate more slowly than Control *S*s, this difference was not reliable. To determine if a group effect was present early in conditioning, the three base trials and first nine conditioning trials were blocked into four blocks of three-trial blocks. The same effects were found as when all trials were analyzed—a seconds main effect and a Trial Blocks X Seconds interaction, indicating HR deceleration to the tone that habituated for both groups.

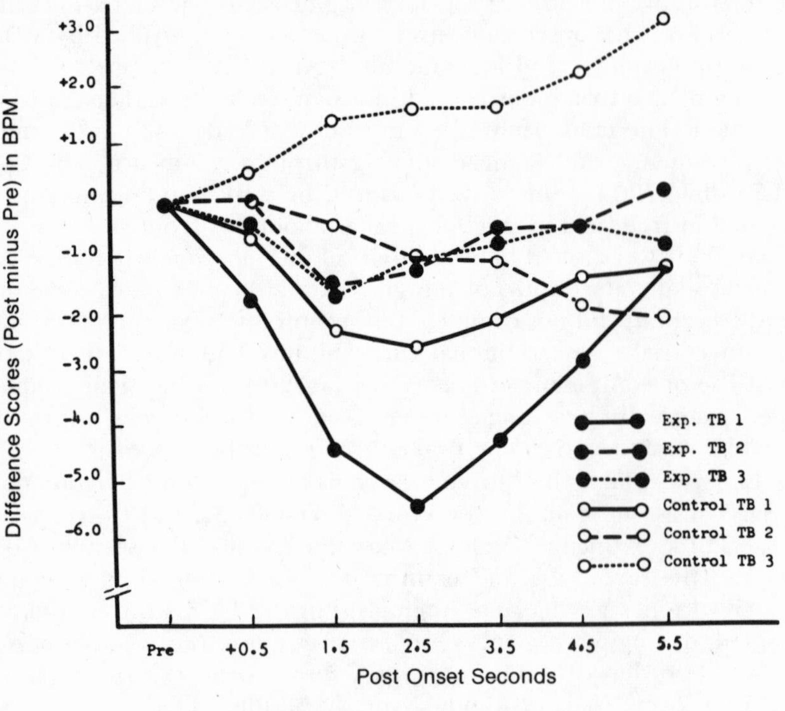

FIGURE 24.7.   *Response of older infants to the CS during conditioning. Each curve is the average of eight trials.*

Note: Data are plotted at midpoint of each interval.

Responses to tone and to absence of rocking during extinction also proved unreliable for the most part. A significant Groups X Trials X Seconds interaction on response to tone during the three extinction trials were uninterpretable, because follow-up analyses on separate groups did not yield the expected effects. No reliable effects were found for Experimental *S*s, while Controls had a seconds main effect. Controls continued to accelerate to tones during extinction as they did on the last block of conditioning trials (see Figure 24.7). In conclusion, the only reliable sources of variance for this study were the response to rocking, response to tone, and habituation to tone.

SUMMARY

The research presented in this chapter offers support for orienting behavior soon after birth, but little evidence for a cardiac CR, even in the older baby. As previously mentioned, the phenomenon of HR deceleration during extinction indicated that both newborns and older infants had developed an expectancy that one event (glucose) would follow another event (tone) after a set interval. It was suggested that a deceleratory OR on probe or extinction trials might be a more sensitive index of learning than the development of a CR to the CS. Cardiac deceleration might also be obtained by using a simple habituation paradigm and omitting an occasional stimulus. Certainly, these CS-CR relationships should be further explored, using different combinations of responses and conditioned stimuli.

The problem of an effective UCS remains. Despite the previous objections raised concerning glucose, it has a long history as an effective reinforcer. Siqueland and Lipsitt (1966), Papousek (1967), Marquis (1931), and many others have reinforced motor behaviors with glucose or formula. Its great advantage may be that the experimenter can judge its reinforcement value for S to some extent, because S must cooperate in receiving it. In the research presented in this chapter, subjects were excluded if they refused the nipple on three consecutive trials. This assurance of some minimal reinforcement value of the UCS does not apply to rocking. Although there is some evidence (Bridger and Birns 1963; Korner and Thoman 1972) and a common-sensical belief that motion is soothing and reinforcing to young infants, more solid evidence is needed as to the particular type most appropriate in the conditioning situation. Operant procedures offer one means of establishing reinforcement values. For example, if sucking or head-turning produced a rocking movement, increased responding under such contingencies would imply reinforcement value.

The failure to find a cardiac CR to the CS could be due to a number of factors. The lack of literature on autonomic conditioning with infants leaves a wide range of choice in selecting ISI length, overlap between CS and UCS, number of conditioning trials given, and relative effectiveness of various CS and UCS combinations. Poor choice on any of these variables may have led to negative results in the present studies. The solution of these methodological problems is important, and would bring joy to the heart of any nit-picker. Yet, I would like to propose a new direction for devotees of infant learning. The excellent review of two-process learning theory by Rescorla and Solomon

(1967) should excite infant researchers to explore the relationships between classical conditioning and instrumental learning. Rescorla and Solomon view classical conditioning procedures as independent variables, to be manipulated and tested in subsequent instrumental learning tasks. Numerous animal studies (Bower and Grusec 1964; Mellgren and Ost 1969; Solomon and Turner 1962) indicate that pairing an instrumental response to be learned with a previously conditioned CS+ will facilitate learning, while pairing the same response with a previous CS− will retard learning. This type of interaction process in learning may occur in a set developmental sequence. For example, the excitatory aspect of the transfer effect probably appears earlier in the baby's development. The newborn is lacking in inhibitory powers, as evidenced by his many reflexive behaviors present at birth. During the first postnatal months as the cortex matures, he develops inhibitory abilities that result in the disappearance of the earlier reflexes (Humphrey 1969; Scheibel and Scheibel 1964). The continued presence of these reflexes after certain ages leads to a diagnosis of brain damage. Thus, the developmental sequence of events most likely in a transfer task would be first excitatory effects (shown by more rapid learning, when a new instrumental response is paired with a previously conditioned CS+), followed at a later age by inhibitory effects (shown by retarded or inhibited learning, when a new response is paired with a previously conditioned CS−).

In conclusion, conditioning in infants has a long history of exploration. Much of the impetus for the 1930s and 1940s research on infant conditioning was founded on the hope that classical conditioning offered a means of assessing CNS maturation and intactness (Morgan and Morgan 1944). Since then, infant conditioning has been demonstrated as a phenomenon, but information has not proceeded much beyond a mere demonstration. Studying more subtle aspects of the conditioning situation may lead to the realization of the full potential of this paradigm's usefulness for the developmental psychologist.

NOTES

1. I wish to thank Ian Thomas for his help in determining the signal's characteristics.

2. These data have been reinterpreted after further analyses. See Pomerleau-Malcuit, Malcuit & Clifton, 1972.

25

ROGERS ELLIOTT

The Motivational Significance
of Heart Rate

INTRODUCTION

My concern in this chapter is to discuss the ways in which statements about heart rate (HR) have been thought to have meaning in descriptive and causal discussions of behavior. Heart rate has been, perhaps, the most popular of the peripheral physiological measures in psychology by history of use, ease of application, and evident importance of the organ being measured. The rate and power of beating of the heart are intimate data in a way that hormones and brainwaves are not, and it is easy to see why they become prominent whenever discussions of motivation and emotion, or activation and arousal, take a physiological turn. The action of the heart has, of course, long been a metaphor of emotion, as in growing heavy and sinking, growing light and singing, breaking, and so on.

In psychology the question is, when we see changes in HR, what do they mean? If a patient or client were sitting silently in a psychotherapeutic session or interview and we could watch changes in his HR, would we learn something useful to us, and if so, what? If in a laboratory we manipulate incentive level but see no change in task performance, would a concurrent change in HR or the absence of such a change tell us something psychologically useful? It has often been the hope that we can learn something from recording HR, and, of course, other physiological events, that would otherwise escape us.

The writing of this paper, and some of the research reported in it, were supported by Grants HD04047 and HD12648 from the National Institute of Child Health and Human Development.

The discussion to follow is organized with reference to the roles that HR changes can take in contributing to our understanding of its behavioral significance. It might serve as an independent variable, affecting other behavior, and thus be, in Mandler's (1967) terms, a psychologically functional physiological variable. The hypothesis developed by the Laceys, which I will refer to in this review simply as the Lacey hypothesis, casts HR in such a role.

Or HR can be, and frequently is, taken as a correlate of other behavior, an index of other events or states of interest. That is the role it takes when it is used as an index of activation level, or of emotional state. Finally, HR may be viewed behaviorally simply as a response in its own right, one whose meaning is known partially by the events that control it, and partly by the events that correlate with it. This latter role as a covariate in a response-response relation is given to it in the cardiac-somatic formulation, although that hypothesis also views HR occasionally as a one-muscle index of total somatic activity. Heart rate takes its clearest role as a dependent variable when it is brought under specific stimulus and reinforcement control, as happens if and when it is operantly conditioned. That area is very well covered in this book and I shall not, except in passing, refer to it.

I will review the Lacey hypothesis, then the activation and emotion positions with reference to HR, and, finally, the cardiac-somatic hypothesis: a decreasing order of imputed behavioral significance for HR, but, as will become clear, an increasing order of degree of testability and empirical support. But even though the cardiac-somatic view has, it seems to me, considerable merit, it too has clear difficulties in testability and limits in applicability, even within the range of conditions to which the various hypotheses apply.

The various views of HR are, indeed, meant to apply only within limits. Effects of exercise, physical pathologies, anoxemia, passive tilting, large postural changes, sinus arrhythmia and other homeostatic reflexes, and so on are not considered—we assume for purposes of this discussion that their effects are absent or random. Generally speaking, we are concerned with seated human Ss doing the sorts of physically untaxing tasks that will be described; or animals most often in classical-conditioning or conditioned emotional response (CER) situations with some operant baseline activity (bar- or pedal-pressing) that can be suppressed.

CARDIOVASCULAR FEEDBACK: THE LACEY HYPOTHESIS

What the Hypothesis States

The Lacey hypothesis has been elaborated at various symposia over more than a decade. For example, in 1959, data are reported showing that some stimulus situations resulted in HR decrease with concomitant skin conductance (SC) increase, while others caused the more frequently reported result of increase in both measures (Lacey 1959). In the former situations, Ss had been attending simple visual or auditory inputs, and, in the latter, they had been solving mental arithmetic problems or enduring cold pressor stress. The early hypothesis was, thus, that "cardiac deceleration accompanied and perhaps even facilitated ease of 'environmental intake,' whereas cardiac acceleration accompanied or facilitated 'rejection of the environment' " (Lacey et al. 1963, p. 165). The "rejection" of the environment implies primarily a filtering out "of irrelevant stimuli that have distraction value for the organism" (Lacey 1967, p. 35). The dimension of intake versus rejection of stimuli was also said to be related to the pleasant-unpleasant dimension, and Lacey (1967) reviewed some of the evidence showing that commerce with pleasant stimuli was often accompanied by cardiac deceleration.

The hypothesis was given further empirical definition with reference to the data reported in 1963. For tasks (e.g., mental arithmetic, reverse spelling) that required "internal manipulation of symbols and retrieval of stored information," HR and SC went up together relative to resting levels or pretask alerting periods. For tasks that did not require "cognitive elaboration," but demanded only that the S receive, by simply noting and detecting, incoming stimuli (e.g., looking at a flashing light), HR went down, although SC went up. The time-base from which measures of the different experimental periods were taken was in most instances 1 minute.

In 1967, Lacey elaborated the neurophysiological evidence for his hypothesis mainly from acute physiological preparations in infrahuman mammals, and that discussion is summarized in Chapter 26. There was some change in emphasis in terms of the data under discussion. Although the data cited in 1963 were tonic—in the sense that the reference time-base was at least 1 minute for the base, alerting-for-task, and task conditions—the data cited in 1967 were primarily phasic, concerning effects occurring over brief durations. (The distinction has meaning, as we shall see, especially when phasic effects in one direction may be superimposed on tonic effects in another.) For instance, the study by Birren, Cardon, and Phillips (1963) was cited to show that reaction time (RT) changed within the period of a single heart cycle as a function of the time at which the reaction signal was presented. RTs were fast when the signal was presented during the P-wave, a cardiac phase occurring just before atria contract and in which aortic pressure is falling to its minimum. And they were slow when signals were presented during contraction, higher aortic pressure, and presumed central inhibition. Moreover, when the RT task used had a fixed, 4-second preparatory interval (PI), Lacey found a marked deceleration occurring during the interval, interpretable as a cardiovascular response facilitating "intake" of the reaction signal by activating the cortex: And the greater the deceleration, the quicker the reaction. And, finally, Lacey cited data on infants gathered at the Fels Research Institute (Kagan and Lewis 1965; Lewis et al. 1966) showing that there was a HR deceleration accompanying attention in children, and that the magnitude of deceleration correlated with the duration of fixation, another case in which "taking in" was accompanied, and presumably facilitated, by HR deceleration.

Lacey (1967) emphasized the high degree of speculativeness associated with any hypothesis extrapolating from acute physiological preparations in animals to the sorts of tasks already mentioned in human experimentation, and mentioned a variety of complicating and possibly confounding factors as he has also done in this book (see Chapter 26). But, despite all these complications, the hypothesis was asserted and it, not its qualifications, needs primarily to be assessed. That is to say, within the range of the psychological events described by the Laceys, the idea is, and is taken by many to be, that lowered HR will facilitate a "taking in" attitude and greater sensitivity to stimuli, while a raised HR will facilitate a "rejection" attitude and cognitive manipulation and elaboration, with a raised threshold for simple incoming stimuli.

One may evaluate the hypothesis in terms of two broad classes of data. First, there are relatively direct tests of various implications of the theory, particularly with respect to sensitivity to external stimuli as measured both by threshold estimation and by reaction time, and with HR responses to pleasant and unpleasant stimuli. Second, there are studies that point up the difficulties of independent definition of the critical terms, intake and rejection, of the hypothesis.

Some Relatively Direct Tests

Various investigations have examined different relatively specific aspects of the hypothesis with a fair degree of directness, and with results that are mixed but generally not encouraging to the hypothesis. Edwards and Alsip (1969b) determined auditory thresholds, presenting test tones under both high and low transient HR. Although the hypothesis seems to predict that there would be lower thresholds during low HR, no difference in threshold was observed, and the authors concluded that signal detection was not related to unprovoked changes in HR.

A recent paper by Saxon and Dahle (1971) reports a within-S design in which auditory sensitivity was better during lower HR than during higher; but, the high HRs were induced by exercise, and it cannot be determined whether the direct aftereffects of the exercise (heavy breathing, "body noise," difficulty in settling down) might have affected sensitivity directly, since the post-exercise period was brief. The method used also precluded any signal detection analysis to determine whether apparent change in threshold was a change in response criterion or not. It might be possible for an incentive manipulation to cause an improvement in apparent threshold by the method employed, for example, even though the typical result of adding incentives is higher HR (Elliott 1969).

Saxon (1970) measured auditory sensitivity for threshold level signals in four Ss and found that sensitivity in the P-wave of the cardiac cycle was, as Lacey would predict, much higher than sensitivity during the QRS complex, which signals high aortic pressure. Elliott and Graf (1972) repeated Saxon's design testing visual sensitivity in 25 Ss. There was no significant variation in sensitivity across four phases of the cardiac cycle. Although the hit rate for the P-wave was slightly higher than that for the QRS complex—49% to 45%—the difference was not significant (t was less than 1), with 13 Ss showing greater sensitivity in the P phase, and 12 showing less.

Delfini and Campos (1971) reported a similar design with similarly negative results in 10 Ss, each given 800 signal and 800 nonsignal trials: Phase of cardiac cycle was unrelated either to sensitivity or to response bias. These authors also reviewed neurophysiological evidence that suggests that afferent baroreceptor discharge correlated with phases of the cardiac cycle is not prominent past the level of nucleus tractus solitarius, and may be "lost" at the reticular cells.

Thompson and Botwinick (1970) presented signals either during the R, T, and P waves, or at different times after the R-wave, but were unable to repeat the earlier finding by Birren, Cardon, and Phillips (1963) of a relation between RT and the phase of heart cycle in which the reaction signal was presented. Even though Callaway and Layne (1964) had also found such a relation, Birren (1965) failed to find one among aged Ss, and we can agree with the suggestion of Thompson and Botwinick that "the relationship between RT and phase in the cardiac cycle, if real, is reproducible only under extraordinarily unique circumstances" (Thompson and Botwinick 1970, p. 64).

By the terms of the Lacey hypothesis, the viewing of pleasant scenes ought to evoke "intake" and HR deceleration, and the viewing of unpleasant scenes, "rejection" and HR acceleration. The recent reports of Hare and his colleagues (Hare et al. 1970; Hare et al. 1971; Craig and Wood 1971) gainsay that prediction. In all these studies, subjects viewed slides of nudes, homicide victims, and common objects. In the first of these (Hare et al. 1970) the nudes were rated as the most pleasant, and the homicide victims as the least pleasant stimuli. In all the studies, the cardiac response to the viewing of the homicide slides was a strong deceleration which was, in males, as strong as or stronger than the deceleration accompanying the viewing of nude slides. The decline in blink rate was also strong in response to pictures of homicide victims (Hare et al. 1970, 1971). It could be argued that the homicides draw attention as much as or more than the nudes, somewhat as listening empathically to a dying man in the Lacey et al. (1963) report produced deceleration. But since two dimensions said to be related to "taking in"—pleasantness-unpleasantness and attention-gettingness—are here opposed, it would be hard to say, in advance, what to predict.

Obrist and his colleagues (Obrist et al. 1970a) blocked the cardiac decelerative response pharmacologically in a group of Ss, and found that such blockage did not affect their RT performance relative to a group of normal controls, that showed the decelerative response.

Johnson and May (1969) compared the HR response during a RT task having a fixed 4-second foreperiod with the HR response during a 4-second time estimation task. They reasoned that since a S estimating time should be rejecting the environment concentrating on some sort of internal cognitive process (probably counting), the HR ought to have gone up. On the contrary, however, it showed reliable deceleration, as did the HR of the RT Ss, shortly before the key-press response common to both groups. Interestingly enough, Lacey and Lacey have recently reported a deceleration "much the same as that found during the anticipatory period of the RT experiment," in a serial time-estimation situation in which the S, "with no external stimulation except his perception of the elapsed period," must decide when to press (Lacey and Lacey 1970, p. 222). This would seem to be an explicit denial that the task requires attention to the external environment or an "intake" attitude. They invoked "response intention" as an explanatory hypothetical term distinct from attention or intake, but since all three states appear to have similar effects on HR, and since, as it will be shown, it is difficult to see how intention to respond (something like *set*, presumably) can be operationally or conceptually distinguished from attention, the finding of deceleration in time-estimation tasks would seem awkward for the Lacey hypothesis to handle.

To return to the RT task, the pattern of results having to do with the HR deceleration response just prior to the reaction signal raises another difficult issue. Subjects in such a task are trying, so they report, to focus on the reaction signal and *nothing else*, particularly when under incentive conditions, and they become quiet both generally throughout the series (Elliott 1964, 1966b) and prior to each signal (Obrist, Webb, and Sutterer 1969; Obrist et al. 1970a). Trying to shut out task-irrelevant stimuli is said (see above) to be characteristic of "rejection," and should be manifest in accelerating HR. It might be argued that the task is so simple that little cognitive elaboration is involved, but in this case one of Lacey's paradigm tasks becomes, in fact, the occasion for competing HR tendencies: decelerative, because the task is simple, and accelerative, because it requires rejection of distracting stimuli. Dengerink (1971) has met a similar difficulty. He noted that the HR levels in his Ss were high both during shock threshold assessment and, after a rest, the giving of task instructions. The second elevation, as noted, as not readily predictable, because Ss "take in" instructions. He speculated that they also, however, had to focus their attention on the instructions.

The studies reviewed have been concerned with the phasic HR response just before an anticipated point in time at which the S will act or react. Some of the studies to be examined next concern tasks (series of stimulus situations demanding continued responses), and the measures reported are average HRs representing all or part of task periods of from 20 seconds to 90 seconds—i.e., tonic measures. It is natural that both sorts of experiment should be done: Lacey's original (1963) data were tonic (1- or 2-minute tasks); his later, RT data, were phasic; and the data reported in this book are both. But the two sorts do not always match. Eason and Dudley (1971) have shown recently that a greater phasic deceleration occurred in a condition of high incentive RT than in one of low, despite higher tonic levels of the former condition. That result matches one of Lacey and Lacey (1970) who showed that phasic HR responses, both accelerative and decelerative, were greater during the PI of "motivated" RT trials than during "unmotivated" trials, but no corresponding difference in tonic level was mentioned by them. It would seem useful to deal explicitly with the distinction between tonic and phasic effects, as Malmo and Belanger (1967) have suggested.

Studies of the anticipation of shock also illustrate the importance of a tonic-phasic distinction, and they also appear to present some difficulties for the Lacey hypothesis. It is a common observation that HR shows phasic deceleration just prior to shock (Zeaman and Smith 1965; Obrist 1968; Obrist, Webb, and Sutterer 1969). One may ask, why should the organism wish to facilitate the "taking in" rather than the "rejection" of such a signal? But there is also good evidence that HR shows tonic acceleration in anticipation of or under threat of shock (e.g., Deane 1969; Elliott 1966a; Granger 1970; Zeaman and Smith 1965), at least for the first few trials, and one might say that Ss are thereby rejecting the environment. Indeed, it has been shown that both HR effects, tonic accelerative and phasic decelerative, occur in anticipation of discrete shock (see Zeaman and Smith 1965).

This author (Elliott 1969) has also produced data that appear to contradict the tonic version of the Lacey hypothesis. Subjects performed three tasks of the Stroop test: reading the names of colors; then, naming the hues of different rectangles of color; and, finally, naming the hue, not the word, in which a color word is printed—the word and hue not being the same. The order just given was reversed for half of the 64 Ss to control for habituation and other order effects. Although the final task described is, by comparison with the first two, very difficult, requiring continuous resolution of response conflicts (cognitive processing) and evoking tendencies on the part of Ss to reject the textual environment, HR was lowest on this task. My own interpretation is that there being fewer responses per unit time in the hardest task, there is less somatic involvement, and thus lower HR. (Although response rate was not a sufficient explanation, as another experiment showed, when all tasks were done at a rate controlled by a metronome, *then* the hard task produced the highest HR.)

Problems of Testability and Definition

Studies of tonic HR responses to various tasks of the sort just discussed fall within an established convention of assessing motivation-performance relations with psychophysiological data. There are a number of studies that have been done with the Lacey hypothesis as a point of reference or a framework for interpretation, and some will be cited here to illustrate the difficulty of giving independent definition of the intake-rejection dimension, a difficulty that has resulted, as we shall see, in awkward distinctions among such terms as attention, verbalization requirement, and task difficulty. The lack of a clear independent definition of what an "intake" task is and what a "rejection" task is makes it difficult to make predictions, although post hoc use of the intake-rejection dimension is, as with all theories, alarmingly easy. The Laceys themselves, in a recent statement (1970), have illustrated an application of their hypothesis to data where the relevance seems quite tenuous. They discussed an experiment by Craig and Wood (1969) on vicarious affective experiences, in which all HR effects were measured relative to the last minutes of a 5-minute adaptation period. In one sequence, a S put his hand in very cold water, and showed an acceleration of 12 bpm. A few minutes later he watched another S put his hand into the water, and, while watching, his HR was 7 bpm *below* the reference level. The Laceys interpreted this as deceleration as a result of vicarious (a "taking in") experience. But the HR of Ss in the minute before they were to watch the other S was already nearly 7 bpm below reference level: The Ss were finished with their own stress and were, presumably, simply relaxing. One might well have produced such a result without any vicarious experience at all, simply by resting one's Ss for an equivalent time after stress.

Some of the difficulties in bringing the hypothesis to test are manifest in studies addressing the question of "verbalization." Campos and Johnson (1966, 1967) performed a series of investigations testing whether the intake-rejection dimension is confounded with a verbalization requirement, one which might itself account for HR increases for those tasks in which it was present. For example, doing mental arithmetic almost certainly involves a covert verbal process, as does reverse spelling and making up sentences, all tasks used by Lacey to induce "rejection."

Although there was no consistent anticipatory HR deceleration to simple viewing of various sorts of slides when there was no requirement to describe them, instructions to describe the viewed scenes (or prepare a description for later use) accelerated HR. The former result might be difficult for the Lacey hypothesis, but the hypothesis could account for the latter, possibly by pointing out that a requirement to verbalize requires "cognitive elaboration." Hence, the Campos and Johnson reports are only partly negative with respect to the hypothesis, and, certainly, they did not succeed in their effort to test "whether verbalization instructions can produce shifts in direction of HR with attention held constant." Instructions on how to interact with stimuli (e.g., verbalization instructions) must surely have some effect on attention to them.

If a requirement to verbalize requires "cognitive elaboration" perhaps the converse is also partly true—i.e., tasks said to involve cognitive elaboration must often depend on covert verbalization. If so, one can understand the failure of the attempt by Edwards and Alsip (1969a) to unconfound the verbalization from the intake-rejection dimension. It is possible to look at a pictorial scene (one of their intake tasks) and either verbalize it or not. But it is very difficult to do the following "rejection" task—"see how many three-letter words you can make from *HALLMARK*"—without some form of verbalization, even though the instruction quoted is a nonverbalization instruction.

Similar considerations may be applied to a similar effort by Adamowicz and Gibson (1970). They had college students simply listen to recordings of comedy or of textual material in one condition, and listen with intent to present a viva voce summary in the other. There was deceleration in the former condition, and acceleration in the latter. But the deceleration cannot be attributed to "intake," it being most unlikely that students were taking in less when they were preparing a précis of what they were hearing than when they were merely listening more or less passively.

Dahl and Spence (1971) had judges rate a variety of tasks on each of nine items of a "Task Demand Scale." Judges showed good agreement on total scale scores, and total scores were highly correlated with tonic HR for the different tasks. Only one of the items in the scale failed to correlate with tonic HR significantly in any of the three groups assessed, and that was the item, derived from the Lacey's formulation, concerning direction of attention. The authors pointed out that on the tasks they used, the dimension could be applied only with relative difficulty, but the tasks were fairly common, like the three parts of the Stroop test, digit symbol, listening to white noise, discrimination of blank versus signal stimuli, and so on.

Porges and Raskin (1969) used a set of tasks in which Ss in different groups were required either to watch a flashing light, or to count the number of its flashes in a trial, or to match the rate of flashing to the rate of presentation of intermittent tones, or to match the rate of flashing to their own HR. They found that during the first few seconds of the 26-second trials, average HR rose for the group estimating its own HR, and fell for the other three groups. Their interpretation was that the estimation of own HR required internal observation and rejection of the environment, thus evoking cardiac acceleration. It may be observed, though, that estimating one's own HR, especially at the beginning of a trial when one needs to "home in" on it, is harder than matching tones, a point noted by Porges and Raskin and consistent with the fact that errors of estimation were greater among those Ss estimating HR than among those estimating tone rate. Unconfounding the task difficulty and direction of attention dimensions is not altogether simple: For example, making the judging of one's own HR easy by amplifying its beat through use of a stethoscope would be, of course, to make the task stimuli external as well.

It is possible that the difficulty of a task might be represented by the amount of energy a person typically applies to its completion, as many of the items in the Dahl and Spence (1971) paper implied, and that possibility will be considered in the final section on cardiac-somatic coupling.

The foregoing discussion can be summarized as showing that the Laceys' hypothesis, in its more testable implications having to do with HR and sensitivity to stimuli, has received only mixed and generally unencouraging support, and that in wider applications to more complex behaviors, the conceptual confusion arising from lack of independent definition of the critical terms of the hypothesis has rendered it virtually untestable. A recent critique of the Laceys' hypothesis by Hahn (1973, p. 60) comes to a similar conclusion: namely, that "the hypothesis is of dubious testability by current methods."

The kind of question asked by a cardiovascular feedback hypothesis is how change in HR might facilitate taking in or rejecting stimuli of many degrees of complexity. Putting the question that way leaves out questions about what caused the HR to change in the first place. When that latter question is considered it may be possible to account for the changes in HR without any postulation of afferent feedback effects.

The virtues of simplicity would not justify such ignoring of feedback effects if there was substantial evidence for them in the kinds of human, perceptual-motor performance data reviewed; but, there is none, at least not of the sort that cannot be readily employed to support a variety of other hypotheses, aside from the RT data of Birren, Cardon, and Phillips (1963) and Callaway and Layne (1964) and the sensitivity data of Saxon (1970). Even if there was such evidence, it would be essential to try to assess the degree to which the kinds of HR effects surveyed here can be accounted for by viewing HR changes as responses rather than causes. Such an assessment might permit an estimate of how much might remain for a visceral afferent feedback position to account for uniquely.

Addendum: Response to the Conference Presentation

The Laceys' interesting contribution seems to me to highlight, but not to dispose of, many of the issues drawn above.

Consider first their experiment on task difficulty and divided set, wherein doing a difficult tone discrimination task was rated difficult but was accompanied by a lowered HR, while doing simple serial adding was rated easy and was accompanied by raised HR (relative to an alert-for-task HR). There are two issues here: one is the multidimensional nature of the notion "difficulty," and the other is the nature of verbalization and its effect on HR. In a sense, it is more difficult to ponder the solution to a difficult equation, or do the *Times* crossword puzzle, than to recite the alphabet, sing a familiar song, or play a familiar tune. Nevertheless, the HR would be higher during the latter set of activities because they require more activity, including rapid verbalization in two instances. (The covert verbal activity involved in doing difficult equations and crossword puzzles occurs at a relatively slow rate.) The result is, in fact, reminiscent of one of my own (see above) in which the most difficult part of the Stroop test was accompanied by a slower response rate and a relatively slow HR. When doing mental arithmetic, subjects are busily talking to themselves—when doing tone discrimination, Ss are quietly (but not flaccidly—presumably they are not curarized) listening. When listening to instructions (or Rules of the Game) with the prospect of having later to repeat them, subjects no doubt engage in covert verbal echoic behavior, but at a rate lower than what occurs during serial adding. These references to the degree of activity of the organism as a result of task requirements can serve to account reasonably well for the results without any reference to internal state. "Intentions" are simply an inference from, primarily, "instructions."

In discussing their experiment (with Libby) on looking at pictures varying in pleasantness, the Laceys deal with the apparent problem of HR deceleration to very unpleasant pictures. I think they are correct in noting that subjects must frequently be fascinated (orient steadily and without interruption) by pictures of, for example, homicide victims. But to say that Ss *intend* "to note and detect" fascinating stimuli is only really to observe that Ss *do* note and detect, usually very quietly, fascinating pictorial stimuli. The relative somatic quieting suits pretty well as an explanation, without reference to states of mind. These remarks would apply to important incentive stimuli, such as the shocks that occasionally followed slow reaction times in one of the experiments reported by Obrist and his colleagues (see Chapter 8), or the rewards following accurate time estimations in the experiment reported by the Laceys (see Chapter 26). There is little question that most Ss would orient quietly to the source of such stimuli, with accompanying low HR.

AROUSAL AND HEART RATE

Activation

The activation hypothesis is one that relates quality of performance to arousal (or activation, or drive), usually taken to be degree of nonspecific afferent stimuli affecting the cortex via the ascending reticular arousal system. The view discussed by Malmo (1962) is Hebbian, and suggests that the neural organization responsible for some behavior will function more efficiently, up to a point, with increased toning up of the cortex by summation. But that, beyond that point, more stimulation may result in refractory cells, inappropriate timing, and so on, and hence, degraded performance.

In its role as a physiological version of drive, the concept of activation has been applied often to studies of water and food deprivation in rats. As motivational concept in human performance, it has been applied to predict or account for changes in quality of performance with changes in instructions designed to be more or less activation-inducing. In both cases, HR has been a very common measure for indexing activation and drive. As such, it is taken to be one of many possible measures, all correlated. The others most often used are various electrodermal measures, electroencephalogram (EEG) measures, electromyogram (EMG) measures, and blood pressure. As we shall see, the assumption of correlation among these measures does not hold, as Lacey has pointed out for some time (1959, 1967), and it has, therefore, become difficult to maintain that any one of them is a measure of general arousal or drive.

The more fundamental difficulty with the interpretation of HR (or any other index) as drive is that studies are usually done in such a way that an experimental manipulation has an effect on a peripheral physiological measure, and an effect on performance. Then, rather than consider each effect the result of the prior manipulation, the activation theorist relates one effect to the other in a fixed order: activation, then performance. Equally plausible assumptions are that the autonomic responses are concurrent and partially correlated with the overt behavioral response, or that the behavioral response affects the autonomic response.

This line of argument was made by Kendler (1959) in his comment on Stennet's (1957) well-known paper, and by me in discussing my own (1964) data also taken in Malmo's laboratory:

Perhaps the simplest way to conceptualize the results of this study, or any study in which covert physiological and overt motor variables are concurrently measured, is to assume that both the overt and covert behaviors are affected chiefly not by each other, but by whatever antecedent manipulations have been made. . . . What is being maintained is that under normal conditions the two sets of measures can be parsimoniously considered as responses which are largely independent, not related by any given function, and not so organized that one set has any special influence over the other.

Over and above the questionable utility of the hypothetical construct, the data taken to assess it have seldom actually had any logical relation to it. Thus, one wants to see performance plotted against some measure of arousal, but what one typically sees is each plotted separately against some independent variable, and then interpreted one in terms of the other. The famous study of Belanger and Feldman (1962) is a case in point; HR rose monotonically with hours of deprivation, and bar-pressing described an inverted-U. But if one arrays the data of each rat, with bar-pressing plotted against HR, there may be no consistent relationship. I analyzed human data in that way (1964), testing two predictions from activation theory. First, the worst performance should be associated with either the highest individual physiological level (overactivation), or with the lowest (underactivation). For four physiological variables in adults, and five in children, the association of the worst performance with extreme ranks of physiological activity did not exceed chance level. Second, activation levels associated with extreme differences in performance should themselves be quite different; but the proportion of cases in which there were very small differences in physiological activity associated with best versus worst performance was close to what might be expected by chance, and certainly was higher than the hypothesis can comfortably allow.

Finally, it turns out that one can produce a great variety of relations between a physiological measure and a measure of performance efficiency. Granger, Ducharme, and Belanger (1969) have reported that *both* HR and change in running speed were monotonic functions of the same water deprivation series that produced inverted-U bar-pressing data; and they cited work in which bar-pressing itself, if sufficiently well practiced, was monotonic with deprivation. Malmo (1966) showed a large performance difference in tracking, comparing a divided set with a unified set condition, but it was not accompanied by differences in physiological measures. I have shown the same effect in RT, in well-practiced Ss, who change speed but not HR with changes in incentive (Elliott 1966b). In another experiment (Elliott, 1969), one group showed improvement in RT performance with rising HR, and another no change with change in HR—it depended upon what order the different incentives were presented in. We will discuss below another example of equal improvements in RT performance with different patterns of change in HR, among children, depending again on incentive order. There are also reports of large changes in HR with incentive, but no changes in performance (Evans 1971, 1972).

There seems little doubt, from the review by Malmo and Belanger (1967), that water deprivation will predispose rats to show HRs whose levels vary with hours of deprivation, provided that incentive-motivational cues are present. There is equally little doubt that deprivation alone, presumably an antecedent of drive, will *not* raise the HR of rats in their home cages without the presence of cues to the consummatory response (cf. Malmo and Belanger 1967; also Hahn, Stern and McDonald 1962; and, for a similar result from the use of a dehydrating stomach load of hypertonic saline, O'Kelly et al. 1965). Malmo and Belanger state that HR also rises monotonically with food deprivation in an incentive-cue situation (with bar-pressing a concomitant inverted-U function), but that function appears to be less well documented. A recent paper by Doerr and Hokanson (1968) found a relationship between HR and hours of deprivation, for example, only in the last 5 minutes of a 30-minute session of bar-pressing.

In the two of these studies of HR and food or water deprivation that dealt with the question, there was no relation between force of bar-pressing, varied by the force required to activate the magazine, and HR (Hahn, Stern, and Fehr 1964; Doerr and Hokanson 1968). Beyond that, Ducharme (1966) has shown that HR of thirsty rats was higher when the lever was retracted than it was when they were pressing it. He proposed that appropriate organized activity can under some conditions play a deactivating, regulating role, with reduced HR. More than that, Ouellet and Ducharme (1965) showed that rats pressed faster for water on an FR6 schedule (in which every sixth response was reinforced) than did rats on a CRF schedule (in which every response was reinforced), but the HR in the FR6 group was lower; and that, in a same subjects design, rats pressed faster for smaller drops of water than they did for large ones, but that their HR was lower when they pressed at the higher rate.

On their face, these data certainly go against a notion relating physical activity and exertion to HR. The problem is that we do not know very much about what the rat is doing besides bar-pressing and drinking. There are many movements apart from the instrumental-consummatory sequence that go unrecorded unless special efforts are made to measure movement by ratings, stabilimeters, and so on. It may be that organized appropriate activity reduces HR because it reduces other task-inappropriate movement—only appropriate measurement will tell us.

In a study by Venderwolf and Vanderwort (1970), the investigators quite deliberately assessed the different overt behaviors of their rats including both instrumental food-taking behaviors and other behaviors (sniffing, scratching, rearing, licking, etc.), and their concomitant HRs. Different behaviors had reliably different rates associated with them, and the highest rates were associated with the most vigorous activities. There was no general effect of food deprivation on either behavior or HR. The authors suggest that drive operations, when they do affect HR, may do so because they affect rate and nature of motor activities as well.

In the same vein, we have attempted to repeat some of Ducharme's observations, but have added a measure of general movement—namely, vibrations of the wire mesh in the bottom of the experimental space, recorded by a Korotkoff sound microphone. In our first experiment, 12 rats 120-days-old were trained to press for water under a CRF schedule and 23 hours' water deprivation. They were then operated for electrode placement and reshaped for baseline rates of about 20 presses per minute. We did not use a retractable lever, as Ducharme did: Rather, we used a plexiglass shield to block off the entire wall of the box in which the lever and water cup were placed. Otherwise, we used Ducharme's schedule of conditions, with 1 minute of lever availability, 1 of time out, another of availability, and so on for 5 minutes. The HR score was the rate for the minute; movement was measured in six, 2-second samples, every 10 seconds starting with the fourth, the highest deflection being taken. We found a nearly 20 bpm difference between lever available and lever-not-available, with the latter showing the higher rate over 11 sessions. This result very nearly duplicated Ducharme's. But we also found a dramatic increase in gross movement when the lever was not available. Figure 25.1 illustrates these data.

Correlational analyses indicated the degree with which changes in movement and HR were related. For five sessions (2, 5, 8, 10, and 11) the product-moment correlations, across 12 animals, of the differences in the two measures between lever available and lever-not-available were .64, .61, .73, .37, and .77 ($p < .05$ in all but one case).

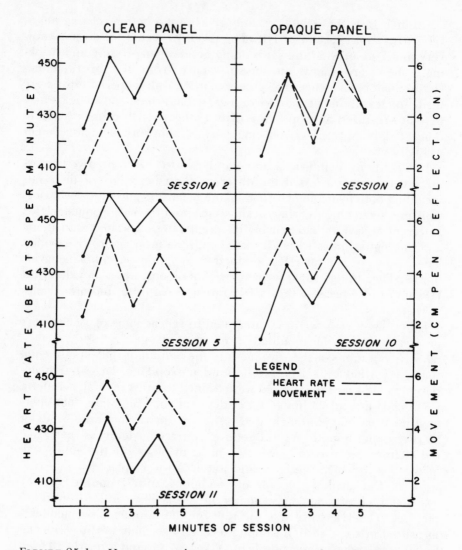

FIGURE 25.1.   *Heart rate and gross movement scores of rats during 5-minute sessions. In the second and fourth minutes, a panel (clear or opaque) prevented the rats from access to lever and cup.*

Within subject correlations were done, relating movement and HR scores over each of the 5 minutes of the session. These averaged .89, .80, .77, .69, and .75 for the five sessions (p<.001 in each case). It is evident that, with our conditions, the HR effects are more simply viewed as somatomotor correlates than the results of the regulation of activation by task appropriate behavior. It seems preferable to say that task appropriate behavior regulates *activity*, not activation.

We may end this section, and introduce the next, with a note on "drive" as a general personality variable. Assuming that such a variable exists as a reliable differentiator of individuals, Hokanson and his colleagues (Burgess and Hokanson 1964; Hokanson and Burgess 1964; Doerr and Hokanson 1965) have attempted to index it by measuring a 5-minute "resting" HR of adult subjects. But the possibility of specific situational determinants is strong. For example, subjects are told in advance that the study concerns various intellectual tasks which will be presented following the rest period, and that information is very likely to affect Ss differently. Some will be highly involved and anticipate their task-to-come; others will be apprehensive; others will not care. To the degree that such reactions affect HR differentially, what is being measured is at least as much a conditioning history with respect to evaluation in educational settings as a dimension of generalized drive. (That there is some effect of the prerest information on "rest" is indicated by the "resting" rates, which are high by comparison with many other studies (Elliott 1970a). A more persuasively nonreactive allocation of Ss to drive categories could be accomplished by asking Ss simply to rest—nothing more—and later selecting Ss for task performance from such an initially established pool of HR scores.

Social and Emotional Arousal

This reference to personality characteristics may serve to introduce the topic of HR as a measure of emotional arousal. If one is emotionally aroused (in fear, frustration, anger, anxiety, or uncertainty) is one's HR a feature that distinguishes these states in general from nonarousal states, and does one state tend to have associated with it levels of HR different from other states? Also, does HR indicate much about the quality of interpersonal relations? These are the general sorts of questions now to be addressed.

There are a number of recent reviews of this general area (Martin and Sroufe 1970; Shapiro and Crider 1969; Shapiro and Schwartz 1970), and it is not necessary to cover all of that already competently covered ground. I will emphasize what I can conclude from those reviews about HR, as well as some of my own work in this area and other recent papers not yet covered in reviews.

Martin (1961; Martin and Sroufe, 1970) has reviewed the question of different emotions producing different physiological effects. There is no question whether HR will rise under threat of shock or anger-induction. For Ss awaiting initial shock, a rise from base rate of 20 bpm is not uncommon (see below). Hokanson and Burgess (1964) have reported a similar rise consequent to their simple frustration manipulation. But whether HR will differentiate fear from anger probably depends on what Martin and Sroufe (1970) refer to as the strength of arousal to each, a factor that may reduce in part to the degree to which the S is instigated to action. In Ax's famous (1953) study, for example, fear of electrocution may have been a greater incentive to action than anger toward an insulting assistant.

As for anxiety, and quite apart from traditional difficulties in defining it, I reviewed three papers in 1969 in which self-reported or rated anxiety did not correlate with task HR—although in one of those studies (Hodges and Spielberger 1966), the HR response to threat of shock did relate to self-reported fear of shock (a result repeated by Pearson and Thackray 1970). There are two more recent papers that report relations between HR and self-reported anxiety (Dengerink 1971; Hare 1971), but in each case the major results tend to consist of interactions with such variables as time or sex, and are very complex. In comparing persons diagnosed as anxious with normals, there appear to be many physiological differences, particularly in size and persistence of response to stressors (Malmo 1957), and HR is sometimes one of them. So, often, are measures of movement, tremor, and muscle tension.

For other emotions, Damaser, Shor, and Orne's (1963) paper is perhaps instructive. They induced them by describing them and asking Ss to "really feel" them, explicitly including body and face in "really" feeling. Fear-panic descriptions evoked greatest HR, with exuberant happiness next, followed by physical and mental exhaustion ("depression"), followed by calmness. The effects are significant, but we cannot say to what degree somatic involvement entered the states differentially. Frontalis muscle action differentiated the states, and general bodily activity may also have done so had it been measured. Furthermore, had there not been an instruction not to thrash around in the chair, it seems possible the exuberant joy may have produced a HR as high as that produced in fear.

The roughly obverse case, in which each of two conditions is unpleasant but distinct in HR level, was suggested by a study by Gottlieb, Gleser, and Gottschalk (1967) in which the subjects were hypnotized twice and the suggestion was made each time that their hand would be burned by the experimenter and they would feel mistreated. After the suggested (but not actual) burning, the further suggestion was made to the subject in dramatic terms that, in one instance, he wanted to assault his tormentor, and that, in the other, although he felt mistreated, he was a helpless victim of injustice and there was nothing he could do or even wanted to do about his misfortune. No overt action was taken in either case. There was a significant (p<.01) rise in HR over resting level under the active attitude, and no significant increase under the passive attitude. The differences in changes was itself significant. The difference in the conditions seems predominantly to have been in action instigation, not in "emotionality," since it can be assumed that the subjects found both suggestions unpleasant.

The foregoing considerations do nothing to contradict the judgment that HR is not useful in the differentiation of emotion. There is a somewhat more specific concept, uncertainty, about which there has been considerable research effort. Some years ago, I designed a variety of tests of a prediction that uncertainty, interruption, and conflict would result in arousal, measurable as HR increase. Included among the failures of this prediction were those studies reported in 1969. In summary, when subjects had control (an escape response) over shock, they had a higher, not lower, HR than when they didn't; Ss awaiting a shock whose time of onset was unknown had lower, not higher HRs than Ss awaiting a shock whose onset was certain; Ss doing the parts of the Stroop color-word interference test had lower, not higher HRs in the most difficult, conflict-producing part of it; and, in a group given tone discrimination tasks that were difficult and became impossible, HR went down slightly, not up.

Two recent investigations, however, have reported a relation between the size of the *phasic* components of the HR responses in anticipation of signal stimuli on the one hand, and the importance and probability (hence, uncertainty) of those signals on the other. Higgins (1971) sought to differentiate the anticipatory autonomic effects associated with response uncertainty from those associated with simple motor set in two tasks, RT and vigilance. He arranged that in both tasks the probability of stimulus presentation on any trial in a series vary from 0.0 to 1.0. The main result was that the size of the phasic HR changes during the foreperiod was closely correlated with degrees of stimulus uncertainty, describing an inverted-U function with a maximum about a probability of a "go" signal of 0.5. At the same time Ss were obviously best prepared to respond (were fastest) at the probability of 1.0, and such preparation was monotonically related to the probability of the "go" stimulus. Also, the size of the phasic acceleratory and deceleratory responses were greater to the RT signal, which demanded a quick reaction, than to the vigilance signal, which needed only detection. Jennings et al. (1971) manipulated the probability both of the arrival of shock and of making a particular response, and also found larger phasic anticipatory HR responses with greater uncertainty in each kind of manipulation.

Conclusions in these studies are very similar, to the effect that, in Higgins' case, HR changes reflected attentional requirements of the task, and that, in the Jennings et al. case, they are produced by factors that increase the intensity of attention. While the use of the concept attention, rather than uncertainty, does not seem required, the interpretations seem plausible. What is missing, and what might help to discriminate a recourse to an explanation in terms of a less measurable hypothetical construct (attention) from recourse to a more measurable one (cardiac-somatic coupling), is some measure of phasic somatic effects, particularly general effects independent of the limited motor organization involved in the response.

My own work on the effect of uncertainty about the time and/or the probability of arrival of shocks suffers the same lack. There is a very large HR acceleration in Ss awaiting their first, unknown shock (Elliott 1966a; Deane 1961; Bankart and Elliott 1972; Averill, Olbrich, and Lazarus 1972; Pearson and Thackray 1970), very often of the order of 20 bpm or more. Such large accelerations diminish greatly after one experience with shock (Elliott 1966a; Bankart and Elliott 1972). Is this a reduction in nonsomatic arousal per se, perhaps as a result of knowing what the shock is like; or is it also a reduction in somatic activity, including muscle tension? We did not, unfortunately, take the appropriate measures of movement and tension.

It is, of course, possible to assess HR as a measure of uncertainty where the uncertainty refers to the probability that a shock will occur after some waiting period. A very cursory summary of results would be this: Average anticipatory tonic HR is inversely related to shock probability (Deane 1969), directly related to shock probability (Bankart and Elliott 1972), or lower for a 50% probability than for 100% or 0% probabilities (Bowers 1971a,b). That last result would seem to support a view that HR might reflect uncertainty (inversely in this case), but Bowers confounded two uncertainties in his 50% groups—*when* the shock might come, as well as *whether* it would come. That shock might come at almost any time throughout the anticipation period in the 50% condition is a circumstance almost certainly predisposing somatically quiet alertness. In an experiment only now being analyzed, my subjects (N = 32) had significantly higher HR in anticipation of shock than no-shock and slightly, but not significantly, higher HR when anticipating 100% probability rather than 50% probability of shock. In this case we did use measures of movement. Only blinking activity parallels HR substantially, and even it does not show anything like the large elevation to the first anticipation of shock that HR shows.

Another set of studies we had done was related to the work on uncertainty, but was cast in a social psychological framework. In these experiments, interviewers adopted various roles toward Ss who had all just read the same material (a "transcript" of a young college man telling his many troubles to a counselor). The Ss were asked three questions about the case (summarize it, suggest solutions, and tell how it relates to your own life), and given 5 to 6 minutes to answer each. The three interviewers were in some cases "passive friendly," in Rogerian style; and, in others, "deadpan," sitting attentively but in silence, with as little nonverbal responding as possible. In a second experiment, a third role was added, called "ambiguous-nervous," in which the interviewer's comments consisted of "perhaps," "maybe," "that's one way of looking at it," and so on; his manner was hesitant and stiff, and he might interrupt but trail off, forgetting what he was about to say. My prediction was that uncertainty and ambiguity would create stress, and this stress would appear as higher HR.

The general course of HR in the two experiments is shown in Figure 25.2. There are many reliable characteristics of the curves, including the rise from Rest to Reading, the dip in the beginning of Reading, the strong acceleration to the first minute of the interview, and the regular decline within and across questions. Note, with reference to the unconnected dots prior to Question 1, that HR accelerated in the half-minute period just before the interviewer asked the first question—in this period the interviewer had reentered the room and was connecting his own HR leads and checking his record.

But there were scarcely any role effects during any of the question periods in either of the experiments: a sex by role effect in Question 1 of Experiment I, and two different triple interactions in different questions of Experiment II. This lack of effect on HR could not be attributed to a general lack of psychological effect. Just after the third question period, subjects in Experiment I in the passive-friendly role rated it as significantly ($p<.01$) more certain than did Ss in the deadpan role, and somewhat ($p<.10$) more comfortable. In Experiment II, Ss rated passive-friendly as most certain, ambiguous-nervous as next most, and deadpan as least, to a marginally significant degree ($p<.10$). They rated passive-friendly as more comfortable than either ambiguous-nervous ($p<.01$) or deadpan ($p<.10$).

We pursued the question of HR and emotional arousal in these experiments in another way by asking whether the characteristic acceleration in the fourth minute of the reading period had anything to do with what was read. The transcript took just under 6 minutes to read (as an average of a separate sample of 12), and we wondered whether the discussion of particularly bitter problems with parents in the fourth minute might have touched an especially sensitive area in most of our Ss, women as well as men (there were no interactions between sex and minutes during the reading period). We altered the material in two ways: first by simply altering the original transcript so that the parental problems came near the beginning of the transcript, at the point of the dip; second, by using a wholly new transcript, based on an interview with a man with several problems reported in Rogers (1942) and edited to be as long as the others. Fourteen Ss read the "new" transcript, and 14 read the "altered" transcript. The results, with the HR patterns of Experiment I and II for reference, appear in Figure 25.3. The time effect was significant for the "altered" group ($p<.05$), although not for the "new" group. The question whether the

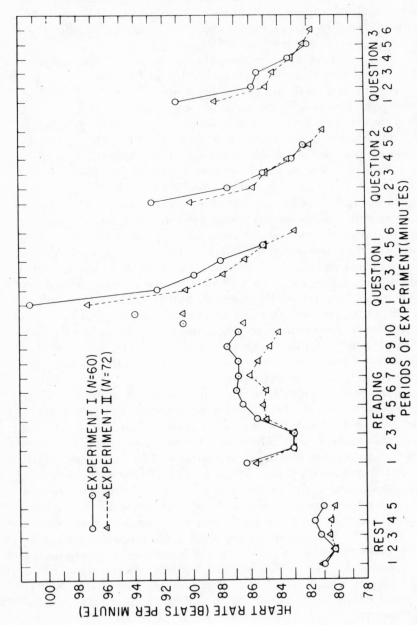

FIGURE 25.2. *Average HRs for male and female Ss in an interview study while they rested, read the transcript of a case, and answered three questions about it. Unconnected data points between Reading and Question 1 were taken in two 15-second periods just prior to asking the first question.*

changes in material affected the pattern of HR was assessed by choosing the 10 male Ss already seen by this same interviewer in Experiment I, and analyzing the resulting data in groups (three) by trial (10 minutes) analysis of variance. There was no groups effect; there was a trials effect (p<.001), and there was no interaction: Thus, the patterns of HR must be considered the same, despite the changes in content.

One might suspect by now that there is no obvious mandate in evidence for using HR to measure complex variables in social psychology and personality. The reviews of Shapiro and Crider (1969) and Shapiro and Schwartz (1970) certainly do not offer grounds for optimism as far as HR goes, although other variables, such as electrodermal or pupillary responses, seem more hopeful. There is no doubt, as already mentioned, that a particular stressor-threat of shock, for example—will have a reliable acceleratory effect on HR, but there is considerable question whether individual differences in such effects will correlate substantially or at all with other traits or behaviors. The question is much like that posed by Mischel (1968) concerning the relations between specific behaviors and traits, or traits with other traits, or the same trait with itself when assessed by different methods. Thus, Averill, Olbrich, and Lazarus (1972) are pessimistic about stability of any relation between autonomic responses to threat and personality variables, citing three studies on the topic from their laboratories on the personality correlates of response to threat, no two of which agree.

A recent study by Gormly (1971) comes to a similar conclusion with respect to HR and reactions to disagreement. He found that there was no significant difference in the HRs of Ss between occasions when they were agreed with by a peer on attitudes toward significant issues, and occasions when they were disagreed with. Nor were differences in the characteristic manner in which they resolved disagreements reflected in differences in HR, although they were in SC. Finally, in a review of the use of physiological measures of sexual arousal, Zuckerman (1971) arrived at this conclusion: "The research using heart rate as a measure of sexual arousal indicates that this measure is not very sensitive to sexual arousal prior to intromission or genital manipulation."

THE CARDIAC-SOMATIC HYPOTHESIS

Among the most prominent hypotheses about the significance of HR, and one that illustrates the conception of HR changes primarily as effect rather than cause, is one that has been called by Obrist and his colleagues (Obrist et al. 1970b) the cardiac-somatic relationship. Their work and that of many others is well summarized elsewhere in this volume (see Chapter 8). In general, the view is that HR is not primarily

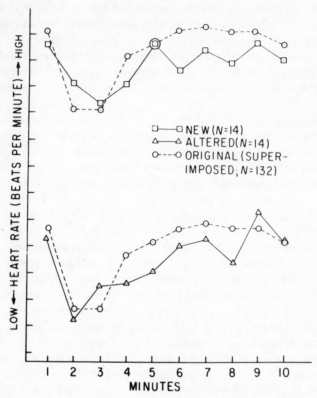

FIGURE 25.3.   *Heart rate during reading of the original transcript, an altered version of it, and an entirely different transcript.*

a psychologically functional physiological variable. The HR deceleration in the RT task, for example, is seen not as a feedback mechanism but as part of a general quieting response that often accompanies close attention. The general conclusion from their results is the central assertion that HR in the intact organism, in the settings in which we usually study it, is primarily controlled by the same set of events that govern somatic (striate, skeletal) activity. The reader will have noticed recourse to this view in critical comments elsewhere in this review.

There are difficulties in testing the cardiac-somatic view. Since, in the hypothesis, HR change is related to metabolic requirements involved in action, and since action includes everything the organism is doing, then no measurement system so far reported can be taken to be completely suitable—strain gauges beneath the floor of a chamber, for example, Obrist (Obrist et al. 1972a) picked up a dog's body movements, but not his barking. And, as we have already noted, the hypothesis cannot be evaluated by measuring only the rate and amplitude of instrumental responding.

A variety of investigators have data that support the cardiac-somatic hypothesis. Many of their reports are summarized in this volume by Obrist et al. (see Chapter 8). Roberts (see Chapter 9) and Black (see Chapter 12) also offer dramatic illustrations. But there are a few studies that offer either mixed or no support for the hypothesis, and some will be reviewed to illustrate both its difficulties of measurement and the probably real limitations of its scope. For example, Teyler (1971), in a classical conditioning paradigm with shock as the unconditioned stimulus (UCS), had groups of animals either free or restrained, and a shock locus either at the feet or the chest in a 2 by 2 design. Heart rate dropped more during a 7-second conditioned stimulus (CS) period in restrained than unrestrained animals, and more to chest-shocked than foot-shocked animals: i.e., the less the situation stimulated and permitted movement, the greater the conditioned HR deceleration. But the size of the HR conditioned response was correlated significantly with the change in movement in only 1 of 4 groups.

Cohen and Johnson (1971b) had three groups of human Ss either tense all their muscles, relax all their muscles, or simply continue uninstructed in a classical conditioning (shock as UCS) paradigm. Anticipatory HR and EMG during the CS was much higher in the group under tension instructions than in the other two groups, which did not differ. To that degree the study supported the cardiac-somatic hypothesis. But there was no deceleration in EMG prior to UCS, and there was a striking deceleration in HR. This discordance may have been the result of the special effects of instructions to tense muscles on certain muscle groups and not others, but it illustrates again the problem of measurement with this hypothesis: It is sometimes difficult to tell what is a limitation of the hypothesis (i.e., where nonsomatic effects on HR appear) and what is a limitation of the adequacy of its test.

Another example of this sort comes from my own data. Changes upward in incentive usually result in HR elevation (Elliott 1969). But they also, in my first studies of HR and RT (Elliott 1964, 1966b), result in reduced general bodily movement in an RT task. In order to account for the increase in tonic HR, one would need to show increases in muscular *tension* that would more than compensate for declines in overt movement. There were significant EMG increases accompanying the rise in HR with incentive in adults, but there were not in five-year-old children. Such a discrepancy might be resolved with more careful and extensive analysis of both overt movement and muscular tension. In these two studies, EMG was measured from the nonresponding arm only, and general bodily movement was indexed by artifacts in the EEG and respiration polygraph recordings.

There are a few reports of the relation between somatic activity and HR that seem quite negative with respect to the cardiac-somatic hypothesis. Smith and his associates (Stebbins and Smith 1964; Smith and Stebbins 1965; Nathan and Smith 1968) have shown that in the CER situation with monkeys, HR and blood flow increase during the period of aversive stimulation, without any change in gross activity. DiCara and Weiss (1969) reported that rats that had been conditioned under curare to speed their HR in the presence of a tone CS, also speeded it later in the normal state when presented with the same CS, and that slow HR learners did the opposite. But the measured activity of the animals in response to the CS in the normal state was just the opposite of what the cardiac-somatic formulation holds: Activity went down to the CS in those animals whose HR went simultaneously up, and vice versa. They speculated that very strong shocks, and inferentially very strong fear, breaks down the relationship between HR deceleration and anticipation of shock.

These studies, particularly the one by DiCara and Weiss, argue for HR as an index of what it is often thought to be an index of— emotional arousal. To the degree that such nonsomatic effects continue to be reliably demonstrated, a clear limit on the cardiac-somatic hypothesis will be established. That sort of result has been the expectation of tradition, and no one holds that HR change can be accounted for *exclusively* in terms of change in general activity, and, by inference, the current needs of the musculature for blood. Obrist et al. (See Chapter 8) have also discovered a few instances, typically marked by stress and uncertainty, in which HR and somatic activity were uncoupled.

Habituation, as well as fear, has some claim to status as an effect on HR not paralleled in movement. A perusal of Figure 25.1 will illustrate the decline of HR over the sessions, when at the same time general movement was increasing. A separate experiment has also shown the same general effects *within* a session when conditions are constant, whether movement is measured as vibration of the experimental space, or as a specific set of behaviors. Roberts and Young (1971) have shown a similar independence of HR and movement over trials.

There may be other HR effects that are relatively independent of movement and tension changes. Orienting and defensive responses are candidates. Heart rate change is also known to anticipate change in overt movement, as when it goes up prior to actual speech in an interview situation (see above); or up in dogs just before they exercise (Rushmer, Smith, and Lasher 1960, cited in Black and DeToledo, 1972); or up during the minute prior to a task during which the S has been "alerted" that the task will be coming (Lacey et al. 1963). In these cases, given a thorough attempt to sample tension and movement (or some other correlate of cardiac output like O_2 consumption), the less the relation to HR, the more the likelihood that other variables will be required to account for its variation. It is in this sense that any limitation in the cardiac-somatic hypothesis is a source of strength to other hypotheses about the control of HR. The most important contribution of taking measures of movement, tension, or metabolic activity may be to delimit, clarify, and probably reduce nonsomatic interpretation of one's results.

The same remarks apply to HR changes under curare, and to HR changes as a result of direct operant conditioning. In all these cases a conditioning history will undoubtedly be required along with a measure of current metabolic demand, to render a reasonably complete account of HR change in the tasks that have been discussed. Such a history is, of course, observable in a sense in which "intention" to take in or reject the environment, along with cardiovascular feedback effects, is not. There are awkward measurement problems with the cardiac-somatic formulation, but they are difficulties of method, not conception, and presumably are tractable. There seems nothing in the formulation as difficult so far as the problems of independent definition and measurement of such terms as intake, rejection, activation, or emotion.

A recent study on reaction time in children will perhaps serve to illustrate some of the foregoing points. We used 48 children, 24 in each of two groups—each group containing about the same proportions of boys and girls, with an average age of about 6.5 years. The task was simple RT (a key-lift to a loud tone) under two incentive levels. In low incentive, the S was given 25 cents before the trials, and then simply encouraged noncontingently and without feedback throughout the trials. In high incentive, the child was again given 25 cents; in addition, he or she was given a nickel each time that his or her RT was judged good (about 60% of the trials were so judged), the judgment depending on performance in previous trials, including practice trials. The two groups were defined by order: low, then high (LH), and HL, with a brief rest in between incentive conditions. The tasks in each condition were to perform in trials with foreperiods of 4, 6, 8, and 12 seconds, presented in irregular (random) order; in regular presentation, 11 trials each at foreperiods of 4 and 12 seconds.

We recorded HR, eyeblink, head movements, and the vibrations of S's chair using a Korotkoff sound microphone taped to the bottom of it. The phasic measures for the movement variables were taken for the second prior to the ready signal, for each second of the anticipation period, and for 4 seconds after it. The deflections in each of the three movement variables were measured alike: i.e., the greatest deflection in each second, measured in .5 cm steps. For HR, since we did not have a cardiotachometer in this study, we measured the R-R intervals at the ready signals (the S presses his key down after being told that he may), at the response and for the two beats before it, and at the four beats following it. Other beats between the ready and respond beats were measured as indicated in Figure 25.4: These represented approximately the peak of the acceleratory limb of the biphasic HR response, and one or two intermediate beats.

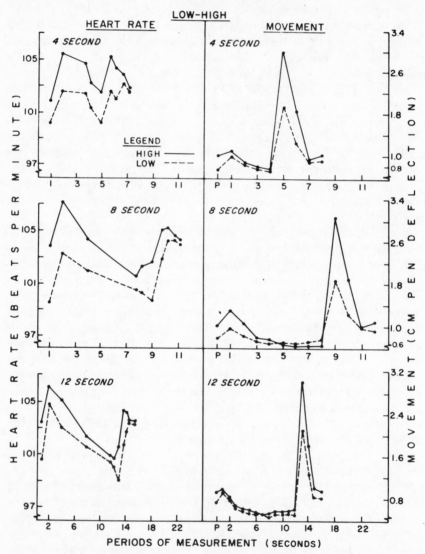

FIGURE 25.4. *Phasic HR (left) and phasic movement (right) during the different preparatory intervals in the RT task for the LH group. The letter P stands for the second prior to the ready signal. Incentive level is a parameter of these figures.*

The left panels of Figure 25.4 show the anticipatory HR response in the LH group in each of three preparatory intervals, divided by incentive condition, which tended to have significant or near significant effects. (Levels of significance of the F-ratios for incentive were, reading top to bottom, .07, .01, and .06.) The curves are based on measures taken for each occurrence of the preparatory interval during random presentation and for alternate trials during regular presentation. Difference in mode of presentation (random or regular) for any interval did not affect deceleration in any systematic or statistically reliable way. The right panels show the corresponding phasic somatic effects, including the second prior to the ready signal, for chair vibration, also divided according to incentive level. The measure of head movement closely paralleled that of chair vibration; and eyeblink activity tended to parallel HR. These latter two are, therefore, not shown.

All the curves shown are highly reliable—i.e., there were significant effects associated with periods of measurement. There are, of course, marked similarities, and also some interesting differences, between phasic HR and phasic movement. The initial upward rise in gross movement peaks as the S presses the key down at the ready signal—the peak in HR then follows. Incentive does not affect movement prior to response, even though it does affect HR. With the movement measure, but not HR, incentive markedly affects the magnitude of the response itself.

Figure 25.5 illustrates the same data for the HL group. The sensitivity of the movement measure to incentive during response appears again, as well as the fact that phasic changes in HR lag those in movement by a short time. (Cardiotachometer delay is not an issue here, since we didn't use one.) The incentive effect on preparatory HR in the single case where it existed was opposite to what one usually expects: That is, the low incentive HR was significantly higher (p<.05) than the high incentive HR in the preparatory phase of the 8-second foreperiods. We have no ready explanation for this lack of and even inversion of typical incentive effects.

In general, then, the pattern of *phasic* changes in gross movement and HR was similar in both groups, similar enough to support a hypothesis of cardiac-somatic linkage. But differences in features of the patterns argue for limits to the applicability of that hypothesis.

There was less encouragement for a cardiac-somatic view when we examined tonic effects. We measured 3 minutes (one each during the random, 4-second regular, and 12-second regular tasks) in each incentive condition. We measured the largest deflection in each 5-second period for the head movement and chair vibration, and the total number of eyeblinks. Among the LH Ss, the results, illustrated in the left panel of Figure 25.6, were much as we expected, as far as direction

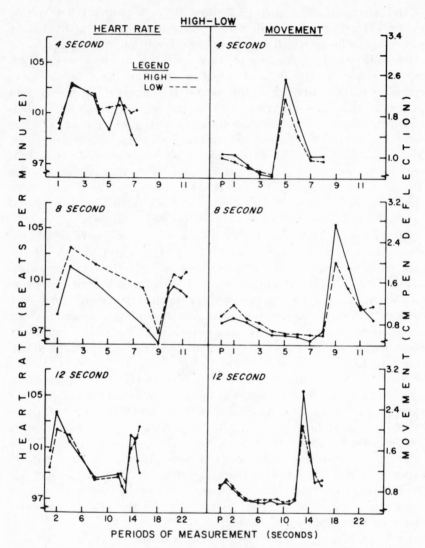

FIGURE 25.5.   *Phasic HR (left) and phasic movement (right) during the different preparatory intervals in the RT task for the HL group. The letter P stands for the second prior to the ready signal. Incentive level is a parameter of these figures.*

went, although the decline in number of blinks is anomalous and significant (p<.05): HR and head movement increased marginally (p<.10), and chair vibration (Korotkoff) increased reliably (p<.01) with high incentive. In the HL group, however, the HR was significantly *lower* (p<.05) in high incentive than in low; blink rate was this time significantly higher in high incentive (p<.05); and, of the incentive differences in head movement and chair vibration (Korotkoff), only the latter was close to significant (p<.10).

We remeasured in an attempt to rid the data of response correlated movement effects, sampling six 5-second periods in the intertrial intervals for each task condition of each incentive level, measuring in the phasic way—i.e., second-by-second—and then adding. Analysis of these data indicated *no* incentive effects even of a marginally significant sort on HR in either group, a significant (p<.05) increase in chair vibration with high incentive in the LH group, a significant (p<.05) decrease in size of blinks with low incentive in the HL group, and a near-significant (p<.10) decrease in head movement with low incentive in the HL group. This pattern of results still leaves HR somewhat disconnected from movement indices, but the other results are slightly more coherent.

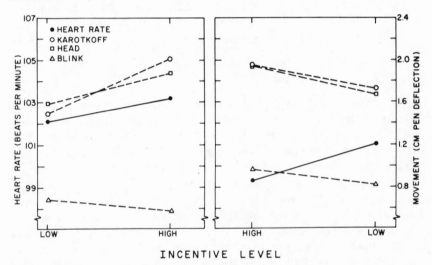

FIGURE 25.6. *Tonic movement and HR as a function of incentive level in the LH group (left) and the HL group (right).*

At the moment, I am not quite sure how to consider these data. In part the problem may be that there is too small a range of movement and of HR. For example, when we asked the children to rest for a minute, before and after the trials, they didn't really rest very quietly, so we began to insert a "quiet" period at the end of the session ("Sit just as quietly as you possibly can"). Figure 25.7 shows the data. It is obvious that the tonic HR and tonic movement measures in this case are more covariant.

On the other hand, even though the incentive difference did not produce consistent effects on HR, it certainly had significant effects

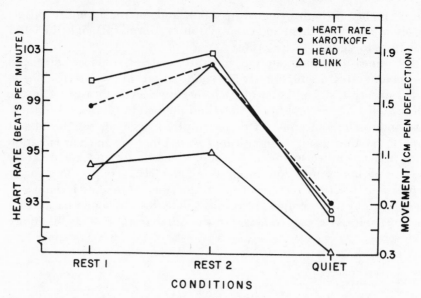

FIGURE 25.7. *Effect of "rests" and an instruction to sit very quietly on HR and movement scores of children.*

on performance. Figure 25.8 illustrates the data. Separate analyses of variance of the regular and irregular data revealed highly significant incentive and preparatory intervals effects in both analyses ($p<.01$), and no significant main effects of group (HL or LH) or significant interactions. Additional analyses showed that the speeds to the 4-second preparatory interval were reliably ($p<.001$) faster when it was regular than when it was irregular, even though the corresponding phasic anticipatory HR decelerations were not different. In addition, although HR decelerations were greater for the 12-second preparatory intervals than for the 4-second intervals in both modes of presentation, the RTs were significantly faster for 12 seconds in the regular mode, and significantly slower in the irregular mode than the RTs for 4 seconds.

To be sure of this independence of deceleration and speed, we assessed the RTs accompanying the largest and smallest HR deceleration in each condition: e.g., 4-second, random, low incentive; 4-second, fixed, low incentive, and so on. In each major group there were, thus, 10 comparisons for each S. Of the 20 dependent t-tests, only two were significant, but these were in opposite directions. It would be difficult to argue from these data that deceleration had much to do with performance.

There are in these data, in short, grounds for skepticism about *any* view of the motivational significance of HR. The data at the phasic level are compatible enough with the cardiac-somatic view. And the

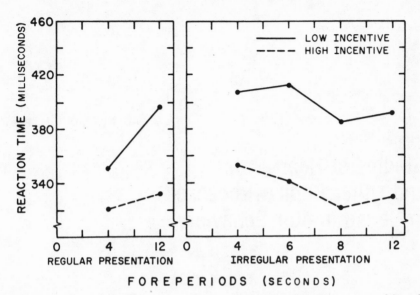

FIGURE 25.8. *Reaction time as a function of mode of presentation and length of foreperiod. The two groups are combined so that N = 48. Incentive level is the parameter.*

difficulties at the tonic level *may* be primarily a problem of restriction of range and error of measurement. That is, the average excursion of HR and movement measures in the phasic intervals was greater than in the tonic intervals, except in the one instance—comparing the ordinary rest periods with the "quiet" condition—in which the tonic measures covaried quite well. And, of course, we cannot say we have sampled somatic activity adequately. But I would feel more content if we had produced large incentive shifts in HR.

In the meantime, and as a conclusion, it may be worth considering that the cardiac-somatic hypothesis, to the degree that it is sound and comprehensive, makes HR changes relatively uninteresting to the psychologist. If HR does, as Obrist et al. (1972a) have suggested "provide in one muscle a picture of the total somatic involvement at any given time," it is a picture too simple for use by most psychologists (although to check whether one's S is resting during rest, or generally involved during tasks, a summary index would be useful). The heart has few direct effects on the environment, and it is not the totality, but the particularity of striate muscle activity that most of us are concerned with most of the time. If HR is not, in short, a good index of classically conditioned effects and motivational-emotional effects, independent of somatic effects, much of our interest in it will diminish. For me, that is all the more reason to test the limits of the cardiac-somatic hypothesis.

26

BEATRICE C. LACEY and JOHN I. LACEY

Studies of Heart Rate
and Other Bodily Processes
in Sensorimotor Behavior

INTRODUCTION

Heart rate and blood pressure may increase or decrease, or, indeed, may exhibit no change in response to stimulation or as concomitants of the performance of various tasks. These changes themselves may be correlated, both positively and negatively, or uncorrelated. Most importantly, the direction of blood pressure and heart rate changes may reveal parasympathetic-like responses while other simultaneously recorded responses reveal sympathetic-like responses, such as digital vasoconstriction, pupillary dilation, and decrease in skin resistance. To this phenomenon, we have applied the term "directional fractionation" (Lacey 1959), to imply that different fractions of the total somatic response pattern may respond in *opposite* directions; opposite, that is, from the point of view of the notion that autonomic "arousal" is characterized by a mélange of positively correlated sympathetic-like changes.

Directional fractionation is only a special form of a more general phenomenon of stereotypy or specificity of autonomic response patterns. Autonomic responses are poorly correlated. The lack of correlation is not due to unreliability of measurement. As a consequence, different tasks and stimuli produce reliably different patterns of response, with large responses in some variables and small responses in others. Different individuals, too, show reliably different patterns of response, over times as long as four years and over such diverse tasks as hyper-

Supported by grants MH000623 and FR00222 from the National Institute of Mental Health and the National Institutes of Health, United States Public Health Service.

ventilation, mental arithmetic, and the cold pressor test (e.g., Lacey, Bateman, and Van Lehn 1953; Lacey and Lacey 1958; Lacey and Lacey 1962; Lacey et al. 1963). In this paper, we will report additional examples of these phenomena.

Our first studies of directional fractionation suggested to us that momentary bradycardia and hypotension occurred when the subject intended to note and detect external events. This we characterized earlier (Lacey et al. 1963) as a first level of inference from the empirical data. It seemed to us (Lacey 1959; Lacey et al. 1963) that, despite a wide variety of specific parameters of stimuli and tasks, attention to external events contributed a deceleratory and hypotensive component to the final resulting cardiovascular response; cognitive work, inferentially involving motivated inattention (the intention by the subject to ignore or reject intrusive and disturbing external events) contributed an acceleratory and hypertensive component. Only heart rate and blood pressure differentiated these two kinds of tasks; respiratory and skin conductance measures did not.

The general formulation has been successful, both in our hands and in the hands of others: Simple attention produces cardiac deceleration; simple cognitive work produces acceleration. Shifting from one to the other produces a shift from deceleration to acceleration. We will see again, in new experiments to be reported in the current paper, the successful operation of this behavioral manipulation of the direction of heart rate change.

This is not to say that the attentional dimension—motivated attention versus motivated inattention—totally accounts for changed directions of cardiovascular response. There has been misunderstanding by some of our position. For one thing, our first tentative attempts to deal with heart rate as a factor in the control and regulation of brain and behavior showed greater relationship of fluctuating heart rate to impulsive *motor* responses than to perceptual discrimination. And, indeed, today we will have occasion to reemphasize the motor end of sensorimotor behavior, because we have found that response-intention also may contribute a deceleratory component to the cardiovascular accompaniment of behavior.

There is a higher level of inference—or, more properly stated, a speculation—underlying our research. This is that many of the phenomena uncovered in the study of the bradycardia of attention and response-intention can be explained as the consequences of the neurophysiological fact that increases of blood pressure and of heart rate determine the frequency of impulses along visceral afferent feedback pathways from the baroreceptors of the carotid sinus, aortic arch, and other structures. This visceral afferent feedback is *negative* and *inhibitory* of motor behavior and of electroencephalographic activity.

Increased input from the baroreceptors has been shown to produce decreased muscle tone, increased slow activity in the electroencephalogram and electrocorticogram, diminutions in the duration of stimulus-produced increases in neural and muscle activities, cessation of drug-induced convulsions, termination of episodes of sham rage, and elevations of the threshold for a monosynaptic reflex. Decreased input would have the opposite effects.

The operation of these pathways, however, is not automatic and invariant. Baroreceptors, like other sensory receptors, respond variably. Their response to stimuli is subject to control from higher levels of the nervous system, particularly limbic lobe structures and the cerebellum, and, since their adequate stimulus is rate of deformation, they will respond differently to different stimulus rise times. The response, furthermore, depends on the variable stiffness of the deformed structure (e.g., the carotid sinus) in which the receptors are embedded, and on a host of other variables. These complications led us to caution that the acute neurophysiological results could not be generalized to the behavior of intact man, nor even to lower animals, without attention to many variables. "Our task," we said, after reviewing most of the then available neurophysiological literature, "is to formulate specific statements, so that under specific circumstances a reliable and specifiable set of consequences will follow" (Lacey 1967, p. 31).

Our experiments constitute a series devoted to this task of specification. Some of the phenomena are totally unexpected, and at least suggest the heuristic value of thinking about the consequences of visceral afferent feedback from the baroreceptors to the higher levels of the nervous system.

THE EFFECTS OF TASK-DIFFICULTY AND OF DIVIDED SET ON HEART RATE AND PLANTAR CONDUCTANCE

Attention to external environmental events, we have said, produces bradycardia, but mental "work" produces tachycardia. But, in our early studies the tasks requiring simple environmental intake, such as looking at a flickering light or listening to a dramatic recitation, might be judged to be less difficult than tasks such as mental arithmetic or reversed spelling, and our results might be attributable to task difficulty rather than to the intended difference in the transaction between the subject and the environment. For this new study, therefore, we chose tasks in which the order of difficulty would be reversed. The Mental Arithmetic task was simplified by eliminating a requirement for multiplication and substituting a requirement for simple successive additions. Starting with a two-digit number, the subject summed the digits, then added the sum to the number. The answer provided the next digits to be summed, and the operation was repeated throughout the 1-minute long stimulus period, at which time the subject announced his last answer.

To represent the intake extreme of our postulated behavioral continuum we chose a more demanding task, one of Tone Detection. Subjects were required to attend carefully to a series of standard tones of 500 Hz. Embedded in this series was a number of "signal tones" of 513 Hz. The subject's task was to try to detect each "signal tone," noting such detections by depressing a telegraph key.

Two other tasks were included in the experiment to study the effect on heart rate response of a divided set, requiring both attention to the external environment and cognitive processing. We included the task Rules of the Game, shown in our earlier study to produce intermediate effects on heart rate. These intermediate results, which we wished to replicate, had been interpreted as the "vectorial" resultant of the opposing demands for attention to the external environment and for mental work. In Rules of the Game, the demands for attention and for cognitive work were integrated. The subject had to be highly attentive to a verbally delivered set of rules for a fictitious card game. Simultaneously, however, he had to store and organize the input for retrieval, because he was to be tested on his knowledge of the rules as soon as they were given to him. We wondered if simultaneous opposing demands in *nonintegrated* tasks would result also in intermediate effects on heart rate. Thus, we added a fourth task in which the subject was required simultaneously to perform the Tone Detection and the Mental Arithmetic tasks.

Each of the four tasks was presented twice in counterbalanced fashion to each subject, and all possible task sequences were represented in the group of 24 subjects.

At the end of the experimental session, subjects were asked to rate the absolute difficulty of the tasks on a five-point scale and also to rank the tasks in order of relative difficulty. The rankings were significantly concordant. Kendall's W was .51, p<.001, for subject agreement on relative difficulty and .48, p<.001, for subject agreement on absolute difficulty. Paired comparisons of individual tasks showed that ratings for Mental Arithmetic were significantly different from those for any other task, Mental Arithmetic being judged easiest of all. Ratings for the combined Mental Arithmetic-Tone Detection task differed significantly from any of the other tasks, being judged the most difficult. Tone Detection and Rules of the Game were judged to be about equal in difficulty and, on the average, were classified as of moderate difficulty.

Figure 26.1 shows that all four tasks resulted in significant, although small, changes from a 1-minute alert to a 1-minute stimulus period.

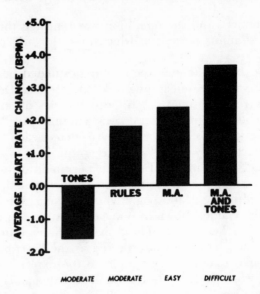

FIGURE 26.1.   *Average heart rate changes from 1 minute of alert to 1-minute periods of task-performance. Rated task difficulty is noted in italics.*

These changes differed significantly among tasks (p<.001) by Friedman's two-way analysis of variance by ranks. As expected, heart rate decreased during Tone Detection and increased during Mental Arithmetic, despite the fact that Tone Detection was significantly the more difficult of the two tasks. The difference in response between these two tasks was significant (p<.01) by Wilcoxon's paired replicates test. The small size of the average cardiac changes is notable. The absence of large average responses may be due to the facts that the cognitive task (Mental Arithmetic) was quite easy, so that heart rate increases were rather small, whereas the Tone Detection task was not purely a measure of attentive behavior, because it involved frequent key presses, a motor activity.

The heart rate response to Rules of the Game, as before, was intermediate between Tone Detection and Mental Arithmetic. It differed significantly from that to Tone Detection but not from that to Mental Arithmetic.

The data from these three tasks replicated and generalized our previous findings, lending further support to the notion that the differential requirements of tasks for attention to external events may be, for appropriately chosen tasks, a more important determinant of heart rate than the comparative difficulty of the tasks.

The divided set task which required that signal detection and mental arithmetic be carried on simultaneously, however, did not produce an intermediate cardiac response. The task resulted in a significant cardiac acceleration. The response was significantly different from that to Tone Detection and to Rules of the Game, but not from that to Mental Arithmetic. It should be noted that the task was accompanied by marked performance decrements from either task performed alone.

The intermediate effects on heart rate, therefore, held only for the divided set condition which itself constituted a unified, integrated task and not for the one in which the demands of the individual components proved distracting and mutually interfering. Apparently we cannot "artificially" combine task demands for attentive observation of external events with those for cognitive elaboration and get a "vectorially" resultant cardiac response. The task itself, like Rules of the Game, must meaningfully integrate and combine the two demands. Failure to do so seems to add an additional variable of distraction or interference.

Skin conductance once again failed to distinguish among tasks. Although each task resulted in a significant increase in conductance, there was no overall significant difference in response among the tasks. Paired comparisons of tasks also showed no significant differences, with the single exception of Mental Arithmetic versus the combined Tone Detection-Mental Arithmetic task for which p = .05.

INDIVIDUAL DIFFERENCES IN DIRECTIONAL FRACTIONATION, AND THE EFFECTS OF TASK DIFFICULTY

The task of tone detection is an example of situational stereotypy, a majority of subjects showing cardiac deceleration while noting and detecting signal tones. The same task was used in this experiment in order to study, among other things, individual differences in the tendency to decelerate. One can frequently find exceptions even to fairly strong group tendencies. In the just-reported study, not all subjects decelerated during tone detection. We had no way of knowing, however, whether this represented random variation from a modal tendency for most people to decelerate under these conditions, most of the time, or whether the exceptions represented reliable idiosyncratic differences in response patterns.

We attempted, at the same time, to study another problem. The first study had shown that cardiac response was related to the set requirements of a task rather than to its difficulty level. We now addressed ourselves to the question of the effect of difficulty level within the context of a single set—in this case, that of noting and detecting environmental events.

In this study, each of 16 subjects participated in four experimental sessions. In each session, four different task difficulties were used and were presented either in ascending or descending order of difficulty.

The orders were counterbalanced over the four daily experimental subsections or sets. Difficulty was varied by changing the difference in frequency between the 500 Hz standard tone and the embedded signal tones. These differences were, in order of difficulty, 16, 8, 4, and 2 Hz. For contrast with cardiac response, measures of finger volume and skin conductance were analyzed as well.

The data again showed a strong group tendency for cardiac deceleration. The overall response of 75% of the subjects (12 of the 16) was deceleratory. For 10 of the 12, the Wilcoxon paired replicates test showed that the deceleration was reliable over time; $p < .01$ for 9 of the 10, $p < .02$ for the remaining case. There were, however, *consistent* exceptions to this tendency. Four subjects accelerated during tone detection, and for 3 of the 4, the acceleration was statistically significant. The experiment thus provides, we believe, a first demonstration of intrastimulus stereotypy with stimuli which characteristically evoke deceleratory responses.

The implications of this atypical acceleratory response under these conditions are as yet unclear. The number of subjects are few, and characteristics which distinguish the two groups are not immediately apparent, with a single exception. Accelerators showed more conductance response and greater digital vasoconstriction than did decelerators. The difference in vasoconstriction between the two groups was significant below the .05 level by Wilcoxon's paired replicates test. It is possible, though purely speculative, that this small subgroup was more "stressed" by some aspect of the situation than were the other subjects. This component may have masked any deceleratory tendency and resulted in greater sympathetic-like responses in all three variables.

The direction of cardiac response, while related to the size of the vasomotor response, was not related to its direction. Fourteen of the 16 subjects showed finger volume constriction. For 10 of the 14, the constriction occurred reliably. Only one subject showed a significant tendency to dilate, but the tendency was not as strong or pervasive as that shown by the constrictors. Conductance response was less systematic, only about half the subjects tending to show increases in conductance.

There was a task-induced decrease in heart rate variability for both accelerators and decelerators alike, 15 of the 16 subjects showing the stabilization, 12 of them reliably. Finger volume variability tended also to decrease systematically during tone detection.

When all subjects were considered as a group, difficulty level and cardiac response did not appear to be related. This proved to be due to an interaction between difficulty level and the type of cardiac response which subjects tended to make during tone detection. Decelerators decelerated more as difficulty increased, $p < .05$, by Friedman's two-way analysis of variance by ranks, and accelerators showed increased acceleration with increasing difficulty, p = .07. In other words the *idiosyncratic response was enhanced by increasing difficulty*. The maximum difference in response to the various difficulty levels was small, although systematic for both groups. On the average it was less than a beat for decelerators and about two beats for accelerators. Peak heart rate response was found with difficulty level 3 rather than 4. Level 4, requiring a discrimination of only 2 Hz, was so very difficult, it is possible that some subjects may have resigned themselves to poor performance in that task and been maximally involved during level 3.

The decrease in heart rate variability, found in both accelerators and decelerators, also became significantly greater as task difficulty increased, p<.05 by Friedman's two-way analysis of variance.

Significant relationships between physiological responses and task difficulty were restricted, however, to the cardiac variables. Neither finger volume nor conductance response bore significant relationships to difficulty level. The nonsignificant trends in both variables were in the direction of increased sympathetic-like activity as difficulty increased.

The fact that there is a small subset of subjects who reliably accelerate during tone detection, the acceleration increasing with increased difficulty level, serves to reemphasize our caution that responses are not invariant. They will be affected by many factors, among them the obvious one that "identical" tasks are not necessarily identically perceived nor identically performed by all subjects.

A STUDY OF THE STIMULUS-DETERMINANTS
OF AND INTERRELATIONSHIPS BETWEEN
PUPILLARY AND HEART RATE RESPONSES

In this experiment we tried to isolate some stimulus characteristics that determine cardiac deceleratory responses, and we compared these responses with simultaneous changes in pupillary diameter. The experiment was conducted in collaboration with Dr. William Libby.

Studies by Hess and Polt, Kahneman and others (Hess and Polt 1960, 1964, 1966; Hess 1965; Kahneman and Beatty 1966; Beatty and Kahneman 1966; Kahneman et al. 1969; Wenger and Videbeck 1969) showed that the pupil dilates both during attentive observation of external stimuli and during problem-solving activities like mental arithmetic. The pupillary response of dilatation, then, does not differentiate attention to external stimuli from mental work. As we have seen, however; heart rate does differentiate these two behaviors. It seemed likely, therefore, that a task demanding attention to external events would produce a simultaneous sympathetic-like response of pupillary dilatation and a parasympathetic-like response of cardiac deceleration. This would be a further example of the phenomenon of directional fractionation and situational stereotypy.

Thirty pictorial slides, rated by a panel of judges using 22 semantic differential scales, were used as stimuli. For each experimental slide there was a control slide containing a dot pattern. Experimental and control slides were matched as closely as possible for luminous flux. These slide-pairs were presented to each of 34 subjects. Each slide was viewed for 15 seconds, with a control slide preceding each experimental slide.

The characteristic response to pictorial stimuli indeed was a sympathetic-like pupillary dilatation and a parasympathetic-like cardiac deceleration, another and a new example of directional fractionation. Twenty-seven of the 34 subjects showed an average deceleration. For 15 subjects p<.05, by Wilcoxon's paired replicates test, including 9 for whom p<.01. No significant differences were found for the 7 subjects who tended to accelerate.

Twenty-five subjects responded with pupillary dilatation (for 13, p<.01 and for an additional 3, p<.05). Seven subjects tended to constrict, 4 of them significantly.

Directional fractionation in response to pictorial stimuli has also been demonstrated by Hare and his colleagues (Hare et al. 1970; Hare et al. 1971) who found cardiac deceleration to coexist with skin conductance increases and vasoconstriction. In our study, pupillary and cardiac responses were not only opposite in direction, they were also quantitatively dissociated, in that the correlation between the two measures was low and variable, *even in direction*. These correlations were computed both within and between subjects and within and between stimuli, and both with and without corrections for unreliability of measurement techniques. They, thus, offer a rather persuasive example of the disagreement afforded by two different physiological indices in estimating the extent of physiological arousal to a given stimulus.

The concept of unidimensionality of physiological responsiveness is further challenged by data from this study which indicated that the pupil and the heart responded differently to different stimulus attributes.

Four factors were identified by a factor analysis of the semantic differential scales: Attention-Interest, Pleasantness-Evaluation, Activity-Potency, and Complexity. Only the first two factors were associated with the autonomic responses.

The linear correlation of pupillary diameter with Attention-Interest was +.43 (p<.05), but with Pleasantness-Evaluation it was only −.10 which was not significant. However, pupillary response was significantly related to Pleasantness-Evaluation in a nonlinear fashion, greater dilatation being evoked by pictures of neutral pleasantness than by pictures of either high or low pleasantness. Only two of the individual scales were significantly correlated with pupillary diameter.

There were many more significant correlations between heart rate responses and stimulus attributes, and there were no nonlinear associations. Heart rate response correlated $-.45$ (p<.05) with Attention-Interest and $+.49$ (p<.01) with Pleasantness-Evaluation. It was also significantly related to 11 individual scales. Greater deceleration was associated with slides that were rated as interesting, attention-getting, unusual, and arousing. This finding has been replicated using entirely different pictures by Collen and Libby (1971) and lends support to our hypothesis concerning the relationship between attention to external events and bradycardia.

The relationship of heart rate response to Pleasantness-Evaluation is one that deserves some extended comment. We previously reviewed reports in the early literature that pleasant stimuli produce deceleration and unpleasant stimuli produce acceleration (Lacey 1967). These reports led us to expect, in our early studies, an intermediate cardiac response when subjects were asked to attend to a loud, markedly unpleasant, fluctuating white noise, or to listen to affectively unpleasant material (Lacey et al. 1963). Instead, these tasks produced highly significant cardiac decelerations—although blood pressure did not decrease—(see Lacey and Lacey 1970). Similar results were found in the current experiment. The more *unpleasant* a picture was rated, the more deceleration it produced. This agrees also with the findings of Hare and his colleagues (Hare et al. 1970, 1971) that cardiac deceleration occurred while viewing gruesome pictures of homicide victims.

These findings are not incompatible, as has been claimed by others, with our hypothesis which expects deceleration to accompany the intention to note and detect external events, and accelerations to accompany motivated inattention to such events. Unpleasantness does not preclude the intention to note and detect. Hare and his colleagues briefly discuss the phenomenon of "morbid fascination," and Hastings and Obrist (1967) have pointed out that attention to unpleasant, aversive, and potentially threatening stimuli may be biologically advantageous. These arguments serve to underline the notion that it is the nature of the total *transaction* of the subject with his environment, rather than isolated stimulus attributes, which will determine physiological responses.

HEART RATE AND ELECTROENCEPHALOGRAPHIC CHANGES IN REACTION TIME AND IN TIMING TASKS

We have, for many years, studied heart rate responses during reaction time experiments, a paradigm which seems particularly appropriate for studies concerned with sensorimotor integration. One might expect, on the basis of some extrapolations from the neurophysiological literature, which we have reviewed elsewhere (Lacey 1967; Lacey and Lacey 1970; Lacey 1972), that the decreases in heart rate seen in states of attention to external events might improve ". . . both the organism's receptivity to afferent stimulation and the organism's readiness to make effective responses to such stimulation" (Lacey 1972, p. 183).

We have reported (Lacey and Lacey 1964, 1966, 1970; Lacey 1972) that sizeable, systematic, beat-by-beat cardiac decelerations occur reliably in most individuals during the preparatory interval of the reaction time experiment, while the subject waits for an imperative stimulus to which he must respond with a rapid motor movement. The nadir of heart rate typically is reached at the time of the imperative stimulus. This implies a temporal targeting by the subject, the target being the anticipated moment of response. This process of temporal targeting was demonstrated ingeniously in a recent experiment by Schwartz and Higgins (1971). However, it cannot totally account for the timing and magnitude of the cardiac deceleration. In "catch" trials in a fixed foreperiod reaction time experiment where the imperative stimulus is omitted, the heart rate continues to decelerate beyond the expected moment of response (Lacey and Lacey 1966, 1970).

The association between cardiac slowing and faster reaction time clearly is not predictable from the notion that increased heart rate is an unequivocal sign of increased behavioral arousal. It is understandable, however, if the concept is correct that decreased visceral afferent feedback from the baroreceptors results in increased receptivity to external stimulation and increased ease of effective motor response, and that heart rate is an effective determinant of this feedback. We hasten to add, as we always do, that proof of the operation of such a mechanism in intact humans still is lacking. As this conference makes clear, our interpretation is controversial. But the explanation that the cardiac slowing is "merely" a consequence of quieting and relaxation leads to an interesting conclusion: that the more relaxed the muscles, the more ready is an organism to make a speedy and effective motor response. This position is contrary to the results of decades of investigation of the relationship between muscle tension and response, particularly with respect to reaction time experiments.

At about the same time we reported the association between cardiac slowing and reaction time, Walter and his colleagues (Walter et al. 1964) reported a slowly increasing vertex negativity, the contingent negative variation (CNV) occurring in the preparatory interval of a reaction time experiment. This newly established, and now well-verified, electroencephalographic phenomenon also was reported to accompany faster reaction time, although the results in the hands of other investigators have been somewhat variable (see Rebert and Tecce, in press, for a review).

The next step seemed obvious. We demonstrated (Lacey and Lacey 1970) a significant relationship ($p<.01$) between cardiac deceleration and the CNV, large decelerations being associated with large CNVs. This has been reported also by Connor and Lang (1969). Our tentative early interpretation of the relationship was that the bradycardia was the now familiar slowing of the heart accompanying attentive behavior. The subject was attending *expectantly* to the external environment. The correlation of heart rate with the CNV was attributable to the common process of *expectant attention*. Indeed, an early synonym for the CNV was the E-wave, "E" standing for "expectancy."

But the reaction time experiment confounds expectant attention to external events with the intention to respond to them, and, even in the first studies of the CNV, the vertex negativity was interpreted also as a sign of *priming of the motor cortex*. Moreover, Low and his collaborators (Low et al. 1966) emphasized that response-intention alone can produce the CNV, and suggested that the "C" stand for "conative" as well as "contingent." Others, too, described a "readiness potential (Bereitschaftspotential) preceding voluntary limb and eye movements (Kornhuber and Deecke 1965; Becker et al. 1972, 1968; Becker et al., in press). This "readiness potential" was seen maximally in the vertex but also elsewhere, particularly in precentral and parietal regions. It is clear that the increased cortical negativity is associated with response-intention. Was this also true for heart rate deceleration? Could we distinguish a bradycardia of attention from a bradycardia of response-intention? We did so in the second of two experiments using so-called drl schedules (differential reinforcement of low rates of responding).

The first experiment was designed only to determine whether cardiac deceleration and the CNV would appear concomitantly in an experiment in which the time of emission of a motor response was determined, not by experimenter-imposed stimuli, but by the subject's volition. The subjects worked on a drl 15″ lh 4″ schedule. This schedule required that a response be made not earlier than 15 seconds nor later than 19 seconds from the last key-press response. Typically, subjects were not efficient at the task and most had little idea that they were to respond within the particular time period. We found that prior to the subject-initiated press there was a gradual increase in cortical negativity and a marked beat-by-beat cardiac deceleration which increased exponentially to the press (Lacey and Lacey 1970). The lowest heart rate was found for the cardiac cycle in which the subject pressed the key!

This experiment, however, only established a concomitance between bradycardia and the CNV in a situation radically different from the reaction time situation. It seemed to emphasize the role of response-intention, but, on second thought, it was clear that this experiment too confused attention and response-intention, because the subject was informed of the correctness of his response, via a visual display, each time he pressed the telegraph key.

In a second experiment (Lacey and Lacey 1970, and in press), therefore, we set out to disentangle the effects of attention and response-intention. Forty-eight subjects were maintained on a drl 30″ schedule, i.e., a successful press was one made no sooner than 30 seconds after the last press. Subjects were informed of the correctness of their response by means of a visual display of "+" (for correct) or "−" (for incorrect). On half the trials the visual reinforcement (signalling 2 cents gained or lost) was delivered immediately upon the subject's key-press. In the other half of the trials the reinforcement was delayed for 4½ seconds. Half of the subjects worked on a block program, half of the blocks with immediate reinforcement. On the other half of the blocks, the reinforcement was delayed. The other group of subjects worked under prearranged haphazard schedules, with immediate and delayed reinforcements mixed in a haphazard sequence.

Both vertex negativity and frontal negativity were seen to develop regularly in advance of the key-press, and a beat-by-beat cardiac deceleration accompanied this negativity. Again, the lowest heart rate was found to occur as the subject emitted his voluntary motor response. For each measure, $p<.01$ in all four experimental groups. On trials with delayed reinforcement, the heart either showed a second highly significant deceleration, or sustained its low rate, while the subject waited for the display which informed him of the correctness of his response. This is the purest example of a simple attentive episode we have been able to devise. No response or decision is required: The response has already been made. The subject is merely expectantly attending to the environment, to receive a signal informing him whether he has won or lost 2 cents. A second wave of negativity did not develop during this purely attentive period, however; nor was the previous one sustained. The heart, then, decelerated as a correlate of both attention and response-intention. The CNV response, under the conditions of this experiment, indexed only response-intention, and, thus, the CNV and cardiac response were dissociable.

Indeed, they were doubly dissociable. The CNV responded to the expected immediacy of reinforcement, because it was significantly greater ($p<.01$) on block administration of trials with immediate reinforcement than on block trials with delayed reinforcement. The heart rate did not show this effect. Perhaps we have discovered something about the physiology of delayed gratification! And, in the process, a new dissociation has been demonstrated between two physiological measures that otherwise seem to covary.

THE PRINCIPLE OF TEMPORAL PROXIMITY: THE RELATIONSHIP
BETWEEN MOMENTARY HEART RATE LEVELS AND BEHAVIOR

Within subject relationships between *momentary* heart rate levels and reaction time are of considerable significance for they show that averaging several heart rates, even over brief periods of time, may conceal important phasic phenomena.

We found, in one of our early reaction time experiments (Lacey and Lacey 1964), that when the single heart period at stimulus was correlated with reaction time, the distribution of obtained rhos was nonnormal and nonsymmetrical. Of the 62 rhos computed (for subjects showing no significant time trends only), 51 were positive (slow heart rate associated with fast reaction time) and 11 negative. Thirteen of the positive rhos were significant (for three, p<.05; for 5, p<.02; for three, p<.01; and for two, p<.001). Two of the negative rhos were significant (for one, p<.05, for the other p<.01). The probability of obtaining 13 positive rhos with p<.05 in an N of 62 is <.001 (Sakoda, Cohen, and Beall 1954).

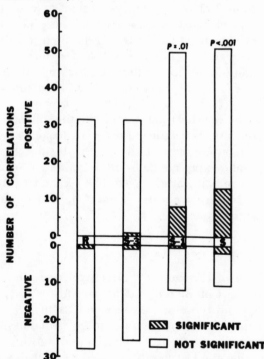

FIGURE 26.2. *Number of subjects showing positive and number showing negative rank order correlations between reaction time and heart rate at four different points in time.*

It is slow heart rate *at the time of the event*, however, which is best associated with fast reaction time; temporally more remote heart rates are not.

Figure 26.2 shows the distribution of *rhos* obtained between reaction time and each of four different heart rates. "S" indicates correlations between reaction time and heart rate at stimulation. These are the correlations which were described above. "S-1" signifies the heart beat just prior to the beat at stimulation. We found a nonsymmetrical distribution of rhos, and a greater-than-chance number of individually significant positive correlations with reaction time, for this proximate heart beat as well. For "S-3," three beats prior to stimulation, and for "R," the heart beat at the time of the ready signal a mere 4 seconds before the imperative stimulus, *there was no systematic relationship to reaction time*. In both distributions, there were approximately as many negative correlations as positive ones. It is, thus, only the low heart rate at, or immediately prior to, stimulation which tends to be associated with faster reaction time.

These data have led us to a formulation which we call "the principle of temporal proximity": The momentary heart rate level is a determinant of the relation of heart rate to reaction time. This principle of temporal proximity has been successfully replicated in our laboratory recently and is currently being studied under markedly different experimental conditions. Among other things, no formal foreperiod was used, so that we had a wider distribution of momentary heart rate levels.

The new results overwhelmingly confirm the phenomenon. The average correlation with the predicted criterion sequence of monotonically increasing magnitude of relationship for 40 subjects was .69 and .74, in two separate experimental determinations. Normal deviate values exceeded six in both cases! As we shall see shortly, this principle assumes additional importance with respect to the distribution of events within a single cardiac cycle.

THREE NEW CARDIAC CYCLE EFFECTS

The main question of cardiac cycle effects on reaction time remains at issue. The findings of Birren and his colleagues (Birren, Cardon, and Phillips 1963) and those of Callaway and Layne (1964), that reaction time varies as a function of cycle time of stimulus presentation, have been challenged recently by Thompson and Botwinick (1970). We doubt, however, that the last word has been said on this subject, and we have a new and thoroughly replicated cycle effect on reaction time to report—one, however, more complex than the Birren-Callaway phenomenon.

In three simple auditory reaction time experiments, without foreperiods, we have found that the relationship between momentary heart rate level and reaction time differs for stimuli presented at different points within the cardiac cycle. We found again that slow heart rates at the time of response were significantly, but modestly, associated with fast reaction time (within subject correlations). But the relationship was *significantly greater* when the stimuli were presented later in the cardiac cycle, during electrical diastole, than when the sensorimotor sequence was elicited early in the cycle. In two of the experiments we presented the stimuli either at the R-wave, so that the response would be made during the period of time when the presumably inhibitory visceral afferent feedback would be occurring, or at 350 msec after the R-wave, a point approximately at the time of ventricular repolarization and the onset of diastole. The association between slow momentary heart rate and fast reaction time was significantly greater when the stimuli were presented at 350 msec after the R-wave than when they were presented at the R-wave. The correlations were observed to increase by as much as .3! For one experiment, with 40 subjects, p was less than 10^{-4}. For two other experiments, with 16 subjects each, p was $<.02$ and $<.01$.

In a fourth experiment, with 16 subjects, stimuli were presented either at the R-wave or 400 msec after the R-wave, a point of time clearly during diastole. *Every one* of the 16 subjects showed an increased correlation of heart rate with reaction time at 400 msec. The increases ranged from .02 to .29, with an average of .14. Any statistical test that can be applied yields extraordinarily high confidence levels. Moreover, for trials at R-wave, only 2 of 16 within subject correlations were significant, whereas for trials 400 msec after the R-wave, 7 were individually significant, a proportion which is of itself significant below the .001 level. The same effects were found in the other experiments.

Our theory, if it can be called that, is evolving slowly and rather painfully, and we have difficulty in conceptualizing this result. The Birren-Callaway effect, if true, could be viewed as support for the visceral afferent feedback hypothesis, but our theory deals with heart *rate*. Our first intuitive attempt at incorporating the alleged cycle effect on reaction time was to refer, vaguely and privately, to some process of temporal summation: Slow heart rates would mean fewer episodes of inhibitory feedback over a period of several (or many) cardiac cycles. But these results, and our results concerning temporal proximity, emphasize heavily the period of a single cardiac cycle. The current effect suggests to us that the events and effects associated with systole *perturb* and *diminish* the events and effects associated with *heart rate*; and, that, in still unperceived ways, heart rate effects and cardiac cycle effects may be separable but interacting. The next experiment to be described, provides another example of this interaction, for in it we found a cycle effect that depends on heart rate.

Callaway and his colleagues, in preliminary communications, reported some pilot work concerning nonrandom distributions within the cardiac cycle of key presses and releases in a time-estimation study. While we looked, from time to time, for such effects we found no evidence for nonrandomness until recently. At this time it occurred to us that cycle effects might interact with the level of heart rate itself, and that the nature of the interaction was predictable, although not rigorously as yet, from studies of input-output relationships in baroreceptor mechanisms.

In a drl experiment, each of 52 subjects worked on a drl 15″ lh 4″ schedule until he had made 60 successful presses within the appropriate time slot. For each of the 60 trials we determined the heart rate of the cardiac cycle which preceded the one in which the press was executed. This gave us a measure of momentary heart rate level uncontaminated by the actual execution of the motor act. The trials were then divided into quintiles of pre-press heart rate level, and the median value of relative time-of-press was determined for each quintile.

Figure 26.3 is an average curve for all subjects. It shows that as heart rate level increases, the subject tends to press later and later in the cycle! The monotonic trend is significant below the 10^{-4} level by Ferguson's nonparametric test (Ferguson 1965), most subjects showing the effect, although not with the smoothness seen in the average curve. We have not yet had the opportunity to generalize and replicate this extraordinary phenomenon. Previous demonstrations of cardiac cycle effects have not been replicable easily, so a degree of caution is in order before accepting and interpreting these data. But some interpretation is desirable, if only for its heuristic value.

Why should it be that as heart rate increases, the time of emission of a voluntary response is delayed until later and later in the cardiac cycle? Such an effect is not explainable by traditional theories. We have a testable working hypothesis, however, which is congruent with the facts of visceral afferent feedback.

Our speculations are based on the verified fact that both the "gain" and the "phase shift" of the carotid sinus feedback loop are *frequency dependent* (Gero and Gerová 1967; Spickler and Kezdi 1967). As the frequency of input to the baroreceptors increases, other variables, such as pulse pressure and pressure levels, hold constant and the number of impulses along the feedback-nerves increases, as does the number of discharging neural fibers. Moreover, the point of maximum increase in whole-nerve impulse frequency and amplitude is *displaced forward in time*. This is the phase shift. As frequency decreases, the baroreceptor reflexes become less vigorous and responsive, and the envelope of impulse discharge becomes more synchronous with the input, and smaller in amplitude.

Our working hypothesis is that, because of this demonstrated frequency-dependency, as heart rate (frequency) increases, stronger

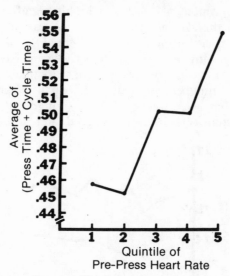

FIGURE 26.3.   *The relationship of heart rate to the relative time within the cardiac cycle at execution of a simple motor response under a drl 15" lh 4" schedule.*

baroreceptor reflexes are initiated and the maximum inhibitory baroreceptor output is displaced forward in time; at any constant point of time, the baroreceptor output is a source of an increasingly effective inhibitory stimulus as heart rate increases. Thus, the inhibitory phase of the early part of the cardiac cycle, is prolonged and stronger. It would then follow that as heart rate increases we might expect that the favored time for emission of response will be displaced to later and later portions of the cardiac cycle. We shall see! The argument is not rigorous as yet, because previous investigations have favored the use of sinusoidal input to the baroreceptors, thus confounding frequency with rate of rise. The latter is known to be a most effective stimulus parameter. We are trying now to disentangle these effects. In the meantime, the results present a challenge to the interpretive and predictive capabilities of any of the current theories—including our own.

In the course of our investigations we have identified still another cycle effect which is perhaps even more difficult to interpret. Studies of cycle effects are usually concerned with the dependence of responses on momentary physiological state. This new effect, however, can best be characterized as a dependence of momentary physiological state on sensorimotor events: A temporal variation has been found in the effect a brief sensorimotor event has on the period of the concurrent cardiac cycle.

In a group of 66 subjects engaged in a fixed foreperiod (4 seconds) reaction time experiment, we found a highly significant relationship between where in the cardiac cycle a stimulus was presented and the duration of *that* cycle. Stimuli were presented according to a pre-arranged schedule with intertrial intervals varying from 6 to 11 seconds. They were not triggered with respect to phase of the cardiac cycle. When such stimuli happened to fall early in the cardiac cycle, the duration of that cycle was significantly longer—that is the heart rate was slower—than when stimuli occurred later in the cycle.

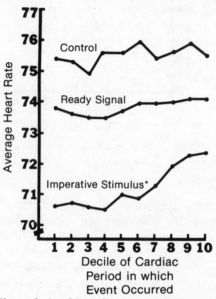

FIGURE 26.4. *The relationship of momentary heart rate level to cardiac cycle time of event occurrence. The asterisk indicates that significance was obtained for imperative stimuli only.*

In Figure 26.4, the abscissa indicates the decile of the cardiac cycle in which an event occurred; the ordinate indicates average heart rate for that cycle, over all subjects. The bottom curve shows a strong tendency for heart rates to increase as the imperative stimulus is presented later and later in the cardiac cycle. The monotonic trend is highly significant, $p < 10^{-8}$ by Ferguson's nonparametric test (Ferguson 1965). The bitonic trend is also significant, $p < .01$. This relationship holds only for the imperative stimulus, to which the subject was to execute a rapid motor response. Identical analyses, one based on time of presentation of the ready signal, one on a control point 4 seconds prior to the ready signal, yielded no significant trends. Real time analyses confirmed these based on relative cycle time.

We have no easy explanation for this nor are we, in fact, sure of precisely what is happening. At first glance it appears that cycle duration is modified by the stimulus (and/or the attendant motor response), with the degree and perhaps the direction of modification dependent on elapsed time from previous systole. For example, early stimuli might lengthen the cycle more than later stimuli or, alternately, shorten it less. Or early stimuli might lengthen and late stimuli abruptly terminate a cycle. The occurrence of preparatory decelerations in the foreperiod, however, and the underlying concept of inhibitory visceral afferent feedback, leads us to suspect that the cycle is *lengthened* by the occurrence of certain sensorimotor events, more so by events which occur early than those which occur late in the cardiac cycle. This would be congruent with recent work by Levy and his collaborators and by Reid which shows temporal variations in the susceptibility of the cardiac pacemaker to vagal stimuli. Stimuli placed early in the cardiac cycle slow that cardiac cycle; stimuli late in the cycle have no effect on that cycle, but may slow the subsequent cycle (Levy et al. 1969, 1970; Levy, Iano, and Zieske 1972; Reid 1969).

Our results can be interpreted as a direct extension (to another species and involving a higher level of the nervous system) of these acute physiological studies. We are currently engaged in studies which, hopefully, will contribute to our understanding of these processes. In the meantime, we must conclude that caution is indicated in experiments predicated on the notion that stimuli, randomly presented, will, in fact, be randomly distributed throughout the cardiac cycle. The evidence points to the fact that they will not, thus adding still another complexity to the many inherent in the studies of cardiac cycle effects.

REACTION TIME STUDIES IN CAT

The experiments discussed so far have all employed human subjects. While the data are congruent with our theorizing, we must look to experiments with animals for eventual proof of the validity of our speculations. We have been concerned, first of all, with trying to demonstrate some of the same sorts of relationships in cats that we have found in our human subjects. If cats were to exhibit the same phenomena in reaction time experiments as do humans, we would then be in a position to attempt modification of these relationships by techniques not possible with human subjects.

We have chosen to work first with an animal analog of the human reaction time experiment. The results of one such study, a collaborative effort with Dr. David Galin, have recently been reported elsewhere (Galin and Lacey 1972). Five cats were implanted with electrodes for recording heart rate, respiration, and the electroencephalogram (EEG), and for stimulating the mesencephalic reticular formation. The animals were trained to work for their entire daily ration of food and water in the reaction time situation. Two of the animals were veterans of many reaction time sessions; three were newly trained.

The animals were trained to press a lever, which was introduced into the experimental box at the onset of the ready signal (a continuing auditory click) and to hold the lever down for the duration of the foreperiod. Foreperiod timing began when the animal pressed the lever. The foreperiod was ended by presentation of the imperative stimulus, a 1 kHz tone, with simultaneous termination of the ready signal. A liquid reinforcement was automatically dispensed as soon as the cat released the lever. Cats learn to work well under these conditions. They have reaction times which approximate those of human subjects, and they show both current and preceding foreperiod effects.

Two of the cats showed a heart rate pattern, during the foreperiod, which is typical of human subjects. There was a slight acceleration followed by a large beat-by-beat deceleration which ended at or close to the time of the imperative stimulus. This pattern persisted in session-after-session, day-after-day. Both of these cats had been newly trained for this experiment. Two other animals, however, one newly trained and one with long experience, showed consistent acceleration. The fifth and most experienced animal showed a variable pattern.

The consistent acceleration in two of the animals suggested the possibility that they were *not* expectantly waiting for the imperative stimulus as we had assumed. This led to a further series of sessions in which it became apparent that the animals were timing the foreperiod, rather than attending to the imperative stimulus. They responded with lever release at the appropriate time *even when the imperative stimulus was eliminated*. A variable foreperiod design was then tried in an attempt to circumvent this behavior. The less experienced cat immediately converted to a deceleratory pattern! The experienced animal, however, one with more than 1,000 sessions over several years time, continued to accelerate during the foreperiod.

We obviously have a way to go in designing a situation in which most cats will consistently decelerate during the foreperiod of a reaction time experiment. The data so far demonstrate clearly, however, that consistent deceleration can and does occur in a situation which must be considered arousing. Further, the demonstration comes from animals that, unlike human subjects, are standing up and making postural adjustments, and are frequently weaving and bobbing about throughout the foreperiod.

In this study we found no clear relationship of cardiac deceleration to reaction time. Cyclic temporal trends and lack of normality in both variables made evaluation of this relationship very complex.

The data concerning reticular stimulation was of considerable interest and should be mentioned here. To avoid cuing the subject, stimulation was not linked to trial presentation, but rather was on and off alternately for 5-minute intervals. The effects of stimulation varied with electrode site and with current level. Of those electrodes for which stimulation was associated both with improved reaction time and with a shift in EEG pattern from high voltage slow to low voltage fast activity, some produced increases, some decreases, and some no effect on phasic heart rate response. Different electrodes also had different effects on tonic heart rate level during the intertrial interval, although the effects tended to be smaller and less consistent than those on phasic response. The effects of reticular stimulation on phasic changes and tonic levels could be dissociated!

The important point, for those interested in the arousing properties of reticular stimulation, is that stimulation associated with increased "behavioral arousal" and with "electroencephalographic arousal," may either have no effect on heart rate or may, indeed, be associated with decreases in heart rate.

SUMMARY

The experiments discussed in this chapter have a communality of purpose and outcome despite the diversity of design and emphasis. Their underlying theme concerns the role of the cardiovascular system in the modification of brain function and behavior. The results are compatible with the neurophysiology of visceral afferent feedback loops and often incompatible with more traditional theories.

Those experiments which had in common a major requirement for sustained attention to external stimuli provide evidence that a majority of individuals show cardiac deceleration while performing such tasks. The experiment on Tone Detection, provided evidence that the response is an individually reliable one, over four separate sessions. This same experiment also demonstrated intrastimulus stereotypy, since reliable cardiac acceleration was found in a small subset of subjects. Further experimentation will be necessary to better understand these atypical responses. It is possible that undefined responses to undefined parameters of the particular situation overwhelmed and masked a usual tendency to decelerate while noting and detecting environmental events. One must inquire, however, whether such individuals characteristically fail to show a decelerative response under more benign conditions requiring environmental intake.

Within the context of a single set, requiring attention to external stimuli, idiosyncratic cardiac response was enhanced as a function of increased task difficulty. In an experiment where set requirements differed from task to task, however, heart rate reflected task set requirements rather than task difficulty.

Directional fractionation was demonstrated in several experiments in that cardiac deceleration was accompanied by simultaneous sympathetic-like responses in finger volume, skin conductance, or pupillary diameter. Furthermore, heart rate and pupillary responses to pictorial stimuli were found to be quantitatively dissociated as well, and the two variables responded differently to different stimulus attributes.

Dissociation between heart rate and the CNV was found in still another study. Heart rate reflected both attention to external events and intention to respond. The CNV reflected only response intention, under the conditions of the experiment. This experiment served to highlight the relevance of cardiovascular activity to both sensory input and motor response, a return to a point we had emphasized in our earliest theoretical formulations (Lacey and Lacey 1958).

The principle of temporal proximity, concerned with the improvement in the ability of single heart beats to predict reaction time as the beats become more proximate to the response-eliciting sensory input, emphasizes the importance of the single cardiac cycle in sensorimotor integration. The importance of phasic events within a given cycle has also been demonstrated in recent experiments. We have found a new cardiac cycle effect which is more complex, but seemingly much more reliable, than the controversial dependency of reaction time on cycle time of stimulation. In three different experiments we have found that when stimuli are presented during electrical diastole, the relationship between reaction time and momentary heart rate level is significantly greater than when stimuli are presented during electrical systole. We have suggested that the events attendant upon systole may perturb the relationship between speed of motor response and heart rate level.

There is still another cycle effect: The point of time in the cardiac cycle at which a subject executes a semi-volitional key-press is related to the existing momentary heart rate level. The link to visceral afferent feedback theory of such a relationship may lie in the demonstrated frequency dependency of the gain and phase shift of baroreceptor output.

Results which indicate that the total duration of the cardiac cycle is related to cycle time of stimulus presentation pose an additional problem for studies in this area. While the phenomenon is not easily explainable, it seems to indicate complex modifying effects of stimulus, response, or both on the cycles in which they occur.

Finally, results from reaction time experiments in cats have provided evidence that heart rate deceleration occurs in these animals in an "arousing" situation, despite postural readjustment and movement. It can also be seen as an accompaniment of behaviorally and electroencephalographically "arousing" reticular stimulation.

The evidence, to date, although rewarding and suggestive, provides no proof of our speculations. We hope to find such proof eventually in critical demonstrations with both chronic and acute animal preparations.

Obrist and his colleagues, in the paper included in this volume and elsewhere, have been critical of our hypothesis that cardiac deceleration may play a role in modifying brain function and, hence, behavior, although they seem to accept our proposition that there is a link between attentive behavior and cardiac deceleration. At the least, they and others have verified our findings that there is an anticipatory cardiac deceleration during the foreperiod of a reaction-time experiment, and that responses are faster, the greater the cardiac deceleration. Elliott also has been very critical of our position, both in this volume and in a recent review (Elliott 1972). His review presents the same arguments he has included in this volume, and some of it rests heavily on the arguments by Obrist and his colleagues. Elliott's position was not debated in the final discussion period of the conference, and the interested reader may wish to refer to our answer in that journal (Lacey and Lacey, in press).

In discussions with Obrist and Howard, we advanced several observations and arguments that seem worthy of brief summary.

We have no quarrel with the notion that at least some task-irrelevant motor activity may be inhibited in preparation for the execution of a reaction-time trial, as part of an attentional episode. Nor do we deny the obvious fact that there is an association between motor activity and heart rate, particularly when truly gross and vigorous motor activity is involved. We do not think, however, that the metabolically relevant association between somatic activity and heart rate provides an explanation for the decreased heart rate during the preparatory interval of a reaction-time trial. The evidence seems clear that the somatic changes reported by Obrist and his colleagues in the reaction-time experiment are small and metabolically trivial—chin electromyogram (EMG), cessation of eyeblinks, and even decreases in "general activity." The latter are measured by an extraordinarily sensitive strain-gauge system, and respond to such things as cessation of occasional foot movements or slight postural changes as the subject is alerted by a ready signal that a stimulus-to-respond is forthcoming. Indeed, the system can even record a ballistocardiographic signal. Many of these changes are conspicuous by their absence, as Obrist et al. specifically state in their discussion in this volume of instances of independence between heart rate and somatic effects under conditions of low "stress." The heart, however, may be observed to slow even in the absence of these bits of "somatic inhibition." Moreover, the somatic sampling employed seems to us severely restricted, considering the large numbers of muscles that would need to be sampled to justify the suggestion (see Chapter 8) that " . . . the cardiovascular system and somatic musculature can be so finely tuned or coupled that the least alteration in somatic activity will be accompanied by an equally discrete alteration of heart rate." Other muscles than the few sampled by Obrist et al. most probably (see below) are increasing in tension.

Obrist et al. ignore one of their own findings (Obrist, Webb, and Sutterer 1969). Subjects were required to tap continually with one finger while they were being conditioned to an aversive stimulus. They recorded EMGs from the muscles involved in the tapping and found that there was an *increase* in muscle activity at the same time that the heart was showing an anticipatory deceleration just before the aversive unconditioned stimulus. It is difficult to fit these results into that version of the Obrist hypothesis that heart rate is completely commensurate with the metabolic demands of the active musculature.

Other evidence indicates clearly that somatic activity and cardiac activity can be dissociated even when more vigorous activity is required than in the usual reaction-time experiment, or greater "stress" is involved. Chase, Graham and Graham (1968) report, for example, on heart rate changes in a reaction-time task when the required response was a vigorous and energetic one—repeated leg lifts. Commensurate with the increased metabolic demands, the major anticipatory response was a cardiac acceleration. But, superimposed on this response was a statistically significant cardiac deceleration of the same timing and magnitude as that observed when the required response was the usual simple key-press. Of similar import are the recent findings by Eason and Dudley (1970). They studied a variety of physiological responses in a reaction-time experiment in which "activation level" was manipulated by having subjects perform both with and without the threat of shock for long reaction times. The overall levels of heart rate were higher under threat of shock ("high activation"). Nevertheless, the anticipatory cardiac deceleration was found in advance of the stimulus-to-respond. Moreover, muscle action potentials from the task-irrelevant left forearm flexor muscles increased significantly in successive 30-second intervals, but heart rate decreased significantly, particularly under conditions of "high activation." Costello, Brown, and Low (1969) report EMG changes in the participating and nonparticipating arm in a pursuit rotor task that were not paralleled by heart rate changes. Hahn, Stern, and Fehr (1964) report no change in heart rate in rats as a function of a marked increase in the force that was required to press a bar.

We also do not understand how the alleged association between somatic inhibition and cardiac slowing explains the association, repeatedly verified, between fast reaction time and slow heart rate. Intuitively, one can appreciate that diminished task-irrelevant somatic activity betrays expectant attention and preparation for a specific task-relevant somatic activity. But, following what may be termed the periphalist Obrist position, do they then claim that the more relaxed and quiescent the organism (and hence the lower the heart rate), the more prompt the resultant motor response? If so, how do we explain the thoroughly documented fact that increased muscle tension results in faster reactions, whether the muscles are task-relevant or task-irrelevant (see reviews by Duffy 1962; Woodworth 1938; Woodworth and Schlosberg 1954)?

The literature shows clearly, in particular, that muscle tension in the responding muscle and in the contralateral muscle increases during the foreperiod of a reaction-time trial. A similar effect has been reported recently by Jennings and his colleagues (Jennings et al. 1971). Reactions were faster when the reaction was preceded by a burst of EMG activity within 5 seconds of the respond signal. There was a concomitant deceleration, smaller, however, than that observed in the absence of EMG activity. (This suggests to us what should be obvious: that somatic activity can be viewed as *one* factor contributing to the resultant cardiac response.)

The failure by Obrist and his colleagues to detect such anticipatory changes in the relevant extensor muscles probably is attributable to a methodological problem. In their experiments, the subject held a tele-graph key closed throughout the experiment, and responded to the reaction signal by a momentary release in pressure. Hence, the flexor muscles were in almost constant tension, antagonizing the extensor muscles. The task they used *required relaxation* of the relevant extensor muscles.

It seems highly probable that different tasks produce different patterns of spatially and temporally varying muscular activity. Some muscles show increases in activity; other muscles, decreases. It may be that the heart rate reflects only the resultant metabolic demand represented by all these changes, but, as yet, there is no evidence for so extreme a position with respect to the reaction-time experiment.

The appeal to such metabolic considerations, moreover, is not totally convincing—at least to us. The metabolically relevant variable is cardiac output, not heart rate. Heart rate is only one factor in the determination of cardiac output, and the two are imperfectly correlated. To quote from Guyton, an eminent cardiovascular authority:

> . . . the decreased cardiac output is not proportional to the decrease in heart rate because the degree of filling of the ventricles becomes enhanced during the prolonged diastolic filling periods, which increases the stroke volume,

and in this way offsets to a great extent the decrease in output that one might predict. (Guyton 1963, pp. 288-289)

The central version of Obrist's position equally gives us trouble. It is quite clear that somatic changes and cardiovascular changes can occur in response to central nervous system (CNS) processes, and that stimulation of one and the same neural locus can produce coordinated somatic and cardiac changes. But the CNS mechanism has to be highly differentiated to cause, for example a cessation of eyeblinks and a preparatory increase in muscle tension in the task-relevant musculature. If the somatic changes and the cardiac changes are caused by an unspecified common central mechanism, reflecting precisely anticipated metabolic needs, how does the CNS compute the net effect and cause a precise correlation between the two changes? What are the determining factors? We think that a more realistic position is that heart rate, indeed, may reflect the actual or anticipated energy requirements, but that other influences are brought to bear on heart rate that can add an acceleratory or deceleratory component to the resultant.

Obrist and his colleagues contend that our position is incomplete because we do not attempt "to explain how heart rate changes come about in the first place." We maintain that their position is incomplete because they do not deal with the possibility that the heart rate changes, even if brought about in the manner they suggest, do not represent the end of the process; there is a distinct possibility that these heart rate changes have secondary effects on brain and behavior via visceral afferent feedback pathways.

Finally, neither their position nor ours accounts for some of the relationships between heart rate and behavior, such as we have described in our paper in this volume. In our view, however, the facts of visceral afferent feedback provide a better preliminary understanding. In a word, even a complete and perfect parallelism between somatic activity and heart rate does not preclude the likelihood of subsequent effects of the heart rate change.

Summary

As is true of most conferences, the papers and discussions at this one dealt with relatively specific issues. More general questions about the proper goals and strategies for research on the psychophysiology of the cardiovascular system were, on the whole, not considered, probably because we had to deal with a large amount of information in a brief period of time. We have, therefore, taken the opportunity to discuss (or perhaps it can be described more accurately as "the opportunity to express our prejudices about") these more general issues in this concluding chapter. In addition, we have attempted to provide statements about some of the more specific issues that the participants considered to be important.

We have not attempted to write one unified concluding chapter. Rather, three of the editors (P. Obrist, A. H. Black, J. Brener) have commented separately on the issues about which they felt moved to comment. The author of each section is identified.

GENERAL ISSUES

The most obvious general issues concern the goals of research on the psychophysiology of the cardiovascular system, and the appropriate strategies for achieving these goals.

Goals (A. H. Black)

By definition, the purpose of research on the psychophysiology of the cardiovascular system is to analyze the relationship between psychological or behavioral processes and the functioning of the cardiovascular system. This more general goal subsumes several closely related but different goals which were discussed by the participants of the conference.

The most obvious and, perhaps, the most popular of these goals is the attempt to understand how the manipulation of psychological or behavioral variables influences the functioning of the cardiovascular system. Much of the research that is directed to this goal concerns the

565

effects of various stimuli—for example, psychologically stressful stimuli—on cardiovascular responding. Even more popular has been an interest in the plasticity of cardiovascular function. What types of changes in cardiovascular functioning are produced by the operant conditioning of cardiovascular and other responses? What changes are produced by classical conditioning? Can these conditioning procedures change the relationship between cardiovascular and other responses? Can they be employed to reduce cardiovascular malfunctioning? If the contributions to this volume are any indication, the analysis of plasticity is one of the major focuses of current research on the psychophysiology of the cardiovascular system.

One especially heartening development is the growing concern with mechanism. Instead of being satisfied with an analysis of the effects of some psychological manipulation on cardiovascular responding, more and more attempts are being made to describe the sequence of physiological events that underlie particular cardiovascular changes. The importance of this development is made clear by Obrist in the next section.

A second goal of research on psychophysiology of the cardiovascular system concerns the inverse problem. The first goal was to determine how the manipulation of psychological and behavioral variables affects cardiovascular functioning. The second goal is to determine how changes in cardiovascular functioning affect psychological or behavioral functioning. Does it make a difference in our ability to process information if heart rates are high or low? Does it make a difference to our psychological functioning if our blood pressure is continually high?

Research that has been designed to attain these two goals will, I think, provide useful information. I do have a question, however, about a third goal of research on the cardiovascular system. This is the attempt to find measures of cardiovascular function which will provide us with an index of some internal psychological state. Consider for example that old chestnut—the attempt to employ heart rate as an index of conditioned fear. The evidence that has accumulated against this simplistic notion is now so overwhelming that to list it would simply take too much time and space. The linkage between change in the cardiovascular system and changes in internal psychological states and in behavior is subtle and complex, as the papers in this book make clear. We are long past the point at which we can assume a one-to-one relationship between a cardiovascular change and a psychological change. I would, therefore, suggest that the attempt to find measures of cardiovascular functioning which can act as indices of internal psychological states is probably the one goal that is most difficult to justify at present.

Research Strategies (P. Obrist)

One of the characteristics of the contributions in this book is the emphasis on a biological strategy. In part this might reflect the selection of contributors. However, in part, I believe this reflects a contemporary trend. Thus, I would like to discuss the justification of such a strategy in psychophysiological research. The major point I wish to make is that a biological strategy is a necessity if we wish to make further progress in studying the interrelationship between behavioral and cardiovascular events. There is a need to discuss such a strategy explicitly since I feel that the justification of the strategy still eludes many investigators.

By a biological strategy, I mean any effort which attempts to depict within a behavioral paradigm any one or more of the following: (1) hemodynamic processes or the relationship among two or more parameters of cardiovascular function; (2) the relationship between hemodynamic processes and other peripheral events, such as somatic activity; and (3) the extent and process by which neural-humoral factors are involved in the control of cardiovascular and other peripheral events. A biological strategy goes beyond establishing a concomitance between stimulus events and some parameter of cardiovascular activity, in that it attempts to depict more completely what else occurs biologically. Until recently, psychophysiological work has not been particularly concerned with the relationship among biological events. Rather attention has been focused on the effects of our experimental manipulations on some one parameter of cardiovascular function. It seemed sufficient that if the experimental manipulation worked in some consistent manner, e.g., modified heart rate (HR), then the investigator was satisfied that something biologically substantial and relevant to behavior had been demonstrated. However, there is a danger in this strategy, particularly if one views it from a biological perspective. This is that between a given stimulus event and a manifestation of some change in cardiovascular activity, a lot occurs biologically. It is risky to leave the in between unexplored and to carry on as if we had demonstrated some significant biological phenomena which provides us with a biological anchor point or basis of a behavioral event.

It appears that one of the principal reasons we were willing to use such an abiological strategy was the way the physiology of the cardiovascular (CV) system was viewed. As has been pointed out elsewhere (Obrist et al. 1970a), it had been implicitly assumed that the CV changes associated with stimulus events are specific to those events and have little to do with the metabolic function the CV system performs. In a sense it was not surprising that such a dualistic conceptualization of the system was maintained, since the size of effects commonly dealt with are hardly of the magnitude seen when an appreciable metabolic load, such as exercise, is placed on the organism.

Initially, our own approach in studying HR effects emphasized a similar strategy. We resorted to a more biological approach only because the data were inconsistent with conceptualizations about learning and motivational processes. The first experiments, where we examined the relationship between HR and somatic activity in dogs during classical conditioning, were not intended for this purpose. But in the pilot studies this relationship seemed obvious just from observing the dogs and the polygraph, and we wondered why no one had reported seeing such effects, i.e., a concomitance between HR and somatic activity. As things stand today, I feel it is not feasible to view some one parameter of CV activity as a simple unidimensional index of behavioral processes unrelated to other peripheral events, nor to ignore the very real likelihood that at least HR is related to somatic activity even when there is little significant metabolic demand placed on the organism.

The purpose of a biological strategy is that by providing a more complete picture of biological events, a clearer perspective is achieved as to the significance of CV activity to behavioral processes. This can be seen in several regards. For one thing, various chapters illustrate the use of a biological strategy, and in different ways. For example, one can single out one parameter of CV function as the Laceys have, and then, on the basis of its relationship to neurophysiological feedback processes, derive a hypothesis as to how this parameter may influence sensorimotor processes. In this case, the neurophysiological mechanism is used to specify both how this CV parameter exerts its influence on behavior and the way one evaluates this influence in a behavioral paradigm. Another approach is illustrated by Cohen's work. Although the purpose of this work is to determine the means by which central nervous system processes control HR, the approach is to work from the periphery, first establishing the respective influence of the neural innervations, then determining the extent the innervations are influenced reflexively by other hemodynamic changes associated with the stimulating events in contrast to more direct central nervous system processes. Roberts's work illustrates still another way a biological strategy can be used. By utilizing a CV parameter in conjunction with sudomotor activity and then evaluating their respective relationship to still a third peripheral measure, i.e., somatic activity, it is quite forcefully shown that in anticipation of an aversive event, the two autonomic events tell us quite different things about preparatory activity.

Several chapters, e.g., Cook, Schneiderman, Schwartz, and Forsyth, emphasize the relationship among cardiovascular events. Schwartz indicates, for example, that by utilizing the relationship that can exist between diastolic blood pressure and HR, biofeedback techniques are more effective in modifying both HR and diastolic blood pressure than when either is reinforced alone. Schneiderman, in another vein, demonstrates that the conditioned and unconditioned decelerations of HR in rabbits have a different biological basis. The unconditioned effect appears to be a reflexive baroreceptor effect triggered by an elevation of blood pressure, while the conditioned deceleration is not so influenced by pressor effects. The fact that the conditioned response (CR) is associated with behavioral freezing suggests that the same types of heart rate effects have a different biological basis, which, in turn, suggests that they have different consequences for behavioral processes. In our own research evaluating the relationship between HR, cardiac contractility, blood pressure, and somatic activity and the respective influence of the neural innervation of the heart, has helped us regarding behavioral processes in two respects. First, the fact that under certain circumstances phasic HR changes are related to somatic activity indicates a means by which the phasic HR changes are initiated. In turn, this suggested how we could understand the observation that performance on a reaction time (RT) task was directly related to the magnitude of the phasic cardiac and somatic effects. Second, a consideration of hemodynamic events and the role of the cardiac innervation has provided us with a new perspective on how behavioral stressors might influence the CV system. It also served to allow us for the first time to demonstrate convincingly an independence of cardiac and somatic events—something most of us believed was possible, but which we had been unable to do prior to obtaining a more complete picture of hemodynamic events.

There are still other examples from the various chapters that could be used to illustrate and justify a biological strategy. However, it might be more profitable to illustrate the value of the strategy by recourse in a somewhat hypothetical manner to a specific problem area, namely essential hypertension.

Blood pressure is a parameter of CV function which has been thought for some time to be related to affective states and/or stress of some nature. Biologically, there are two aspects to the problem: (a) the hemodynamic basis both for the development and maintenance of the hypertension; and, (b) the biological processes that link behavioral processes to these hemodynamic events. There is one current viewpoint as to the hemodynamics of at least certain instances of hypertension which, although still speculative, will serve to make the point. It is that in the development of hypertension the most significant hemodynamic events are an elevation of cardiac output in the presence of a normal peripheral resistance, an effect which is mediated by the beta-adrenergic innervation of the heart. In turn, the elevated cardiac output results in an excessive perfusion of the tissues, with respect to metabolic requirements, which initiates autoregulatory processes in the vascular system to counteract the excess perfusion. This results in an increase in peripheral resistance, a return of cardiac output to normal, and a sustaining of the hypertensive state. This model is in contrast to ones which consider the elevation of total peripheral resistance as the primary causal factor. This sort of hemodynamic information is important in several respects with regard to behavioral processes. It allows one to evaluate what behavioral parameters, e.g., type and intensity of stress or type of coping mechanisms, that are relevant in the etiology of hypertensive conditions, i.e., those conditions which produce an elevated cardiac output which not all stressors do (see Brod 1963). It indicates the type of hemodynamic effect one should look for in trying to predict whether a person is predisposed to hypertension. It guides experimental efforts, such as with animal preparations, in evaluating relevant biological and behavioral parameters. Most important it indicates that therapeutic efforts utilizing behavioral intervention, such as with biofeedback procedures, should focus on the early stages of the hypertension where the neurogenic influence is more significant in contrast to where autoregulation is more dominant.

It is less clear in this model as to the central nervous mechanisms which mediate these hemodynamic effects. Nonetheless, such knowledge would act like knowledge of the hemodynamic processes to specify further the significance of behavioral stress and therapeutic procedures. For example, Brod (1963) has proposed that because the hemodynamic effects seen in hypertension are at times similar to those seen in the exercising organism, hypertension may be likened to an anticipatory exercise response. If this is the case, then the neural mechanisms must involve some sort of short circuiting of the means by which the CV system is normally controlled to meet metabolic requirements. Specifications of such a short circuiting process would surely have therapeutic value.

The point of this example involving hypertension can be restated. For some time, it has been believed that behavioral stressors are significant in the etiology of hypertension. The primary evidence for this has been the concomitance demonstrated between phasic alterations in blood pressure and behavioral stressors. At this point, it has not been very convincing evidence since it has shed little light on the prevention, etiology, or even treatment of hypertension. Similarly, experimental studies using animal preparations have, until recently, shed little light on the problem. What I propose is that, until we understand more about what goes on biologically between behavioral stress and an elevation of blood pressure, we shall remain in the dark concerning both the relevance of behavioral stress in the first place and the means to prevent or treat hypertension by behavioral intervention. Blood pressure is very complexly determined both in regard to hemodynamic processes and the extrinsic, i.e., neural-humoral, and intrinsic mechanisms that control the heart and vasculature. Trying to evaluate or treat only the symptom, i.e., elevated pressure, without regard to the biological mechanisms, is like treating a fever without concern over the infecting organism.

SPECIFIC ISSUES

The Curarized Preparation (A. H. Black)

During this conference, a great deal of attention has been focused on the curarized preparation. This interest has been stimulated in large part by the inability of Miller and DiCara to replicate some of their earlier results on autonomic conditioning in curarized rats. A further question has received less attention, but is, I think, equally important. This is: "Of what use is the curarized preparation in the first place?" I would like to comment on this latter question, and then discuss the failure to replicate.

Uses of the Curarized Preparation. The original use of the curarized preparation in research on operant autonomic conditioning was to block skeletal movement, in order to rule out the possibility that autonomic responses were mediated by peripheral skeletal responses. There is no doubt that the curarized preparation is useful in helping us find out whether overt skeletal responses, and feedback from these skeletal responses, mediate a given autonomic response. The curarized preparation, however, does not provide information on the mediating function of central components of motor circuits that control these peripheral skeletal responses (nor, for that matter, on the central components of the neural systems that control the autonomic responses). That is, it does not rule out the possibility that the curarized subjects produced an autonomic change by attempting to move. Other techniques must be employed to deal with this possibility. Therefore, the curarized preparation is of limited usefulness for those interested in analyzing the central and peripheral mechanisms involved in the performance of operantly conditioned autonomic responses.

As has been made clear in a number of chapters in this book, curare-like drugs have side effects, among which is an interference with cardiovascular functioning. It is obvious that the curarized preparation will not be adequate for studying mechanisms involved in response performance to the extent that it interferes with the response that we want to study. This defect in the curarized preparation also prevents us from employing it for other purposes—for example, for the immobilization of the subject in order to make recording easier, or for the comparison of the form and magnitude of the conditioned autonomic response when an animal is capable of moving and when it is prevented from moving by neuromuscular blocking agents.

There is a further use for the curarized preparation. It is the attempt to provide more data on the phenomena that were demonstrated by Miller and DiCara in the curarized rat. They found in their early work, for example, that the effects of conditioning under curare were much greater than those seen in animals trained in the normal state. Also, there is a suggestion that the training under curare led to a dissociation between the cardiovascular and somatic systems, as seen in data on the transfer from conditioning under curare to the normal state. While results such as these are exciting, it would be unwise to attempt to work out their implications until the replication has been accomplished.

In summary, the curarized preparation is of limited usefulness in studying the mediating mechanisms of operantly conditioned autonomic responses, because it deals only with the peripheral components of the neural circuits that control skeletal responding. Furthermore, its interference with cardiovascular functioning makes its use hazardous, even for this limited purpose. Finally, although the results of Miller, DiCara, and their associates on operant autonomic conditioning in the curarized rat are very interesting, it is not possible to use the curarized preparation to extend these results until the original experiments have been replicated. Therefore, it seems to me, at this time, that the curarized preparation is useful primarily (or, perhaps, only) for those who want to determine the reasons for failure to replicate previously published results on the curarized rat. I would like to turn to this problem next.

Failure of Replication in the Curarized Rat (A. H. Black)

I shall discuss only the conditioning of heart rate, since it is the response for which the replication difficulties have been reported. There are two preliminary comments that I must make. First, I am assuming that heart rate conditioning does occur in the normal animal and in the partially curarized animal on the basis of Engel's and our own data (Engel 1972; Black 1971b). Therefore, the question of replicability, as far as I am concerned, does not involve a question as to whether heart rate can be operantly conditioned. It is concerned only with results on the operant conditioning of heart rate in the apparently completely curarized rat, employing conditioning procedures similar to those of Miller, DiCara, and their associates. Second, the fact that operant conditioning procedures can change heart rate in the normal and partially curarized animal says nothing about the role of central nervous system (CNS) motor control circuits in mediating these changes. Much of the available data indicate that there is a close relationship between skeletal responding and heart rate, but the evidence is not firm enough to permit us to reach a definitive conclusion on this mediation issue at present.

A great deal of effort has been expended in attempting to identify the specific factors that produce a failure of operant conditioning in the curarized rat. The major concern of this effort, to date, has been to determine the specific procedures necessary for maintaining the rat in a healthy alert state while curarized, and to locate and minimize the interfering side effects of the curare-like drugs. This research has not as yet identified the factors responsible for the failure of operant conditioning in the curarized rat, as is made clear by the contributions to this book. Therefore, it might be worthwhile to consider other approaches in attempting to account for this failure.

A reasonable place to begin is to consider the possible causes for the failure to replicate heart rate conditioning in the curarized rat. As I see it, there are four main possibilities.

1. Some inadvertent procedural change which reduced the effectiveness of the operant conditioning procedure may have developed.
2. The heart rate changes during training under curare may have been produced by some factor other than operant conditioning in the first place, and this factor may have been excluded as the training procedures were refined.
3. Some interference with the general functioning of the central nervous system may have developed so that the rats could not learn. Such a general interference could have been produced by the following:
    a) inadvertent changes in the procedures employed to maintain the rat in a healthy alert state while curarized (respiration, adaptation to discomfort, etc.).
    b) changes in the curare-like drugs which produced new or more potent side effects on the CNS.
4. The CNS might be functioning normally, but some interference specific to the functioning of the cardiovascular system may have developed, so that the rat could not perform and learn the cardiovascular response that one wants to reinforce. Such a specific interference could have been produced by either:
    a) inadvertent changes in the maintenance procedures [see 3(a) above].
    b) changes in the curare-like drugs which produced new or more potent side effects on the cardiovascular system.

It is obvious that any combination of these four sources of trouble might be operating in a given experiment. Therefore, rather than studying only the last two possibilities, it might be more useful to go back to the beginning and attempt to deal with each of these variables in a systematic sequence.

It seems to me that one ought to begin by making sure the operant conditioning procedure one employs is a powerful one (Point 1, above). First, one could attempt to develop a more effective operant conditioning procedure for the heart rate response in the normal state. For example, it looks as though shock avoidance may be a less effective reinforcer than electrical stimulation of the brain (ESB). Brener (Chapter 19) and Hahn (Chapter 15) employed ESB in their experiments. DiCara (personal communication) has indicated more success in recent work with ESB than with shock avoidance.

Obviously, one ought to be on the lookout for changes in heart rate produced by variables other than those involved in operant conditioning (Point 2, above). Most of the participants in this conference would consider this an unlikely possibility. Nevertheless, it must be examined. For example, consider the following hypothesis for heart rate avoidance conditioning, which was suggested by S. Clarke (personal communication). If the heart rate response to shock is an acceleration in rate, then, early in training, one might expect shocks to be relatively widely spaced in rats that were being conditioned to accelerate heart rate, and to be densely packed in rats that were being trained to decelerate heart rate. The rats in the deceleration group could enter a protective inhibitory state, similar to that described by Pavlov, if they received too many intense shocks in a short period of time. This inhibitory state could lead to a marked reduction in heart rate, and an absence of shock later in conditioning among rats trained to decrease heart rate. If this happened, the rats trained to increase heart rate and to decrease heart rate would display appropriate cardiac responses at the end of conditioning, and could receive the same total number of shocks during conditioning, even though the density of shock could be different at different stages of conditioning. This hypothesis could account for additional results that have been obtained in heart rate avoidance conditioning in curarized rats. For example, one might expect more decelerators who were subjected to very dense shocks to die than accelerators who were subjected to spaced shocks. Also dense shocks might have a very different effect on skeletal avoidance learning than spaced shocks after recovery from curarization.

Next, one could turn to difficulties with the curarized preparation that were described in Points 3 and 4 above. The first task, it seems to me, should be to determine whether there is a general effect on the CNS, or a specific effect on the cardiovascular system. One simple approach to this question is to condition electroencephalogram (EEG) activity in the same curarized preparation employed for heart rate conditioning. If the EEG can be conditioned, then the problem cannot be an interference with general CNS functioning. We employed this strategy in research on the dog, and successfully conditioned the EEG (Black Chapter 12). In this case, the failure to produce heart rate conditioning was not produced by an interference with general CNS functioning. If the same results are found for the rat, then one more possible source of trouble will be ruled out. [Roberts (Chapter 9) employed the classical conditioning of electrodermal responses for the same purpose.]

The remaining possibility is an interference with the normal functioning of the cardiovascular system. Although many researchers have begun by trying to deal with this factor, it may be more productive in the long run to attempt to rule out the other factors first.

Many of those who have been working in this area feel confident that heart rate conditioning will be demonstrated in the curarized rat. In fact, this discussion may be out of date as I write. At the same time, it is important to note that similar failures to condition have not been encountered by those who have attempted to operantly condition other internal responses. The operant conditioning of a variety of patterns of CNS electrical activity has been demonstrated in normal and curarized animals including the rat (Black 1972a; Olds 1967; Hiatt 1972). Electromyogram (EMG) is easily conditioned in normal subjects and in partially curarized subjects.

One can easily conjure up a number of reasons for this difference between types of internal responses in ease of conditioning. One possibility is that autonomic responses are more difficult to operantly condition than certain EEG responses, because of constraints produced by the neural systems that control autonomic responses. Furthermore, the differences noted by Roberts (Chapter 17) between electrodermal and heart rate responses suggest that there may be differences among autonomic responses in amenability to operant conditioning. The recognition of fundamental differences between autonomic and other responses, and among autonomic responses in amenability to operant conditioning, goes against the view that autonomic and skeletal responses are more or less equally conditionable. It is important, however, to keep this possibility in mind, especially when so much data are accumulating now on such differences in operant conditionability among skeletal responses (Shettleworth 1972).

The Curarized Preparation (J. Brener)

Prior to this conference, it was conspicuously rumored that difficulties were being experienced by a number of investigators in the replication of operant cardiovascular conditioning in curarized rats. I feel that a considerable service has been performed by bringing this issue into the open and enabling the individuals responsible for reporting discrepant results to air their views and present their data to one another. Although the problems surrounding these phenomena have not been solved, it has been agreed that there is, indeed, a problem, and a number of possible factors underlying the replication difficulties have been identified.

Most of these factors relate to the maintenance of curarized animals. The contribution of respiratory factors has been discussed in detail in the contributions of Miller and Dworkin (Chapter 16) and DiCara (Chapter 14), and in the chapter by Eissenberg, Middaugh, and myself (Chapter 13). Given the general instability of the curarized preparation and the close interdependence of respiratory and cardiovascular processes, it would seem imperative that more sophisticated means of artificial respiration be developed.

A second factor that has been identified relates to the ganglionic blocking effects of curare and the influence of such effects on cardiovascular performance. Here we are clearly in need of more data. Whereas Howard et al. have demonstrated convincingly that d-tubocurarine has a profound vagolytic action in cats, an effect substantiated by the work of Black on dogs, Hahn and Miller provide evidence that would indicate that in rats massive doses of curare does not lead to vagal blockade. In any case, it is difficult to assimilate this possibility with the large literature indicating that vagally mediated responses may be conditioned in curarized rats. In the absence of further information relating to this factor, we are forced for the present to assume either that there are substantial species differences in the ganglionic blocking effects of this drug or, as Miller has suggested, that the chemical properties of curare have been altered inadvertently by the manufacturers over the past several years.

It should be noted that the purpose of employing curare in these experiments has changed. Judging from the reactions of conference participants (Obrist et al.; Elliott; Black; Roberts; Brener et al.), the need to demonstrate that cardiovascular learning is independent of peripheral somatomotor activity is now passé. The immediate goal of future research using this drug in the context of operant cardiovascular conditioning would seem to be to define those factors that have made these phenomena so fickle.

The Curarized Preparation (P. Obrist)

I think the justification of a biological strategy is very clearly evidenced by the problems encountered in the curarized preparation. It seems we have failed both to understand what curarization achieves as a means of controlling somatic activity as well as what now appear to be serious side effects of at least some curarizing agents. We have suffered from both conceptual and methodological confusion. I can't help but feel that the current status of the operant and biofeedback work would be clearer if we had known more about the biological properties of the curarizing agent and the associated problems encountered when one curarizes an organism as pointed out by Brener (Chapter 19) and Howard (Chapter 18), and if we understand that curarization controls somatic influences only to the extent that afferent feedback from striate muscular activity influences CV function.

As a final note in regard to the curarization work, I hope that in attempting to resolve the issue of replicability we do not ignore an equally significant issue, namely the theoretical significance of this work. Assuming that the effects seen in both the curarized and non-curarized preparations are the result of the experimental contingencies and not an artifact of the methodologies, we are still faced with the problem of interpretation. It appears that some of the original conceptualizations concerning specificity of effects and the implied power of the contingencies to modify specific visceral functions are still very unsettled. The issue of somatic mediation appears as important as ever. Our suggestion is that we shall likely obtain a better grasp of what has been achieved by recourse to a more biological approach. That is, we need to clarify the hemodynamic picture, the role of the neural innervations, and the mediating mechanisms.

The Nature of Operant and Voluntary Control (A. H. Black)

Most of the discussions of operant autonomic conditioning at this conference were concerned with its use as a technique for analyzing and modifying the normal and abnormal functioning of the cardiovascular system. Questions have arisen in this research about the type of control that is established over cardiovascular functioning, and about the conditions that are necessary for establishing it. Several of the contributors to this volume considered these problems (e.g., Brener, Chapter 19, and Schwartz, Chapter 21). I would like to reinforce their comments, because I think that these problems merit more attention than they have received so far.

The first question that I would like to discuss concerns the relationship between "operant control" and "voluntary control." Although many assume that these terms refer to the same phenomenon, they are not, I think, the same. One can point to several differences between the two types of control.

First, in everyday terms, operant control usually refers to control over behavior which can be exerted either by someone else or by the subject himself. Voluntary control, on the other hand, refers to "self-control" only.

Second, voluntary control seems to be more complex than operant control. Consider the operational criteria that might be employed to demonstrate that control is operant and that it is voluntary. For operant control, the main requirement is to show that the probability of some response in the presence of a discriminative stimulus has been changed by a contingency between response and reinforcer. For voluntary control, we have to do more. Although there is no general agreement about what we mean by the term voluntary, and about the operational criteria for assessing the degree of voluntary control, a "minimal" set of more or less intuitive criteria can be described.

In order to say that we have voluntary control over a response, we should demonstrate not only that we can instruct a subject to make the response to a stimulus which normally does not elicit it, but also that we can instruct him to refrain from making the response to this stimulus, and to other stimuli which normally elicit it. We would be loath to call a response voluntary if a subject could not inhibit as well as initiate its occurrence. Furthermore, the subject should be able to switch back and forth from performance to inhibition of the responses easily. In addition, if a subject can perform or inhibit the response in a variety of situations, we would be more likely to consider that he has voluntary control over the response than if his ability to perform or inhibit the response were limited to one class of situations.

In order to satisfy this set of criteria for voluntary control, we must demonstrate a great deal more than the operant conditioning of the response. This is not to deny that voluntary control may be intimately related to operant control. As we shall see below, one group of researchers holds the position that voluntary control is a special, complex form of operant control. The point is that, even if one accepts this position, the criteria for identifying two types of control would not be identical. As I see it, difficulties in understanding the relationship between the two types of control arise primarily from our lack of agreement concerning the meaning of the term voluntary and the operational criteria for ascertaining the degree of voluntary control.

Next, I would like to discuss the conditions that are sufficient for achieving voluntary control over cardiovascular responses. Although the data are few and provide no clear answers, one can see that two quite distinct accounts of these conditions are beginning to develop.

One account of the sufficient conditions for establishing voluntary control over internal responses goes something like this. Voluntary control depends on an "awareness" of the response to be controlled. For the purpose of this discussion, I shall define awareness as the ability to discriminate between the occurrence and nonoccurrence of a response: That is, when the response, or response-produced stimuli, or internal states that are correlated with the response, can act as a discriminative stimuli, we have "awareness" of the response. If one accepts the definition, the "awareness" hypothesis can be stated as follows: When a subject learns to discriminate the occurrence and non-occurrence of an internal response, he becomes aware of the response, and, therefore, achieves voluntary control over that response.

Three procedures have been proposed for producing awareness and increased voluntary control, as defined above. One is to provide added feedback when some internal response occurs; that is, to make some neutral stimulus (a stimulus which does not act as a primary or secondary reinforcer for other responses) contingent on the response. As Brener (Chapter 19) points out, such feedback can be employed to substitute for interoceptive response-produced stimuli when they do not exist, or to make the subject aware of interoceptive response-produced stimuli when they do exist. This procedure, however, does not seem to be sufficient. Consider, for example, simple operant conditioning. We have added clicks and tones following the occurrence of hippocampal theta waves in rats, and this, by itself, has not produced learning. (It might be that the above procedure would produce savings when a reinforcer is made to follow the internal response subsequently. We have no data on this point.)

One might argue, however, that human subjects are different from infrahuman subjects, and that for human subjects, added feedback is a sufficient condition for establishing voluntary control. Unfortunately, even if one obtained an effect of added informational feedback, the interpretation of the result is equivocal. The added feedback could have an effect, because subtle reinforcers are established by instructions and by the previous history of the subject. Therefore, feedback could help to establish voluntary control, not because it provides information about response state, but because it indicates successful performance. Obviously, it would be extremely useful to have more data in order to determine which of these alternatives is correct.

In a second and more common procedure that has been proposed for establishing voluntary control, one motivates the subject to attempt to achieve voluntary control over a given response, usually by employing instructions, and one makes some stimulus contingent on the response that not only indicates that the correct response has occurred but also provides or leads to some payoff. This, of course, is one statement of the conditions that produce operant conditioning. (The operant procedure is discussed in more detail in a later part of this section.) Those who support the view that awareness is sufficient to establish voluntary control would have to hypothesize that this operant conditioning procedure works because it trains the subject to be aware of the internal response that is reinforced. Obviously, the effectiveness of the operant conditioning procedure cannot provide evidence for or against this hypothesis, because alternative explanations of its effectiveness are equally plausible.

There is a third procedure for producing awareness of internal responses, and the voluntary control that is assumed to follow from such awareness. It is to train subjects directly to discriminate internal responses by employing the internal responses as discriminative stimuli. Kamiya (1969), for example, employed the presence and absence of occipital alpha electroencephalographic activity as discriminative stimuli for verbal responses. Once the subjects had learned to discriminate between the two EEG states, Kamiya asked them to produce alpha and non-alpha, and they did. Brener (Chapter 19) employed an analogous procedure to train subjects to discriminate heart beats, and found that such training enhanced voluntary control. In these cases, voluntary control was increased by making the subjects aware of the response, and not by reinforcing it directly.

This procedure obviously provides a direct test of the awareness hypothesis. There are problems with these experiments, however. First, the subjects may have been reinforced for producing the responses inadvertently while they were being trained to discriminate them. Furthermore, the same procedure has failed for other responses. Reynolds (1966) showed that pigeons that had been trained to discriminate long interresponse times (IRTs), subsequently did not learn to produce those IRTs. Discrimination was not sufficient to establish operant control in this case.

In summary, the hypothesis that awareness is sufficient for the establishment of voluntary control has not been established unequivocally, as Brener has also pointed out in his concluding comments.

A second account of the conditions that are necessary for establishing voluntary control argues that it is produced by a sequence of special types of operant conditioning procedures. This view implies that the contingency between response and reinforcer is essential, and that awareness of the response is not sufficient in itself.

This is a relatively straightforward position. But, again we lack important data. What are the specific operant conditioning procedures that enhance voluntary control? Not all of them do. For example, the operant conditioning of avoidance responses in dogs seems to decrease voluntary control, as defined above, rather than to increase it. Solomon, Kamin, and Wynne (1953) found it extremely difficult to train dogs to inhibit avoidance responding once they had trained them to perform such responses. Also, how would this account handle the experiments in which subjects were trained to discriminate internal responses, and, consequently, achieved voluntary control (if, in fact, no inadvertent reinforcement of the responses occurred in those experiments)? Finally, voluntary control may be achieved for only certain classes of operantly conditionable responses, and what are the identifying features of those responses? In short, this account of the techniques for producing voluntary control is not more firmly established empirically than the first one I described.

One might argue, at this point, that we will not make much headway in this attempt to specify the sufficient conditions for voluntary control, until we reach more agreement about what we mean by voluntary control. In fact, one might argue even further that it might be better to concentrate on a more restricted problem for the moment—on the specification of the conditions that are sufficient for obtaining discriminative stimulus control over internal responses. One promising approach to this question is that taken in analyzing the learning of complex motor skills, and the development of sensory motor coordination (see Chapters 19, 20, and 21 by Brener, Lang, and Schwartz). Motor skills training, for example, can be thought of as a form of operant training in which an analysis is made of the role of both information about response state (e.g., the role of information about magnitude of error in performance) and the role of reinforcement (e.g., the role of magnitude and delay of reinforcement). One advantage of this approach is that it attempts to deal with the two functions of response-contingent stimuli that are emphasized in each of the accounts described above, i.e., providing information about response state, and providing response-contingent payoffs.

In summary, I have outlined two accounts of the conditions that are sufficient for obtaining voluntary control over internal responses, each of which seems to be gaining acceptance at least in some circles. Neither is strongly supported by the available data. It would be valuable if more research were carried out, especially on the conditions sufficient for establishing discriminative stimulus control over internal responses, before each account hardens into dogma and unnecessary conflicts develop.

Conceptual Issues Related to Learned Cardiovascular Control in Humans. (J. Brener)

In the preceding section, Black has provided an evaluation of the concepts of operant and voluntary control and has speculated about the mechanisms involved in the development of voluntary control. Since both of these issues are of fundamental importance to our further understanding of learned cardiovascular control in particular and of voluntary control in general, Black's comments warrant our careful attention.

Behavioral control is generally evidenced in the systematic influence of certain manipulable stimulus events upon the activity of organisms. The classification of forms of behavioral control has not received explicit treatment in the writings of behavioral theorists. In general, however, a major distinction is accepted between reflexive and learned control. In the former case, the behavioral controlling properties of stimuli are attributed to innate structural connections between the receptors receiving the eliciting stimuli and the effectors expressing the motor reflex. In the case of learned forms of behavioral control, response-controlling properties of stimuli are seen as the consequence of certain prior treatments. Thus, the procedures of classical conditioning represent one effective means of generating response-controlling properties in otherwise neutral stimuli, and the operant conditioning procedures, another means. The question raised by Black and of immediate interest here is whether or not a meaningful distinction may be drawn between "operant" and "voluntary" forms of control. Three potential sources of distinction are discernible: (1) the nature of voluntary and operant responses; (2) the stimulus conditions necessary for demonstrating responses of these classes; and, (3) the nature of the procedures necessary for establishing operant and voluntary behavioral controlling properties in such stimuli.

Voluntary and Operant Responses. As has been pointed out in this volume (see Chapter 19, Brener), it is difficult to specify the differences between those responses we traditionally refer to as voluntary responses and those we classify as operants. Skinner explicitly and specifically defined an operant response as an activity, the stimulus antecedents of which are not specifiable. If the eliciting stimuli for a response are specifiable, that response is classified as a respondent. Skinner's use of the term "emitted" to characterize the mode of production of operant responses implies that the antecedent conditions for the occurrence of such behavioral events reside within the organism. Insofar as voluntary responses are also attributed to covert processes within the subject organism, it will be recognized that members of this class of behavior share with operants the characteristic of being of an objectively unspecifiable origin. Traditionally, both operants and voluntary responses have been thought to find their expression in the activities of the striate musculature. However, in the light of the current literature in learned visceral control, this characteristic appears to be an unwarranted attribute of either class. It would appear, therefore, that Skinner's concept of an operant incorporates the least defensible attributes of the traditional mentalistic appreciation of voluntary behavior. Most notably, both operants and voluntary responses are activities of unspecifiable origin that are primarily subject to the influence of a vis a fronte.

The Demonstration of Voluntary and Operant Behaviors. The demonstration of the operant characteristics of a response conventionally resides in the ability of a discriminative stimulus to systematically influence the rate of the response in question. Such discriminative properties are established in a previously neutral stimulus through the procedure of operant conditioning. Black accepts the traditional notion that whereas operant behaviors are subject to control via such external influences, the essential characteristic of voluntary behaviors is that they are self-controlled. By conceptually embedding the antecedent conditions for voluntary behavior within the behaving organism, these conditions are effectively removed from the public domain and, therefore, from scientific scrutiny. It is for this reason that it has been proposed (see Chapter 19, Brener) that a voluntary response be defined as one that is systematically influenced by instructions. Although this definition implies that voluntary behaviors are demonstrable only in verbal organisms, acknowledgment of instructional stimuli of a nonverbal nature circumvents this implication. Self-control of the sort traditionally associated with voluntary behavior could be assimilated by this definition as a case of instructionally controlled behavior where the instructions and the response to the instructions are displayed by the same individual. This would be a case of what Hull referred to as a "pure stimulus act." In cases of such "self-instruction," the task of the researcher remains one of identifying the tangible external factors which gave rise to the "self-instructional" response. It is argued, therefore, that a scientific appreciation of voluntary behavior rests on our ability to specify the external, objectively definable and manipulable factors which give rise to voluntary behaviors. The prevalent concept of "teaching organisms to control their behavior" subverts these fundamental requirements for an objective specification of voluntary behavior, by implying that source of such behavior resides within the organism and is, therefore, indeterminate.

Procedures for Establishing Operant and Voluntary Control. Whereas the procedures for establishing operant controlling properties in otherwise neutral stimulus are well known and have been meticulously examined, the same cannot be said for the procedures responsible for establishing control of voluntary responses in instructional stimuli. It is generally conceded that operant controlling (discriminative) properties are established in a previously neutral stimulus by the consistent pairing of that stimulus with the conjunction between an operant and a consequent reinforcing stimulus. In general reinforcing stimuli are not classified in terms of their intrinsic attributes, but rather in terms of their functional properties, viz, they lead to systematic changes in the rate of responses upon which they are made contingent. Because of the definitional interdependence of "operants and reinforcing stimuli," the principle of reinforcement has a limited heuristic utility.

It will be generally conceded that the only substantial distinction that may be drawn between operant and voluntary control procedures resides in the motivational properties of that class of feedback stimuli (reinforcers) necessary for establishing operant control. Although feedback stimuli do not necessarily incorporate motivational (energizing) properties, operant reinforcing events do necessarily incorporate the informational properties that are implied by the term "feedback stimuli." Insofar as the development of behavioral control refers to the processes whereby previously neutral stimuli (either discriminative or instructional) acquire the ability to elicit specific motor responses, such informational properties are deemed to be of primary importance. The motivational properties implicit in reinforcing stimuli, and presumably acquired by discriminative stimuli, are ancillary to the primary process of learned control and relate more directly to the performance of such learned control.

Critique.   Within this frame of reference we may now consider the points raised by Black. He mentions that "to label a response voluntary, we should demonstrate not only that we can instruct a subject to make a response to a stimulus which does not normally elicit it, but also that we can instruct him to refrain from making the response to this stimulus, and to other stimuli which normally elicit it." It is important to point out that, in terms of the definition of a voluntary response proposed earlier, the instructions themselves represent the stimulus for the voluntary response. Whether we would wish to classify as voluntary responses only those activities which may be demonstrably facilitated *and* inhibited by instructions suggests an additional criterion that one may wish to impose on the classification of voluntary activities, but that is not logically demanded. It is clear that the resolution of this question depends, among other things, on what we mean by a "response." Frequently, increases and decreases in a particular biological function are under the control of differentiable neural circuits and effectors. In view of this, it would seem legitimate to entertain the possibility that increases in such a function may be subject to learned control and decreases not, or vice versa. In any case, it will be recognized that the systematic increases and decreases in the rate of an operant response produced by the presentation and withdrawal of a discriminative stimulus are demonstrative of facilitative and inhibitive control in the case of operant conditioning. Since facilitation and inhibition are relative terms, the baseline rates of activity upon which such forms of control are superimposed must be taken into account. Attention tends to be directed toward inhibitory control in the case of voluntary visceral activity, largely because the intrinsic rates of activity displayed by the viscera are noticeably higher than those displayed by the striate muscles.

It is also doubtful that the ability of instructions to override the influence of reflex-eliciting stimuli is a reasonable criterion to impose on the classification of voluntary behaviors. Thus, we would not disqualify arm movement as a voluntary response if instructions to inhibit arm movement were not effective in suppressing the arm flexion elicited by electric shock to the fingers.

Black correctly points out that voluntary activities tend to be less situation-specific than do operant behaviors. Since the initiating conditions for voluntary responses reside in the auditory characteristics of instructional stimuli rather than in the topographical features of the environment, this is scarcely surprising. However, it is reasonable to assume that if a trans-situational discriminative stimulus, particularly one that could be produced by the organism, were employed in operant conditioning, this apparent difference would recede. The motivational aspects implicit in the operant conditioning procedure are also probably germane to the relatively greater trans-situational control associated with voluntary as opposed to operant processes. Whereas operant conditioning procedures tend to entrench specific drive stimuli in the definition of the preconditions for specific operant responses, voluntary control training procedures generally do not. For this reason, operant control tends to be manifested only in those conditions where the reinforcing stimulus and the deprivation state to which it is relevant are present. In this connection, it would seem reasonable to assume that operant control manifesting all the characteristics deemed by Black to be important criteria for the classification of voluntary behaviors could be demonstrated in rats by employing a nontopographic discriminative stimulus (e.g., a tone) and a reinforcing stimulus, the incentive properties of which are not dependent upon the deprivation state of the organism (e.g., electrical stimulation of the brain). An analog of "self-control" could then be structured by providing the subjects with a means of producing the discriminative stimulus.

Black then goes on to a discussion of the methods for establishing voluntary motor control and a consideration of the possible mechanisms by which these methods may achieve their effect. He distinguishes between "awareness" and reinforcement explanations of the development of voluntary control. In this connection, it will be noted that the principle of reinforcement has a very limited heuristic utility, since it does not attempt to account for the processes whereby the reinforcement of a response establishes response-eliciting properties in the accompanying discriminative stimulus. When the principle of reinforcement is invoked for explanatory purposes, a final explanation incapable of further reduction is implied. The use of the term "awareness" to characterize the type of explanation proposed by me (Chapter 19) is unfortunate, since it invokes a type of mentalism that I am anxious to avoid. Nevertheless, it is true that this model proposes that the ability of subjects to discriminate the consequences of their actions is prerequisite to the development of instructional control over

these actions. The primary advantage of this approach over the reinforcement approach is that it proposes a mechanism to account for
the processes whereby the prior consequences of an act acquire eliciting
properties for that act.

The question of whether or not a motivationally neutral stimulus
which is made to consistently follow a response will by virtue of this
procedure acquire the ability to elicit that response, is by no means
as remote a possibility as Black suggests. For example, during the
1950s, a considerable body of literature attested to the ability of simple
visual and auditory stimuli to maintain bar-pressing in rats. Although
one may attribute reinforcing properties to such stimuli on a post hoc
basis, the understanding of operant control is not facilitated by this
maneuver. More germane to a consideration of the question raised by
Black is an experiment reported by Razran (1961). In this experiment,
subjects were permitted to watch large manometer dials which reflected
their intra-urinary bladder pressures. When the intra-bladder pressure
reached a certain threshold level, the subject would urinate—resulting
in a decrease in the manometer reading. Following extended exposure
to this procedure, the readings on the manometer dials were artificially
increased. This experimental manipulation resulted in an intense urge
to urinate in the subjects, thereby providing a cogent example of the
operation of William James's ideo-motor theory of voluntary action.

The gist of Black's discomfort with the feedback formulation of voluntary control was anticipated by James almost a century ago. He
argued that the activation of the brain circuits representing the affer-
ence previously associated with a response was the necessary and sufficient condition for the occurrence of the response, and provided
extremely compelling arguments to support this assertion. The idea
of having to order ourselves to execute responses (fiat) was, he argued,
more a function of our language and cultural heritage than of the
biology of voluntary control. Reinforcement is essentially a motivational
concept, and it is true that we have not yet adequately come to grips
with the operation of such processes. However, strict attention to the
motivational or incentive properties of reinforcing stimuli has led to
an almost universal neglect of informational and discriminative properties of these events.

Among those investigators engaged in research on learned cardiovascular control in humans (Brener, Engel, Lang, Miller and Dworkin,
Schwartz, and Shapiro), there seems to be general agreement that a
skills-acquisition-feedback approach provides a more powerful conceptual framework than does the traditional operant approach. This preference which is shared by Black appears to be based on considerations
of the sort mentioned above. Given the difficulties of adequately mo-
tivating human subjects in the laboratory, there may be just an element

of sour grapes in the determination of this choice. Nevertheless, it is true that the cybernetic models adopted by investigators in the area of motor skills are readily applicable to the phenomena of learned cardiovascular control. They provide what the operant approach does not, viz, a conceptual system within which the functions of feedback stimuli may be analyzed.

Human research within this framework warrants a few conclusions and identifies a number of areas requiring systematic work. The development of learned cardiovascular control is generally conceded to depend on the provision of exteroceptive feedback of effector activity. It is established that such feedback is necessary during training, but is not essential for the maintenance of cardiovascular control following training. This indicates that exteroceptive feedback serves a calibrating function that enables subjects to identify instances of the required behavior. In elucidating the nature of this process, several lines of inquiry are indicated:

1. What are the effective parameters of exteroceptive feedback, e.g., modality, informational content, discriminability, temporal properties, etc.?
2. Does training in cardiovascular control in fact lead to a demonstrable improvement in the ability of subjects to discriminate occurrences of the activity?
3. If so, what is the basis of these discriminations? Are subjects discriminating cardiovascular afferent events or are they discriminating afferent events associated with the occurrence of somatic correlates?
4. Will training subjects to discriminate the interoceptive consequences of cardiovascular activity lead to reliable improvements in their ability to control such activities?
5. If so, what are the optimal procedures for the training of interoceptive discrimination?

As this list of questions indicates, I consider the study of interoceptive discrimination, which has been so sorely neglected by Western psychophysiology, to be of paramount importance to our further understanding of learned cardiovascular control. In conclusion, it is proposed that in this area of research, we redevelop an interest in the question of what is learned and attempt to specify the mechanisms whereby the procedures that we so freely and occasionally effectively employ, achieve their effects.

Clinical Applications of Operant Autonomic Conditioning (A. H. Black)

Research on clinical application of operant autonomic conditioning is just beginning. Although there are few experimental data (see Engel Chapter 23, and Shapiro Chapter 22), one would expect data on clinical procedures to accumulate over the next few years, and to gradually provide us with a growing repertoire of applied techniques. What worries me is that this normal development might be partially aborted.

First, many applied researchers had great expectations of future success based primarily on the impressive results that had already been obtained in the curarized rat. There is a possibility that researchers in the field will overreact and become discouraged, because the expectation of great success in the future has been withdrawn (even if only temporarily). The second point concerns the overblown claims that have been made for operant autonomic conditioning and biofeedback in the popular press. If the disparity between these claims and what is actually accomplished is great, then some sort of general counter-reaction may develop, and the whole field may be rejected.

It would be regrettable if the normal development of the field were blocked either by discouragement from within or rejection from without. The advantages of the technique, not only as a therapeutic tool, but also as an analytic method for studying relationships between internal processes and behavior, have been demonstrated. The operant conditioning of autonomic responses could have a great deal to offer, even though it is not the panacea that many have claimed it to be.

Cardiac-Somatic Effects (J. Brener)

An almost unanimous consensus seems to have been reached regarding the assumption that in the general case somatomotor and cardiovascular activities are integrally coupled at a central level. Implicit in this recognition is the acknowledgment that the dissociation of cardiovascular and somatomotor activities represents an aberration of function, rather than being indicative of the normal organization of these activities. The latter view, which has been supported by the curare literature, has required that evidence of operant or voluntary cardiovascular control be free of correlated somatomotor activity. In addition to imposing this unreasonable and abiological constraint on the definition of voluntary and operant cardiovascular responses, it has deflected research from the investigation of the clinically significant phenomenon of somatomotor-cardiovascular dissociation.

Several approaches to such phenomena have been identified at this conference. Black has pointed out the utility of dissociative conditioning paradigms in exploring the extent to which somatomotor and cardiovascular events may be amenable to learned dissociation. The work reported by Obrist et al. on the relationship between somatomotor and cardiovascular responses during stressful reaction time tasks identified the importance of sympathetic activity in the dissociation of activities of the two systems. Also relevant to this issue is the observation that rats which have been trained to increase and decrease their heart rates under curare acquire a dissociation of heart rate from general activity and respiration during subsequent noncurarized training (Miller and DiCara 1969). Taken together these studies suggest possible mechanisms underlying learned somatomotor-cardiovascular dissociation and provide the methods whereby this process may be studied.

Cardiac-Somatic Effects (P. Obrist)

This section is in part a reply to the Laceys' critique of our position concerning the relationship between heart rate and somatic activity. We agree with the Laceys that our two positions are not mutually exclusive and may well be complementary. Previous work (Obrist et al. 1969, 1970a, 1970b) has suggested that the hypothesized coupling of cardiac and somatic effects provides a biological basis for why heart rate decelerates in the first place and one explanation of the direct relationship between RT performance and the magnitude of the phasic cardiac deceleration associated with responding. This does not deny that performance might be further facilitated by afferent feedback processes associated with cardiac deceleration, or by events within the cardiac cycle such as the Laceys have proposed. However, we were unable in one experiment to demonstrate such a facilitation when the phasic cardiac deceleration was blocked pharmacologically (Obrist et al. 1970b). On the basis of this result and those of others who have been unable to show any relationship between sensorimotor processes and events within the cardiac cycle (see Chapter 22, Elliott) we have tended to view the role of afferent processes from cardiac events as not too significant in the control of behavioral events. However, the data presented by the Laceys in their chapter appears to add new significance to the role of afferent processes. This is encouraging because it extends the role cardiac events may serve in our understanding of behavioral processes. That is, in our own formulation, these vagally-mediated phasic heart rate changes are primarily an index of somatic quieting or excitation. If phasic heart rate changes or events within the cardiac cycle also influence behavioral processes via afferent mechanisms, then the study of cardiac events has even greater significance in psychophysiological endeavors as Elliott concludes is necessary if heart rate is to be of interest in behavioral research.

The Laceys also question our conceptualization that the cardiac and somatic events are biologically coupled or integrated events. We have based this on two lines of evidence: (a) the physiological evidence indicating that heart rate is directly related to cardiac output and O_2 consumption, and the neurophysiological evidence indicating that cardiac and somatic effects can be integrated within similar areas of the cortex (Obrist et al. 1970a); and, (b) our own data where we have observed a pronounced and consistent relationship between phasic heart rate and somatic activities (Obrist 1968; Obrist et al. 1969; Obrist et al. 1970b; Obrist et al. 1972b; Sutterer and Obrist 1972; Webb and Obrist 1970). In regard to our own experiments, there are two types of data to note. First, various experimental paradigms and manipulations have influenced phasic heart rate and somatic changes in a similar manner. Second, within several experiments the extent heart rate and somatic activity covary has been assessed. For example, in the classical aversive conditioning paradigm (Obrist 1968), momentary bursts of chin EMG activity during a resting period were associated with a significant momentary increase in heart rate. During the pre-conditioned stimulus (CS) base period, trials on which such EMG bursts were present had a significantly higher base level heart rate than trials with no EMG bursts. In turn, the phasic anticipatory deceleration of heart rate was much greater on trials with an elevated base level than on trials with no base level EMG activity, indicating that a significant part of this phasic deceleratory effect could be attributed to the inhibition or cessation of this EMG activity which is concomitant with this deceleratory effect.

In a second experiment in which the CS-UCS interval was shortened from 7.0 to 1.0 seconds, a biphasic deceleration-acceleration was found on nonreinforced test trials. Not only was the briefly sustained deceleration associated with a decrease in chin EMG, but the acceleratory component was found only on trials during which bursts of EMG activity occurred. Similar effects were found in the reaction time paradigm. For example, when trials were dichotomized into those with the lowest and fastest heart rate during the preparatory interval, there were reliably less chin EMG and eye movements on the low heart rate trials (Obrist et al. 1970b). Thus, even though these alterations in somatic activity or in heart rate do not represent appreciable changes in either metabolic activity or in cardiac output, the concomitance between each type of event has been so consistently seen as to suggest that these events must have a common integrating mechanism.

The fact that, during exercise, heart rate is directly related to cardiac output and to O_2 consumption suggests that the same integrating mechanisms involved during exercise could be involved under these less metabolically demanding conditions. We know as yet of no alternative which would explain this apparent coupling. Also, it doesn't seem biologically impossible that the integrating mechanism could compute the net effect of decreases in task irrelevant activities and any increases in task relevant activities. This sort of summation is done during exercise, since the output of the heart is linearly related to O_2 consumption over a wide range of activities.

Admittedly, there are studies which question the validity of the coupling notion, in that they seemingly demonstrate heart rate changes either opposite in direction to or in the absence of somatic changes (e.g., Cohen 1972). However, these studies are hard to evaluate since the quantification techniques or assessment of somatic parameters are not comparable to ours. Moreover, there are studies other than our own which clearly support the coupling notion. There is a danger that we shall get caught up in a controversy over whether somatic activity is present or not, or whether it has been reliably evaluated, etc.

In this regard, we have found that there are two types of somatic activity that are particularly sensitive in human adults to the experimental manipulations used, EMG from the chin, and eye movements and blinks. Chin EMG in some Ss shows a fairly high level of background activity, probably because it reflects activities, such as mouth and tongue movements and swallowing, which Ss can indulge in under the circumstances. Eye movements show even higher levels of background activity and in about all Ss. Thus, conditions which result in an inhibition of task irrelevant activities are more readily detected on these measures than on other aspects of somatic activity which show little background activity. However, unless these other aspects of somatic activity are assessed, there is always the possibility that such activity has gone undetected. This creates a problem in the light of the number of muscles in the body.

The strategy we have used in our more recent studies, where we have observed an independence of cardiac events and somatic changes, would appear to be one way around such a methodological problem. In these studies, we have not only observed heart rate to be accelerated when somatic activity is either decreasing or not changing as assessed by up to four different measures of somatic activity, but we have observed that the biological basis of these cardiac effects differs from situations where somatic and heart rate appear coupled, i.e., sympathetic influences are more apparent when the cardiac effects appear independent of somatic activity. Also, this independence of cardiac and somatic effects appears to occur in more stressful conditions. Finally, the fact that we can observe both an independence and dependence of cardiac and somatic activities at different points in the measurement period in one experiment and on different trials in another study seems to further validate our conclusions.

We do not deny that the phasic decreases in heart rate observed in the reaction time and similar paradigms might be influenced by processes associated with sensorimotor activity independently of somatic activity. It is only that we are not yet convinced that this has been demonstrated. The phenomena of syncope and sudden death involving vagal inhibition of heart rate suggest this possibility, but whether such nonsomatic influences are relevant in the less stressful paradigms is not known. To reiterate, it would be important to show nonsomatic influences on heart rate since, as with the Laceys' recent work with intra-cardiac cycle effects, it also extends the possible usefulness of phasic heart rate changes in behavioral research. But until such time as this nonsomatic influence can be shown, we should not delude ourselves in the light of available evidence that these small vagally-mediated phasic changes in heart rate are something other than an index of somatic inhibition or excitation.

Abrahams, V. C., Hilton, S. M., & Zbrozyna, A. W. Active muscle vasodilatation by stimulation of the brain stem: Its significance in the defense reaction. Journal of Physiology, 1960, 154, 491-513.

Abramson, D. I. Circulation in the Extremities. New York: Academic Press, 1967.

Abramson, D. I., & Ferris, E. B., Jr. Responses of blood vessels in the resting hand and forearm to various stimuli. American Heart Journal, 1940, 19, 541-553.

Abramson, D. I., & Katzenstein, K. H. Spontaneous volume changes in the extremities. American Heart Journal, 1941, 21, 191-198.

Achari, N. K., & Downman, C. B. Autonomic effector responses to stimulation of nucleus fastigius. Journal of Physiology, 1970, 210, 637-650.

Achari, N. K., Downman, C. B., & Weber, W. V. A cardioinhibitory pathway in the brain stem of the cat. Journal of Physiology, 1968, 197, 35P.

Acker, L. E., & Edwards, A. E. Transfer of vasoconstriction over a bipolar meaning dimension. Journal of Experimental Psychology, 1964, 67, 1-6.

Ackner, B. Emotions and the peripheral vasomotor system: A review of previous work. Journal of Psychosomatic Research, 1956, 1, 3-20, (a).

Ackner, B. The relationship between anxiety and the level of peripheral vasomotor activity, Journal of Psychosomatic Research, 1956, 1, 21-48, (b).

Adam, G. Interoception and behaviour. Budapest: Akademiai Kiado, 1967.

Adamowicz, J. K., & Gibson, D. Cue screening, cognitive elaboration, and heart-rate change. Canadian Journal of Psychology, 1970, 24, 240-248.

Adams, D. B., Baccelli, G. Mancia, G., & Zanchetti, A. Cardiovascular changes during preparation for fighting behavior in the cat. Nature, 1968, 220, 1239-1240.

Adams, D. B., Bacelli, G., Mancia, G., & Zanchetti, A. Cardiovascular changes during naturally elicited fighting behavior in the cat. American Journal of Physiology, 1969, 216, 1226-1235.

Agress, C. M., Wegner, S., Bleifer, D. J., Lindsey, A., Van Houten, J., Schroyer, K., & Estin, H. M. The common origin of precordial vibrations. American Journal of Cardiology, 1964, 13, 226-231.

Ahlquist, R. P. A study of the adrenotropic receptors. American Journal of Physiology, 1948, 1531, 586-600.

Alexander, R. H., Nippa, J. H., & Folse, R. Directional transcutaneous assessment of venous inflow. American Heart Journal, 1971, 82, 86-92

Alexander, R. S. Tonic and reflex functions of medullary sympathetic cardiovascular centers. Journal of Neurophysiology, 1946, 9, 205-217.

Alexander, R. S. The peripheral venous system. In W. F. Hamilton & P. Dow (eds.), Handbook of physiology, Section 2: Circulation. Vol. 2. Washington, D. C.: American Physiological Society, 1963. 1075-1098.

Allwood, M. J., Barcroft, H., Hayes, J. P. L. A., & Hirsjarvi, E. A. The effect of mental arithmetic on the blood flow through normal, sympathectomized and hyperhibrotic hands. Journal of Physiology, 1959, 148, 108-116.

Altura, B. M. Chemical and humoral regulation of blood flow through the precapillary sphincter. Microvascular Research, 1971, 3, 361-384.

Ambrosi, C., & Starr, I. Incoordination of the cardiac contraction, as judged by the force ballistocardiogram and the carotid pulse derivative. American Heart Journal, 1965, 70, 761-774.

Amoroso, E. C., Bell, F. R., & Rosenberg, H. The relationship of the vasomotor and respiratory regions in the medulla oblongata of the sheep. Journal of Physiology, 1954, 126, 86-95

Antal, J. The role of the carotid sinus baroreceptors in muscular effort and in food intake. In P. Kezdi (Ed.), Baroreceptors and hypertension. Oxford: Pergamon Press, 1967.

Antal, J., & Gantt, W. H. Blood flow, blood pressure and heart rate changes accompanying hind leg flexion in conditional and unconditional reflexes. Conditional Reflex, 1970, 5, 197-206.

Apgar, V. A proposal for a new method of evaluation of the newborn infant. Current Research in Anesthesia and Analgesia, 1953, 32, 260-267.

Appleton, C. Classical reward conditioning of the heart rate response to auditory stimuli in three month old infants. Unpublished MA thesis, University of Massachusetts, 1972.

Ardill, B. L., Bhatnagar, V. M., Fentem, P. H., & Greenfield, A. D. M. Clinical use of venous occlusion plethysmography. Scandinavian Journal of Clinical and Laboratory Investigation, 1967, 19 (Suppl. 99), 95-100

Armitage, R., & Rose, G. A. The variability of measurements of casual blood pressure: I. A. laboratory study. Clinical Science, 1966, 30, 325-335.

Averill, J. R. Autonomic response patterns during sadness and mirth. Psychophysiology. 1969, 5, 399-414.

Averill, J. R., Olbrich, E. & Lazarus, R. S. Personality correlates of differential responsiveness to direct and vicarious threat: A failure to replicate previous findings. Journal of Personality and Social Psychology, 1972, 21, 25-29.

Ax, A. R. The physiological differentiation between fear and anger in humans. Psychosomatic Medicine, 1953, 15, 433-442.

Bach, L. M. N. Relationships between bulbar respiratory, vasomotor and somatic facilitatory and inhibitory areas. American Journal of Physiology, 1952, 171, 417-435.

Baer, P. E., & Fuhrer, M. J. Cognitive processes in the differential trace conditioning of electrodermal and vasomotor activity. Journal of Experimental Psychology, 1970, 84, 176-178.

Bankart, C. P., & Elliott, R. Heart rate and skin conductance in anticipation of shocks with varying probability of occurrence. Unpublished manuscript, 1972.

Banuazizi, A. Modification of an autonomic response by instrumental learning. Ph.D. Thesis, Yale University, 1968

Banuazizi, A. Discriminative shock-avoidance learning of an autonomic response under curare. Journal of Comparative and Physiological Psychology, 1972, 81, 336-346.

Barber, T. X. LSD, marihuana, yoga and hypnosis. Chicago: Aldine Publishing Co., 1970

Barber, T. X., DiCara, L. V., Kamiya, J., Miller, N. E., Shapiro, D., & Stoyva, J. (Eds.) Biofeedback & self-control. Chicago: Aldine-Atherton, 1971. (a)

Barber, T. X., DiCara, L. V., Kamiya, J., Miller, N. E., Shapiro, D., & Stoyva, J. (Eds.) Biofeedback & self-control 1970. Chicago: Aldine-Atherton, 1971. (b)

Barcroft, H. Sympathetic control of vessels in the hand and forearm skin. Physiological Reviews, 1960, 40 (Suppl. 4), 81-91.

Barcroft, H. Circulation in sketetal muscle. In W. F. Hamilton & P. Dow (eds.), Handbook of physiology, Section 2: Circulation. Vol. 2. Washington, D. C.: American Physiological Society, 1963, 1353-1385.

Barcroft, H., & Swan, H. J. C. Sympathetic control of human blood vessels. London: Arnold, 1953.

Bard, P. A diencephalic mechanism for the expression of rage with special reference to the sympathetic nervous system. American Journal of Physiology, 1928, 84, 490-519.

Bard, P. Anatomical organization of the central nervous system in relation to control of the heart and blood vessels. Physiological Reviews, 1960, Suppl. 4, 3-26.

Bard, P. Control of systemic blood vessels. In V. B. Mountcastle (Ed.), Medical Physiology (12th ed.) Vol. 1. St. Louis: C. V. Mosby, 1968, 150-177

Bartoshuk, A. K. Human neonatal cardiac acceleration to sound: Habituation and dishabituation. Perceptual and Motor Skills, 1962, 15, 15-27 (a).

Bartoshuk, A. K. Response decrement with repeated elicitation of human neonatal cardiac acceleration to sound. Journal of Comparative and Physiological Psychology, 1962, 55, 9-13 (b).

Baxter, C. F., Tewari, S., & Raeburn, S. The possible role of gamma-aminobutyric acid in the synthesis of protein. In advances in biochemical pharmacology, Vol. 4. New York: Raven Press, 1972, 211.

Bayliss, W. M. The Vasomotor System. New York: Longmans and Green, 1923

Beacham, W. S., & Perl, E. R. Background and reflex discharge of sympathetic preganglionic neurones in the spinal cat. Journal of Physiology, 1964, 172, 400-416.

Beattie, J., Brow, G. R., & Long, C. N. H. Physiological and anatomical evidence for existence of nerve tracts connecting the hypothalamus with spinal sympathetic centres. Proceedings of the Royal Society, Series B, 1930, 106, 253-275.

Beatty, J., & Kahneman, D. Pupillary changes in two memory tasks. Psychonomic Science, 1966, 5, 371-372.

Becker, W., Deecke, L., Hoehne, O., Iwase, K., Kornhuber, H. H., &
    Scheid, P. Bereitschaftspotential, Motor-potential und prae-
    motorische Positivierung der menschlichen Hirnrinde vor Willkur-
    bewegungen. Naturwissenschaften, 1968, 55, 550.
Becker, W., Iwase, K., Hoehne, O., & Kornhuber, H. H. Cerebral and
    ocular muscle potentials preceding voluntary eye-movements in man.
    Electroencephalography and Clinical Neurphysiology. 1972, in press.
Belanger, D., & Feldman, S. M. Effects of water deprivation upon
    heart rate and instrumental activity in the rat. Journal of
    Comparative and Physiological Psychology, 1962, 55, 220-225.
Bell, I. R., & Schwartz, G. E. Individual and situational factors
    in bidirectional voluntary control and reactivity of human heart
    rate. Unpublished manuscript, 1972. (a)
Bell, I. R., & Schwartz, G. E. Cognitive and somatic mechanisms in
    voluntary control of human heart rate. Paper presented at the Bio-
    feedback Research Society Meetings, Boston, Massachusetts, 1972. (b)
Benson, H., & Herd, J. A. Oscillometric measurement of arterial
    blood pressure. Circulation, 1969, 40 (Suppl. 3).
Benson, H., Herd, J. A., Morse, W. H., & Kelleher, R. T. The be-
    havioral induction of arterial hypertension and its reversal.
    American Journal of Physiology, 1969, 217, 30-34.
Benson, H., Shapiro, D., Tursky, B., & Schwartz, G. E. Through
    operant conditioning techniques in patients with essential hy-
    pertension. Science, 1971, 173, 740-742.
Berg, K. M., Berg, W. K., & Graham, F. K. Infant heart rate response
    as a function of stimulus and state. Psychophysiology, 1971, 8,
    30-44.
Berg, W. K. Habituation and dishabituation of cardiac responses in
    4-month-old, alert infants. Journal of Experimental Child Psy-
    chology, 1972, 14, 92-107.
Bergman, J. S., & Johnson, H. L. Sources of information which affect
    training and raising of heart rate. Psychophysiology, 1972, 9,
    30-39.
Bernstein, A. S. To what does the orienting response respond?
    Psychophysiology, 1969, 6, 338-350.
Bernstein, A. S., Taylor, K., Austen, B. G., Nathanson, M., & Scarpelli,
    A. Orienting response and apparent movement toward or away from the
    observer. Journal of Experimental Psychology, 1971, 87, 37-45.
Bilodeau, E. A. Acquisition of Skill. New York: Academic Press, 1966.
Bilodeau, E. A., & Bilodeau, I. M. Variable frequency of knowledge
    of results and the learning of a simple skill. Journal of Ex-
    perimental Psychology, 1958, 55, 379-383.
Bilodeau, I. McD. Information feedback. In E. A. Bilodeau and I.
    McD Bilodeau (Eds.), Principles of skill acquisition. New York:
    Academic Press, 1969.
Birren, J. E. Age changes in speed of behavior: Its central nature
    and physiological correlates. In A. T. Welford & J. E. Birren
    (Eds.) Behavior, aging and the nervous system. Springfield,
    Illinois: Charles C. Thomas, 1965.
Birren, J. E., Cardon, P. V., & Phillips, S. L. Reaction time as a
    function of the cardiac cycle in young adults. Science, 1963,
    140, 195-196.
Black, A. H. Cardiac conditioning in curarized dogs: The relation-
    ship between heart rate and skeletal behavior. In W. F. Prokasy

(Ed.), Classical conditioning: A symposium. New York: Appleton-Century-Crofts, 1965, 20-47.

Black, A. H.   A comment on yoked control designs. Technical Report
No. 11. Department of Psychology, McMaster University, Hamilton,
Ontario, September 1967. (a)

Black, A. H.   Operant conditioning of heart rate under curare. Technical Report No. 12, Department of Psychology, McMaster University, Hamilton, Ontario, October 1967. (b)

Black, A. H.   Autonomic aversive conditioning in infrahuman subjects.
In F. R. Brush (Ed), Aversive conditioning and learning. New
York: Academic Press, 1971, 3-104.

Black, A. H.   The direct control of neural processes by reward and
punishment. American Scientist, 1971, 59, 236-245. (b)

Black, A. H.   The operant conditioning of central nervous system electrical activity.   In G. H. Bower (Ed.), The psychology of learning and motivation. Vol. 6. New York: Academic Press, 1972. (a)

Black, A. H.   The operant conditioning of the electrical activity of
the brain as a method for controlling neural and mental processes.   In F. J. McGuigan (Ed.), The Psychophysiology of Thinking.   New York: Academic Press, 1973 (b) 35-68.

Black, A. H., Carlson, N., & Solomon, R.   Exploratory studies of the
conditioning of autonomic responses in curarized dogs. Psychological Monographs, 1962, 76 (29, Whole No. 548), 1-31.

Black, A. H., & DeToledo, L.   The relationship among classically conditioned responses: Heart rate and skeletal behavior.   In A. H.
Black and W. F. Prokasy (Eds.), Classical conditioning II: Current theory and research. New York: Appleton-Century-Crofts,
1972.   290-311.

Black, A. H., & Lang, W. M.   Cardiac conditioning and skeletal responding in curarized dogs. Psychological Reviews, 1964, 71,
80-85.

Black, A. H., & Young, G. A.   The electrical activity of the hippocampus and cortex in dogs operantly trained to move and to hold
still. Journal of Comparative and Physiological Psychology,
1972, 79, 128-141. (a)

Black, A. H., & Young, G. A.   Constraints on the operant conditioning of drinking.   In R. M. Gilbert and J. R. Millenson (Eds.),
Reinforcement: Behavioral analyses. New York: Academic Press,
1972.   Pp 35-50. (b)

Black, J. W., Duncan, W. A. M., & Shanks, R. G.   Comparison of some
properties of pronethalol and propranolol. British Journal of
Pharmacology, 1965, 25, 577-591.

Blair, D. A., Glover, W. E., Greenfield, A. D. M., & Roddie, I. C.
Excitation of cholinergic vasodilator nerves to human skeletal
muscles during emotional stress. Journal of Physiology, 1959,
148, 633-647.

Blanchard, E. B., & Young, L. B.   Self-control of cardiac functioning: A promise as yet unfulfilled. Psychological Bulletin,
1973, 79, 145-163.

Blanchard, E. B., Young, L. B., & McLeod, P.   Awareness of heart
activity and self-control of heart rate. Psychophysiology, 1972,
9, 63-68.

Bleecker, E. R., & Engel, B. T.   Learned control of ventricular rate
in patients with atrialfibrillation. Psychosomatic Medicine,
1973, 35, 161-175.

Bleecker, E. R. and Engel, B. T.   Learned control of cardiac rate
    and cardiac conduction in the Wolff-Parkinson-White syndrome.
    New England Journal of Medicine, 1973, 288, 560-562.
Blood, F. R., Elliott, R. V. & D'Amour, F. E.   The physiology of the
    rat in extreme anoxia. American Journal of Physiology, 1946,
    146, 319-329.
Bolme, P., Ngai, S. H., Uvnas, B., & Wallenberg, L. R.   Circulatory
    and behavioral effects on electrical stimulation of the sympa-
    thetic vasodilator areas in the hypothalamus and the mesencepha-
    lon in unanesthetized dogs. Acta Physiologica Scandinavica,
    1967, 70, 334-346.
Bolme, P., & Novotny, J.   Conditional reflex activation of the sympa-
    thetic cholinergic vasodilator nerves in the dog. Acta Physio-
    logica Scandinavica, 1969, 77, 58-67.
Bolton, B., Carmichael, E. A., Sturup, G., Vaso-constriction follow-
    ing deep inspiration. Journal of Physiology, 1936, 86, 83-94.
Bond, D. D.   Sympathetic and vagal interaction in emotional responses
    of the heart rate. American Journal of Physiology, 1943, 138,
    468-478.
Bovet, D., & Longo, V. G.   Action of natural and synthetic curares on
    the cortical activity of the rabbit. Electroencephalography and
    Clinical Neurophysiology, 1953, 5, 225-234.
Bower, G., & Grusec, T.   Effect of prior Pavlovian discrimination
    training upon learning an operant discrimination. Journal of
    Experimental Analysis of Behavior, 1964, 7, 401-404.
Bowers, K. S.   The effects of UCS temporal uncertainty of heart rate
    and pain. Psychophysiology, 1971, 8, 382-389. (a)
Bowers, K. S.   Heart rate and GSR concomitants of vigilance and
    arousal. Canadian Journal of Psychology, 1971, 25, 175-184. (b)
Brackbill, Y.   Developmental studies of classical conditioning: Be-
    havioral state and temporal conditioning of heart rate. Paper
    presented at Society for Psychophysiological Research, Boston,
    1972.
Brackbill, Y., Fitzgerald, H., & Lintz, L.   A developmental study of
    classical conditioning. Society for Research in Child Develop-
    ment Monographs, 1967, 32 (8, Serial No. 116).
Brady, J. V.   Emotion revisited. Journal of Psychiatric Research, 1971,
    8, 363-384.
Brady, J. V., Kelly, D., & Plumlee, L.   Autonomic and behavioral re-
    sponses of the rhesus monkey to emotional conditioning. Annals
    of the New York Academy of Sciences, 1969, 159, 959-975.
Braunwald, E., Epstein, S. E., Glick, G., Wechsler, A. S., & Braun-
    wald, N. S.   Relief of angina pectoris by electrical stimulation
    of the carotid-sinus nerves. The New England Journal of Medicine,
    1967, 277, 1278-1283.
Brener, J.   Heart rate as an avoidance response. Psychological Record,
    1966, 16, 329-336.
Brener, J.   Some curious concepts concerning cardiovascular control.
    Paper presented at a Symposium at the Society for Psychophysi-
    ology Research Meetings, New Orleans, 1972. (a)
Brener, J.   Some experiments on the relationship between somatic-
    motor and heart rate conditioning. Paper prepared for workshop
    at Winter Conference on Brain Research, Aspen, Colorado, January
    1970. (b)
Brener, J., & Goesling, W. J.   The effects of instruction on heart

rate control. Papers read at SEPA conference, Atlanta, 1967.

Brener, J. & Goesling, W. J. Heart rate and conditioned activity. Paper read at Society for Psychophysiological Research Meeting, Washington, D. C., October 1968

Brener, J. & Goesling, W. J. Avoidance conditioning of activity and immobility in rats. Journal of Comparative and Physiological Psychology, 1970, 70, 276-280.

Brener, J. & Hothersall, D. Heart rate control under conditions of augmented sensory feedback. Psychophysiology, 1966, 3, 23-28.

Brener, J. & Hothersall, D. Paced respiration and heart rate control. Psychophysiology, 1967, 4, 1-6.

Brener, J. & Kleinman, R. A. Learned control of decreases in systolic blood pressure. Nature, 1970, 226, 1063-1064.

Brener, J., Kleinman, R. A., & Goesling, W. J., The effects of different responses to augmented sensory feedback on the control of heart rate. Psychophysiology, 1969, 5, 510-516.

Brener, J., & Shanks, E. The interaction of instructions and feedback in the training of cardiovascular control. In preparation, 1972.

Bridger, W. H. Sensory habituation and discrimination in the human neonate. American Journal of Psychiatry, 1961, 117, 991-996.

Bridger, W. H., & Birns, B. Recent Advances in Biological Psychiatry. Vol. 5. Neonates' behavioral and autonomic responses to stress during soothing. New York: Plenum Press, 1963, 1-6.

Brod, J. Essential Hypertension. Haemodynamic observations with a bearing on its pathogenesis. The Lancet, 1960, 2, 773-778.

Brod, J. Haemodynamic basis of acute pressor reactions and hypertension. British Heart Journal, 1963, 25, 227-245.

Brod, J., Fencl, V., Hejl, L., Jirka, J., & Ulrych, M. General and regional haemodynamic pattern underlying essential hypertension. Clinical Science, 1962, 23, 339-349.

Brod, J., Hejl, Z., & Ulrych, M. Metabolic changes in the forearm muscle and skin during emotional muscular vasodilation. Clinical Science, 1963, 25, 1-10.

Brown, A. M. Sympathetic ganglionic transmission and the cardiovascular changes of the defense reaction in the cat. Circulation Research, 1969, 24, 843-849

Brown, C. C. The techniques of plethysmography. In C. C. Brown (Ed.), Methods in psychophysiology. Baltimore: William & Wilkins, 1967, 54-74.

Browse, N. L., Shepherd, J. T., & Donald, D. E. Differences in response of veins and resistance vessels in limbs to the same stimulus. American Journal of Physiology, 1966, 211, 1241-1247.

Bruner, A. Reinforcement strength in classical conditioning of leg flexion, freezing, and heart rate in cats. Conditional Reflex, 1969, 4, 24-31.

Buchwald, J. S., & Eldred, E. Activity in muscle spindle circuits during conditioning. In D. Barker (Ed.), Symposium on muscle receptors. Hong Kong: Hong Kong University Press, 1962, 175-183.

Buchwald, J. S., Standish, M., Eldred, E. & Halas, E. S. Contribution of muscle spindle circuits to learning as suggested by training under Flaxedil. Electroencephalography and Clinical Neurophysiology, 1964, 16, 582-594.

Budzynski, T., Stoyva, J. & Adler, C. Feedback-induced muscle relaxation: Application to tension headache. Journal of Behavior Therapy and Experimental Psychiatry, 1970, 1, 205-211.

Bulbring, E., & Burn, J. H. The sympathetic dilator fibres in the muscles of the cat and dog. Journal of Physiology, 1935, 83, 483-501.

Bunag, R. D., Page, I. H., & McCubbin, J. W. Inhibition of renin release by vasopressin and angiotensin. Cardiovascular Research, 1967, 1, 67-73.

Bunzl-Federn, E. Der centrale Ursprung des Nervus Vagus. Monatsschrift fur psychiatrie und Neurologie, 1899, 5, 1-22.

Burch, G. E. Digital plethysmography. New York: Grune & Stratton, 1954, (a)

Burch, G. E. A method for measuring venous tone in digital veins of intact man: Evidence for increased digital venous tone in congestive heart failure. Archives of Internal Medicine, 1954, 94, 724-742. (b)

Burch, G. E. Influence of the central nervous system on veins in man. Physiological Reviews, 1960, 40 (Suppl. 4), 50-56.

Burch, G. E., & DePasquale, N. P. Methods for studying the influence of higher central nervous centers on the peripheral circulation of intact man. American Heart Journal, 1965, 70, 411-422.

Burgess, M., & Hokanson, J. E. Effects of increased heart rate on intellectual performance. Journal of Abnormal and Social Psychology, 1964, 65, 85-91

Burki, N., & Guz, A. The distensibility characteristics of the capacitance vessels of the forearm in normal subjects. Cardiovascular Research, 1970, 4, 93-98.

Burton, A. C. The range and variability of the blood flow in the human fingers and the vasomotor regulation of body temperature. American Journal of Physiology, 1939, 127, 437-453.

Burton, A. C. Physiology and biophysics of the circulation. Chicago: Year Book Medical Publishers, 1965.

Burton, A. C., Editorial - The criterion for diastolic pressure revolution and counterrevolution, Circulation, 1967, 34, 805-809. (a)

Burton, A. C. Report of a Subcommittee of the Postgraduate Education Committee, American Heart Association, "Recommendations for human blood pressure determination by sphygmomanometers, Circulation, 1967, 34, 980-988. (b)

Calaresu, F. R., & Henry, J. L. The mechanism of the cardio-acceleration elicited by electrical stimulation of the parahypoglossal area in the cat. Journal of Physiology, 1970, 210, 107-120.

Calaresu, F. R., & Pearce, J. W. Effects on heart rate of electrical stimulation of medullary vagal structures. Journal of Physiology, 1965, 176, 241-251. (a)

Calaresu, F. R., & Pearce, J. W. Electrical activity of efferent vagal fibers and dorsal nucleus of the vagus during reflex bradycardia in the cat. Journal of Physiology, 1965, 176, 228-240. (b)

Calaresu, F. R., & Thomas, M. R. The function of the paramedian reticular nucleus in the control of heart rate in the cat. Journal of Physiology, 1971, 216, 143-158.

Callaway, E., & Layne, R. S. Interaction between the visual evoked response and two spontaneous biological rhythms: The EEG alpha cycle and the cardiac arousal cycle. Annals of the New York Academy of Sciences, 1964, 112(1), 421-431.

Campbell, D., Sanderson, R. E., & Laverty, S. G. Characteristics of a conditioned response in human subjects during extinction trials following a single traumatic conditioning trial. Journal of Abnormal and Social Psychology. 1964, 68, 627-639.

Campos, J. J., & Johnson, H. J. The effects of verbalization instructions and visual attention on heart rate and skin conductance. Psychophysiology, 1966, 2, 305-310.

Campos, J. J., & Johnson, H. J. Affect, verbalization, and directional fractionation of autonomic response. Psychophysiology, 1967, 3, 285-290.

Campos, J., Langer, A., & Krowitz, A. Cardiac responses on the visual cliff in pre-locomotor human infants. Science, 1970, 170, 196-197.

Cannon, W. B. Bodily changes in pain, hunger, fear, and rage. (2nd ed.) New York: Appleton-Century, 1936.

Cannon, W. B., & Britton, S. W. Studies on the conditions of activity in endocrine glands. American Journal of Physiology, 1925, 72, 283-294.

Capps, R. B. A method for measuring tone and reflex constriction of the capillaries, venules and veins of the human hand with the results in normal and diseased states. Journal of Clinical Investigation, 1936, 15, 229-239.

Carlton, P. L. Some behavioral effects of atropine and Methylatropine. Psychological Reports, 1962, 10, 579-582.

Carmona, A. Trial and error of the cortical EEG activity, Unpublished Ph.D. Thesis, Yale University, 1967.

Carmona, A. Sistema nervioso viscersal. Rev. Medica de Chile, 1971, 99, 15-26.

Carmona, A., Demierre, T., & Miller, N. E. Instrumental learning of gastric vascular tonicity (GVT) responses. Submitted manuscript 1972.

Celander, O. The range of control exercised by the "sympathico adrenal system." Acta Physiologica Scandinavica, 1954, 32 (Suppl. 116). 1-132.

Chai, C. Y., Share, N. N., & Wang, S. C. Central control of sympathetic cardiac augmentation in lower brain stem of the cat. American Journal of Physiology, 1963, 205, 749-753.

Chai, C. Y. & Wang, S. C. Localization of central cardiovascular control mechanism in lower brain stem of the cat. American Journal of Physiology, 1962, 202, 25-30.

Chai, C. Y., & Wang, S. C. Integration of sympathetic cardiovascular mechanisms in medulla oblongata of the cat. American Journal of Physiology, 1968, 215, 1310-1315.

Chase, M. H., & Harper, R. M. Somatomotor and visceromotor correlates of operantly conditioned 12-14 c/sec censorimotor cortical activity. Electroencephalography and Clinical Neurophysiology, 1971, 31, 85-92.

Chase, W. G., Graham, F. K., & Graham, D. T. Components of HR response in anticipation of reaction time and exercise tasks. Journal of Experimental Psychology, 1968, 76, 642-648.

Chen, M. P., Lim, R. K. S., Wang, S. C., & Yi, C. L. On the question of a myelencephalic sympathetic centre. I. The effect of stimulation of the pressor area on visceral function. Chinese Journal of Physiology, 1936, 10, 445-472

Chen, M. P., Lim, R. K. S., Wang, S. C., & Yi, C. L. On the question of a myelencephalic sympathetic centre. II. Experimental evidence for a reflex sympathetic centre in the medulla. Chinese Journal of Physiology, 1937, 11, 355-366. (a)

Chen, M. P., Lim, R. K. S., Wang, S. C., & Yi, C. L. On the question
    of a myelencephalic sympathetic centre. III. Esperimental locali-
    zation of the centre. Chinese Journal of Physiology, 1937, 11,
    367-384. (b)
Chen, M. P., Lim, R. K. S., Wang, S. C., & Yi, C. L. On the question
    of a myelencephalic sympathetic centre. IV. Experimental locali-
    zation of its descending pathways. Chinese Journal of Physiology,
    1937, 11, 385-408. (c)
Chiang, B. N., Perlman, L. V., Ostander, L. D., Jr., & Epstein, F. H.
    Relationship of premature systoles to coronary heart disease and
    sudden death in the Tecumseh epidemiologic study. Annals of
    Internal Medicine, 1969, 70, 1159-1166.
Church, R. M. LoLordo, V., Overmier, J. B., & Solomon, R. L. Cardiac
    responses to shock in curarized dogs: Effects of shock intensity
    and duration, warning signal, and prior experience with shock.
    Journal of Comparative and Physiological Psychology, 1966, 62,
    1-7.
Cicardo, V. H., & Garcia, J. C. Neurogenic arterial hypertension by
    the corticospinal pathway. Archives Internationales de Physiologie
    et de Biochimie, 1958, 66, 309-317
Clarke, N. P., Smith, O. A., Jr., & Shearn, D. W. Topographical
    representation of vascular smooth muscle of limbs in the primate
    motor cortex. American Journal of Physiology, 1968, 214, 122-129.
Clifton, C. An economical system for collecting and reducing heart-
    rate data, using someone else's small computer. Behavioral
    Research Methods and Instrumentation, 1971, 3, 261-263.
Clifton, R. K. Heart rate conditioning in the newborn infant.
    Journal of Experimental Child Psychology, 1974. In Press.
Clifton, R. K., Graham, F. K., & Hatton, H. M. Newborn heart-rate
    response and response habituation as a function of stimulus du-
    ration. Journal of Experimental Child Psychology, 1968, 6,
    265-278.
Clifton, R. K., & Meyers, W. J. The heart-rate response of four-
    month-old infants to auditory stimuli. Journal of Experimental
    Child Psychology, 1969, 7, 122-135.
Cochrane, R. High blood pressure as a psychosomatic disorder: A
    selective review. British Journal of Social and Clinical Psy-
    chology, 1971, 10, 61-72.
Coffman, J. D., & Cohen, A. S. Total and capillary fingertip blood
    flow in Raynaud's phenomenon. New England Journal of Medicine,
    1971, 285, 259-263.
Cohen, D. H. Development of a vertebrate experimental model for
    cellular neurophysiologic studies of learning. Conditional
    Reflex, 1969, 4, 61-80.
Cohen, D. H. The informational flow and central pathways mediating
    a conditioned autonomic response. In L. V. DiCara (Ed.),
    Advances in Autonomic and Limbic System Research. New York:
    Plenum Press, 1972, in press.
Cohen, D. H., & Pitts, L. H. Vagal and sympathetic components of
    conditioned cardioacceleration in the pigeon. Brain Research,
    1968, 9, 15-31.
Cohen, D. H., and Durkovic, R. G. Cardiac and respiratory condition-
    ing, differentiation, and extinction in the pigeon. Journal of
    the Experimental Analysis of Behavior, 1966, 9, 681-688.

Cohen, D. H., & Schnall, A. M. Medullary cells of origin of vagal cardioinhibitory fibers in the pigeon. II. Electrical stimulation of the dorsal motor nucleus. Journal of Comparative Neurology, 1970, 140, 321-342.

Cohen, D. H., Schnall, A. M., Macdonald, R. L., & Pitts, L. H. Medullary cells of origin of vagal cardioinhibitory fibers in the pigeon. I. Anatomical studies of peripheral vagus nerve and the dorsal motor nucleus. Journal of Comparative Neurology, 1970, 140, 299-320.

Cohen, M. J. The relation between heart rate and electromyographic activity in a discriminated escape-avoidance maradigm. Psychophysiology, 1972, in press.

Cohen, M. J., & Johnson, H. J. Effects of intensity and the signal value of stimuli on the orienting and defensive responses. Journal of Experimental Psychology, 1971, 88, 286-288. (a)

Cohen, M. J., & Johnson, H. J. Relationship between heart rate and muscular activity within a classical conditioning paradigm. Journal of Experimental Psychology, 1971, 90, 222-226. (b)

Collen, A., & Libby, W. L., Jr. Effects of hunger upon the cardiac deceleratory response to food pictures. Paper presented at the meeting of the Society for Psychophysiological Research, Clayton, Missouri, October, 1971.

Conel, J. Histologic development of the cerebral cortex. In The biology of mental health and disease. New York: P. B. Hoeber, Inc., 1952, 1-10.

Connor, W. H., & Lang, P. J. Cortical slow-wave and cardiac rate responses in stimulus orientation and reaction time conditions. Journal of Experimental Psychology, 1969, 82(2), 310-320.

Cook, M. R. The cutaneous vasomotor orienting response and its habituation. Unpublished doctoral disseration, University of Oklahoma, 1970.

Cook, M. R. The cephalic vasomotor orienting response. Paper presented at the meeting of the Society for Psychophysiological Research, St. Louis, October, 1971. (a)

Cook, M. R. Criteria for habituation of the vasomotor orienting response. Paper presented at the meeting of the Eastern Psychological Association, New York, April 1971. (b)

Coote, J. H., & Perez-Gonzalez, J. F. The baroreceptor reflex during stimulation of the hypothalamic defense region. Journal of Physiology, 1972, 224, 74-75.

Costello, C. G., Brown, P. A., & Low, K. Some physiological concomitants of pursuit rotor performance and reminiscence. Journal of Motor Behavior, 1969, 1, 181-194.

Craig, K. D., & Wood, K. Physiological differentiation of direct and vicarious affective arousal. Canadian Journal of Behavioral Science, 1969, 2, 98-105.

Craig, K. D. & Wood, K. Autonomic components of observers' responses to pictures of homicide victims and nude females. Journal of Experimental Research in Personality, 1971, 5, 304-309.

Crider, A., Schwartz, G. E., & Shapiro, D. Operant suppression of electrodermal response rate as a function of punishment schedule. Journal of Experimental Psychology, 1970, 83, 333-334.

Crider, A., Schwartz, G. E., & Shnidman, S. On the criteria for instrumental autonomic conditioning. Psychological Bulletin, 1969, 71, 455-461.

Crosby, E. C., Humphrey, T., & Lauer, E. W. Correlative Anatomy of the Nervous System. New York: The Macmillan Co., 1962.

Culp, W. C., & Edelberg, R. Regional specificity in the electrodermal reflex. Perceptual and Motor Skills, 1966, 23, 623-627.

Cummings, G. R., & Carr, W. Hemodynamic response to exercise after beta-adrenergic and parasympathetic blockade. Canadian Journal of Physiological Pharmacology, 1967, 45, 813-819.

Cyon, E. de, & Ludwig, C. Die Reflexe eines der sensiblen Nerven des Herzen auf die motorischen der Blutgefasse. Bericht uber die Verhandlungen der Sachsischen Akademie der Wissenschaften zu Leipzig, 1866, 18, 307-328.

Dahl, H., & Spence, D. P. Mean heart rate predicted by task demand characteristics. Psychophysiology, 1971, 7, 369-376.

Dahl, L. K., Heine, M., & Tassinari, L. Effects of chronic excess salt ingestion. Evidence that genetic factors play an important role in susceptibility to experimental hypertension. Journal of Experimental Medicine, 1962, 115, 1173-1190.

Damaser, E. C., Shor, R. E., & Orne, M. T. Physiological effects during hypnotically requested emotions. Psychosomatic Medicine, 1963, 25, 334-343.

Danilewsky, B. Experimentelle Beitrage zur Physiologie des Gehirns. Pflugers Archiv, 1875, 11, 128-138.

Datey, K. K., Deshmukh, S. N. Dalvi, C. P., & Vinekar, S. L. "Shavasan": A Yogic exercise in the management of hypertension. Angiology, 1969, 20, 325-333.

Davidoff, R. A., & McDonald, D. G. Alpha blocking and autonomic responses in neurological patients. Archives of Neurology, 1964, 10, 283-292.

Davis, D. L., & Hammond, M. C. Blood flow redistribution in the dog paw. American Journal of Physiology, 1968, 215, 496-501.

Davis, R. C. Continuous recording of arterial pressure: An analysis of the problem. Journal of Comparative and Physiological Psychology, 1957, 50, 524-529.

Deane, G. E. Human heart responses during experimentally induced anxiety. Journal of Experimental Psychology, 1961, 61, 489-493.

Deane, G. E. Human heart rate responses during experimentally induced anxiety: A follow-up with controlled respiration. Journal of Experimental Psychology, 1964, 67, 193-195.

Deane, G. E. Cardiac activity during experimentally induced anxiety. Psychophysiology, 1969, 6, 17-30.

Delfini, L. F., & Campos, J. J. Signal detection and the "cardiac arousal cycle." Paper presented at the meeting of the Society for Psychophysiological Research, St. Louis, October 1971.

Delgado, J. M. R. Circulatory effects of cortical stimulation. Physiological Reviews, 1960, 40(Suppl. 4), 146-171.

Dengerink, H. A. Anxiety, aggression, and physiological arousal. Journal of Experimental Research in Personality, 1971, 5, 223-232.

DeSanctis, R. W., Block, P., & Hutter, A. M., Jr., Tachyarrhythmias in myocardial infarction. Circulation, 1972, 45, 681-702.

DeToledo, L. Changes in heart rate during conditioned suppression in rats as a function of US intensity and type of CS. Journal of Comparative and Physiological Psychology, 1971, 77, 528-538.

DeToledo, L., & Black, A. H. Heart rate: Changes during conditioned suppression in rats. Science, 1966, 152, 1404-1406.

DiCara, L. V. Analysis of arterial blood gases in the curarized, artificially respirated rat. Behavior Research Methods and Instrumentation, 1970, 2, 67-70. (a)

DiCara, L. V. Learning in the autonomic nervous system. Scientific American, 1970, 222, 30-39. (b)

DiCara, L. V. Learning of cardiovascular responses: A review and a description of physiological and biochemical consequences. Transactions of the New York Academy of Sciences, 1971, 33, 417-422.

DiCara, L. V., Braun, J. J., & Pappas, B. A. Classical conditioning and instrumental learning of cardiac and gastrointestinal responses following removal of neocortex in rats. Journal of Comparative & Physiological Psychology, 1970, 73, 208-216.

DiCara, L. V., & Miller, N. E. Changes in heart rate instrumentally learned by curarized rats as avoidance responses. Journal of Comparative and Physiological Psychology, 1968, 65, 8-12. (a)

DiCara, L. V., & Miller, N. E. Instrumental learning of peripheral vasomotor responses by the curarized rat. Communications in Behavioral Biology, Part A, 1968, 1, 209-212. (b)

DiCara, L. V., & Miller, N. E. Instrumental learning of systolic blood pressure responses by curarized rats: Dissociation of cardiac and vascular changes. Psychosomatic Medicine, 1968, 30, 489-494. (c)

DiCara, L. V., & Miller, N. E. Long term retention of instrumentally learned heart-rate changes in the curarized rat. Communications in Behavioral Biology, Part A, 1968, 2, 19-23. (d)

DiCara, L. V., & Miller, N. E. Heart-rate learning in the non-curarized state, transfer to the curarized state, and subsequent retraining in the noncurarized state. Physiology and Behavior, 1969, 4, 621-624. (a)

DiCara, L. V., & Miller, N. E. Transfer of instrumentally learned heart rate changes from curarized to noncurarized state. Journal of Comparative and Physiological Psychology, 1969, 68, 159-162. (b)

DiCara, L. V., & Stone, E. A. The effect of instrumental heart rate training on rat cardiac and brain catecholamines. Psychosomatic Medicine, 1970, 32, 359-368.

DiCara, L. V., & Weiss, J. M. Effect of heart rate learning under curare on subsequent noncurarized avoidance learning. Journal of Comparative and Physiological Psychology, 1969, 69, 368-374.

Dittmar, C. Ueber die Lage des sogenannten Gefasscentrums in der Medulla oblongata. Berict uber die Verhandlungen der Sachsischen Akademie der Wissenschaften zu Leipzig, 1873, 25, 449-469.

Doba, N., & Reis, D. J. Cerebellum: Role in reflex cardiovascular adjustment to posture. Brain Research, 1972, 39, 495-500.

Doba, N., & Reis, D. J. Acute fulminating neurogenic hypertension produced by brainstem lesions in the rat. Circulation Research, 1973, 32, 584-593.

Doerr, H. O., & Hokanson, J. E. A relation between heart rate and performance in children. Journal of Personality and Social Psychology, 1965, 2, 70-76.

Doerr, H. O., & Hokanson, J. E. Food deprivation performance and heart rate in the rat. Journal of Comparative and Physiological Psychology, 1968, 65, 227-231.

Donald, D. E., & Samueloff, S. L. Exercise tachycardia not due to blood-borne agents in canine cardiac denervation. American Journal of Physiology, 1966, 211, 703-711.

Donald, D. E., & Shepherd, J. T.   Response to exercise in dogs with
    cardiac denervation. American Journal of Physiology, 1963, 205,
    393-400.
Douglas, W. W.   Autocoids.   In L. S. Goodman and A. Gillman (Eds.)
    Pharmacological basis of therapeutics. New York: McMillan,
    1970, 620-662.
Downs, D., Cardozo, C., Schneiderman, N., Yehle, A. L., VanDercar, D.
    H., & Zwilling, G.   Central effects of atropine upon aversive
    classical conditioning in rabbits. Psychopharmacologia, 1972,
    23, 318-333.
Doyle, A. E., Fraser, J. R. E., & Marshall, R. J.   Reactivity of fore-
    arm vessels to vasoconstrictive substance in hypertensive and
    normotensive subjects. Clinical Science, 1959, 18, 441-454.
Drazen, J. M., & Herd, J. A.   Cardiac output at rest in the squirrel
    monkey: Role of β-adrenergic activity. American Journal of
    Physiology, 1972, 222, 988-993.
Drill, U. A. Pharmacology in Medicine. (3rd ed.) Ed. by J. R. Di
    Plama. New York: Blakistan, 1965.
Ducharme, R.   Activite physique et deactivation: Baisse du rhythme
    cardiaque au cours de l'activite instrumentale. Canadian Jour-
    nal of Psychology, 1966, 20, 445-454.
Duffy, E. Activation and behavior. New York: John Wiley & Sons, 1962.
Duggan, J. J., Love, V. L., & Lyons, R. H.   A study of reflex veno-
    motor reactions in man. Circulation, 1953, 7, 869-873
Dunlop, D., & Shanks, R. G.   Inhibition of the carotid sinus reflex
    by the chronic administration of propranolol. British Journal
    of Pharmacology, 1969, 36, 132-143.
Durrer, D., Schuilenberg, R. N., & Willens, H. S.   Pre-excitation re-
    visited. American Journal of Cardiology, 1970, 25, 690-697.
Dustan, H. P., Tarazi, R. C., & Bravo, E. L.   Physiologic character-
    istics of hypertension. The American Journal of Medicine, 1972,
    52, 610-622.
Dykman, R.   On the nature of classical conditioning. In C. C. Brown
    (Ed.), Methods in Psychophysiology. Baltimore: Williams & Wil-
    kins, 1967.
Dykman, R. A., & Gantt, W. H.   The parasympathetic component of un-
    learned and acquired cardiac responses. Journal of Comparative
    and Physiological Psychology, 1956, 52, 163-167.
Dykman, R. A., Mack, R. L., & Ackerman, P. T.   The evaluation of auto-
    nomic and motor components of the nonavoidance conditioned re-
    sponse in the dog. Psychophysiology, 1965, 1, 209-230.
Eason, R. G., & Dudley, L. M.   Physiological and behavioral indicants
    of activation. Psychophysiology, 1971, 7, 223-232.
Edelberg, R.   The relationship between the galvanic skin response,
    vaso-constriction, and tactile sensitivity. Journal of Experi-
    mental Psychology, 1961, 62, 187-195.
Edelberg, R.   Mechanisms of electrodermal adaptations for locomotion,
    manipulation or defense.   In E. Stellar & J. M. Sprague (Eds.),
    Progress in physiological psychology. New York: Academic Press,
    1972, in press.
Edwards, D. C., & Alsip, J. E.   Intake-rejection, verbalization, and
    affect: Effects on heart rate and skin conductance. Psycho-
    physiology, 1969, 6, 6-12. (a)
Edwards, D. C., & Alsip, J. E.   Stimulus detection during periods of
    high and low heart rate. Psychophysiology, 1969, 5, 431-434. (b)

Eich, R. H., Cuddy, R. P., Smulyan, H., & Lyons, R. H. Hemodynamics in labile hypertension. A follow-up study. Circulation, 1966, 34, 299-307.

Eisenberg, R. B., Griffin, E. J., Coursin, D. B., & Hunter, M. A. Auditory behavior in the human neonate: A preliminary report. Journal of Speech and Hearing Research, 1964, 7, 245-269.

Eliasson, S., Folkow, B., Lindgren, P., & Uvnas, B. Activation of sympathetic vasodilator nerves to the skeletal muscles in the cat by hypothalamic stimulation. Acta Physiologica Scandinavica, 1951, 23, 333-351.

Eliasson, S., Lindgren, P., & Uvnas, B. Representation in the hypothalamus and the motor cortex in the dog of the sympathetic vasodilator outflow to the skeletal muscle. Acta Physiological Scandinavia, 1952, 27, 18-37.

Eliasson, S., Lindgren, P., & Uvnas, B. The hypothalamus, a relay station of the sympathetic vasodilator tract. Acta Physiologica Scandinavica, 1954, 31, 290-300.

Elliott, R. Physiological activity and performance: A comparison of kindergarten children with young adults. Psychological Monographs, 1964, 78(10, Whole No. 587).

Elliott, R. Effects of uncertainty about the nature and advent of a noxious stimulus (shock) upon heart rate. Journal of Personality and Social Psychology, 1966, 3, 353-356. (a)

Elliott, R. Physiological activity and performance in children and adults: A two-year follow-up. Journal of Experimental Child Psychology, 1966, 4, 58-80. (b)

Elliott, R. Reaction time and heart rate as functions of magnitude of incentive and probability of success: A replication and extension. Journal of Experimental Research in Personality, 1966, 1, 174-178. (c)

Elliott, R. Tonic heart rate: Experiments on the effects of collative variables lead to a hypothesis about its motivational significance. Journal of Personality and Social Psychology, 1969, 12, 211-288.

Elliott, R. Comment on the comparability of measures of heart rate in cross-laboratory comparison. Journal of Experimental Research in Personality, 1970, 4, 156-158. (a)

Elliott, R. Simple reaction time: Effects associated with age, preparatory interval, incentive-shift, and mode of presentation. Journal of Experimental Child Psychology, 1970, 9, 86-107. (b)

Elliott, R. The significance of heart rate for behavior: A critique of Lacey's hypothesis. Journal of Personality and Social Psychology, 1972, 22, 398-409.

Elliott, R., Bankart, B., & Light, T. Differences in the motivational significance of heart rate and palmar conductance: Two tests of a hypothesis. Journal of Personality and Social Psychology, 1970, 14, 166-172.

Elliott, R., & Graf, U. Visual sensitivity as a function of phase of cardiac cycle. Psychophysiology, 1972, 9, 3-16.

Elster, A. J. Cardiovascular responses to intracranial microinjection of acetylcholine or nonepinephrine in unanesthetized rabbits. Unpublished doctoral dissertation, Department of Biology, University of Miami, 1971.

Elster, A. J., VanDercar, D. H., & Schneiderman, N. Classical conditioning of heart rate discriminations using subcortical electrical stimulations as conditioned and unconditioned stimuli. Physiology and Behavior, 1970, 5, 503-508.

Engel, B. T. Operant conditioning of cardiac function: A status report. Psychophysiology, 1972, 9, 161-177.

Engel, B. T., & Chism, R. A. Operant conditioning of heart rate speeding. Psychophysiology, 1967, 3, 418-426. (a)

Engel, B. T., & Chism, R. A. Effect of increases and decreases in breathing rate or heart rate and finger pulse volume. Psychophysiology. 1967, 4, 83-89. (b)

Engel, B. T., & Hansen, S. P. Operant conditioning of heart rate slowing. Psychophysiology, 1966, 3, 176-187.

Enoch, D. M., & Kerr, F. W. L. Hypothalamic vasopressor and vesicopressor pathways. II. Anotomic study of their course and connections. Archives of Neurology, 1967, 16, 307-320.

Epstein, S. E., Robinson, B. F., Kahler, R. L., & Braunwald, E. Effects of beta-adrenergic blockade on the cardiac response to maximal and submaximal exercise in man. Journal of Clinical Investigation, 1965, 44, 1745-1753.

Erlanger, J. Blood volume and its regulation. Physiological Reviews, 1921, 1, 177-207.

Estes, W. K. Reinforcement in human behavior. American Scientist, 1972, 60, 723-729.

Estes, W. K., & Skinner, B. F. Some quantitative properties of anxiety. Journal of Experimental Psychology, 1941, 29, 390-400.

Evans, J. F. Social facilitation in a competitive situation. Canadian Journal of Behavioral Science, 1971, 3, 276-281.

Evans, J. F. Resting heart rate and the effects of an incentive. Psychonomic Science, 1972, 26, 99-100.

Evans, S. H., & Anastasio, E. J. Misuse of analysis of covariance when treatment effect and covariate are confounded. Psychological Bulletin, 1968, 69, 225-234.

Everett, G. M. Pharmacological studies of d-tubocurarine and other curare fractions. Journal of Pharmacology and Experimental Therapeutics, 1948, 92, 236-248.

Farmer, J. B., & Levy, G. P. A comparison of some cardiovascular properties of propranolol, MJ1999 and quinidine in relation to their effects in hypertensive animals. British Journal of Pharmacology, 1968, 34, 116-126.

Fehr, F., & Stern, J. Heart rate conditioning in the rat. Journal of Psychosomatic Research, 1965, 8, 441-453.

Feigl, E. O. Carotid sinus reflex control of coronary blood flow. Circulation Research, 1968, 23, 223-237.

Feigl, E., Johansson, B., & Lofving, B. Renal vasoconstriction and the 'defense reaction.' Acta Physiologica Scandinavica, 1964, 62, 429-435.

Ferguson, G. A. Nonparametric trend analysis. Montreal: McGill University Press, 1965.

Ferrario, C. M., Gildenberg, P. L., & McCubbin, J. W. Cardiovascular effects of angiotensin mediated by the central nervous system. Circulation Research, 1972, 30, 257-262.

Festinger, L., & Canon, L. K. Information about spatial location based on knowledge about efference. Psychological Review, 1965, 72, 373-384.

Festinger, L., Ono, H., Burnham, C. A., & Bamber, D. Efference and the conscious experience of perception. Journal of Experimental Psychology, 1967, 74, (4, Pr. 2).

Fetz, E. D., & Finocchio, D. V. Operant conditioning of specific patterns of neural and muscular activity. Science, 1971, 174, 431-435.

Fields, C. I. Instrumental conditioning of cardiac behavior. Unpublished Ph.D. thesis, Rockefeller University, 1970. (a).

Fields, C. I. Instrumental conditioning of the rat cardiac control systems. Proceedings of the National Academy of Science, 1970, 65, 293-299. (b)

Figar, S. Conditional circulatory responses in men and animals. In W. F. Hamilton & P. Dow (Eds.)·, Handbook of physiology, Section 2: Circulation. Vol. 3. Washington, D. C.: American Physiological Society, 1965, 1991-2035.

Fitts, P. M., & Posner, M. I. Human Performance. Belmont, California: Brooks/Cole Publishing, 1968.

Fitzgerald, H., Lintz, L., Brackbill, Y., & Adams, G. Time perception and conditioning of an autonomic response in young infants. Perceptual and Motor Skills, 1967, 24, 479-486.

Fitzgerald, R. D., & Walloch, R. A. Changes in respiration and the form of the heart-rate CR in dogs. Psychonomic Science, 1966, 5, 425-426.

Fitzgerald, R. D., Martin, G. K., and O'Brien, J. H. Influence of vagal activity on classically conditioned heart rate in rats. Journal of Comparative and Physiological Psychology, 1973, 83, 485-491.

Flynn, J. P. Discussion: Papers by W. G. Reese and W. H. Gantt. Physiological Reviews, 1960, (Suppl. 4), 419-431.

Foerster, O., & Gagel, O. Die Vorderseitenstrangdurchschneidung beim Menschen. Eine Kinisch-patho-physiologisch-anatomische Studie. Zentralblatt fur die Gesante Neurologie und Psychiatrie, 1932, 138, 1-92.

Folkow, B. Nervous control of the blood vessels, Physiological Reviews, 1955, 35, 629-663.

Folkow, B. Regulation of the peripheral circulation. British Heart Journal, 1971, 33, 27-31

Folkow, B., Haeger, K., & Unvas, B. Cholinergic vasodilator nerves in the sympathetic outflow to the muscles of the hind limbs of the cat. Acta Physiologica Scandinavica, 1948, 15, 401-411.

Folkow, B., & Neil, E. Circulation, New York: Oxford University Press, 1971.

Folkow, B., & Uvnas, B. The distribution and functional significance of sympathetic vasodilators to the hind limbs of the cat. Acta Physiologica Scandinavica, 1948, 15, 389-400.

Forbes, E. J., & Porges, S. W. Heart rate classical conditioning with a noxious auditory stimulus in human newborns. Paper presented at Society for Psychophysiological Research, Boston, 1972.

Foreman, R., & Wurster, R. D. Electrophysiological characteristics of the descending sympathetic spinal pathways. The Physiologist, 1972, 15, 137.

Forsyth, R. P. Blood pressure responses to long-term avoidance schedules in the restrained rhesus monkey. Psychosomatic Medicine, 1969, 31, 300-309.

Forsyth, R. P. Hypothalamic control of the distribution of cardiac output in the unanesthetized rhesus monkey. Circulation Research, 1970, 26, 783-794.

Forsyth, R. P. Regional blood flow changes during 72-hour avoidance schedules in the monkey. Science, 1971, 173, 546-548.

Forsyth, R. P. Sympathetic nervous system control of the distribu-
    tion of cardiac output in the unanesthetized monkey. Federation
    Proceedings, 1972, 31, 1240-1244.
Forsyth, R. P., Hoffbrand, B. I., & Melmon, K. L. Redistribution of
    cardiac output during hemorrhage in the unanesthetized monkey.
    Circulation Research, 1970, 27, 311-320.
Forsyth, R. P., Hoffbrand, B. I., & Melmon, K. L. Hemodynamic effects
    of angiotensin in normal and environmentally stressed monkeys.
    Circulation, 1971, 44, 119-129.
Forsyth, R. P., & Rosenblum, M. A. A restraining device and proce-
    dure for continuous blood pressure recordings in monkeys. Jour-
    nal of the Experimental Analysis of Behavior, 1964, 7, 367-368.
Francis, J. S., Sampson, L. D., Gerace, T., & Schneiderman, N. Cardio-
    vascular responses of rabbits to ESB: Effects of anesthetization,
    stimulus frequency and pulse-train duration. Physiology and Be-
    havior, 1973, 11, 195-203.
Franke, E. K. Physiologic pressure transducers. Methods in Medical
    Research, 1966, 11, 137-161.
Franklin, D. L., Elis, R. M., & Rushmer, R. F. A pulsed untrasonic
    flowmeter. I. R. E. Transactions on Medical Electronics, Medi-
    cal Electronics, 1959, 6, 204-206.
Freeman, G. L. The energetics of human behavior. Ithaca: Cornell
    University Press, 1948.
Freyschuss, U. Cardiovascular adjustment to somatomotor activation:
    The elicitation of increments in heart rate, aortic pressure and
    venomotor tone with the initiation of muscle contraction. Acta
    Physiologica Scandinavica, 1970 (Supple. 342). Pp. 1-63.
Frohlich, E. D., Tarazi, R. C., & Dustan, H. P. Hyperdynamic β-adren-
    ergic circulatory state: Increased β-receptor responsiveness.
    Archives of Internal Medicine, 1969, 123, 1-7.
Frohlich, E. K., Ulrych, M., Tarazi, R. C., Dustan, H. P., & Page, I.
    H., A hemodynamic comparison of essential and renovascular hyper-
    tension. Circulation, 1967, 35, 289-297.
Frumin, M. J., Ngai, S. H., & Wang, S. C. Evaluation of vasodilator
    mechanisms in the canine hind leg; question of dorsal root par-
    ticipation. American Journal of Physiology, 1953, 173, 428-436.
Fuhrer, M. Differential verbal conditioning of heart rate with mini-
    mization of changes in respiratory rate. Journal of Comparative
    and Physiological Psychology, 1964, 58, 283-289.
Furedy, J. J. Electrodermal and plethysmographic OR components:
    Repetition of and change from UCS-CS trials with surrogate UCS.
    Canadian Journal of Psychology, 1969, 23, 127-135.
Furedy, J. J., & Gagnon, Y. Relationships between and sensitivities
    of the galvanic skin reflex and two indices of peripheral vaso-
    constriction in man. Journal of Neurology, Neurosurgery and
    Psychiatry, 1969, 32, 197-201.
Gaebelein, C. J., Howard, J. L., Galosy, R. A., & Obrist, P. A.
    Classical aversive conditioning in cats under various neuromus-
    cular blocking drugs. Paper presented at the 12th annual meet-
    ing of the Society for Psychophysiological Research, Boston,
    1972.
Galin, D., & Lacey, J. I. Reaction time and heart rate response pat-
    tern: Effects of mesencephalic reticular formation stimulation
    in cats. Physiology & Behavior, 1972, 8, 729-739.
Gantt, W. H. Cardiovascular component of the conditional reflex to

pain, food and other stimuli, Physiological Reviews, 1960, 40 (Suppl. 4), 266-291.

Gaskell, P., & Burton, A. C. Local postural vasomotor reflexes arising from the limb veins. Circulation Research, 1953, 1, 27-39.

Gasser, H. S., & Meek, W. J. A study of the mechanism by which muscular exercise produces acceleration of the heart. American Journal of Physiology, 1914, 34, 48-72.

Gauer, O. H., Henry, J. P., & Behn, C. The regulation of extra-cellular fluid volume. Annual Review of Physiology, 1970, 32, 547-595.

Gauer, O. H., & Thron, H. C. Postural changes in the circulation. In W. F. Hamilton & P. Dow (Eds.), Handbook of Physiology, Section 2, Vol. III. Washington, D. C.: American Physiological Society, 1965, 2409-2439.

Gebber, G. L., & Klevans, L. R. Central nervous system modulation of cardiovascular reflexes. Federation Proceedings, 1972, 31, 1245-1252.

Gebber, G. L., & Snyder, D. W. Hypothalamic control of baroreceptor reflexes. American Journal of Physiology, 1970, 218, 124-131.

Geddes, L. A. The direct and indirect measurement of blood pressure. Chicago: Year Book Medical Publishers, Inc., 1970.

Geddes, L. A., Hoff, H. E., Valbona, G., Harrison, G., Spencer, W. H., & Canzanero, J. Numerical indication of indirect systolic and diastolic blood pressure, heart, and respiration rates. Anesthesiology, 1964, 25, 861-866.

Geddes, L. A., Knight, W., Posey, J., & Sutherland, M. Indirect determination of the rate of rise of arterial pressure, Cardiovascular Research Bulletin, 1968, 7, 71-78.

Geddes, L. A., Spencer, W. A., & Hoff, H. W. Graphic recording of Korotkoff sounds. American Heart Journal, 1959, 57, 361-370.

Geer, J. H. Measurement of the conditioned cardiac response. Journal of Comparative and Physiological Psychology, 1964, 57, 426-433.

Gelder, M. G., & Mathews, A. M. Forearm blood flow and phobic anxiety. British Journal of Psychiatry, 1968, 114, 1371-1376.

Gellhorn, E. The influence of curare on hypothalamic excitability and the electroencephalogram. Electroencephalography and Clinical Neurophysiology, 1958, 10, 697-703.

Gellhorn, E. Motion and emotion: The role of proprioception in the physiology and pathology of the emotions. Psychological Review, 1964, 71, 457-472.

Germana, J. Central efferent processes and autonomic behavioral integration. Psychophysiology, 1969, 6, 78-90.

Gero, J., & Gerova, M. Significance of the individual parameters of pulsating pressure in stimulation of baroreceptors. In P. Kezdi (Ed.), Baroreceptors and hypertension. Oxford: Pergamon Press, 1967, 17-30.

Getz, B., & Sirnes, T. The localization within the dorsal motor vagal nucleus. Journal of Comparative Neurology, 1949, 90, 95-110.

Giarman, H. J., & Pepeu, G. The influence of centrally acting cholinolytic drugs on brain acetycholine levels. British Journal of Pharmacology, 1964, 23, 123-130.

Ginsberg, S., & Furedy, J. J. Comparisons among an electrodermal and two plethysmographic components of the orienting reaction. Paper presented at the meeting of the Society for Psychophysiological Research, Boston, November, 1972.

Girden, E. The EEG in curarized mammals. Journal of Neurophysiology, 1948, 11, 169-173.

Goesling, W. J. The effects of prior skeletal conditioning on the conditioning of heart rate changes in curarized subjects. Unpublished doctoral dissertation, University of Tennessee, 1969.

Goesling, W. J., & Brener, J. Effects of activity and immobility conditioning upon subsequent heart rate conditioning in curarized rats. Journal of Comparative and Physiological Psychology, 1972, 81, 311-317.

Goetz, R. H. Effect of changes in posture on peripheral circulation, with special reference to skin temperature readings and the plethysmogram. Circulation, 1950, 1, 56-75.

Goldblatt, H., Lynch, J., Hanzal, R. F., & Summerville, W. W. Studies on experimental hypertension. I. The production of persistent elevation of systolic blood pressure by means of renal ischemia. Journal of Experimental Medicine, 1934, 59, 347-379.

Golenhofen, K. Blood flow of muscle and skin studied by the local heat clearance technique (Warmeleitmessung). Scandinavian Journal of Clinical and Laboratory Investigation, 1967, 19 (Suppl. 99), 79-85.

Goodman, L. S. & Gilman, A. (Eds.) Pharmacological Basis of Therapeutics. New York: Macmillan, 1970, 601-619.

Gootman, P. M., & Cohen, M. I. Evoked splanchnic potentials produced by electrical stimulation of medullary vasomotor regions. Experimental Brain Research, 1971, 13, 1-14.

Gorlin, R., Brachfeld, N., Turner, J. D., Messer, J. V., & Salazar, E. The idiopathic high cardiac output state. Journal of Clinical Investigation, 1959, 38, 2144-2153.

Gormly, J. Sociobehavioral and physiological responses to interpersonal disagreement. Journal of Experimental Research in Personality, 1971, 5, 216-222.

Gorski, R. A., & Shryne, J. Intracerebral antibiotics and androgenization of the neonotal female rat. Neuroendocrinology, 1972, 10, 109-120.

Gottlieb, A. A., Gleser, G. C., & Gottschalk, L. A. Verbal and physiological responses to hypnotic suggestion of attitudes. Psychosomatic Medicine, 1967, 29, 172-183.

Gottlieb, G., & Simner, M. Relationship between cardiac rate and nonnutritive sucking in human infants. Journal of Comparative and Physiological Psychology, 1966, 61, 128-131.

Graham, F. K., & Clifton, R. K. Heart rate change as a component of the orienting response. Psychological Bulletin, 1966, 65, 305-320.

Graham, F. K., & Jackson, J. C. Arousal systems and infant heart rate responses. In H. Reese, L. Lipsitt, (Eds.), Advances in Child Development and Behavior. Vol. 5. New York: Academic Press, 1970, 59-117.

Granger, L. Variation de la frequence cardiaque dans different types de situations de'attention visuelle. Canadian Journal of Psychology, 1970, 24, 370-379.

Granger, L., Ducharme, R., & Belanger, D. Effects of water deprivation upon heart rate and running speed of the white rat in a straight alley. Psychophysiology, 1969, 5, 638-643.

Green, H. D., & Kepchar, J. H. Control of peripheral resistance in major systemic vascular beds. Physiological Reviews, 1959, 39, 617-686.

Green, J. H.   Blood pressure follower for continuous blood pressure re-
cording in man. Journal of Physiology (London), 1955, 130, 37-38.
Greene, W. A.   Operant conditioning of the GSR using partial rein-
forcement. Psychological Reports, 1966, 19, 571-578.
Greenfield, A. D. M.   The circulation through the skin.   In W. F.
Hamilton & P. Dow (Eds.), Handbook of physiology, Section 2:
Circulation. Vol. 2. Washington, D. C.: American Physiologi-
cal Society, 1963, 1325-1351.
Greenfield, A. D. M., & Patterson, G. C.   The effect of small degrees
of venous distension on the apparent rate of blood inflow to the
forearm. Journal of Physiology, 1954, 125, 525-533.
Greenfield, A. D. M., Whitney, R. J., & Mowbray, J. F.   Methods for
the investigation of peripheral blood flow. British Medical
Bulletin, 1963, 19, 101-109.
Gregg, C., Clifton, R. K., & Heith, M.   Heart rate change as a function
of visual stimulation in the newborn. Paper presented at Society
for Research in Child Development, Philadelphia, 1973.
Grings, N.   Preparatory set variables related to classical conditioning
of autonomic responses. Psychological Review, 1960, 67, 243-252.
Grings, W. W., & Carlin, S.   Instrumental modification of autonomic
behavior. Psychological Record, 1966, 16, 153-159.
Grob, D.   Neuromuscular blocking drugs.   In W. S. Root and F. G. Hoffman (Eds.), Physiological Pharmacology. Vol. 3.   The Nervous
System - Part C: Autonomic Nervous System Drugs.   New York:
Academic Press, Inc., 1967, 389-460.
Grose, S. A., Herd, J. A., Morse, W. H. & Kelleher, R. T.   Behavioral
hypertension in the squirrel monkey. Federation Proceedings, 1971,
30, 549. (Abstract).
Grossman, W., Brooks, H., Meister, S., Sherman, H., & Dexter, L.   New
techniques for determining instantaneous myocardial forcevelocity
relations in the intact heart. Circulation Research, 1971, 28, 290-297.
Guberina, P.   Use of the tactile sense in understanding speech.   Journal
Francais d'oto-rhini-laryngologie et chirurgie Maxillo-Faciale,
1955, 4.
Gunn, C. G., Sevelius, G., Puiggari, M. J., & Myers, F. K.   Vagal cardiomotor mechanisms in the hindbrain of the dog and cat.   American
Journal of Physiology, 1968, 214, 258-262.
Gutmann, M. C., & Benson, H.   Interaction of environmental factors and
systemic arterial blood pressure: A review. Medicine, 1971, 50, 543-553.
Guyton, A. C.   Circulatory physiology: Cardiac output and its regula-
tion.   Philadelphia: W. B. Saunders Company, 1963.
Guyton, A. C., Coleman, T. G., Bower, J. D., & Granger, H. J.   Circu-
latory control in hypertension. Circulation Research, 1970, 26
(Suppl. 11), 135-147.
Guyton, A. C., & Reeder, R. C.   Quantitative studies on the automatic
actions of curare. Journal of Pharmacology and Experimental Thera-
peutics, 1950, 98, 188-193.
Hagbarth, K. E., Hallin, R. G., Hangell, A., Torebjork, H. E., & Wallin,
B. G.   General characteristics of sympathetic activity in human
skin nerves. Acta Physiologica Scandinavica, 1972, 84, 164-176.
Hahn, W. W.   Apparatus and technique for work with the curarized rat.
Psychophysiology, 1970, 7, 283-286.
Hahn, W. W.   The hypothesis of Lacy: A critical appraisal.   Psycholo-
gical Bulletin, 1973, 79, 59-70.

Hahn, W. W. and Slaughter, J.   Heart rate responses of the curarized
    rat.   Psychophysiology, 1970, 7, 429–435.
Hahn, W. W., Slaughter, J. S., and Rinaldi, P.   Some methodological
    difficulties in obtaining heart rate responses in the curarized
    rat.   Paper presented at the meeting of the Rocky Mountain Psy-
    chological Association, Albuquerque, New Mexico, 1969.
Hahn, W. W., Stern, J. A., & Fehr, F. S.   Generalizability of heart
    rate as a measure of drive state.   Journal of Comparative and
    Physiological Psychology, 1964, 58, 305–309.
Hahn, W.W., Stern, J. A., & McDonald, D. G.   Effects of water depri-
    vation and bar pressing activity on heart rate of the male al-
    bino rat.   Journal of Comparative and Physiological Psychology,
    1962, 55, 786–790.
Hamilton, W. F.   Role of Starling concept in regulation of the nor-
    mal circulation.   Physiological Reviews, 1955, 35, 160–168.
Hamilton, W. F.   Measurement of the cardiac output.   In W. F. Hamil-
    ton & P. Dow (Eds.), Handbook of Physiology, Section 2: Circu-
    lation, Vol. 1.   Washington, D. C.: American Physiological
    Society, 1962, 551–584.
Hamlin, R. L., & Smith C. R.   Effects of vagal stimulation on S-A
    and A-V nodes.   American Journal of Physiology, 1968, 215, 560–
    568.
Harding, D. C., Rushmer, R. F., & Baker, D. W.   Thermal transcutaneous
    flowmeter.   Medical and Biological Engineering, 1967, 5, 623–626.
Harding, G., & Punzo, F.   Response uncertainty and skin conductance.
    Journal of Experimental Psychology, 1971, 88, 265–272.
Hare, R. D.   Anxiety (APQ) and autonomic responses to affective visual
    stimulation.   Journal of Experimental Research in Personality
    1971, 5, 233–241.
Hare, R. D.   Orienting and defensive responses to visual stimuli.
    Psychophysiology, 1973, 10, 453–464.
Hare, R., Wood, K., Britain, S., & Frazelle, J.   Autonomic responses
    to affective visual stimulation: Sex differences.   Journal of
    Experimental Research in Personality, 1971, 5, 14–22.
Hare, R. D., Wood, K., Britain, S. & Shadman, J.   Autonomic responses
    to affective visual stimulation.   Psychophysiology, 1970, 7,
    408–417.
Harlow, H. F., & Stagner, R.   Effect of complete striate muscle paral-
    ysis upon the learning process.   Journal of Experimental Psy-
    chology, 1933, 16, 283–294.
Harman, M. A., & Reeves, T. J.   Effects of efferent vagal stimulation
    on atrial and ventricular function.   American Journal of Physi-
    ology, 1968, 215, 1210–1217.
Harper, M., Gurney, C., Savage, R. D., & Roth, M.   Forearm blood flow
    in normal subjects and patients with phobic anxiety states.
    British Journal of Psychiatry, 1965, 111, 723–731.
Harris, R. E., & Forsyth, R. P.   Personality and emotional stress in
    essential hypertension in man.   In J. H. Moyer, G. Onesti, & K.
    E. Kim (Eds.), High blood pressure.   New York: Grune and Stratton,
    1972, in press.
Harrison, J. V., Adams, R. D., Bennett, I. L., Resnik, W. H., Thorn,
    G. W., & Winthrobe, M. M., (Eds.) Principles of internal medicine.
    New York: McGraw Hill, 1966.
Hastings, S., & Obrist, P.   Heart rate during conditioning in humans:
    Effect of varying the interstimulus (CS-UCS) interval.   Journal
    of Experimental Psychology, 1967, 74,431–442.

Hatton, H. M. Developmental change in infant heart rate response during sleeping and waking states. Unpublished doctoral dissertation, University of Wisconsin, 1969.

Headrick, M., & Graham, F. K. Multiple-component heart rate responses conditioned under paced respiration. Journal of Experimental Psychology, 1969, 79, 486–494.

Hecht, H. H. Physiological seminar: Atrioventricular & Intraventricular Conduction. Circulation, 1971, 43, 944–982.

Hefferline, R. F., & Bruno, L. J. The psychophysiology of private events. In A. Jacobs and L Sachs (Eds.), Psychology of private events. New York: Academic Press, 1971.

Hefferline, R. F., & Perera, T. B. Proprioceptive discrimination of a covert operant without its observation by the subject. Science, 1963, 139, 834–835.

Hein, P. L. Heart rate conditioning in the cat and its relationship to other physiological responses. Psychophysiology, 1969, 5, 455–464.

Held, R. Plasticity in sensory-motor systems. Scientific American. 1965, 213, 84–94.

Henning, M. Studies on the mode of action of α-methyldopa. Acta Physiologica Scandinavica, 1969 (Suppl. 322), 1–37.

Henry, J. P., Meehan, J. P., & Stephens, P. M. The use of psychosocial stimuli to induce prolonged systolic hypertension in mice. Psychosomatic Medicine, 1967, 29, 408–432.

Herd, J. A. Overall regulation of the circulation. Annual Review of Physiology, 1970, 32, 289–312.

Herd, J. A., Morse, W. H., Kelleher, R. T., & Jones, L. G. Arterial hypertension in the squirrel monkey during behavioral experiments. American Journal of Physiology, 1969, 217, 24–29.

Hering, H. W. Die Anderung der Herzschlagzahl durch Anderung arteriellen Blutdruckes erfolgt auf reflectorischen Wege. Pflugers Archiv, 1924, 206, 721–723.

Herting, R. L., & Hunter, H. L. The physiologic and pharmacologic basis for the clinical treatment of hypertension. Medical Clinics of North America, 1967, 51, 25–37.

Hertzman, A. B. The blood supply of various skin areas as estimated by the photoelectric plethysmograph. American Journal of Physiology, 1938, 124, 328–340.

Hertzman, A. B. Photoelectric Plethysmography of the skin. Methods in Medical Research, 1948, 1, 177–182.

Hertzman, A. B. Vasomotor regulation of cutaneous circulation. Physiological Reviews, 1959, 39, 280–306.

Hertzman, A. B., & Dillon, J. B. Selective vascular reaction patterns in the nasal septum and skin of the extremities and head. American Journal of Physiology, 1939, 127, 671–684.

Hertzman, A. B., Randall, W. C., & Jochim, K. E. The estimation of the cutaneous blood flow with the photoelectric plethysmograph. American Journal of Physiology, 1946, 145, 716–726.

Hertzman, A. B., Randall, W. C., & Jochim, K. E. Relations between cutaneous blood flow and blood content in the finger pad, forearm, and forehead. American Journal of Physiology, 1947, 150, 122–132.

Hertzman, A. B., & Roth, L. W. The absence of vasoconstrictor reflexes in the forehead circulation. Effects of cold. American Journal of Physiology, 1942, 136, 692–697.

Hess, E. H. Attitude and pupil size. Scientific American, 1965, 212, 46-54.

Hess, E. H., & Polt, J. M. Pupil size as related to interest value of visual stimuli. Science, 1960, 132, 349-350.

Hess, E. H., & Polt, J. M. Pupil size in relation to mental activity during simple problem-solving. Science, 1964, 140, 1190-1192.

Hess, E. H., & Polt, J. M. Changes in pupil size as a measure of taste difference. Perceptual and Motor Skills, 1966, 23, 451-455.

Hess, W. R., & Brugger, M. Das subkortikale Zentrum der affektiven Abwehrreaktion. Helvetica Physiologica et Pharmaeologica Acta, 1943, 1, 33-52.

Heymans, C., & Neil, E. Reflexogenic areas of the cardiovascular system. Boston: Little, Brown, and Co., 1958.

Hiatt, D. E. Investigations of Operant Conditioning of Single Unit Activity in the Rat Brain. Unpublished doctoral dissertation, California Institute of Technology, 1972.

Higgins, J. D. Set and uncertainty as factors influencing anticipatory cardiovascular responding in humans. Journal of Comparative and Physiological Psychology, 1971, 74, 272-283.

Hill, L., & Barnard, H. A simple and accurate form of sphygmomanometer of arterial pressure gauge contrived for clinical use. British Medical Journal, 1897, 2, 904.

Hill, R. V., Jansen, J. C., & Fling, J. L. Electrical impedance plethysmography: A critical analysis. Journal of Applied Physiology, 1967, 22, 161-168.

Hilton, S. M. Inhibition of baroreceptor reflexes on hypothalamic stimulation. Journal of Physiology, 1962, 165, 56-57.

Hilton, S. M. Hypothalamic regulation of the cardiovascular system. British Medical Bulletin, 1966, 22, 243-248.

Hilton, S. M. Central nervous regulation of skeletal muscle circulation. In Symposium on Circulation in Skeletal Muscle. Oxford: Pergamon Press, 1968, 5-9.

Hilton, S. M., & Zbrozyna, A. W. Amygdaloid region for defense reactions and its efferent pathway to the brain stem. Journal of Physiology, 1963, 165, 160-173.

Hinman, A. T., Engel, B. T. and Bickford, A. F. Portable blood pressure recorder: Accuracy and preliminary use in evaluating intra daily variations in pressure. American Heart Journal, 1962, 63, 663.

Hnatiow, M., & Lang, P. J. Learned stabilization of cardiac rate. Psychophysiology, 1965, 1, 330-336.

Hodes, R. Electrocortical synchronization resulting from reduced proprioceptive drive caused by neuromuscular blocking agents. Electroencephalography and Clinical Neurophysiology, 1962, 14, 220-232.

Hodges, W. F., & Spielberger, C. D. The effects of threat of shock on heart rate for subjects who differ in manifest anxiety and fear of shock. Psychophysiology, 1966, 2, 287-294.

Hofer, M. A. Cardiac and respiratory function during sudden prolonged immobility in wild rodents. Psychosomatic Medicine, 1970, 32, 633-647.

Hoff, E. C., Kell, J. F., Jr. & Carroll, M. N., Jr. Effects of cortical stimulation and lesions on cardiovascular function. Physiological Reviews, 1963, 43, 68-114.

Hoffbrand, B. I., & Forsyth, R. P. Validity studies of the radio-active microsphere method for the study of the distribution of cardiac output, organ blood flow and resistance in the conscious rhesus monkey. Cardiovascular Research, 1969, 3, 426-432.

Hoffbrand, B. I., & Forsyth, R. P. The hemodynamic consequences of moderate postoperative anemia in monkeys. Surgery, Gynecology, & Obstetrics, 1971, 132, 61-66.

Hokanson, J. E., & Burgess, M. Effects of physiological arousal level, frustration, and task complexity on performance. Journal of Abnormal and Social Psychology, 1964, 68, 698-702.

Hokanson, J. E., Burgess, M., & Cohen, M. F. Effect of displaced aggression on systolic blood pressure. Journal of Abnormal and Social Psychology, 1963, 67, 214-218.

Holland, W. W., & Humerfelt, S. Measurement of blood pressure: Comparison of intra-arterial and cuff values. British Medical Journal, 1964, 2, 1241-1243.

Holling, H. E., & Verel, D. Circulation in the elevated forearm. Clinical Science, 1957, 16, 197-213.

Holloway, F. A., & Parsons, O. A. Physiological concomitants of reaction time performance. Psychophysiology, 1972, 9, 189-198.

Horrobin, D. F. A theory of hypertension. The Lancet, 1966, I, 574-579.

Hothersall, D. Operant conditioning of heart rate changes in curarized rats with brain stimulation reinforcement. Unpublished doctoral dissertation, University of Tennessee, 1968.

Hothersall, D., & Brener, J. Operant conditioning of changes in heart rates in curarized rats. Journal of Comparative and Physiological Psychology, 1969, 68, 338-342.

Hovland, C. I., & Riesen, A. H. Magnitude of galvanic and vasomotor responses as a function of stimulus intensity. Journal of General Psychology, 1940, 23, 103-121.

Howard, J. L., & Obrist, P. A. Gaebelein, C. J. & Galosy, R. A. Multiple somatic measures and heart rate during classical aversive in the cat. Journal of Comparative and Physiological Psychology, 1974, in press.

Humphrey, D. R. Neuronal activity in the medulla oblongata of cat evoked by stimulation of the carotid sinus nerve. In P. Kezdi (Ed.), Baroreceptors and hypertension. Oxford: Pergamon Press, 1967, 131-168.

Humphrey, T. The embryologic differentiation of the vestibular nuclei in man correlated with functional development. In International symposium on vestibular and oculomotor problems. Tokyo: Japan Society for Vestibular Research, 1965, 51-56.

Humphrey, T. Postnatal repetition of human prenatal activity sequences with some suggestions on their neuroanatomical basis. In R. Robinson (Ed.), Brain and early behavior. New York: Academic Press, 1969, 43-71.

Humphrey, T. The development of human fetal activity and its relation to postnatal behavior. In H. Reese, & L. Lipsitt (Eds.) Advances in child development and behavior. Vol. 5. New York: Academic Press, 1970, 1-57.

Humphreys, P. W., Joels, N., & McAllen, R. M. Modification of the reflex response to stimulation of carotid sinus baroreceptors during and following stimulation of the hypothalamic defense area in the cat. Journal of Physiology, 1971, 216, 461-482.

Hunt, R.   Direct and reflex acceleration of the mammalian heart with some observations on the relations of the inhibitory and accelerator nerves. American Journal of Physiology, 1899, 2, 395-470.

Hurst, V. W., & Logue, R. B.   The heart. (2nd ed.)   New York: McGraw-Hill, 1970.

Hutt, S. J., Hutt, C., Lenard, H. G., Von Bernuth, H.,' & Muntjewerff, W. F.   Auditory responsivity in the human neonate. Nature, 1968, 218, 888-890.

Illert, M., & Gabriel, M.   Descending pathways in the cervical cord of cats affecting blood pressure and sympathetic activity. Pflugers Archiv, 1972, 335, 109-124.

Illert, M., & Seller, H.   A descending sympathoinhibitory tract in the ventrolateral column of the cat. Pflugers Archiv, 1969, 313, 343-360.

Iriuchijima, J., & Kumada, M.   Activity of single vagal fibers efferent to the heart. Japanese Journal of Physiology, 1964, 14, 479-487.

Jacklin, C. N.   The pattern of cardiac response of olfactory stimulation in neonates. Unpublished doctoral dissertation, Brown University, 1972.

Jackson, B. T., & Barry, W. F.   The vasomotor component of the orientation reaction as a correlative of anxiety. Perceptual and Motor Skills, 1967, 25, 514-516.

Jackson, J., Kantowitz, S., & Graham, F. K.   Can newborns show cardiac orienting? Child Development, 1971, 42, 107-121.

Jacobs, R. R., Schmitz, V., Heyden, W. C., Roding, B., & Schenk, W. G., Jr.   Determination of the accuracies of the dye-dilution and electromagnetic flowmeter methods of measuring blood flow. Journal of Thoracic and Cardiovascular Surgery, 1969, 58, 601-608.

Jacobson, E.   Progressive relaxation. Chicago: University of Chicago Press, 1938.

James, T. N.   Cardiac innervation: Anatomic and pharmacologic relations. Bulletin of the New York Academy of Medicine, 1967, 43, 1041-1086.

James, T. N.   The Wolff-Parkinson-White Syndrome: Evolving concepts of its pathogenesis. Progress in Cardiovascular Diseases, 1970, 13, 159-180.

James, W.   Principles of Psychology, new edition. Vol. 2.   New York: Dover, 1950.   Chapter 26.

James, W.   Principles of Psychology.   New York: Holt, 1890.

Janig, W., & Schmidt, R. F.   Single unit responses in the cervical sympathetic trunk upon somatic nerve stimulation. Pflugers Archiv, 1970, 314, 199-216.

Jaworska, K., Kowalska, M., & Soltysik, S.   Studies on the aversive classical conditioning. 1. Acquisition and differentiation of motor and cardiac conditioned classical defensive reflexes in dog. Acta Biologiae Experimentalis, 1962, 22, 23-24.

Jennings, J. R., Averill, J. R., Opten, E. M., & Lazarus, R. S.   Some parameters of heart rate change: Perceptual versus motor task requirements, noxiousness, and uncertainty. Psychophysiology, 1971, 7, 194-212.

Jewett, D. L.   Activity of single efferent fibres in the cervical vagas nerve of the dog, with special reference to possible cardioinhibitory fibres. Journal of Physiology, 1964, 175, 321-357.

Johns, T. R.   Heart rate control in humans under paced respiration
    and restricted movement: The effect of instructions and extero-
    ceptive feedback.   Paper presented at the meeting of the Ameri-
    can Psychological Association, Washington, 1971.

Johnson, D. A., Roth, G. M., Cray, W. M.   Autonomic pathways in the
    spinal cord.   Journal of Neurosurgery, 1952, 9, 599–605.

Johnson, H. J., & Campos, J. J.   The effect of cognitive tasks and
    verbalization instructions on heart rate and skin conductance.
    Psychophysiology, 1967, 4, 143–150.

Johnson, H. J., & May, J. R.   Phasic heart rate changes in reaction
    time, and time estimation.   Psychophysiology, 1969, 6, 351–357.

Johnson, H. J., & Schwartz, G. E.   Suppression of GSR activity through
    operant reinforcement.   Journal of Experimental Psychology, 1967,
    75, 307–312.

Johnson, L. C.   A psychophysiology for all states.   Psychophysiology,
    1970, 6, 501–516.

Johnson, L. C., & Lubin, A.   The orienting reflex during waking and
    sleeping.   Electroencephalography and Clinical Neurophysiology,
    1967, 22, 11–21.

Jones, S. E., MacGrath, B. B., & Aculthorpe, H. H.   Pathological pro-
    cesses in disease.   II.   Blood of the albino rat.   Approximate
    physico-chemical description.   Annals of Tropical Medicine and
    Parasitology, 1950, 44, 168–186.

Jose, A. D., & Taylor, R. R.   Autonomic blockade by propranolol and
    atropine to study intrinsic myocardial function in man.   Jour-
    nal of Clinical Investigation, 1969, 48, 2019–2031.

Jose, A. D.   Effect of combined sympathetic and parasympathetic
    blockade on heart rate and cardiac function in man.   American
    Journal of Cardiology, 1966, 18, 476–478.

Julius, S., & Conway, J.   Hemodynamic studies in patients with border-
    line blood pressure elevation.   Circulation, 1968, 38, 282–288.

Kaada, B. R.   Cingulate, posterior, orbital, anterior insular and
    temporal pole cortex.   In J. Field, H. W. Magoun, & V. E. Hall
    (Eds.), Handbook of Physiology.   Vol. 2.   Baltimore: Williams
    and Wilkins, 1960.

Kabat, H., Magoun, H. W., & Ranson, S. W.   Electrical stimulation of
    points in the forebrain and midbrain.   The resultant alterations
    in blood pressure.   Archives of Neurology and Psychiatry, 1935,
    34, 931–955.

Kagan, J., Henker, B., Hen-Tov, A., Levine, J., & Lewis, M.   Infants'
    differential reactions to familiar and distorted faces.   Child
    Development, 1966, 37-519–532.

Kagan, J., & Lewis, M.   Studies of attention in the human infant.
    Merrill-Palmer Quarterly, 1965, 11, 95–127.

Kahneman, D., & Beatty, J.   Pupil diameter and load on memory, Science,
    1966, 154, 1583.

Kahneman, D., Tursky, B., Shapiro, D., & Crider, A.   Pupillary, heart
    rate, and skin resistance changes during a mental task.   Journal
    of Experimental Psychology, 1969, 79(1), 164–167.

Kaihara, S., van Heerden, P. D. Migita, T., & Wagner, H. M., Jr.
    Measurement of distribution of cardiac output.   Journal of Applied
    Physiology, 1968, 25, 696–700.

Kamiya, J.   Operant control of the EEG alpha rhythm and some of its
    reported effects on consciousness.   In Charles Tart, (Ed.), Al-
    tered States of Consciousness.   New York: John Wiley & Sons, 1969.

Kannel, W. B., Gordon, T., & Schwartz, M. J.   Systolic versus dia-
    stolic blood pressure and risk of coronary heart disease. Ameri-
    can Journal of Cardiology, 1971, 27, 335-343.
Kao, F. F., & Ray, L. H.   Regulation of cardiac output in anesthe-
    tized dogs during induced muscular work.   American Journal of
    Physiology, 1954, 179, 255-260.
Karplus, J. P., & Kreidl, A.   Gehirn und Sympathicus. I. Zwischen-
    hirnbasis und Halssympathicus.   Pflugers Archiv, 1909, 129, 138-
    144.
Katcher, A. H., Solomon, R. L., Turner, L. H. Lolordo, V., Overmier,
    J. B., & Rescorla, R. A.   Heart rate and blood pressure responses
    to signaled and unsignaled shocks: Effects of cardiac sympa-
    thectomy.   Journal of Comparative and Physiological Psychology,
    1969, 68, 163-174.
Katkin, E. S., & Murray, E. N.   Instrumental conditioning of auto-
    nomically mediated behavior: Theoretical and methodological
    issues.   Psychological Bulletin, 1968, 70, 52-68.
Katkin, E. S., Murray, E. N., & Lachman, R.   Concerning instrumental
    autonomic conditioning: A rejoinder.   Psychological Bulletin,
    1969, 71, 462-466.
Katona, P. G., Poitras, J. W., Barnett, G. O., & Terry, B. S.   Cardiac
    vagal efferent activity and heart period in the carotid sinus re-
    flex.   American Journal of Physiology, 1970, 218, 1030-1037.
Kazis, E., & Powell, D. A.   Cholinergic and adrenergic control of
    heart-rate changes in the rabbit.   Paper presented at the meet-
    ings of the Southeastern Psychological Association, Miami Beach,
    Florida, 1971.
Kearsley, R.   Neonatal response to auditory stimulation: A demonstra-
    tion of orienting behavior.   Child Development, 1973, 44, 582-
    590.
Keefe, F. B.   Cardiovascular responses to auditory stimuli.   Psycho-
    nomic Science, 1970, 19, 335-337.
Keen, R. E., Chase, H. H. & Graham, F. K.   Twenty-four hour retention
    by neonates of an habituated heart rate response.   Psychonomic
    Science, 1965, 2, 265-266.
Kell, J. F., & Hoff, E. C.   Descending spinal pathways mediating pres-
    sor responses of cerebral origin.   Journal of Neurophysiology,
    1952, 15, 299-311.
Kelleher, R. T., Morse, W. H., & Herd, J. A.   Effects of propranolol,
    phentolamine, and methyl atropine on cardiovascular function in
    the squirrel monkey during behavioral experiments.   Journal of
    Pharmacology, and Experimental Therapeutics, 1972, 182, 204-217.
Kelly, D. H. W.   Measurement of anxiety by forearm blood flow.   British
    Journal of Psychiatry, 1966, 112, 789-798.
Kelly, D., Brown, C. C., & Shaffer, J. W.   A comparison of physiologi-
    cal and psychological measurements on anxious patients and normal
    controls.   Psychophysiology, 1970, 6, 429-441.
Kelly, D. H. W., & Walter, C. J. S.   The relationship between clinical
    diagnosis and anxiety, assessed by forearm blood flow and other
    measurements.   British Journal of Psychiatry, 1968, 114, 611-626.
Kendler, H. H.   Learning.   Annual Review of Psychology, 1959, 10, 43-
    88.
Kerr, F. W. L.   Preserved vagal visceromotor function following de-
    struction of the dorsal motor nucleus.   Journal of Physiology,
    1969, 202, 755-769.

Kerr, F. W. L., & Alexander, S. Descending autonomic pathways in the spinal cord. Archives of Neurology, 1964, 10, 249-261.

Kety, S. S. The cerebral circulation. In J. Field (Ed.), Handbook of physiology, Section 1: Neurophysiology. Vol. 3. Washington, D. C.: American Physiological Society, 1960, 1751-1760.

Khachaturian, A. A., Kerr, J., Kruger, R. and Schachter, J. A methodological note: Comparison between period and rate data in studies of cardiac function. Psychophysiology, 1972, 9, 539-545.

Khayutin, V. M., & Lukoshkova, E. V. Spinal mediation of vasomotor reflexes in animals with intact brain studied by electrophysiological methods. Pflugers Archiv, 1970, 321, 197-222.

Kimble, G. A., & Perlmuter, L. C. The problem of volition. Psychological Review, 1970, 77, No. 5, 361-384.

Kimmel, H. D. Instrumental conditioning of autonomically mediated behavior. Psychological Bulletin, 1967, 67, 337-345.

King, G. E. Errors in clinical measurement of blood pressure in obesity. Clinical Science, 1967, 32, 223-237.

King, T. K. C., & Bell, D. Arterial blood gases in specific pathogen free and bronchitic rats. Journal of Applied Physiology, 1966, 146, 319-329.

Kirchner, F., Sato, A., & Weidinger, H. Bulbar inhibition of spinal and supraspinal sympathetic reflex discharges. Pflugers Archiv, 1971, 326, 324-333.

Koelle, G. B. Neuromuscular blocking agents. In L. S. Goodman and A. Gilman (Eds.), The pharmacological basis of therapeutics. New York: MacMillan, 1965.

Koelle, G. B. Neuromuscular blocking agents. In L. S. Goodman and A. Gilman (Eds.), The pharmacological basis of therapeutics. (4th ed.) New York: McMillan, 1970, 601-619.

Koepke, J. E., & Pribram, K. H. Habituation of the vasoconstriction responses as a function of stimulus duration and anxiety. Journal of Comparative and Physiological Psychology, 1967, 64, 502-504.

Kolin, A. Blood flow determination by electromagnetic method. In O. Glasser (Ed.), Medical Physics. Vol. 3. Chicago: Year Book, 1960, 141-155.

Korner, A. F. & Thoman, E. B. The relative efficacy of contact and vestibular-proprioseptive stimulation in soothing neonates. Child Development, 1972, 43, 443-453.

Korner, P. I. Integrative neural cardiovascular control. Physiological Reviews, 1971, 51, 312-367.

Korner, P. I., Langford, G., & Starr, D. The effects of chloralose urethane and sodium pentobarbitone anesthesia on the local and autonomic components of the circulatory response to arterial hypoxia. Journal of Physiology (London) 1968, 199, 283-325.

Korner, P. I., Uther, J. B., & White, S. W. Circulatory effects of chloralose-urethane and sodium pentobarbitone anesthesia in the rabbit. Journal of Physiology (London) 1968, 199, 253-265.

Kornhuber, H. H., & Deecke, L. Hirnpotentialandererungen bei Willkurbewegungen und passiven Bewegungen des Menschen: Bereitschaftspotential und reafferente Potentiale. Pflugers Arch. Physiol., 1965, 284, 1-17.

Korotkoff, N. S. A contribution to the problem of methods for the determination of the blood pressure. Rep. Imper. Melt.-Med. Acad. St. Petersburg, 1905, 11, 365.

Kramer, K., Lochner, W., & Wetterer, E.   Methods of measuring blood
    flow.   In W. F. Hamilton (Ed.), Handbook of Physiology, Section
    2: Circulation.   Vol. 2.   Washington, D. C.: American Physiologi-
    cal Society, 1963, 1277-1324.
Kuo, J. S., Chai, C. Y., Lee, T. M., Liu, C. N., & Lim, R. K. S.
    Localization of central cardiovascular control mechanism in the
    brain stem of the monkey.   Experimental Neurology, 1970, 29,
    131-141.
Lacey, B. C., &'Lacey, J. I.   Cardiac deceleration and simple visual
    reaction time in a fixed foreperiod experiment.   Paper presented
    at the meeting of the Society for Psychophysiological Research,
    Washington, D. C., October, 1964.
Lacey, B. C., & Lacey, J. I.   Change in cardiac response and reaction
    time as a function of motivation.   Paper presented at the meeting
    of the Soceity for Psychophysiological Research, Denver, Colo-
    rado, October 1966.
Lacey, J. I.   Psychophysiological approaches to the evaluation·of
    psychotherapeutic process and outcome.   In E. A. Rubenstein &
    M. B. Parloff (Eds.), Research in psychotherapy, Washington, D.
    C.: American Psychological Association, 1959, 160-208.
Lacey, J. I.   Somatic response patterning and stress: Some revisions
    of activation theory.   In M. H. Appley & R. Trumball (Eds.),
    Psychological stress: Issues in research.   New York: Appleton-
    Century-Crofts, 1967, 14-44.
Lacey, J. I.   Some cardiovascular correlates of sensorimotor behavior:
    Examples of visceral afferent feedback.   In C. H. Hockman (Ed.),
    Limbic system mechanisms and autonomic function.   Springfield,
    Ill.: Charles C. Thomas, 1972, 175-196.
Lacey, J. I., Bateman, D. E., & VanLehn, R.   Autonomic response
    specificity: An experimental study.   Psychosomatic Medicine,
    1953, 15, 8-21.
Lacey, J. I., Kagan, J., Lacey, B. C., & Moss, H. A.   The visceral
    level: Situational determinants and behavioral correlates of
    autonomic response patterns.   In P. H. Knapp (Ed.), Expression
    of the emotions in man.   New York: International Universities
    Press, 1963, 161-196.
Lacey, J. I., & Lacey, B. C.   Verification and extension of the prin-
    ciple of autonomic response stereotypy.   American Journal of
    Psychology, 1958, 71, 50-73.
Lacey, J. I., & Lacey, B. C.   The law of initial value in the longi-
    tudinal study of autonomic constitution: Reproducibility of
    autonomic responses and response pattern over a four-year inter-
    val.   Annals of the New York Academy of Sciences, 1962, 98,
    1257-1290; 1322-1326.
Lacey, J. I,, & Lacey, B. C.   Some autonomic-central nervous system
    interrelationships.   In P. Black (Ed.), Physiological correlates
    of emotion.   New York: Academic Press, 1970, 205-227.
Lacey, J. I., & Lacey, B. C.   Experimental association and dissocia-
    tion of phasic bradycardia and vertex-negative waves: A psycho-
    physiological study of attention and response-intention.   Elec-
    troencephalography and Clinical Neurophysiology, 1972, in press.
Lacey, J. I. & Lacey, B. C.   On heart rate responses and behavior: A
    reply to Elliott.   Journal of Personality and Social Psychology.
    in press.

Lachman, S. J. _Psychosomatic disorders: A behavioristic interpre-tation._ New York: Wiley, 1972.

Lader, M. H. Pneumatic plethysmography. In P. H. Venables & I. Martin (Eds.), _A manual of psychophysiological methods._ New York: Wiley, 1967, 159-183.

Landis, C. Electrical phenomena of the skin (galvanic skin responses). _Psychological Bulletin,_ 1932, _29,_ 693-752.

Lang, P. J. Autonomic control or learning to play the internal organs. _Psychology Today,_ October 1970, 37-41.

Lang, P. J., Geer, J., & Hnatiow, M. Semantic generalization of con-ditioned autonomic responses. _Journal of Experimental Psychology,_ 1963, 65, 552-558.

Lang, P. J., Sroufe, L. A., & Hastings, J. E. Effects of feedback and instructional set on the control of cardiac rate variability. _Journal of Experimental Psychology,_ 1967, _75,_ 425-431.

Lansdowne, M., & Katz, L. N. A critique of the plethysmographic method of measuring blood flow in the extremities of man. _Ameri-can Heart Journal,_ 1942, _23,_ 644-675.

Lapides, J., Sweet, R. B., & Lewis, L. W. Role of striated muscle in urination. _Journal of Urology,_ 1957, _77,_ 247-250.

Laragh, J. H., Baer, L., Brunner, H. R., Buhler, F. R., Sealey, J. E., & Vaughan, E. D., Jr., Renin, angiotensin and aldosterone sys-tem in pathogenesis and management of hypertensive vascular dis-ease. _The American Journal of Medicine,_ 1972, _52,_ 633-652.

Laszlo, J. I. The performance of a simple motor task with kinaes-thetic sense loss. _Experimental Psychology,_ 1966, _18,_ 1-8.

Lawler, J. E. Cardiovascular Integration and Somatic Activity during Pre-avoidance, Sidman Avoidance, and Post-avoidance in Dogs. Doctoral dissertation, University of North Carolina, 1973.

Lawler, J. E., & Obrist, P. A. Indirect indices of cardiac contrac-tility: Their utility for cardiovascular psychophysiologists. Submitted for publication, 1972.

Lawson, H. _A manual of popular physiology._ New York: G. P. Putnam's Sons, 1873.

Lawson, H. C. The volume of blood - a critical examination of meth-ods for its measurement. In W. F. Hamilton (Ed.), _Handbook of physiology, Section 2: Circulation._ Vol. I. Washington, D. C.: American Physiological Society, 1962, 23-49.

Lazarus, R. S. _Psychological stress and the coping process._ New York: McGraw-Hill, 1966.

Lenard, H. G., Von Bernuth, H., & Prechtl, H. F. R. Reflexes and their relationship to behavioral state in the newborn. _Acta Paediatrica,_ 1968, _57,_ 177-185.

Leuba, C., Birch, L. & Appleton, J. Human problem solving during complete paralysis of the voluntary musculature. _Psychological Reports,_ 1968, _22,_ 849-855.

Levander, S. E., Lidberg, L., & Schalling, D. Habituation of finger volume and pulse volume responses. _Reports from the Psycholgi-cal Laboratories,_ The University of Stockholm, April 1969, Number 275.

Levenson, R. W. & Strupp, H. H. Simultaneous feedback and control of heart rate and respiration rate. Paper presented at the twelfth annual meeting of the Society for Psychophysiological Research, Boston, 1972.

Levy, M. N., DeGeest, H., & Zieske, H. Effects of respiratory cen-ter activity on the heart. _Circulation Research,_ 1966, _18,_ 67-78.

Levy, M. N., Martin, P. J., Iano, T., & Zieske, H.   Paradoxical effect of vagus nerve stimulation. Circulation Research, 1969, 25, 303-314.

Levy, M. N., Martin, P. J., Iano, T., & Zieske, H.   Effects of single vagal stimuli on heart rate and atrioventricular conduction. American Journal of Physiology, 1970, 218, 1256-1262.

Levy, M. N., Iano, T., & Zieske, H.   Effects of repetitive bursts of vagal activity on heart rate. Circulation Research, 1972, 30, 186-195.

Lewis, M.   The cardiac response during infancy. In R. Thomson, & M. Patterson, (Eds.), Methods in physiological psychology. Vol. 1. Recording of bioelectric activity. New York: Academic Press, 1972.

Lewis, M., Bartels, B., & Goldberg, S.   State as a determinant of infant's heart rate response to stimulation. Science, 1967, 155, 486-488.

Lewis, M., Kagan, J., Cambell, H., & Kalafat, J.   The cardiac response as a correlate of attention in infants. Child Development, 1966, 37, 63-71.

Lidberg, L., Schalling, D., & Levander, S. E.   Some characteristics of digital vasomotor activity. Psychophysiology, 1972, 9, 402-411.

Lim, R. K. S., Wang, S. C., & Yi, C. L.   On the question of a myel-encephalic sympathetic centre. VII. The depressor area - a sympathoinhibitory centre. Chinese Journal of Physiology, 1938, 13, 61-78.

Lincoln, R. S.   Learning a rate of movement. Journal of Experimental Psychology, 1954, 47, 465-470.

Lind, A. R., Taylor, S. H., Humphreys, P. W., Kennelly, B. M., & Donald, K. W.   The circulatory effects of sustained voluntary. muscle contraction. Clinical Science, 1964, 27, 222-244.

Linden, R. J.   The control of output of the heart. In R. Creese (Ed.), Recent Advances of Physiology. Boston: Little, Brown & Co., 1963, 330-381.

Lindgren, P.   The mesencephalon and the vasomotor system. Acta Physiologica Scandinavica, 1955, 35 (Suppl. 121), 1-189.

Lindgren, P.   Localization and function of the medullary vasomotor center in infracollicularly decerebrated cats. Circulation Research, 1961, 9, 250-255.

Lindgren, P.   The autonomic nervous system and the peripheral circulation. International Anesthesiology Clinics, 1969, 7, 215-237.

Lindgren, P., Rosen, A., Strandberg, P., & Uvnas, B.   The sympathetic vasodilator outflow--a cortico-spinal autonomic pathway. Journal of Comparative Neurology, 1956, 105, 95-109.

Lindgren, P., & Uvnas, B.   Vasodilator response in the skeletal muscles of the dog to electrical stimulation in the oblongate medulla. Acta Physiologica Scandinavica, 1953, 29, 137-144. (a)

Lindgren, P., & Uvnas, B.   Activation of sympathetic vasodilator and vasoconstrictor neurons by electric stimulation in the medulla of dog and cat. Circulation Research, 1953, 1, 479-485. (b)

Lindgren, P., & Uvnas, B.   Postulated vasodilator center in the medulla oblongata. American Journal of Physiology, 1954, 176, 68-76.

Lintz, L., Fitzgerald, H., & Brackbill, Y.   Conditioning the eyeblink response to sound in infants. Psychonomic Science, 1967, 7, 405-406.

Lipsitt, L. Learning in the first year of life. In L. Lipsitt, & C.
    Spiker, (Eds.), Advances in Child Development and Behavior. Vol.
    1. New York: Academic Press, 1963, 147-195.
Lipsitt, L. Learning capacities of the human infant. In R. Robinson,
    (Ed.), Brain and early behavior. New York: Academic Press,
    1969, 227-245.
Lipsitt, L. Learning in the human infant. In H. Stevenson, E. Hess,
    & H. Rheingold, (Eds.), Early behavior: Comparative and develop-
    mental approaches. New York: Wiley, 1967, 225-247.
Lipsitt, L., & Jacklin, C. Cardiac deceleration and its stability in
    human newborns. Developmental Psychology, 1961, 5, 535,
Lipsitt, L., Kaye, H., & Bosack, T. Enhancement of neonatal sucking
    through reinforcement. Journal of Experimental Child Psychology,
    1966, 3, 163-168.
Lipton, E. L., Steinschneider, A., & Richmond, J. B. Autonomic func-
    tion in the neonate: II. Physiologic effects of motor restraint.
    Psychosomatic Medicine, 1960, 22, 57-65.
Lipton, E. L., Steinschneider, A., & Richmond, J. B. Autonomic func-
    tion in the neonate: III. Methodological considerations.
    Psychosomatic Medicine, 1961, 23, 461-471.
Lipton, E. L., Steinschneider, A., & Richmond, J. B. Autonomic func-
    tion in the neonate: VIII. Cardio-pulmonary observations.
    Pediatrics, 1964, 33, 212-215
Lipton, E. L., Steinschneider, A., & Richmond, J. B. Swaddling, child
    care practice: Historical, cultural, and experimental observa-
    tions. Pediatrics, 1965, 35, (Suppl.) 519-567.
Lipton, E. L., Steinschneider, A., & Richmond, J. B. Autonomic func-
    tion in the neonate: VII. Maturational changes in cardiac
    control. Child Development, 1966, 37, 1-16.
Lisander, B. Factors influencing the autonomic component of the
    defence reaction. Acta Physiologica Scandinavica, 1970, 42,
    (Suppl. 351), 1-42.
Lisander, B., & Martner, J. Interaction between the fastigial pressor
    response and the baroreceptor reflex. Acta Physiological Scandi-
    navica, 1971, 83, 505-514.
Lisina, M. I. The role of orienting in the conversion of involuntary
    into voluntary reactions. In L. G. Voronin et al. (Eds.), The
    Orienting Reflex and Exploratory Behavior. Moscow: Academy of
    Pedagogical Science, 1958.
Lofving, B. Cardiovascular adjustments induced from the rostral cin-
    gulate gyrus. Acta Physiologica Scandinavica, 1961, 53, (Suppl
    181), 1-82.
London, S. B., & London, R. E. Blood pressure survey of physicians.
    Journal of The American Medical Association, 1966, 198, 981-984.
London, S. B., & London, R. E. Critique of indirect diastolic end
    point. Archives of Internal Medicine, 1967, 119, 39-43.
Love, W. D. Isotope clearance and myocardial blood flow. American
    Heart Journal, 1964, 67, 579-582.
Low, M. D., Borda, R. P., Frost, J. D., & Kellaway, P. Surface-
    negative, slow-potential shift associated with conditioning in
    man. Neurology, 1966, 16, 777-782.
Lown, B., & Wolf, M. Approaches to sudden death. Circulation, 1971
    46, 130-142.
Luborsky, L. Individual differences in cognitive style as a determi-
    nant of vasoconstrictive orienting responses. In I. Ruttkay-

Nedecky, L. Ciganek, V. Zikmund, & E. Kellerova (Eds.), Mechanisms of orienting reaction in man. Bratislava: Publishing House of the Slovak Academy of Sciences, 1967.

Lund-Johansen, P. Hemodynamics in early essential hypertension. Acta Medica Scandinavica, 1967 (Suppl. 482), 1-101.

Luria, A. R. The Mind of a Mnemonist (L. Solotaroff, translator). New York: Basic Books, 1968, 139.

Luria, A. R., & Vinogradova, O. S. An objective investigation of the dynamics of semantic systems. British Journal of Psychology, 1959, 50, 89-105.

Luthe, W. Autogenic training: Method, research and application in medicine. American Journal of Psychotherapy, 1963, 17, 174-195.

Lykken, D. T., Rose, R., Luther, B., & Maley, M. Correcting psychophysiological measures for individual differences in range. Psychological Bulletin, 1966, 66, 481-484.

Lynch, J. J., & Paskewitz, D. A. On the mechanisms of the feedback control of human brain wave activity. Journal of Nervous and Mental Diseases, 1971, 153, 205-217.

Lywood, D. W. Blood Pressure - Manual of psycho-physiological methods. New York: John Wiley & Sons, 1967, 135-158.

MacDonald, H. R., Sapru, R. J. Taylor, S. H., and Donald, K. W. Effect of intravenous propranolol on the systemic circulatory response to sustained handgrip. American Journal of Cardiology, 1966, 18, 333-343.

MacDonald, R. L., & Cohen, D. H. Cells of origin of sympathetic prepostganglionic cardioacceleratory fibers in the pigeon. Journal of Comparative Neurology, 1970, 140, 343-358.

MacDonald, R. L., & Cohen, D. H. Central control of heart rate and blood pressure in the pigeon (Columa livia), Anatomical Record, 1971, 169, 479-480.

MacDonald, R. L., & Cohen, D. H. Heart rate and blood pressure responses to electrical stimulation of the central nervous system of the pigeon (Columba livia). Journal of Comparative Neurology, 1973, 150, 109-136.

Magnus, D., & Lammers, H. J. The amygdaloid-nuclear complex. Folia Psychiatrica, Neurologica et Neurochirurgica Neerlandica, 1956, 59, 555-582.

Magoun, H. W., Ranson, S. W., & Hetherington, A. Descending connections from the hypothalamus. Archives of Neurology and Psychiatry, 1938, 39, 1127-1149.

Maisson, W. H. Effects of curare on elastic properties of chest and lungs of the dog. Journal of Applied Physiology, 1957, 11, 309-312.

Malmo, R. B. Anxiety and behavioral arousal. Psychological Review, 1957, 64, 276-287.

Malmo, R. B. Activation. In A. J. Bachrach (Ed.), Experimental foundations of clinical psychology. New York: Basic Books, 1962.

Malmo, R. B. Cognitive factors in impairment: A neuropsychological study of divided set. Journal of Experimental Psychology, 1966, 71, 184-189.

Malmo, R. B., & Belanger, D. Related physiological and behavioral changes: What are their determinants? In Sleep and altered states of consciousness. Association for Research in Nervous and Mental Disease. Vol. 45. Baltimore: Williams & Wilkins Company, 1967, 288-318.

Maloney, J. V., & Hanford, S. H. Circulatory responses to intermittent positive and alternating positive-negative pressure respirations. *Journal of Applied Physiology*. 1954, 6, No. 8, 453-459.

Maltzman, I., Harris, L., Ingram, E., & Wolff, C. A primacy effect in the orienting reflex to stimulus change. *Journal of Experimental Psychology*, 1971, 87, 202-206.

Mandler, G. The conditions for emotional behavior. In D. C. Glass (Ed.), *Neurophysiology and emotion*. New York: Rockefeller University Press, 1967.

Manning, J. C. Intracranial representation of cardiac innervation. In W. C. Randall (Ed.), *Nervous control of the heart*. Baltimore: The Williams and Wilkins Co., 1965. 16-33.

Marquis, D. Can conditioned responses be established in the newborn infant? *Journal of Genetic Psychology*, 1931, 39, 479-492.

Martin, B. The assessment of anxiety by physiological-behavioral measures. *Psychological Bulletin*, 1961, 58, 234-255.

Martin, B., & Sroufe, L. A. Anxiety. In C. G. Costello (Ed.), *Symptoms of psychopathology*. New York: Wiley, 1970.

Maslach, C., Marshall, G., & Zimbardo, P. G. Hypnotic control of peripheral skin temperature: A case report. *Psychophysiology*, 1972, 9, 600-605.

Mason, D. R., & Bartter, F. C. Autonomic regulation of blood volume. *Anesthesiology*, 1968, 29, 681, 692.

Mason, D. T., & Braunwald, E. The effects of nitroglycerin and amyl nitrite on arteriolar and venous tone in the human forearm. *Circulation*, 1965, 32, 755-766.

Mason, J. W. Organization of the multiple endocrine responses to avoidance in the monkey. *Psychosomatic Medicine*, 1968, 30, 774-790.

Massion, W. H. Effects of curare on elastic properties of chest and lungs of the dog. *Journal of Applied Physiology*, 1957, 11, 309-312.

Mathews, A. M., & Lader, M. H. An evaluation of forearm blood flow as a psychophysiological measure. *Psychophysiology*, 1971, 8, 509-524.

May, J. R., & Johnson, H. J. Positive reinforcement and suppression of spontaneous GSR activity. *Journal of Experimental Psychology*, 1969, 80, 193-195.

McCall, R., & Kagan, J. Stimulus schema discrepancy and attention in the infant. *Journal of Experimental Child Psychology*, 1967, 5, 381-390

McCubbin, J. W., & Page, I. H. Renal pressor system and neurogenic control of arterial pressure. *Circulation Research*, 1963, 12, 553-559.

McGavock, H. An evaluation of the heated thermocouple method of recording skin blood flow. *Irish Journal of Medical Science*, 1966, 6, 287-295.

McGiff, J. C. Tissue hormones: Angiotensin, bradykinin and the regulation of regional blood flows. *The Medical Clinics of North America*, 1968, 52, 263-281.

Mc Ginn, N. F., Harburg, E., Julius, S., & McLeod, J. M. Psychological correlates of blood pressure. *Psychological Bulletin*, 1964, 61, 209-219.

McIntyre, A. R., Bennett, A. L., & Hamilton, C. Recent advances in the pharmacology of curare. *Annals of the New York Academy of Science*, 1951, 54, 301-305.

Mellander, S., & Johansson, B.   Control of resistance, exchange, and capacitance functions in the peripheral circulation. Pharmacological Reviews, 1968, 20, 117-196.

Mellgren, R., & Ost, J.   Transfer of Pavlovian differential conditioning to an operant discrimination. Journal of Comparative and Physiological Psychology, 1969, 67, 390-394.

Mendlowitz, M., Gitlow, S. E., Wolf, R. L., & Naftohi, N. E.   Pathophysiology of essential hypertension. In A. N. Brest and J. H. Moyer (Eds.), Cardiovascular drug therapy. New York: Grine and Stratton, 1964, 1-8.

Merritt, F. L., & Weissler, A. M.   Reflex venomotor alterations during exercise and hyperventilation. American Heart Journal, 1959, 58, 382-387.

Middaugh, S. J. Operant conditioning of heart rate: The curarized rat as a subject. Unpublished doctoral dissertation, University of Tennessee, 1971.

Miller, N. E.   Some reflections on the law of effect produce a new alternative to drive reduction. In M. R. Jones (Ed.), Nebraska Symposium on Motivation. Lincoln, Nebraska: University of Lincoln Press, 1963, 65-112.

Miller, N. E.   Experiments relevant to learning theory and psychopathology. In Proceedings XVIII International Congress Psychology, Moscow, 1966. Pp. 146-148. (Also in W. S. Sahakian (Ed.), Psychopathology Today: Experimentation, Theory and Research. Itasca, Illinois: F. E. Peacock, 1970. Pp 138-166) (a)

Miller, N. E.   Extending the domain of learning. Science, 1966, 152, 676. (b)

Miller, N. E.   Learning of visceral and glandular responses. Science, 1969, 163, 434-445.

Miller, N. E.   Learning of glandular and visceral responses: Postscript. In D. Singh & C. T. Morgan (Eds.), Current Status of Physiological Psychology: Readings. Monterey, California: Brooks/Cole, 1972, 245-250. (a)

Miller, N. E.   A psychologist's perspective on neural and psychological mechanisms in cardiovascular disease. In Neural and Psyc logical Mechanisms in Cardiovascular Disease. Milano, Italy: Il Ponte, 1972, in press. (b)

Miller, N. E. Interactions between learned and physical factors in mental illness. Seminars in Psychiatry, 1972, 4, 239-254. (c)

Miller, N. E. Experiments on psychosomatic interactions. Invited address, Annual meetings of the Eastern Psychological Association, Boston, Massachusetts, April 29, 1972. (d)

Miller, N. E., & Banuazizi, A. Instrumental learning by curarized rats of a specific visceral response, intestinal or cardiac. Journal of Comparative and Physiological Psychology, 1968, 65, 1-7.

Miller, N. E., & Carmona, A. Modification of a visceral response, salivation in thirsty dogs, by instrumental training with water reward. Journal of Comparative and Physiological Psychology, 1967, 63, 1-6.

Miller, N. E., & DiCara, L. V. Instrumental learning of heart rate changes in curarized rats: Shaping and specificity to discriminative stimulus. Journal of Comparative and Physiological Psychology, 1967, 63, 12-19.

Miller, N. E., DiCara, L. V., Solomon, H., Weiss, J. M., & Sworkin, B.

Learned modifications of autonomic functions: A review and some
new data. Circulation Research, 1970, 26 & 27 (Suppl. 1), 3-11.

Miner, R. W. (Ed.). Curare and anti-curare agents. Annals of the New
York Academy of Sciences, 1951, 54, 297-530.

Mischel, W. Personality and assessment. New York: Wiley, 1968.

Mitchell, G. A. G., & Warwick, R. The dorsal vagal nucleus. Acta
Anatomica, 1955, 25, 371-395.

Miura, M., & Reis, D. J. Termination and secondary projections of
carotid sinus nerve in the cat brain stem. American Journal of
Physiology, 1969, 217, 142-153.

Miura, M., & Reis, D. J. A blood pressure response from fastigial
nucleus and its relay pathway in brainstem. American Journal of
Physiology, 1970, 219, 1330-1336.

Miura, M., & Reis, D. J. The paramedian reticular nucleus: A site of
inhibitory interaction between projections from fastigial nucleus
and carotid sinus nerve acting on blood pressure. Journal of
Physiology, 1971, 216, 441-460.

Miura, M., & Reis, D. J. The role of the solitary and peramedian reticular nuclei in mediating cardiovascular reflex responses from
carotid baro- and chemoreceptors. Journal of Physiology, 1972,
223, 525-548.

Molina, A. F. de, & Hunsperger, R. W. Central representation of affective reactions in forebrain and brain stem: Electrical stimulation of amygdala, stria terminalis, and adjacent structures.
Journal of Physiology, 1959, 145, 251-265.

Monnier, M. Les centres vegetatifs bulbaires. Archives Internation-
ales de Physiologie, 1939, 49, 455-463.

Moran, W. C. Beta adrenergic blockade: An historical review and
evaluation. In A. A. Kattus, G. Ross, & V. E. Hall (Eds.), Cardiovascular beta adrenergic responses. Los Angeles: University
of California Press, 1970, 1-20.

Morgan, B. C., Martin, W. E., Hornbein, T. F., Crawford, E. W., &
Gunteroth, W. G. Hemodynamic effects of intermittent positive
pressure respiration. Anesthesiology, 1966, 27, 584.

Morgan, J., & Morgan, S. Infant learning as a developmental index.
Journal of Genetic Psychology, 1944, 65, 281-289.

Morlock, N., & Ward, A. A. The effects of curare on cortical activity.
Electroencephalography and Clinical Neurophysiology, 1961, 13,
60-67.

Morse, W. H., & Kelleher, R. T. Schedules using noxious stimuli. I.
Multiple fixed-ratio and fixed-interval termination of schedule
complexes. Journal of Experimental Analysis of Behavior, 1966,
9, 267-290.

Moruzzi, G. Azione del paleocerebellum su riflessi vasomotori.
Bollettino della Societa Italiana di Biologia Sperimentale, 1937,
12, 676-677.

Moruzzi, G. Paleocerebeller inhibition of vasomotor and respiratory
carotid sinus reflexes. Journal of Neurophysiology, 1940, 3,
20-32.

Mott, F. W., & Sherrington, C. S. Experiments upon the influences
of sensory nerves upon movement and nutrition of the limbs.
Proceedings of the Royal Society, London, 1895, 57, 481-488.

Mowrer, O. H. On the dual nature of learning: A reinterpretation
of "conditioning" and "problem-solving". Harvard Educational
Review, 1947, 17, 102-148.

Murray, H. A.   Studies of stressful interpersonal disputations.   American Psychologist, 1963, 18, 28-36.

Mushin, W. M., Rendell-Baker, L., Thompson, P. W., & Mapleson, W. W. Automatic Ventilation of the Lungs.   2nd ed.   Blackwell Scientific Publications: Oxford and Edinburgh, 1969

Muzzin, L.   Aversive classical conditioning on different operant base lines.   Unpublished Bachelor's thesis, McMaster University, 1970.

Nachev, C., Collier, J., & Robinson, B.   Simplified method for measuring compliance of superficial veins.   Cardiovascular Research, 1971, 5, 147-156.

Nakano, J., & Kusakari, T.   Effect of beta adrenergic blockade on the cardiovascular dynamics.   American Journal of Physiology, 1966, 210, 833-837.

Nathan, M. A., & Smith, O. A.   Differential conditional emotional and cardiovascular responses--A training technique for monkeys.   Journal of Experimental Analysis of Behavior, 1968, 11, 77-82.

Nathan, M. A., & Smith, O. A.   Conditional cardiac and suppression responses after lesions in the dorsomedial thalamus of monkeys. Journal of Comparative and Physiological Psychology, 1971, 76, 66-73.

Nauta, W. J. H.   Hippocampal projections and related neural pathways to the midbrain in the cat.   Brain, 1958, 81, 319-340.

Nauta, W. J. H.   Fibre degeneration following lesions of the amygdaloid complex in the monkey.   Journal of Anatomy, 1961, 95, 515-531.

Neutze, J. M., Wyler, F., & Rudolph, A. M.   Use of radioactive microspheres to assess distribution of cardiac output in rabbits. American Journal of Physiology, 1968, 215, 486-495.

Nicotero, J. A., Beamer, V., Moutsos, S. E., & Shapiro, A. P.   Effects of propranolol on the pressor response to noxious stimuli in hypertensive patients.   American Journal of Cardiology, 1968, 22, 657-666.

Noble, M. I. M., Trenchard, D., & Guz, A.   Left ventricular ejection in conscious dogs: I.   Measurement and significance of the maximum acceleration of blood from the left ventricle.   Circulation Research, 1966, 19, 139-147.

Nyboer, J.   Electrical impedance plethysmography.   Springfield, Illinois: Charles C. Thomas, 1959.

Obrist, P. A.   Heart rate during conditioning in dogs: Relationship to respiration and gross bodily movements.   Proceedings of 73rd Annual Convention of the American Psychological Association, 1965, 165-166.

Obrist, P. A.   Heart rate and somatic-motor coupling during classical aversive conditioning in humans.   Journal of Experimental Psychology, 1968, 77, 180-193.

Obrist, P. A.   The operant modification of cardiovascular activity -- a biological perspective.   Paper presented at a Symposium at the Society for Psychophysiology Research Meetings, New Orleans, 1970.

Obrist, P. A., & Webb, R. A.   Heart rate during conditioning in dogs: Relationship to somatic-motor activity, Psychophysiology, 1967, 4, 7-34.

Obrist, P. A., Webb, R. A., & Sutterer, J. R.   Heart rate and somatic changes during aversive conditioning and a simple reaction time task.   Psychophysiology, 1969, 5, 696-723.

Obrist, P. A., Webb, R. A., Sutterer, J. R., & Howard, J. L. Cardiac deceleration and reaction time: An evaluation of two hypotheses. Psychophysiology, 1970, 6, 695-706. (a)

Obrist, P. A., Webb, R. A., Sutterer, J. R., & Howard, J. L. The cardiac-somatic relationship: Some reformulations. Psychophysiology, 1970, 6, 569-587. (b)

Obrist, P. A., Wood, D. M., & Perez-Reyes, M. Heart rate during conditioning in humans: Effects of UCS intensity, vagal blockade and adrenergic block of vasomotor activity. Journal of Experimental Psychology, 1965, 70, 32-42.

Obrist, P. A., Sutterer, J. R., & Howard, J. L. Preparatory cardiac bhanges: A psychobiological approach. In A. H. Black and W. F. Prokasy (Eds.), Classical Conditioning II: Current theory and research. New York: Appleton-Century-Crofts, 1972, 312-340. (a).

Obrist, P. A., Howard, J. L., Lawler, J. E., Sutterer, J. R., Smithson, K. W., & Martin, P. L. Alterations in cardiac contractility during classical aversive conditioning in dogs: Methodological and theoretical implications. Psychophysiology, 1972, 9, 246-261. (b).

Obrist, P. A., Howard, J. L., Sutterer, J. R., Hennis, H. S., & Murrell, D. J. Cardiac-somatic changes during a simple reaction time task: A developmental study. Journal of Experimental Child Psychology, 1973, 16, 346-362.

Obrist, P. A., Howard, J. L., Lawler, J. E., & Galosy, R. A. Operant conditioning of heart rate: Somatic correlates. Submitted for publication, 1973. (b)

Obrist, P. A., Lawler, J. E., Howard, J. L., Smithson, K. W., Martin, P. L., & Manning, J. Sympathetic influences on cardiac rate and contractility during acute stress in humans. Psychophysiology, 1973, In press. (c)

Ogden, E., & Shock, N. W. Voluntary hypercirculation. The American Journal of the Medical Sciences, 1939, 198, 329-342.

O'Kelly, L., Hatton, G. I., Tucker, L., & Westall, D. Water regulation in the rat: Heart rate as a function of hydration, anesthesia, and association with reinforcement. Journal of Comparative and Physiological Psychology, 1965, 58, 159-165.

Okuma, T., Fujimori, M., & Hayashi, A. The effect of environmental temperature on the electrocortical activity of cats immobilized by neuromuscular blocking agents. Electroencephalography and Clinical Neurophysiology, 1965, 18, 392-400.

Olds, J. The limbic system and behavioral reinforcement. In W. R. Adey & T. Tokizane (Eds.), Progress in brain research. Vol. 27. Structure and function of the limbic system. Amsterdam: Elseview, 1967.

Orial, A., Sekelj, P., & McGregor, M. Limitations of indicatordilution methods in experimental shock. Journal of Applied Physiology, 1967, 23, 605-608.

Ouellet, B., & Ducharme, R. Physical activity as related to a deactivation mechanism. Paper presented at Canadian Psychological Association Meeting, Vancouver, June 1965.

Overmier, J. B. Instrumental and cardiac indices of pavlovian fear conditioning as a function of US duration. Journal of Comparative and Physiological Psychology, 1966, 62, 15-20.

Owsjannikow, Ph. Die tonischen und reflektorischen Centren der Gefassnerven. Beright uber die Verhandlungen der Sachsischen Akademie der Wissenschaften zu Leipzig, 1871, 23, 135-147.

Page, E. B., Hickam, J. B., Sieker, H. O., McIntosh, H. D., & Pryor, W. W. Reflex venomotor activity in normal persons and in patients with postural hypotension. Circulation, 1955, 11, 262-270.

Page, I. H. A unifying view of renal hypertension. In I. H. Page and J. W. McCubbin (Eds.), Renal hypertension. Chicago: Year Book Medical Publishers, 1966, 391-396.

Panisset, J. C., Biron, P., & Beaulnes, A. Effects of angiotensin on the superior cervical ganglion of the cat. Experientia, 1966, 22, 394-395.

Papousek, H. Experimental studies of appetitional behavior in human newborns and infants. In H. Stevenson, E. Hess, & H. Rheingold, (Eds.), Early behavior: Comparative and developmental approaches. New York: Wiley, 1967, 249-277.

Pappas, B. A., DiCara, L. V., & Miller, N. E. Learning of blood pressure responses in the noncurarized rat: Transfer to the curarized state. Physiology & Behavior, 1970, 5, 722-725.

Pappas, B. A., DiCara, L. V., & Miller, N. E. Acute sympathectomy by 6-hydroxydopamine in the adult rat: Effects on cardiovascular conditioning and fear retention. Journal of Comparative and Physiological Psychology, 1972, 79, 230-236. (a)

Pappas, B. A., Di Cara, L. V. & Miller, N. E. Instrumental learning of heart rate in the weanling rat and long term retention. Submitted manuscript, 1972. (b)

Pappas, B. A., DiCara, L. V., & Miller, N. E. Punishment of uterine motility in the curarized rat. Submitted manuscript, 1972. (c)

Parrish, J. Classical discrimination conditioning of heart rate and bar-press suppression in the rat. Psychonomic Science, 1967, 9, 267-268.

Pearson, D. W., & Thackray, R. I. Consistency of performance change and autonomic response as a function of expressed attitude toward a specific stress situation. Psychophysiology, 1970, 6, 561-568.

Peiper, A. Cerebral function in infancy and childhood. New York: Consultant Bureau, 1963.

Peiss, C. N. Cardiovascular responses to electrical stimulation of the brain stem. Journal of Physiology, 1958, 141, 500-509.

Peiss, C. N. Central control of sympathetic cardioacceleration in the cat. Journal of Physiology, 1960, 151, 225-237.

Peiss, C. N. Concepts of cardiovascular regulation: Past, present and future. In W. C. Randall (Ed.), Nervous Control of the Heart. Baltimore: Williams and Wilkins, 1965, 154-197.

Peper, E. Feedback regulation of the alpha electroencephalogram activity through control of the internal and external parameters. Kybernetik, 1970, 7, 107-112.

Perez-Cruet, J., & Gantt, W. H. Relation between heart rate and "spontaneous" movements. Bulletin of the Johns Hopkins Hospital, 1959, 6, 315-321.

Peterson, L. H. Systems behavior, feed-back loops, and high blood pressure research. Circulation Research, 1963, 12, 585-594.

Petras, J. M., & Cummings, J. F. Anatomical basis of visceral reflexes in the spinal cord. Anatomical Record, 1971, 169, 401.

Petras, J. M., & Cummings, J. F. Autonomic neurons in the spinal cord of the Rhesus monkey: A correlation of the findings of cytoarchitectonics and sympathectomy with fiber degeneration following dorsal rhizotomy. Journal of Comparative Neurology, 1972, 146, 189-218.

Pickering, G. High blood pressure. (2nd ed.) New York: Grune and Stratton, 1968.

Pinneo, L. R. The effects of induced muscle tension during tracking on level of activation and on performance. Journal of Experimental Psychology, 1961, 62, 523-531.

Plumlee, L. A. Operant conditioning of increases in blood pressure. Psychophysiology, 1969, 6, 283-290.

Polikanina, R. The relationship between autonomic and somatic components during development of a defensive conditioned reflex in premature children. Pavolv Journal of Higher Nervous Activity, 1961, 11, 72-82.

Polikanina, R., & Probatova, L. On the problem of formation of the orienting reflex in prematurely born children. In The Orientation reaction and orienting-investigating activity. Moscow: Academy of Pedagogical Sciences, RSFSR, 1958.

Pomerleau-Malcuit, A., Malcuit, G., & Clifton, R. An evidence of cardiac orienting in human newbcrns: Heart rate response to facial stimulations eliciting approach and escape behaviors. Unpublished manuscript. 1972.

Pomerleau-Malcuit, A., & Clifton, R. Neonatal heart rate response to tactile, auditory and vestibular stimulation in different states. Child Development, 1973, 44, 485-496.

Porges, S. W., & Raskin, D. C. Respiratory and heart rate components of attention. Journal of Experimental Psychology, 1969, 81, 497-503.

Perszasz, J., Barankay, T., Szolcsanyi, J., Proszasz-Gibiszer, K., & Madarasz, K. Studies on the neural connection between the vasodilator and vasoconstrictor centres in the cat. Acta Physiologica Academiae Scientiarum Hungaricae, 1962, 22, 29-41.

Powell, D. A., Schneiderman, N., Elster, A. J., & Jacobson, A. Differential classical conditioning in rabbits (oryctolagus cuniculus) to tones and changes in illumination. Journal of Comparative and Physiological Psychology, 1971, 76, 267-274.

Powell, D. A., Goldberg, S. R., Dauth, G. W., Schneiderman, E., & Schneiderman, N. Adrenergic and cholinergic blockade of cardiovascular responses to subcortical electrical stimulation in unanesthetized rabbits. Physiology and Behavior, 1972, 8, 927-936

Prechtl, H. F. R. The directed head turning response and allied movements in the human body, Behavior, 1958, 13, 212-242.

Pribram, K. H. The biology of mind: Neurobehavioral foundations. In Contemporary scientific psychology. New York: Academic Press, 1970, 45-70.

Przybyla, A. C., & Wang, S. C. Neurophysiological characteristics of cardiovascular neurons in the medulla oblongata of the cat. Journal of Neurophysiology, 1967, 30, 645-660.

Randall, W. C., & Priola, D. V. Sympathetic influences on synchrony of myocardial contraction. In W. C. Randall (Ed.), Nervous control of the heart. Baltimore: Williams and Wilkins, 1965.

Ranson, S. W., & Billingsley, P. R. Vasomotor reactions from stimulation of the floor of the fourth ventricle. Studies in vasomotor reflex arcs. III. American Journal of Physiology, 1916, 41, 85-90.

Raskin, D. C. Semantic conditioning and generalization of autonomic responses. Journal of Experimental Psychology, 1969, 79, 69-76.

Raskin, D. C., Kotses, H., & Bever, J. Autonomic indicators of orienting and defensive responses. Journal of Experimental Psychology, 1969, 80, 423-432. (a)

Raskin, D. C., Kotses, H., & Bever, J. Cephalic vasomotor and heart rate measures of orienting and defensive reflexes. Psychophysiology, 1969, 6, 149-159. (b)

Rawitscher, R. E., Lefer, A. M., & Dammann, J. F. Influence of artificial respiration on cardiovascular performance after open-heart surgery. Journal of Thoracic and Cardiovascular Surgery, 1967, 53, 685-694.

Razran, G. The observable unconscious and the inferable conscious in current Soviet psychophysiology: Interoceptive conditioning, semantic conditioning, and the orienting reflex. Psychological Review, 1961, 68, 81-147.

Rebert, C. S., & Tecce, J. J. A summary of CNV and reaction time. Electroencephalography and Clinical Neurophysiology, 1972, in press.

Reeve, E. B., Gregersen, M. I., Alden, T. H., & Sear, H. Distribution of cells and plasma in the normal and splenectomized dog and its influence on blood volume estimates with p^{32} and T-1824. American Journal of Physiology, 1953, 175, 195-203.

Reid, J. V. O. The cardiac pacemaker: Effects of regularly spaced nervous input. American Heart Journal, 1969, 78, 58-64.

Reis, D. J., & Cuenod, M. Tonic influence of rostral brain structures on blood pressure regulatory mechanisms in cat. Science, 1964, 145, 64-65.

Reis, D. J., & Cuenod, M. Central neural regulation of carotid baroreceptor reflexes in the cat. American Journal of Physiology, 1965, 209, 1267-1277.

Rescorla, R. A., & Solomon, R. L. Two-process learning theory: Relationships between Pavlovian conditioning and instrumental learning. Psychological Review, 1967, 74, 151-182.

Reynolds, G. S. Discrimination and emission of temporal intervals by pigeons. Journal of the Experimental Analysis of Behaviour, 1966, 9, 65-68.

Richards, D. W. Circulatory effects of hyperventilation and hypoventilation. In W. F. Hamilton & P. Dow (Eds.), Handbook of physiology, Section 2: Circulation. Vol. 3. Washington, D. C.: American Physiological Society, 1965, 1887-1897.

Riva-Rocci, S. Un hudvo sfigmomanometro. Gazz. Med. Di Torino, 1896, 47, 981-1001.

Robard, S., Rubinstein, H. M., & Rosenblum, S. Arrival time and calibrated contour of the pulse wave, determined indirectly from recordings of arterial compression sounds, American Heart Journal, 1957, 53, 205-212.

Roberts, L. E. Comparative studies of electrodermal and heart-rate conditioning in rats. Technical Report #47, Department of Psychology, McMaster University, 1972.

Roberts, L. E., & Young, R. Electrodermal responses are independent of movement during aversive conditioning in rats, but heart rate is not. Journal of Comparative and Physiological Psychology. 1971, 77, 495-512.

Roberts, L. N., Smiley, J., & Manning, G. W. Comparison of direct and indirect blood pressure determination, Circulation, 1953, 8, 232.

Robinson, B. F., Epstein, S. E., Beiser, G. D., & Braunwald, E. Control of heart rate by the autonomic nervous system. Studies in man on the interrelation between baroreceptor mechanisms and exercise. Circulation Research, 1966, 19, 400-411.

Rochmis, P. G.   Conference on Automated Indirect Blood Pressure Measurement, May 1969, Arlington, Virginia. U. S. Public Health Service Heart Disease and Stroke Control Program.

Roddie, I. C., Shepherd, J. T., & Whelan, R. F. The vasomotor nerve supply to the skin and muscle of the human forearm. Clinical Science, 1957, 16, 67-74.

Rogers, C. R. Counselling and psychotherapy. New York: Houghton Mifflin, 1942.

Rose, G. A., Holland, W. W., & Crowley, E. A. A sphygmomanometer for epidemiologists. Lancet, 1964, 1, 296-300.

Rose, G. Standardization of observers in blood pressure measurement. Lancet, 1965, 1, 673-674.

Rosen, A. Augmented cardiac contraction, heart acceleration and skeletal muscle vasodilatation produced by hypothalamic stimulation in cats. Acta Physiologica Scandinavica, 1961, 52, 291-308. (a)

Rosen, A. Augmentation of cardiac contractile force and heart rate by medulla oblongata stimulation in the cat. Acta Physiologica Scandinavica, 1961, 53, 255-269. (b)

Rosenberg, C. M. Forearm blood flow in response to stress. Journal of Abnormal Psychology, 1970, 76, 180-184.

Ross, G., & Mulder, D. G. Effects of right and left cardiosympathetic nerve stimulation on blood flow in the major coronary arteries of the anesthetized dog. Cardiovascular Research, 1969, 3, 22-29.

Rotman, M., Wagner, G. S., & Wallace, A. G. Bradyarrhythmias in acute myocardial infarction. Circulation, 1972, 45, 703-722.

Rowell, L. B., Brengelmann, G. L., Detry, J-M. R., & Wyss, C. Venomotor responses to local and remote thermal stimuli to skin in exercising man. Journal of Applied Physiology, 1971, 30, 72-77. (a)

Rowell, L. B., Brengelmann, G. L., Detry, J-M. R., & Wyss, C. Venomotor responses to rapid changes in skin temperature in exercising man. Journal of Applied Physiology, 1971, 30, 64-71. (b)

Rubenstein, J. J., Schulman, C. L., Yurchak, P. M., & DeSanctis, R. W. Clinical spectrum of the sick sinys syndrome. Circulation, 1972, 46, 5-13.

Rudolph, A. M., & Heymann, M. A. The circulation of the fetus in utero. Methods for studying distribution of blood flow, cardiac output and organ blood flow. Circulation Research, 1967, 21, 163-184.

Rushmer, R. F. Cardiovascular dynamics. (2nd. ed.) Philadelphia: W. B. Saunders, 1961.

Rushmer, R. F. Effects of nerve stimulation and hormones on the heart: The role of the heart in general circulatory regulation. In W. F. Hamilton (Ed.), Handbook of Physiology, Section 2: Circulation. Vol. 1. Washington: American Physiology Society, 1962, 533-550.

Rushmer, R. F. Initial ventricular impulse: A potential key to cardiac evaluation. Circulation, 1964, 29, 268-283.

Rushmer, R. F. Control of cardiac output. In T. C. Ruch and H. D. Patton (Eds.), Physiology and Biophysics. Philadelphia: W. B. Saunders, 1965, 644-659.

Rushmer, R. F. Cardiovascular dynamics. (3rd ed.) Philadelphia: W. B. Saunders, 1970.

Rushmer, R. F., & Smith, O. A. Cardiac control Physiological Reviews, 1959, 39, 41-68.

Rushmer, R. F., Smith, O. A., & Franklin, D. Mechanisms of cardiac control in exercise. Circulation Research, 1959, 7, 602-627.

Rushmer, R. F., Smith, O. A., & Lasher, E.   Neural mechanisms of car-
    diac control during excitation. Physiological Review, 1960, 40,
    27-34.
Safar, P., & Bachman, L.   Compliance of the lungs and thorax in dogs
    under the influence of muscle relaxants. Anesthesiology, 1956,
    17, 334-346.
Sainte-Anne Dargassies, S.   Le nouveau-ne a terme: Aspect neurologique.
    Biologia Neonatorum, 1962, 4, 174-200.
Sakoda, J. M., Cohen, B. H., & Beall, G.   Test of significance for a
    series of statistical tests. Psychological Bulletin, 1954, 51,
    172-175.
Salmoiraghi, G. C.   'Cardiovascular' neurons in brain stem of cat.
    Journal of Neurophysiology, 1962, 25, 182-197.
Samaan, A.   Muscular work in dogs submitted to different conditions of
    cardiac and splanchnic innervations. Journal of Physiology, 1935,
    83, 313-331.
Sameroff, A.   Can conditioned responses be established in the newborn
    infant: 1971? Developmental Psychology, 1971, 5, 1-12.
Sameroff, A.   Learning and adaptation in infancy: A comparison of
    models. In H. W. Reese (Ed.), Advances in child development and
    behavior. Vol. 7. New York: Academic Press, 1972.
Sameroff, A., Cashmore, T. F., & Dykes, A.   Heart rate deceleration
    during visual fixation in human newborns. Developmental Psychol-
    ogy, 1973, 8, 117-119.
Sampson, L. D., Francis, J. S., and Schneiderman, N.   Selective auto-
    nomic blockade: Effects upon classical conditioning of heart
    rate and level-lift suppression in rabbits. Journal of Compara-
    tive and Physiological Psychology, in press.
Sannerstedt, R.   Hemodynamic response to exercise in patients with
    arterial hypertension. Acta Medica Scandinavica, 1966, 180,
    (Suppl. 458).
Sapirstein, L. A.   Regional blood flow by fractional distribution of
    indicators. American Journal of Physiology, 1958, 193, 161-168.
Saunders, K. B., Hoffman, J. I. E., Noble, M. I. M., & Domenech, R. J.
    A source of error in measuring flow with indocyanine green. Jour-
    nal of Applied Physiology, 1970, 28, 190-198.
Saxon, S. A.   Detection of near threshold signals during four phases
    of cardic cycle. The Alabama Journal of Medical Sciences, 1970,
    7, 427-430.
Saxon, S. A., & Dahle, A. J.   Auditory threshold variation during
    periods of induced high and low heart rate. Psychophysiology,
    1971, 8, 23-29.
Scandinavian Journal of Clinical and Laboratory Investigation, 1967,
    19 (Suppl. 99).
Scheibel, M., & Scheibel, A.   Some neural substrates of postnatal
    development. In Review of child development research. Vol. I.
    New York: Russell Sage Foundation, 1964, 481-519.
Scher, A. M.   Control of arterial blood pressure: Measurement of
    pressure and flow. In T. C. Ruch & H. D. Patton (Eds.), Physi-
    ology and biophysics. Philadelphia: Saunders, 1966.
Scherlag, B. J., Samet, P., & Helfant, R. H.   His bundle electrogram:
    A critical appraisal of its use and limitations. Circulation,
    1972, 46, 601-613.
Schiff, M.   Untersuchungen uber die motorischen Functionen des Gross-
    hirns. Archiv fur Experimentelle Pathologie und Pharmakologie,
    1875, 3, 171-179.

Schneiderman, N. Response system divergences in aversive classical conditioning. In A. H. Black and W. F. Prokasy (Eds.), <u>Classical Conditioning II</u>. New York: Appleton-Century-Crofts, 1972, 341-348.

Schneiderman, N., VanDercar, D. H., Yehle, A. L., Manning, A. A., Golden, T., & Schneiderman, E. Vagal compensatory adjustment: Relationship to heart rate classical conditioning in rabbits. <u>Journal of Comparative and Physiological Psychology</u>, 1969, <u>68</u>, 175-183.

Schouten, J. F., Ritsma, R. J., & Cardozo, B. L. Pitch of the residue. <u>Journal of Acoustical Society of America</u>, 1962, <u>34</u>, 1418-1424.

Schramm, L. P., & Bignall, K. E. Central neural pathways mediating active sympathetic muscle vasodilation in cats. <u>American Journal of Physiology</u>, 1971, <u>221</u>, 754-767.

Schramm, L. P., Honig, C. R., & Bignall, K. E. Active muscle vasodilation in primates homologous with sympathetic vasodilation in carnivores. <u>American Journal of Physiology</u>, 1971, <u>221</u>, 768-777.

Schultz, J. H., & Luthe, W. <u>Autogenic training</u>. New York: Grune and Stratton, 1959.

Schwartz, G. E. Cardiac responses to self-induced thoughts. <u>Psychophysiology</u>, 1971, <u>8</u>, 462-467. (a)

Schwartz, G. E. Operant conditioning of human cardiovascular integration and differentiation. Unpublished doctoral dissertation, Harvard University, 1971. (b)

Schwartz, G. E. Voluntary control of human cardiovascular integration and differentiation through feedback and reward. <u>Science</u>, 1972, <u>175</u>, 90-93.

Schwartz, G. E. Biofeedback as therapy: Some theoretical and practical issues. <u>American Psychologist</u>, in press, 1973. (a)

Schwartz, G. E. Voluntary control of patterns of cardiovascular activity: Implications for learned behavioral-physiological coordination. <u>Proceedings of the XXth International Congress of Psychology</u>, Tokyo, Japan. Abstract in press, 1973. (b)

Schwartz, G. E., & Higgins, J. D. Cardiac activity preparatory to overt and covert behavior. <u>Science</u>, 1971, <u>173</u>, 1144-1146.

Schwartz, G. E., Shapiro, D., & Tursky, B. Learned control of cardiovascular integration in man through operant conditioning. <u>Psychosomatic medicine</u>, 1971, <u>33</u>, 57-62.

Schwartz, G. E., Shapiro, D., & Tursky, B. Self control of patterns of human diastolic blood pressure and heart rate through feedback and reward. <u>Psychophysiology</u>, 1972, <u>9</u>, 270 (abs.).

Scott, J. M. D. The part played by the ala cinerea in vasomotor reflexes. <u>Journal of Physiology</u>, 1925, <u>59</u>, 443-454.

Scott, J. M. D., & Roberts, F. J. Localization of the vasomotor center. <u>Journal of Physiology</u>, 1924, <u>58</u>, 168-174.

Scroop, G. C., & Lowe, R. D. Central pressor effect of angiotensin mediated by the parasympathetic nervous system. <u>Nature</u>, 1968, <u>220</u>, 1331-1332.

Sejrsen, P. Cutaneous blood flow in man studied by freely diffusible radioactive indicators. <u>Scandinavian Journal of Clinical and Laboratory Investigation</u>, 1967, <u>19</u>(Suppl. 99), 52-59.

Seligman, M. E. P. On the generality of the laws of learning. <u>Psychological Review</u>, 1970, <u>77</u>, 406-418.

Senter, R. J., & Hummel, W. F. Suppression of an autonomic response through operant conditioning. <u>Psychological Record</u>, 1965, <u>15</u>, 1-5.

Seward, J. P., & Braude, R. M. Changes in heart rate during discriminative reward training and extinction in the cat. Journal of
Comparative and Physiological Psychology, 1968, 66, 396-401.

Shapiro, A., & Cohen, H. D. The use of mercury capillary length gauges
for the measurement of the volume of thoracic and diaphragmatic
components of human respiration: A theoretical analysis and a
practical method. Transactions of the New York Academy of Sciences, 1965, 27, 634-649.

Shapiro, D., & Crider, A. Operant electrodermal conditioning under
multiple schedules of reinforcement. Psychophysiology, 1967, 41,
168-175.

Shapiro, D., & Crider, A. Psychophysiological approaches in social
psychology. In G. Lindzey and A. Oronson (Eds.), The Handbook of
social psychology. Vol. 3 (2nd ed.), Reading, Massachusetts:
Addison, Wesley, 1969, Ch. 19.

Shapiro, D., Crider, A., & Tursky, B. Differentiation of an autonomic
response through operant reinforcement. Psychonomic Science,
1964, 1, 147-148.

Shapiro, D., & Schwartz, G. E. Psychophysiological contributions to
social psychology. Annual Review of Psychology, 1970, 21, 87-112.

Shapiro, D., & Schwartz, G. E. Biofeedback and visceral learning;
Clinical applications. Seminars in Psychiatry, 1972, 4, 171-184.

Shapiro, D., Schwartz, G. E., Shnidman, S., Nelson, S., & Silverman, S.
Operant control of fear-related electrodermal responses in snake-
phobic subjects. Psychophysiology, 1972, 9, 271. (Abstract.)

Shapiro, D., Schwartz, G. E., & Tursky, B. Control of diastolic blood
pressure in man by feedback and reinforcement. Psychophysiology,
1972, 9, 296-304.

Shapiro, D., Tursky, B., Gershon, E., & Stern, M. Effects of feedback and reinforcement on the control of human systolic blood
pressure. Science, 1969, 163, 588-590.

Shapiro, D., Tursky, B., & Schwartz, G. E. Control of blood pressure
in man by operant conditioning. Circulation Research, 1970, 27,
(Suppl. 1), I-27-32. (a)

Shapiro, D., Tursky, B., & Schwartz, G. E. Differentiation of heart
rate and blood pressure in man by operant conditioning. Psychosomatic Medicine, 1970, 32, 417-423. (b).

Shapiro, D., & Watanabe, T. Timing characteristics of operant electrodermal modification: Fixed-interval effects. Japanese Psychological Research, 1971, 13, 123-130.

Sharpey-Shafer, E. P. Effect of respiratory acts on the circulation.
In W. F. Hamilton & P. Dow (Eds.), Handbook of physiology, Sec-
tion 2: Circulation. Vol. 3. Washington, D. C.: American
Physiological Society, 1965. 1875-1886.

Shean, G. D. Vasomotor conditioning and awareness. Psychophysiology,
1968, 5, 22-30.

Shearn, D. W. Operant conditioning of heart rate. Science, 1962,
137, 530-531.

Sherrington, C. S. The Integrative Action of the Nervous System.
Cambridge: Cambridge University Press, 1906.

Shettleworth, S. J. Constraints on learning. In D. S. Lehrman, R. A.
Hindle & E. Shaw (Eds.), Advances in the study of behavior, 4,
New York: Academic Press, 1972, 1-68.

Shinebourne, E., Fleming, J., & Hamer, J. Effects of beta-adrenergic
blockade during exercise in hypertensive and ischaemic heart disease. Lancet, 1967, 2, 1217-1220.

Sideroff, S., Elster, A. J., & Schneiderman, N. Cardiovascular clas-
    sical conditioning in rabbits (Oryctolagus cuniculus), using
    appetitive or aversive hypothalamic stimulation as the US. Jour-
    nal of Comparative and Physiological Psychology, 1972, 81, 501-508.
Sideroff, S., Schneiderman, N., & Powell, D. A. Motivational proper-
    ties of septal stimulation as the US in classical conditioning
    of heart rate in rabbits. Journal of Comparative and Physiologi-
    cal Psychology, 1971, 74, 1-10.
Siegel, S. Conditioning of insulin-induced glycemia. Journal of
    Comparative and Physiological Psychology, 1972, 78, 233-241.
Sigdell, J. E. A critical review of the theory of the mercury strain-
    gauge plethysmograph. Medical and Biological Engineering, 1969,
    7, 365-371
Silverman, A. J., & McGough, W. E. Perceptual relationships to pe-
    ripheral venous tone. Journal of Psychosomatic Research, 1971,
    15, 199-205.
Simonson, E., & Brozek, J. Russian research on arterial hypertension.
    Annals of internal medicine, 1959, 50, 129-193.
Siqueland, E., & Lipsitt, L. Conditioned head turning in newborn
    infants. Journal of Experimental Child Psychology, 1966, 3, 356-376.
Sirota, A., Schwartz, G. E., & Shapiro, D. Effects of feedback con-
    trol of heart rate on judgments of electric shock intensity.
    Paper read at Annual Meeting of the Biofeedback Research Society,
    November 1972, Boston, Massachusetts.
Sivertsson, R. The hemodynamic importance of structural vascular
    changes in essential hypertension. Acta Physiologica Scandina-
    vica, 1970 (Suppl. 343), 1-56.
Skinner, B. F. Science and human behavior. New York: Macmillan,
    1953.
Slaughter, J., Hahn, W., & Rinaldi, P. Instrumental conditioning of
    heart rate in the curarized rat with varied amounts of pretrain-
    ing. Journal of Comparative and Physiological Psychology, 1970,
    72, 356-359.
Sleight, P. What is hypertension? Recent studies in neurogenic
    hypertension. British Heart Journal, 1971, 33 (Suppl.), 109-112.
Smith, K. Conditioning as an artifact. Psychological Review, 1954,
    61, 217-225.
Smith, K. Curare drugs and total paralysis. Psychological Review,
    1964, 71, 77-79.
Smith, K. Conditioning as an artifact. In G. A. Kimble (Ed.),
    Foundations of conditioning and learning. New York: Appleton-
    Century-Crofts, 1967, 100-111.
Smith, O. A., Jr., Rushmer, R. F., & Lasher, E. P. Similarity of
    cardiovascular responses to exercise and to diencephalic stimu-
    lation. American Journal of Physiology, 1960, 198, 1130-1142.
Smith, O. A., & Stebbins, W. C. Conditioned blood flow and heart
    rate in monkeys. Journal of Comparative and Physiological Psy-
    chology, 1965, 59, 432-436.
Smith, R. W. Discriminative heart rate conditioning with sustained
    inspiration as respiratory control. Journal of Comparative and
    Physiological Psychology, 1966, 61, 221-226.
Smith, S. M., Brown, H. O., Toman, J. E. P., & Goodman, L. S. The
    lack of cerebral effects of d-tubocurarine. Anesthesiology,
    1947, 8, 1-14.

Smith, W. K. The functional significance of the rostral cingular cortex as revealed by its responses to electrical excitation. Journal of Neurophysiology, 1945, 8, 241-255.

Snyder, F., Hobson, J. A., & Goldfrank, F. Blood pressure changes during human sleep. Science, 1963, 142, 1313-1314.

Sokolov, E. N. Perception and the conditioned reflex. New York: Mac-
Millan, 1963.

Sokolow, M., Werdegar, D., Kain, H. K., & Hinman, A. T. Relationship
between level of blood pressure measured casually and by portable
recorders and severity of complications in essential hypertension.
Circulation, 1966, 34, 279-298.

Solomon, R. L., Kamin, L. J., & Wynne, L. C. Traumatic avoidance learning: The outcome of several extinction procedures with dogs.
Journal of Abnormal and Social Psychology, 1953, 48, 291-302.

Solomon, R. L., & Turner, L. H. Discriminative classical conditioning
in dogs paralyzed by curare can later control discriminative
avoidance responses in the normal state. Psychological Review,
1962, 69, 202-219.

Sonnenblick, E. H. Implications of muscle mechanics in the heart.
Federation Proceedings, 1962, 21, 975-990.

Spickler, J. W., & Kezdi, P. Dynamic response characteristics of the
carotid sinus baroceptors. American Journal of Physiology, 1967,
212, 472-476.

Sroufe, L. A. Age changes in cardiac deceleration within fixed foreperiod reaction time task: An index of attention. Developmental
Psychology, 1971, 5, 338-343. (a)

Sroufe, L. A. Effects of depth and rate of breathing on heart rate
and heart rate variability. Psychophysiology, 1971, 8, 648-655. (b)

Starling, E. H. The Linacre lecture on the law of the heart. London:
Longmans, Green, & Co., 1918.

Starr, I. Progress towards a physiological cardiology. Annuals of
Internal Medicine, 1965, 63, 1079-1105.

Starr, I. Further experience with simultaneous records of ULF force
and carotid pulse derivative. Bibliography of Cardiology, 1967,
99-102.

Starr, I., & Ogawa, S. Incoordination of the cardiac contraction in
clinical conditions; as judged by the ballistocardiogram and the
pulse derivative. American Journal of the Medical Sciences, 1962,
244, 663-680.

Starr, I., & Ogawa, S. A clinical study of the first derivative of the
brachial pulse. Normal standards and abnormalities encountered
in heart disease. American Heart Journal, 1963, 65, 482-494.

Stebbins, W. C., & Smith, O. A. Cardiovascular concomitants of the
conditioned emotional response in the monkey. Science, 1964, 144,
881-883.

Stegall, H. F., Kardon, M. B., & Kemmerer, W. T. Indirect measurement of arterial blood pressure by doppler ultrasonic sphyg-
momanomety. Journal of Applied Physiology, 1968, 25, 793-798.

Steinschneider, A. Developmental psychophysiology, in Y. Brackbill,
(Ed.), Infancy and early childhood. New York: Free Press, 1967,
3-47.

Steinschneider, A., Lipton, E., & Richmond, J. Auditory sensitivity
in the infant: Effect of intensity on cardiac and motor responsivity. Child Development, 1966, 37, 233-252.

Stennet, R. G. The relationship of performance level to level of arousal. Journal of Experimental Psychology, 1957, 54, 54-61.

Stern, R. M., & Anschel, C. Deep inspirations as stimuli for responses of the autonomic nervous system. Psychophysiology, 1968, 5, 132-141.

Stone, E. A. The effect of emotionality on thermoregulation during stress. Unpublished Ph.D. Thesis, Yale University, 1970.

Strandness, D. E., Jr., Kennedy, J. W., Judge, T. P., & McLeod, F. D. Transcutaneous directional flow detection: A preliminary report. American Heart Journal, 1969, 78, 65-74.

Subkov, A. A., & Zilov, G. N. The role of conditioned reflex adaptation in the origin of hyperergic reactions. Bulletin de Biologie et Medecine Experimentale, 1937, 4, 294-296.

Sutterer, J. R. Alterations of heart rate and general activity during several aversive conditioning procedures. Unpublished doctoral dissertation, University of North Carolina, 1970.

Sutterer, J. R., & Obrist, P. A. Heart rate and general activity alterations in dogs during several aversive conditioning procedures. Journal of Comparative and Physiological Psychology, 1972, 80, 314-326.

Tart, C. T. States of consciousness and specific state sciences. Science, 1972, 176, 1203-1210.

Taub, E., Bacon, R. C., & Berman, A. J. Acquisition of a trace-conditioned avoidance response after deafferentation of the responding limb. Journal of Comparative and Physiological Psychology, 1965, 59, 275-279.

Taub, E., & Berman, A. J. Movement and learning in the absence of sensory feedback. In S. J. Freedman (Ed.), The Neuropsychology of specially oriented behavior. Homewood, Illinois: Dorsey Press, 1968, 173-192.

Teyler, T. J. Effects of restraint on heart rate conditioning in rats as a function of US location. Journal of Comparative and Physiological Psychology, 1971, 77, 31-37.

Thauer, R. Circulatory adjustments to climatic requirements. In W. F. Hamilton & P. Dow (Eds.), Handbook of physiology, Section 2: Circulation. Vol. 3. Washington, D. C.: American Physiological Society, 1965, 1921-1966.

Thompson, L. W., & Botwinick, J. Stimulation in different phases of the cardiac cycle and reaction time. Psychophysiology, 1970, 7, 57-65.

Tobian, L., Jr., & Binion, J. T. Tissue cations and water in arterial hypertension. Circulation, 1952, 5, 754-758.

Trowbridge, M.H., & Cason, H. An experimental study of Thorndike's theory of learning. Journal of General Psychology, 1932, 7, 245-258.

Trowill, J. A. Instrumental conditioning of the heart rate. Ph.D. Thesis, Yale University, 1966.

Trowill, J. A. Instrumental conditioning of heart rate in the curarized rat. Journal of Comparative Physiological Psychology, 1967, 63, 7-11.

Truex, R. C., & Carpenter, M. B. Human Neuroanatomy. 6th ed. Baltimore: The Williams & Wilkins Co., 1969.

Turnewitz, G., Moreau, T., Birch, H., & Davis, L. Relationships among responses in the human newborn: The non-association and non-equivalence among different indicators of responsiveness. Psychophysiology, 1970, 7, 233-247.

Turkewitz, G., Moreau, T., Davis, L., & Birch, H.   Factors affecting lateral differentiation in the human newborn. Journal of Experimental Child Psychology, 1969, 8, 483-493.

Turner, R. H., Burch, G. E., & Sodeman, W. A.   Studies in the physiology of blood vessels in man. III. Some effects of raising and lowering the arm upon the pulse volume and blood volume of the human finger tip in health and in certain diseases of the blood vessels. Journal of Clinical Investigation, 1937, 16, 789-798.

Tursky, B., Schwartz, G. E., & Crider, A.   Differential patterns of heart rate and skin resistance during a digit-transformation task. Journal of Experimental Psychology, 1970, 83, 451-457.

Tursky, B., Shapiro, D., & Schwartz, G. E.   Automated constant cuff pressure system to measure average systolic and diastolic pressure in man.   Transactions on Bio-medical Engineering, 1972, 19, 271-275.

Ulrych, M.   Changes of general hemodynamics during stressful mental arithmetic and non-stressing quiet conversation and modifcation of the latter by beta-adrenergic blockade. Clinical Science, 1969, 36, 453-461.

Ulrych, M., Frohlich, E. D., Dustan, H. P., & Page, I. H.   Immediate hemodynamic effects of beta-adrenergic blockade with propranolol in normotensive and hypertensive man. Circulation, 1968, 37, 411-416.

Ulrych, M., Hofman, J., & Hejl, Z.   Cardiac and renal hyperresponsiveness to acute plasma volume expansion in hypertension. American Heart Journal, 1964, 68, 193-203.

Unger, S. M.   Habituation of the vasoconstrictive orienting reaction. Journal of Experimental Psychology, 1964, 67, 11-18.

Unna, K. R., & Pelikan, E. W.   Evaluation of curarizing drugs in man. IV. Critique of experiments on unanesthetized subjects. Annals of the New York Academy of Sciences, 1951, 54, 480-489.

Uno, T., & Grings, W. W.   Autonomic components of orienting behavior. Psychophysiology, 1965, 1, 311-321.

Urbach, J. R., Grauman, E. E., & Straus, S. H.   Quantitative methods for the recognition of atrioventricular junctional rhythms in atrial fibrillation. Circulation, 1969, 39, 803-817.

Ursin, H., & Kaada, B. R.   Functional localization within the amygdaloid complex in the cat. Electroencephalography and Clinical Neurophysiology, 1960, 12, 1-20.

Ulvnas, B.   Sympathetic vasodilator outflow. Physiological Reviews, 1954, 34, 608-618.

Uvnas, B.   Central cardiovascular control. In J. Field, H. W. Magoun, & V. E. Hall (Eds.), Handbook of physiology, Section I: Neurophysiology, Vol. 2. Washington, D. C.: American Physiological Society, 1960, 1131-1162. (a).

Uvnas, B.   Sympathetic vasodilator system and blood flow. Physiological Reviews, 1960, 40 (Suppl. 4), 69-76. (b)

Uvnas, B.   Cholinergic vasodilator nerves. Federation Proceedings, 1966, 25, 1618-1622.

Van Citters, R. L., & Franklin, D. L.   Radio-telemetry techniques for study of cardiovascular dynamics in ambulatory primates. Annals of the New York Academy of Science, 1969, 162, 137-155.

Van Holst, E., von.   Relations between the central nervous system and the peripheral organs. British Journal of Animal Behavior, 1954, 2, 89-94.

VanDercar, D. H., Elster, A. S., & Schneiderman, N. Heart-rate classical conditioning in rabbits to hypothalamic or septal US stimulation. Journal of Comparative and Physiological Psychology, 1970, 72, 145-152.

Vanderhoff, E., & Clancy, J. Peripheral blood flow as an indicator of emotional reaction. Journal of Applied Physiology, 1962, 17, 67-70.

Vanderwolf, C. H. Hippocampal electrical activity and voluntary movement in the rat. Electroencephalography and Clinical Neurophysiology, 1969, 26, 407-418.

Vanderwolf, C. H. Limbic-diencephalic mechanisms of voluntary movement. Psychological Review, 1971, 78, 83-113.

Vanderwolf, C. H., & Vanderwart, M. L. Relations of heart rate to motor activity and arousal in the rat. Canadian Journal of Psychology, 1970, 24, 434-441.

Von Euler, U. S. Autonomic neuroeffector transmission. In J. Field, H. W. Magoun, & V. E. Hall (Eds.), Handbook of Physiology, Section 1: Neurophysiology. Vol. 1. Washington, D. C.: American Physiological Society, 1959, 215-237.

Wallace, J. M., & Stead, E. A. Spontaneous pressure elevations in small veins and effects of norepinephrine and cold. Circulation Review, 1957, 5, 650-656.

Wallace, R. K. Physiological effects of transcendental meditation. Science, 1970, 167, 1751-1754.

Wallace, R. K., Benson, H., & Wilson, A. F. A wakeful hypometabolic physiologic state. American Journal of Physiology, 1971, 221, 795-799.

Walter, W. G., Cooper, R., Aldridge, V. J., McCallum, W. C., & Winter, A. L. Contingent negative variation: An electric sign of sensorimotor association and expectancy in the human brain. Nature, 1964, 203, 380-384.

Wang, G. H. Galvanic skin reflex and the measurement of emotions. Canton, China: Sun Yat Sen University Press, 1930.

Wang, S. C., & Chai, C. Y. Central control of sympathetic cardioacceleration in medulla oblongata of the cat. American Journal of Physiology, 1962, 202, 31-34.

Wang, S. C., & Chai, C. Y. Central control of baroreceptor reflex mechanism. In P. Kezdi (Ed.), Baroreceptors and hypertension. New York: Pergamon Press, 1965, 117-130.

Wang, S. C., & Ranson, S. W. Autonomic responses to electrical stimulation of the lower brain stem. Journal of Comparative Neurology, 1939, 71, 437-455. (a)

Wang, S. C., & Ranson, S. W. Descending pathways from the hypothalamus to the medulla and spinal cord. Observations on blood pressure and bladder response. Journal of Comparative Neurology, 1939, 71, 457-472. (b)

Ware, R. W. New approaches to the indirect measurement of human blood pressure. Third National Biomedical Sciences Symposiu, Dallas, Texas, 1965.

Ware, R. W. Doppler ultrasonic indirect blood pressure measurement. Proceedings of Symposium on Objective Recording of Blood Pressure, Northwestern University, Chicago, 1966, 37-49.

Waud, D. R. Pharmacological receptors. Pharmacological Review, 1968, 20, 49-88.

Webb, R. A., & Obrist, P. A. Heart rate change during complex oper-
   ant performance in the dog. Proceedings American Psychological
   Association, 1967, 3, 137-138.
Webb, R. A., & Obrist, P. A. The physiological concomitants of reac-
   tion time performance as a function of preparatory interval and
   preparatory interval series. Psychophysiology, 1970, 6, 389-403.
Webb-Peploe, M. M., & Shepherd, J. T. Veins and their control. New
   England Journal of Medicine, 1968, 278, 317-322.
Weininger, O., McClelland, W. J., & Arima, R. K. Gentling and weight
   gain in the albino rat. Canadian Journal of Psychology, 1954,
   8, 147-151.
Weinman, J. Photoplethysmography. In P. H. Venables and I. Martin
   (Eds.), A manual of psychophysiological methods. New York: Wiley,
   1967, 185-217.
Weinman, J., & Manoach, M. A photoelectric approach to the study of
   peripheral circulation. American Heart Journal, 1962, 63, 219-
   231.
Weisbard, C., & Graham, F. K. Heart rate change as a component of
   the orienting response in monkeys. Journal of Comparative and
   Physiological Psychology, 1971, 76, 74-83.
Weiss, T., & Engel, B. T. Operant conditioning of heart rate in
   patients with premature ventricular contractions. Psychosomatic
   Medicine. 1971, 33, 301-321.
Wenger, M. A. An investigation of conditioned responses in human infants. In Wenger, Smith, Hazard, & Irwin (Eds.), Studies in
   infant behavior III. University of Iowa Studies in Child Welfare,
   1936, 12, No. 1, 9-90.
Wenger, M. A., Clemens, T. L., Darsie, M. L., Engel, B. T., Estess, F.
   M., & Sonnenschein, R. R. Autonomic response patterns during
   intravenous infusion of epinephrine and norepinephrine. Psychosomatic Medicine, 1960, 22, 294-307.
Wenger, W. D., & Videbeck, R. Eye pupillary measurement of aesthetic
   response to forest scenes. Journal of Leisure Research, 1969,
   48, 149-163.
Werdegar, D., Johnson, D. G., & Mason, J. W. A technique for continuous
   measurement of arterial blood pressure in unanesthetized monkeys.
   Journal of Applied Physiology, 1964, 19, 519-521.
Wescott, M. R., & Huttenlocher, J. Cardiac conditioning: The effects
   and implications of controlled and uncontrolled respiration.
   Journal of Experimental Psychology, 1961, 61, 353-359.
White, E. H. Subjectively equated stimulus intensities and autonomic
   reactivity. Journal of Experimental Psychology, 1964, 68, 297-300
Whitney, R. J. The measurement of volume changes in human limbs.
   Journal of Physiology, 1953, 121, 1-27.
Wickens, E., & Wickens, C. A study of conditioning in the neonate.
   Journal of Experimental Psychology, 1940, 26, 40-120.
Wiggers, C. J. Circulatory dynamics: Physiologic studies. New York:
   Grune & Stratton, 1952.
Wiggers, C. J. The circulation and circulation research in perspec-
   tive. In W. F. Hamilton & P. Dow (Eds.), Handbook of physiology,
   Section 2: Circulation. Vol. 1. Washington, D. C.: American
   Physiological Society, 1962, 1-10.
Wilder, J. The law of initial values in neurology and psychiatry.
   Facts and problems. Journal of nervous and mental diseases, 1957,
   125, 73-86.

Williams, J. L. Response contingency and effects of punishment: Changes in autonomic and skeletal responses. Journal of Comparative and Physiological Psychology, 1969, 68, 118-125.

Williams, R. B., Bittker, T. E., Buchsbaum, M. S., & Wynne, L. S. Effect of sensory intake and sensory rejection on cardiovascular (CV) function. Paper presented at the meeting of the Society for Psychophysiological Research, Boston, November 1972.

Wilson, R. S. Cardiac response: Determinants of conditioning. Journal of Comparative and Physiological Psychology Monograph, 1969, 68, 1-23.

Wolferth, C. C., & Wood, F. C. The mechanism of production of short P-R intervals and prolonged QRS complexes in patients with presumably undamaged hearts: Hypothesis of an accessory pathway of AV conduction. American Heart Journal, 1933, 8, 297-311.

Wood, D. M., & Obrist, P. A. Effects of controlled and uncontrolled respiration on the conditioned heart rate response in humans. Journal of Experimental Psychology, 1964, 68, 221-229.

Wood, J. E., & Eckstein, J. W. A tandem forearm plethysmograph for study of acute responses of the peripheral veins of man: The effect of environmental and local temperature change, and the effect of pooling blood in the extremities. Journal of Clinical Investigation, 1958, 37, 41-50.

Woodworth, R. S. Experimental psychology, New York: Henry Holt & Co., 1938.

Woodworth, R. S., & Schlosberg, H. Experimental psychology. New York: Henry Holt & Co., 1954.

Woodworth, R. S., & Sherrington, C. S. A pseudaffective reflex and its spinal path. Journal of Physiology, 1904, 31, 234-243.

Yamori, Y., Lovenberg, W., & Sjoerdsma, A. Norepinephrine metabolism in brainstem of spontaneously hypertensive rats. Science, 1970, 170, 544-546.

Yehle, A. L., Dauth, G. W., & Schneiderman, N. Correlates of heart rate classical conditioning in curarized rabbits. Journal of Comparative and Physiological Psychology, 1967, 64, 98-104.

Zbrozyna, A. W. The organization of the defence reaction elicited from amygdala and its connections. In B. E. Eleftherious (Ed.), The Neurobiology of the Amygdala. New York: Plenum Press, 1972, 597-606.

Zeaman, D., & Smith, R. Review of some recent findings in human cardiac conditioning. In W. F. Prokasy (Ed.), Classical conditioning: A symposium. New York: Appleton-Century-Crofts, 1965, 378-418.

Zeiner, A. R., Nathan, M. A., & Smith, O. A. Conditioned emotional responding (CER) mediated by interference. Physiology and Behavior, 1969, 4, 645-648.

Zierler, K. L. Circulation times and the theory of indicator-dilution methods for determining blood flow and volume. In W. F. Hamilton (Ed.), Handbook of physiology, Section 2: Circulation. Vol. 1. Washington, D. C.: American Physiological Society, 1962, 585-615.

Zimmerman, B. G. Evaluation of peripheral and central components of action on the sympathetic nervous system. Journal of Pharmacology and Experimental Therapeutics, 1967, 158, 1-10.

Zimny, G. H., & Miller, F. L. Orienting and adaptive cardiovascular responses to heat and cold. Psychophysiology, 1966, 3, 81-92.

Zinner, S. H., Levy, P. S., & Kass, E. H. Family aggregation of blood pressure in childhood. The New England Journal of Medicine, 1971, 284, 401-404.

Zitnik, R. S., Ambrosioni, E., & Shepherd, J. T. Effect of temperature on cutaneous venomotor reflexes in man. Journal of Applied Physiology, 1971, 31, 507-512.

Zuckerman, M. Physiological measures of sexual arousal in the human. Psychological Bulletin, 1971, 75, 347-356.

Zweifach, B. W. Functional behavior of the microcirculation. Springfield, Illinois: Charles C. Thomas, 1961.

Author Index

Subject Index